Retinal Disorders

Genetic Approaches to Diagnosis and Treatment

A subject collection from *Cold Spring Harbor Perspectives in Medicine*

OTHER SUBJECT COLLECTIONS FROM *COLD SPRING HARBOR PERSPECTIVES IN MEDICINE*

Human Fungal Pathogens
Tuberculosis
The Biology of Heart Disease
The Skin and Its Diseases
MYC *and the Pathway to Cancer*
Bacterial Pathogenesis
Transplantation
Cystic Fibrosis: A Trilogy of Biochemistry, Physiology, and Therapy
Hemoglobin and Its Diseases
Addiction
Parkinson's Disease
Type 1 Diabetes
Angiogenesis: Biology and Pathology
HIV: From Biology to Prevention and Treatment
The Biology of Alzheimer Disease

SUBJECT COLLECTIONS FROM *COLD SPRING HARBOR PERSPECTIVES IN BIOLOGY*

Innate Immunity and Inflammation
The Genetics and Biology of Sexual Conflict
The Origin and Evolution of Eukaryotes
Endocytosis
Mitochondria
Signaling by Receptor Tyrosine Kinases
DNA Repair, Mutagenesis, and Other Responses to DNA Damage
Cell Survival and Cell Death
Immune Tolerance
DNA Replication
Endoplasmic Reticulum
Wnt Signaling
Protein Synthesis and Translational Control
The Synapse
Extracellular Matrix Biology
Protein Homeostasis
Calcium Signaling
The Golgi
Germ Cells
The Mammary Gland as an Experimental Model

Retinal Disorders

Genetic Approaches to Diagnosis and Treatment

A subject collection from *Cold Spring Harbor Perspectives in Medicine*

EDITED BY

Eric A. Pierce

Massachusetts Eye and Ear
Department of Ophthalmology
Harvard Medical School

Richard H. Masland

Massachusetts Eye and Ear
Departments of Ophthalmology and Neurobiology
Harvard Medical School

Joan W. Miller

Massachusetts Eye and Ear
Department of Ophthalmology
Harvard Medical School

COLD SPRING HARBOR LABORATORY PRESS
Cold Spring Harbor, New York • www.cshlpress.org

Retinal Disorders: Genetic Approaches to Diagnosis and Treatment
A Subject Collection from *Cold Spring Harbor Perspectives in Medicine*
Articles online at www.perspectivesinmedicine.org

Executive Editor	Richard Sever
Managing Editor	Maria Smit
Senior Project Manager	Barbara Acosta
Permissions Administrator	Carol Brown
Production Editor	Joanne McFadden
Production Manager/Cover Designer	Denise Weiss
Publisher	John Inglis

Front cover artwork: The iris of a human eye, slightly enhanced to emphasize the stromal fibers. (Photo provided by Dr. Richard Masland and the Massachusetts Eye and Ear Infirmary Fluorescein Laboratory. Image processing by Haobing Wang, Massachusetts Eye and Ear Infirmary.)

Library of Congress Cataloging-in-Publication Data

Retinal disorders: genetic approaches to diagnosis and treatment: a subject collection from cold spring harbor perspectives in medicine/edited by Eric A. Pierce, Massachusetts Eye and Ear Infirmary, Richard H. Masland, Massachusetts Eye and Ear Infirmary, and Joan W. Miller, Massachusetts Eye and Ear Infirmary.

pages cm

Includes bibliographical references and index.

ISBN 978-1-62182-017-8 (hardcover: alk.paper)

1. Retina--Diseases. 2. Retina--Diseases--Treatment. I. Pierce, Eric A., editor. II. Masland, Richard H., editor. III. Miller, Joan W. (Joan Whitten) editor.

RE551.R485 2014
617.7′35--dc23

2014033172

10 9 8 7 6 5 4 3 2 1

All World Wide Web addresses are accurate to the best of our knowledge at the time of printing.

For a complete catalog of all Cold Spring Harbor Laboratory Press publications, visit our website at www.cshlpress.org.

Contents

Preface

Because they afflict so specialized a tissue, retinal diseases have been approached late by research using molecular genetic techniques. The baffling complexity of the eye, however, has made the recent discoveries these studies have yielded even more exciting. Sometimes these seem to have come out of the blue, unanticipated by more traditional methodologies. In this book, we provide a survey of the new field that has emerged. Our first goal has been simply to collect essays describing the cutting edge of work on retinal disorders. But we have also sought to go beyond the traditional approaches usually taken by such collections and tried to present work that also reaches those working scientists at the margins of the field, including postdocs and faculty working more generally in neurobiology or cell biology, residents, and investigators from related scientific areas.

To accomplish this, we first asked colleagues with a broad general perspective to write chapters that survey the various areas of the field. These chapters introduce the first three sections of the volume and have a broader scope than the others. The authors were charged with introducing the material to readers who are not trained in ophthalmology—basic scientists and physicians from other specialties. The subsequent chapters in each section are more focused, covering specific areas in greater detail.

It will be clear to readers that the application of new molecular approaches is bringing new life to the pathobiology of retinal disease. Perhaps most gratifyingly, they have led directly to potential new treatments for conditions affecting the retina—most notably various forms of gene therapy—and these are covered in other chapters within the book. For a variety of reasons, implementation of these therapeutic approaches is progressing deliberately; but they have enormous promise because of their broad applicability. Here we have tried to compile, as completely as possible, a handbook of the approaches currently in play.

We thank Richard Sever, the initiator of this project at Cold Spring Harbor Laboratory Press, and especially the patient and ever-cheerful Barbara Acosta, who was its main shepherd. Anne Goodwin and Wendy Chao labored long and well to improve the readability, style, and accessibility of the chapters. The production staff at Cold Spring Harbor Laboratory Press labored to make all the chapters look nice, as they emphatically do. Finally, we thank the MEE Fluorescein Laboratory, Haobing Wang, and Michael Becker for creating the cover image.

Eric A. Pierce
Richard H. Masland
Joan W. Miller

Clinical Characteristics and Current Therapies for Inherited Retinal Degenerations

José-Alain Sahel[1,2,3,4,5,6,7], Katia Marazova[1,2,3], and Isabelle Audo[1,2,3,4,7]

[1]Institut de la Vision, Sorbonne Universités, UPMC Univ Paris 06, UMR_S 968, Paris, F-75012, France

[2]INSERM, U968, Paris, F-75012, France

[3]CNRS, UMR 7210, Paris, F-75012, France

[4]Centre Hospitalier National d'Ophtalmologie des Quinze-Vingts, DHU ViewMaintain, INSERM-DHOS CIC 1423, Paris, F-75012, France

[5]Fondation Ophtalmologique Adolphe de Rothschild, Paris, F-75019, France

[6]Académie des Sciences-Institut de France, Paris, F-75006, France

[7]Institute of Ophthalmology-University College London, London EC1V 9EL, United Kingdom

Correspondence: j.sahel@gmail.com

Inherited retinal degenerations (IRDs) encompass a large group of clinically and genetically heterogeneous diseases that affect approximately 1 in 3000 people (>2 million people worldwide) (Bessant DA, Ali RR, Bhattacharya SS. 2001. Molecular genetics and prospects for therapy of the inherited retinal dystrophies. *Curr Opin Genet Dev* **11:** 307–316.). IRDs may be inherited as Mendelian traits or through mitochondrial DNA, and may affect the entire retina (e.g., rod–cone dystrophy, also known as retinitis pigmentosa, cone dystrophy, cone–rod dystrophy, choroideremia, Usher syndrome, and Bardet-Bidel syndrome) or be restricted to the macula (e.g., Stargardt disease, Best disease, and Sorsby fundus dystrophy), ultimately leading to blindness. IRDs are a major cause of severe vision loss, with profound impact on patients and society. Although IRDs remain untreatable today, significant progress toward therapeutic strategies for IRDs has marked the past two decades. This progress has been based on better understanding of the pathophysiological pathways of these diseases and on technological advances.

ROD–CONE DYSTROPHY

Rod–cone dystrophies, also known as retinitis pigmentosa (RP), is a highly heterogeneous group of IRDs characterized by progressive bilateral degeneration of rod and cone photoreceptors. At present, there is no uniformly accepted classification of RP. The main criteria to classify RP include: (i) topography of the retinal involvement (central, pericentral, sector, or peripheral); (ii) age of onset; (iii) inheritance mode; and (iv) predominant type of photoreceptors involved. Many investigators divide RP into three main groups: nonsyndromic or "typical, classical, simple" (affecting the eye alone), syndromic (affecting other systems, such

Cite this article as *Cold Spring Harb Perspect Med* doi: 10.1101/cshperspect.a017111

as hearing), and systemic (affecting multiple tissues and organs). It is generally considered that 70%–80% of all RP cases fall in the category of nonsyndromic rod–cone dystrophy (Ayuso and Millan 2010).

In most forms of typical RP, degeneration of rod photoreceptors and loss of rod function precedes and exceeds cone degeneration. This is why the initial symptoms in RP, usually noted in childhood, are impaired dark adaptation and visual disturbances in dim light (nyctalopia). However, the age of onset may range widely, from early childhood to mid-30s to 50s or even later (Tsujikawa et al. 2008) and, in general, early-onset disease has worse prognosis. As RP advances, patients progressively lose their peripheral vision, while their central vision usually remains preserved until the late stages of the disease. This phenomenon is known as "tunnel vision." Light sensitivity (photophobia) may be present at a later stage of the disease. ~35% of patients experience light flashes (photopsia) (Heckenlively et al. 1988), described as small, blinking lights that are often continuous but tend to decrease over the years as scotomas become denser. Loss of central vision usually occurs by age 60, although most patients are legally blind by the age of 40 yr because of severely constricted visual fields (Hartong et al. 2006).

Clinical Characteristics of RP

Clinical assessment of patients with RP (reviewed in Hartong et al. 2006) starts with complete past medical history and family history. Clinical tests that can reveal features of RP include psychophysical tests, slit lamp examination, fundus examination, electroretinogram (ERG), fundus autofluorescence, and spectral domain optical coherence tomography (OCT). Adaptive optics (described below) is a new tool for imaging cone photoreceptor matrix and is under evaluation for following-up cone disease in retinal dystrophies. Since the advent of fundus autofluorescence imaging, fluorescein angiography is no longer a diagnostic test for RP. Systemic evaluation and additional nonophthalmologic assessments (e.g., audiometric and vestibular tests, neurological examination, kidney function, and ultrasound) may be necessary to rule out syndromes and systemic disorders presenting with RP.

Psychophysical tests include best-corrected visual acuity measurement, which is usually normal in typical cases, even in advanced RP as long as a small area of central visual field is preserved. Kinetic and static perimetry typically show scotomas in the midperiphery that enlarge over years. Color vision (Farnsworth D15 panel or other tests) is usually preserved until advanced stages, when macular blue cone dysfunction (acquired tritanopia) may be apparent. Decline in contrast sensitivity (measured with a contrast chart) and fatigue are common complaints.

The early development of cataract is a common feature in RP, although the reasons for the capsular opacification remain poorly understood and may be because of vitreous changes and modification of blood-ocular barrier (reviewed in Jackson et al. 2001). Slit lamp examination reveals cataract, mainly of posterior subcapsular type, in up to 50% of adult RP patients and its incidence increases with age (Heckenlively 1982; Fishman et al. 1985). The mean age of surgery, as reported by Jackson et al. (2001) is 47.5 yr versus 72.5 yr for age-related cataract. In addition, RP patients tend to develop more posterior capsular opacification requiring YAG laser and zonular instability compared with age-related cataract (Dikopf et al. 2013). Keratoconus is rare and is usually encountered in early onset disease. Cells within the vitreous are common.

Results of fundus examination may vary with the stage of the disease and may initially be normal. The earliest changes are associated with fine, dust-like granularity of the retinal pigment epithelium (RPE), pigmentary mottling but with normal vasculature. In the middle stage of the disease, patchy loss of RPE and the beginning of retinal vessel attenuation are apparent. Advanced RP is characterized by arteriolar narrowing, waxy pallor of the optic nerve head, and migration of intraretinal pigment (termed bone spicule deposits) secondary to photoreceptor cell death. Cystoid macular edema is reported in >40% of cases (Adackapara et al. 2008). Epimacular membrane is not uncommon. In addition, atrophic changes in the macula may also be observed early in some cases and represent another cause of earlier decrease in visual acuity in RP along with cystoid macular edema, epimacular membrane, and cataract.

Full-field Electroretinogram (ERG) is an objective method that records the electrical responses of the retina to light stimuli and is critical for the diagnosis of IRDs. The International Society for Clinical Electrophysiology of Vision (ISCEV) has elaborated recommendations for standardized minimal recording protocols (see http://www.iscev.org/), allowing for accurate diagnosis and inter-laboratory comparison. Full-field (Ganzfeld) ERG allows precise recording of both rod (after dark adaptation, scotopic conditions) and cone (after light adaptation, photopic conditions) photoreceptor function as well as response summation at the inner retinal level. ERG has not only diagnostic but also prognostic value, based on amplitude and implicit time preservation. In the early stages of RP, scotopic responses are more affected than photopic responses, involving both the a-wave (hyperpolarization of photoreceptors—mostly rods—under dark adaptation) and the b-wave (generated at the inner retinal level on visual signal transmission from the photoreceptors). In case of sector RP (disease restricted to a retinal area, usually inferior), there is no implicit time shift. This is not the case in classical RP, which involves the entire retina. ERG abnormalities vary with the underlying genetic defect. X-linked RP is associated with more severely affected ERG responses in comparison with autosomal recessive and dominant RP, these two subgroups being characterized by a wider functional heterogeneity (Hartong et al. 2006). In later stages of the disease, the ERG responses become progressively lower to the point of being undetectable—even though visual acuity can be preserved, the electrical contribution of the macula to full-field ERG is negligible. In these cases, multifocal ERG or pattern ERG can be used to better assess macular function and objectively document disease progression toward the fovea (Hood et al. 1998; Robson et al. 2003). Special recording techniques have been developed to better document cone responses in case of submicrovolt photopic ERG responses (Andreasson et al. 1988; Birch and Sandberg 1996; Sieving et al. 1998).

Fundus autofluorescence is an efficient, noninvasive imaging method for topographic mapping of lipofuscin changes in the RPE and monitoring of retinal degeneration. In RP, decreased or absent fundus autofluorescence, usually observed in periphery, indicates loss of RPE/photoreceptor cells. A peculiar parafoveal ring of hyperautofluorescence was first reported by Robson et al. (2003) and may be present in >60% of patients (Murakami et al. 2008). Its diameter correlates with preservation of macular (Fig. 1) function (Robson et al. 2003) and tends to constrict with disease progression (Robson et al. 2011). This ring, as functional correlate, may be used as a noninvasive outcome measurement in future clinical trials aimed at slowing disease progression.

Spectral domain OCT is now an established method for assessing retinal thickness and photoreceptor layer architecture. For example, the presence of the inner segment ellipsoid and interdigitation zone on OCT images highly correlates with normal visual function (Witkin et al. 2006; Mitamura et al. 2012). Spectral domain OCT is useful for detecting and monitoring macular edema as well as detecting epimacular membrane in RP patients (Koizumi et al. 2008; Hagiwara et al. 2011).

An adaptive optics fundus camera enables observation of cone photoreceptor mosaics in vivo (Fig. 2) (Gocho et al. 2013). The blurred areas of cone mosaics (heavily decreased density) in adaptive optics images correspond to the high-density fundus autofluorescence ring in fundus autofluorescence images and to the border of the external limiting membrane and the ellipsoid zone in OCT images (Tojo et al. 2013). Adaptive optics can therefore be useful in monitoring progression of RP and therapeutic intervention (Talcott et al. 2011).

Epidemiology and Genetics of RP

RP has an estimated worldwide prevalence of 1:3000–1:7000 persons (Bunker et al. 1984;

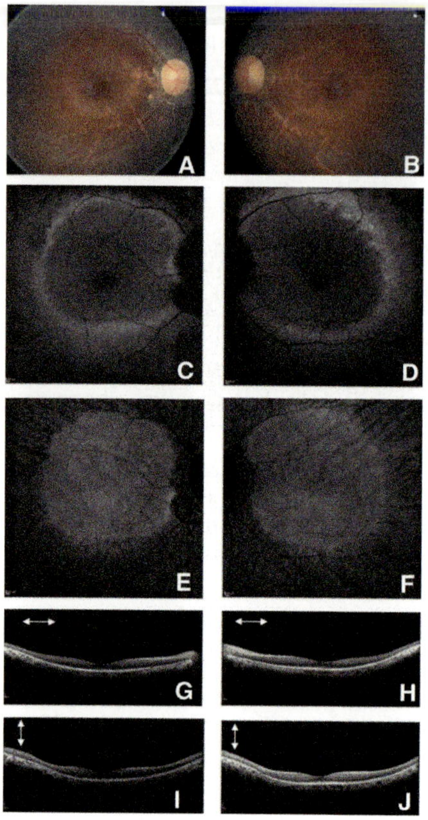

Figure 1. Fundus photographs, autofluorescence and spectral domain optical coherence tomography of a patient with rod–cone dystrophy (retinitis pigmentosa). Fundus photography (*A* right eye and *B* left eye), Fundus autofluorescence blue (*C* right eye and *D* left eye) and near infrared (*E* right eye and *F* left eye) as well as Sd-OCT (*G* horizontal scan, *I* vertical scan of the right eye, *H* horizontal scan and *K* vertical scan of the left eye) of a patient with rod–cone dystrophy (retinitis pigmentosa). On the color pictures note the waxy disc pallor of the optic disc, narrowed retinal vessels and preserved macular region with a high density ring of hyperautofluorescence around the macula associated with relatively preserved macular lamination on Sd-OCT.

Haim 2002). The substantial differences in epidemiological data reflect not only the variable criteria applied in different surveys, but also the substantial genetic diversity between populations in terms of prevalence of specific mutations and proportion of specific genetic types. On the basis of visual field criteria and ophthalmoscopic fundus appearance, the prevalence of RP in adult population (aged ≥30 yr) of rural Central India was estimated at 1:750 (Nangia et al. 2012). High prevalence of 1:930 and 1:372 was reported in the urban and rural South Indian population aged above 40 yr (Sen et al. 2008). The Beijing Eye Study reported RP in about one in 1000 elderly Chinese (aged ≥40 yr) in North China (Jonas et al. 2009), whereas the Beijing Eye Public Health Care Project, a population-based study designed to screen all inhabitants aged of 55 to 85 yr and living in the rural regions of the Beijing municipality, reported prevalence of RP of about 1:4000 (You et al. 2013). RP inheritance can be autosomal dominant, autosomal recessive, or X-linked, in addition to rare mitochondrial and digenic forms, and there is genetic heterogeneity within each group. Of the total number of nonsyndromic, nonsystemic cases, ~19% are autosomal dominant, 65% are autosomal recessive or simplex cases, and ~8% are X-linked (Bunker et al. 1984). Population-based epidemiological and genetic study of X-linked RP (XLRP) in Denmark reported estimated prevalence of affected males of approximately 1:15,000 (Prokisch et al. 2007). The great success in identifying genes and mutations causing RP during the past two decades has revealed the tremendous genetic complexity of IRDs such as RP. According to the Retinal Information Network, RetNet, 232 genes causing IRDs have been mapped to a specific chromosomal site to date and 192 of these have been identified (see https://sph.uth.edu/retnet/sum-dis.htm, accessed May 30, 2013).

The first causative gene for RP, the rhodopsin gene (*RHO*), was discovered in 1990 in autosomal dominant RP (Dryja et al. 1990). A majority of RP mutations affect rods selectively. However, the initial rod photoreceptor death is followed by secondary loss of cone photoreceptors that occurs regardless of the underlying mutation. The strikingly heterogeneous etiology of RP is complicated by the fact that mutations in many distinct genes can cause the same phenotype, mutations in the same gene may cause different diseases, and the same mutation in different individuals may be associated with wide range of phenotypic expressivity, even

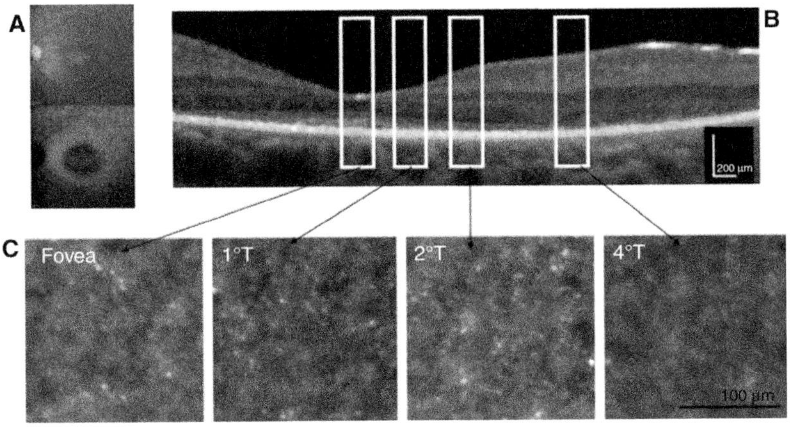

Figure 2. Adaptive optic images from the left eye of a patient with rod–cone dystrophy and perifoveal macular atrophy. (*A*) Infrared and blue autofluorescence from the left eye of the patient showing perifoveal loss of autofluorescence with relatively normal autofluorescence in the foveal region. (*B*) Sd-OCT horizontal scan of the left eye showing thinning of the outer retina with relatively normal foveal lamination with inner segment preservation up to 2°; white rectangles represent retinal location of the corresponding adaptive optics pictures. (*C*) Adaptive optics imaging reveals that cones are still present around the fovea, but the cone mosaic is nearly absent at 4°. (Image courtesy of Kiyoko Gocho and Michel Paques.)

within the same family. For example, autosomal recessive RP can be caused by mutations in more than 44 genes identified so far; these include *RHO* (Rosenfeld et al. 1992), the *PDE-β* gene (encoding the β subunit of rod cGMP phosphodiesterase) (McLaughlin et al. 1993) and the gene encoding the α subunit of the rod cGMP-gated channel (Dryja et al. 1995). At least 23 autosomal dominant RP genes have been identified to date and three of them, *RHO*, *RP1*, and *PRPH2*, account for approximately 25%–30%, 5%–10%, and 5%–10% of all autosomal dominant RP cases, respectively. Similarly to *RHO*, mutations in *NRL* can also cause either dominant or recessive disease. Mutations in the *RPGR* gene are associated with X-linked RP (Roepman et al. 1996) and account for 70%–90% of X-linked cases; another 10%–20% are caused by *RP2* mutations. Mutations in some genes (e.g., *PRPH2*) can cause dominant RP, dominant macular degeneration or other distinct forms of retinopathy (Daiger et al. 2007). The functions of the genes involved in the pathogenesis of RP are highly variable. A majority of causative mutations are directly involved in the phototransduction cascade, for instance, rhodopsin (*RHO*), the genes for the catalytic unit and subunits of PDE6 (*PDE6A* and *PDE6B*, respectively), the subunit of the rod cyclic nucleotide gated channel (*CNGA1*), and arrestin (*SAG*). Some of these mutations cause not only RP but also other IRDs, including congenital stationary night blindness and cone dystrophies. Other mutated genes alter the function of proteins crucially involved in maintaining the visual cycle (e.g., *RPE65*, *RLBP1*, *RGR*, *ABCA4*) or photoreceptor structure (*PRPH2*, *ROM1*), as well as transcription factors (e.g., *NR2E3*, *NRL*, *CRX*).

Syndromic and Systemic Forms of RP

Approximately 20%–30% of RP patients have associated syndromic nonocular disease or systemic conditions involving multiple organs and pleiotropic effects (>30 different syndromes).

Usher syndrome is the most frequent form of syndromic RP, in which RP is associated with hearing impairment. It accounts for ~18% of RP cases (Boughman et al. 1983). The disease is inherited in an autosomal recessive manner and is the most frequent cause of combined deafness and blindness in humans. It has a prevalence of about one in 20,000 in the Caucasian population, but the estimations vary (e.g., 1:12,500 in Germany and 1:29,000 in persons of Scandinavian descent). Fifteen chromosomal loci and 12 genes have been identified so far and assigned to three major clinical types, depending on the severity and progression of the hearing loss, the coexistence with vestibular dysfunction and the age of onset of RP (Petit 2001) (RetNet database, see https://sph.uth.edu/retnet/). Symptoms vary from person to person and progress at different rates. Usher syndrome type I is the most severe form of the disease. It is characterized by congenital, bilateral, severe-to-profound, sensorineural hearing impairment associated with vestibular dysfunction. By the age of ~10 yr, children experience progressive vision loss caused by RP. Balance disturbances result in retarded motor development. Usher syndrome type II is a less severe subtype, with moderate-to-severe hearing impairment from birth, late onset of RP (after puberty), and normal vestibular function. In Usher syndrome type III, hearing loss begins in the first two decades of life and worsens over time, vision loss is progressive and variable in severity (starting around puberty), and vestibular dysfunction is variable.

Another major form of syndromic/systemic RP is Bardet-Biedl syndrome, in which RP is associated to varying degrees with polydactyly, obesity, type 2 diabetes, hypogonadism, cognitive impairment, and renal abnormalities that can be a major cause of morbidity and mortality in this syndrome (Forsythe and Beales 2012). The prevalence of Bardet-Biedl syndrome varies markedly between populations, from 1:160,000 in northern European populations to 1:13,500 in Kuwait (Forsythe and Beales 2012), and this form accounts for about 5%–6% of RP cases (Haim 2002). Currently, 16 genes are known to be associated with Bardet-Biedl syndrome, accounting for approximately 80% of clinically diagnosed cases (Forsythe and Beales 2012).

Recent evidence indicate that a number of multisystemic diseases, collectively termed ciliopathies, result from mutations in ciliary genes, including Joubert syndrome, nephronophthisis, Senior-Løken syndrome, orofaciodigital syndrome, Jeune syndrome, autosomal dominant and recessive polycystic kidney disease, Leber congenital amaurosis, Bardet-Biedl syndrome, Meckel-Gruber syndrome, and Usher syndrome (Novarino et al. 2011). These clinically and genetically heterogeneous disorders share substantially overlapping clinical features, such as renal cysts, hepatic disease, retinal degeneration, polydactyly, cognitive impairment, sinus inversus, cerebellar hypoplasia, and obesity (Waters and Beales 2011).

Joubert syndrome (reviewed in Romani et al. 2013) is a complex ciliopathy, characterized by hypotonia progressing to ataxia, global developmental delay, ocular motor apraxia, breathing dysregulation, and, often renal defects and congenital liver fibrosis. The hallmark of the disease is the "molar tooth sign" visible on cerebral magnetic resonance imaging. Joubert syndrome is commonly associated with retinal defects that range in severity from Leber congenital amaurosis to slowly progressive retinopathies with partially preserved vision. Estimates of the incidence of Joubert syndrome range between 1:80,000 and 1:100,000 live births, but this is probably an underestimate. In the Askhenazi Jewish population, the predicted prevalence of Joubert syndrome is as high as one per 34,000 people. Today, 21 causative genes with autosomal or X-linked recessive inheritance have been identified, all of which encode for proteins of the primary cilium or its apparatus.

Senior-Løken syndrome is an autosomal recessive disease characterized by retinal dystrophy and a medullary cystic kidney disease, nephronophthisis. RP in Senior-Løken syndrome may present either as congenital retinal blindness caused by retinal dysplasia or as progressive retinal degeneration later in childhood (Waters and Beales 2011). So far, mutations in 13 genes coding for proteins in the connecting cilium of photoreceptor cells and in the primary cilium of kidney cells have been shown to cause Senior-Løken syndrome (reviewed in Ronquillo et al. 2012). Most of these mutations are also associated with pathologies in other organs, besides kidneys and retina.

Until now, >80 loci have been reported to be associated with ciliary disorders (van Reeuwijk et al. 2011). Intriguingly, mutations in *CEP290* have been described in ~50% of Joubert syndrome subgroup of ciliopathies and up to 20% of cases of Leber congenital amaurosis, and found to be associated with a wide variety of distinct phenotypes, including Senior-Løken syndrome, nephronophthisis, Bardet-Biedl syndrome, and Meckel-Gruber syndrome (for review Coppieters et al. 2010; Waters and Beales 2011; Drivas et al. 2013). At present, despite the identification of more than 100 *CEP290* mutations (Coppieters et al. 2010), no clear genotype–phenotype correlations could be established and the mechanisms underlying the highly variable phenotypes associated with ciliary dysfunction remain to be elucidated.

CONE–ROD DYSTROPHIES

Although most cases of RP are characterized by typical initial rod loss followed by the loss of cone photoreceptors, there are many inherited retinal diseases in which cone degeneration precedes the rod degeneration. These conditions are referred to as cone–rod degenerations/dystrophies (CORDs). Loss of visual acuity, color vision, and photophobia are characteristic early manifestations of the disease, with onset usually occurring in late childhood or early adult life, followed by night blindness and loss of peripheral visual fields (for a detailed review of clinical manifestations, see Michaelides et al. 2004). Macular pigment deposits and atrophy or a bull's-eye maculopathy are visible on fundus examination in the early stages. Peripheral RPE atrophy, retinal pigmentation, arteriolar attenuation, and optic disc pallor can be seen in the late stages of the disease process. Full-field ERG reveals a predominant alteration of photopic (absent or severely impaired cone function) over scotopic (rod) responses. The rate of disease progression varies widely between families. Visual acuity usually deteriorates severely over time, to the "counting fingers" level. Sometimes the loss of cones and rods is concomitant. CORDs can be inherited as autosomal recessive, autosomal dominant, X-linked, or mitochondrial traits. Most cases of progressive cone dystrophy and CORD are sporadic; autosomal dominant is the most common mode of inheritance in familial cases (Michaelides et al. 2004). So far, mutations causing autosomal dominant CORDs have been identified in 10 genes, including two major genes being *CRX* (which also causes LCA7) and *GUCY2D* (which also causes LCA1), as well as *AIPL1* (which also causes LCA4), *GUCA1A*, *PITPNM3*, *PROM1*, *PRPH2*, *RIMS1*, *SEMA4A*, and *UNC119*, and four loci: *CORD4* (17q), *RCD1* (6q25–q26), *CORD16* (2q24.2–2q33.1), and 10q26 (Kamenarova et al. 2013). Most of the sporadic cases probably represent autosomal recessive inheritance, but some may represent new autosomal dominant mutations and, in severely affected males, X-linked disease. Mutations in *ABCA4* (also known to cause Stargardt disease 1) are responsible for 30%–60% of cases of autosomal recessive CORD; other genes associated with autosomal recessive CORDs include *ADAM9*, *RPGRIP1*, *CDHR1*, and *HRG4*. Mutations in *RPGR*, the gene encoding the protein that interacts with RPGRIP1, have been associated with X-linked CORD families. One additional chromosomal locus for X-linked CORD has been identified to date: CORDX3 (Xp11.4–q13.1). CORDs are usually nonsyndromic, but they may also be associated with several syndromes, including Bardet-Biedl syndrome or spinocerebellar ataxia type 7 (Michaelides et al. 2004).

LEBER CONGENITAL AMAUROSIS (LCA)

LCA is a rare, infantile-onset retinal dystrophy with prevalence at birth of 1:30,000–1:80,000, accounting for ~5% of all inherited retinopathies (reviewed in den Hollander et al. 2008). It is most commonly inherited as an autosomal recessive trait, but autosomal dominant forms have been linked to mutations in *CRX* and less commonly in *IMPDH1* and OTX2. Two types of LCA exist with either rod–cone or cone–rod dysfunction in correlation with the underlying genetic defect. The constellation of severe and early visual loss, nystagmus, sluggish pupils and nondetectable ERG responses is pathognomic. Children with LCA may present with an oculo-digital reflex and, in some cases, neurodevelopmental delay. Rare associated ocular features are strabismus, high hyperopia, high myopia, cataracts, keratoconus/keratoglobus, macular pseudocoloboma, pigmentary retinopathy and maculopathy, disc edema, and retinal vascular attenuation (Koenekoop 2004). LCA is caused by mutations in any one of at least 18 genes (Falk et al. 2012; Koenekoop et al. 2012), (see https://sph.uth.edu/retnet/). At present, more than 400 mutations have been identified and associated with ~70% of all LCA cases. LCA is currently considered to be the most severe retinal dystrophy without major systemic features.

X-LINKED RETINOSCHISIS

X-linked retinoschisis is an inherited retinal disorder with estimated prevalence between 1:5,000 and 1:25,000 (George et al. 1995, 1996; The Retinoschisis Consortium 1998). X-linked retinoschisis accounts for almost all cases of congenital retinoschisis and is the leading cause of macular degeneration in young males. It is characterized by a splitting of the inner layers of the neurosensory retina, resulting in characteristic foveal schisis and vision loss. ERG has a characteristic "electronegative" appearance with relative loss of the positive, rod-driven b-wave and preservation of the negative a-wave (Sieving et al. 1999). X-linked retinoschisis is a clinically heterogenous disease (reviewed in George et al. 1996; Pimenides et al. 2005). It may be diagnosed either in infancy (with squinting, rarely nystagmus and severe vision loss) or at school age (with decreased visual acuity). The disease course may be variable and is usually mild until age 40 yr. The visual acuity thereafter declines progressively. Peripheral retinal abnormalities are seen in more than half of cases. Vitreous hemorrhage, retinal detachment, and neovascular glaucoma may occur. The disease is caused by mutations in the *RS1* gene encoding retinoschisin, an important protein for cell adhesion (Sauer et al. 1997). More than 100 different mutations have been identified so far. Wide variations in clinical phenotype described between and within families are independent of the mutation type. Females who are homozygous for an *RS1* mutation show similar symptoms and signs to affected males.

STARGARDT DISEASE

Stargardt disease, together with its phenotypic variant fundus flavimaculatus, is the most common macular degenerative disease in patients under 50 yr of age. It is characterized by juvenile-onset, progressive, bilateral macular atrophy with subretinal deposition of lipofuscin-like material. Stargardt disease affects approximately one in 10,000 individuals (Blacharski 1988). However, the carrier frequency for a mutation in the causative gene may be as high as 1:20 (Yatsenko et al. 2001), thus explaining why pseudodominant cases are not uncommon. Typical Stargardt disease with macular atrophy is usually diagnosed before the age of 20 with impaired central and detailed vision and decreased visual acuity. Fundus flavimaculatus is usually diagnosed later. Later ages of onset have been associated with a more favorable visual prognosis. The disease manifests with decreased central vision that gradually worsens. Color vision may be variably affected with typical red-green defect. Diagnosis is based on fundus examination, full-field and multifocal or pattern ERG, and fundus imaging (fundus autofluorescence and OCT). Fundus autofluorescence shows typically a loss of foveal autofluorescence, a patchy appearance of autofluorescence in the macular region with alternating hypo- and hyperautofluorescence dots and a peripapillary sparing of the autofluorescence (Fig. 3). Another historical hallmark feature of Stargardt disease is the presentation of a dark choroid during fluorescein angiography examination, which is not necessary for diagnosis since the advent of autofluorescence imaging. Full-field ERG has a prognostic value with three functional groups reported by the Moorfields team: group 1, characterized by restricted macular dysfunction, as documented with multifocal or pattern ERG, with normal scotopic and photopic full-field ERG; group 2, characterized by generalized cone dysfunction on the full-field ERG (abnormal photopic responses, but normal scotopic responses); and group 3, characterized by both cone and rod dysfunction on full-field ERG (both photopic and scotopic response abnormalities) (Lois et al. 2001). The three groups

 Cite this article as *Cold Spring Harb Perspect Med* doi: 10.1101/cshperspect.a017111

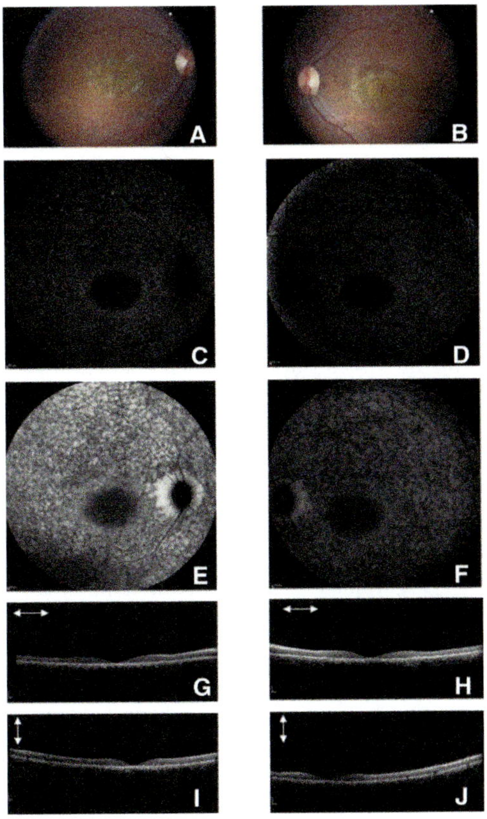

Figure 3. Fundus photographs, autofluorescence and spectral domain optical coherence tomography of a patient with Stargardt disease. Fundus photography (*A* right eye and *B* left eye), fundus autofluorescence blue (*C* right eye and *D* left eye), and near infrared (*E* right eye and *F* left eye) as well as Sd-OCT (*G* horizontal scan, *I* vertical scan of the right eye, *H* horizontal scan and *K* vertical scan of the left eye) of a patient with Stargardt disease. On the color pictures, note central macular atrophy with yellow dots in the mid-periphery. Fundus autofluorescence both on the blue and near infrared autofluorescence shows punctuate loss of autofluorescence in the mid-periphery with peripapillary sparing and loss of foveal autofluorescence in relation with macular atrophy; Sd-OCT reveal thinning of the outer retina in the foveal and parafoveal region.

illustrate the phenotypic variability associated with *ABCA4* mutations. Group 2 and group 3 are the most severe, with not only loss of central vision, but also progressive loss of peripheral visual fields and complete blindness. Such forms really represent a type of cone–rod dystrophy linked to *ABCA4* mutation.

Typically, Stargardt disease, reported for the first time by Karl Stargardt in 1909 (Stargardt 1909), is inherited as an autosomal recessive trait (Stargardt Disease 1, MIM #248200) with mutations in the *ABCA4* gene on chromosome 1p13–p21 (Gerber et al. 1995; Allikmets et al. 1997). More than 600 disease-causing mutations have been identified so far. The *ABCA4* (photoreceptor-specific ATP-binding cassette transporter 4) gene encodes for a retinal protein that is localized at the rims of the outer segments of both rod and cone photoreceptors (Sun and Nathans 1997). The retinal-specific ATP-binding cassette transporter protein has an essential role in the clearance of all-*trans*-retinal from the disk membranes after photoexcitation of rhodopsin (reviewed in Tsybovsky et al. 2010). Loss of protein function results in impaired transport of retinoids, accumulation of toxic substances (of which the best studied is A2E), and death of RPE cells and photoreceptors. As mentioned above, mutations in *ABCA4* are not only responsible for Stargardt disease, but are also a major cause of autosomal recessive CORD, and possibly also autosomal recessive RP (Sun and Nathans 1997; Cremers et al. 1998). The effects of the various mutations on ABCA4 protein function may be responsible for this phenotypic variability; nonsense or frameshift mutations with protein truncation being more commonly involved in CORD or RP than in typical Stargardt disease 1 (Sun and Nathans 1997). More recently, a few rare families have been reported with an autosomal dominant maculopathy with yellow flecks in the fundus resembling Stargardt disease (Stargardt disease, 3, MIM #600110). This is caused by mutations in the *ELOVL4* gene on chromosome 6q14.1 (Zhang et al. 2001).

CHOROIDEREMIA

Choroideremia is an X-linked retinal dystrophy that is characterized by progressive degeneration of the choriocapillaris, RPE, and photoreceptors, and progressive vision loss. Choroideremia typically affects males. Female carriers are usually asymptomatic, but retinal exams may show a characteristic fundus appearance with irregular pigmentation on the fundus. Despite these widespread changes in the fundus, ERG is normal in female carriers ("dirty fundus, normal function"), although some cases of retinal degeneration have been reported (Potter et al. 2004). Night blindness occurring in early childhood is usually the first symptom of the disease. It is followed by progressive loss of the peripheral visual field (tunnel vision) and later decreased visual acuity. The disease is progressive, but, compared with X-linked RP, visual prognosis is more favorable and patients usually maintain good central vision until their 50s or 60s. Full-field ERGs reveal rod–cone dysfunction: Scotopic responses with a reduction of the a-wave amplitude originating from rod photoreceptors are more severely affected than photopic responses. Fundus examination shows typical signs that distinguish choroideremia from RP: There is usually large scalloped chorioretinal atrophy with bare sclera in the periphery spreading toward the macula with little or no pigment migration. Unlike in RP, the optic nerve maintains its normal color until late in the course of the disease, and there is no narrowing of retinal blood vessels. Fundus autofluorescence reveals loss of autofluorescence in chorioretinal atrophic area with island of persistent autofluorescence, which, however, has a salt-and-pepper speckled appearance (Renner et al. 2006). OCT reveals thinning of both outer retinal structures and choriocapilaris that are sharply demarcated with evidence of retinal tabulation on the atrophic areas (Goldberg et al. 2013).

Choroideremia prevalence is estimated to be 1 in 50,000 to 100,000 people, accounting for ~4% of all blindness (see http://ghr.nlm.nih.gov/condition/choroideremia). The disease is caused by mutations in the *CHM* gene (encoding Rab Escort Protein 1, REP-1) (Cremers et al. 1990) and more than 100 causative mutations have been described so far. REP-1 is involved in posttranslational lipid modification of Rabs (small Ras superfamily GTPases), which are key regulators of phagocytosis, secretion, and intracellular trafficking in a variety of tissues throughout the body (reviewed in Preising and Ayuso 2004).

CONGENITAL STATIONARY NIGHT BLINDNESS

Congenital stationary night blindness (CSNB) is a nonprogressive retinal degenerative disorder characterized by lifelong night blindness. The Schubert-Bornschein type is the most common type of CSNB, characterized by an electronegative response of the ERG to a bright white flash in the dark-adapted eye, with a normal a-wave and selective reduction of the b-wave amplitude resulting on a reduced b/a ratio. Electrophysiology is therefore critical for the diagnosis of CSNB. The disease is most commonly inherited as an X-linked recessive trait, but can also have autosomal recessive and rarely autosomal dominant inheritance. Clinically, Schubert-Bornschien CSNB may present in two forms: complete and incomplete, according to whether there is a rod-specific ERG response to a dim light under dark adaptation (Miyake et al. 1986). Complete CSNB is characterized by severe night vision disturbances, nystagmus, high myopia and strabismus, reduced visual acuity, and severely reduced b-wave amplitude, with cone-specific ERG waveform abnormalities (Audo et al. 2008). Complete CSNB is caused by mutations in the gene *NYX* for X-linked forms, and in *GRM6*, *TRPM1*, *GPR179*, or *LRIT3* for autosomal recessive inheritance. Incomplete CSNB has a more variable clinical manifestation, and light sensitivity is usually the main complaint, along with nystagmus, strabismus, and low vision. This form of CSNB is characterized by a reduced rod b-wave and substantially reduced cone responses. Incomplete CSNB has been associated with mutations in *CACNA1F* for the X-linked forms and in *CABP4* and *CACNA2D4* for the autosomal recessive forms (reviewed in Zeitz et al. 2013). To date, more than 300 mutations have been identified in the genes underlying CSNB. A less common form of CSNB has been reported by Riggs and is associated with severe rod photoreceptor dysfunction in association with mutations in genes involved in rod phototransduction cascade such as rhodopsin and the β subunit of rod phosphodiesterases. This Riggs-type of CSNB is usually inherited as a dominant trait with normal daylight vision (reviewed by Dryja 2000).

 Cite this article as *Cold Spring Harb Perspect Med* doi: 10.1101/cshperspect.a017111

ACHROMATOPSIA

Achromatopsia, also called rod monochromacy or total congenital color blindness, is a congenital disorder with estimated prevalence of 1:30,000 (Michaelides et al. 2004). It is an autosomal recessive or X-linked disorder of the cone photoreceptors characterized by inability to distinguish colors, severely impaired visual acuity, photophobia, and nystagmus. The clinical manifestations occur early in infancy, and the disease course is usually nonprogressive. Spectral domain OCT may reveal foveal cone abnormalities (Genead et al. 2011). Five known autosomal recessive achromatopsia genes, *CNGA3*, *CNGB3*, *GNAT2*, *PDE6C*, and *PDE6H* (Kohl et al. 2012; Kohl and Hamel 2013), encode proteins in the cone phototransduction cascade, whereas the X-linked form is associated with mutations in the gene encoding L- and M-opsin. Achromatopsia is characterized by phenotypic variability in terms of visual acuity, residual color vision, and some investigators have proposed the term "dysfunction syndrome" to encompass this phenotypic variability (Michaelides et al. 2004). Clinical diagnosis is established by standard ophthalmologic examination showing decreased visual acuity, usually around 20/200, complete loss or only some residual color perception, normal fundus appearance or some foveal RPE changes, and, more importantly, by ERG recordings showing normal rod and nondetectable cone responses (Michaelides et al. 2004). The majority of human achromatopsia cases are caused by mutations in the *CNGB3* gene (reported prevalence 50%–90% in patients of Northern European descent) (Komaromy et al. 2010).

CURRENT THERAPIES FOR INHERITED RETINAL DISEASES

General Recommendations

Currently, there is no effective treatment that can prevent or reverse vision loss in IRDs. General recommendations include supportive measures to maintain the activities of daily living and improve quality of life. Low vision rehabilitation (orientation and mobility training, educational support, physical and occupational therapy) and optical and nonoptical corrective interventions (appropriate spectacles, high-intensity lamps, contrast-enhancing filters, near- and far magnification devices) should be proposed to all affected individuals. Limited exposure to sunlight and the use of green/blue-blocking sunglasses are recommended. Avoiding smoking and retino-toxic medications such as Plaquenil® is highly advisable. Cystoid macular edema in patients with RP can be treated with oral or topical (less effective) carbonic anhydrase inhibitors (e.g., acetazolamide) (Fishman et al. 1989; Grover et al. 1997). As a general guideline, cataract surgery is indicated in individuals with lens opacities and should be performed as soon as it causes significant impairment of vision and before the disease evolves to a point at which it could limit postoperative recovery. In general, RP patients experience significant improvements in visual acuity after cataract surgery (reviewed in Bayyoud et al. 2013; Dikopf et al. 2013). However, patients should be informed that postoperative visual acuity cannot be accurately predicted before surgery because the part of cataract versus the part of macular dysfunction in the decrease of vision is sometime difficult to evaluate.

Vitamin A +/− lutein and omega-3 DHA can be used as nutritional supplements for patients with retinal degenerations, including RP, in the absence of contraindications (Berson et al. 1993; Berson et al. 2004; Hoffman et al. 2004). Lutein and/or zeaxanthin (macular pigments from dietary sources) alone or in combination with vitamin A have shown some benefits in individuals with RP (e.g., increased macular pigment, decreased loss of visual field) (Aleman et al. 2001; Bahrami et al. 2006; Berson et al. 2010).

Although the general recommendations mentioned above may help, to some extent, to slow down the disease, there are, so far no curative treatment. Active research is being conducted to develop innovative treatments that address different aspects of the disease. These therapies aim to efficiently stop disease progression or restore some visual perception through gene-targeting therapies or neuroprotection, or seek to actively regenerate visual function through retinal prosthesis, optogenetics, cell based-therapies, or sensory substitution devices.

Gene Therapy

The past two decades have been marked by exceptional progress in understanding the biology and pathophysiology of the retina and identifying genes and mutations underlying IRDs. Despite this significant progress, the genetics of ~50% of IRDs remain to be established (Hartong et al. 2006). With the first success of gene therapy for LCA, finding the genetic cause of IRD becomes increasingly important—not only for the correct diagnosis of retinal disease, but also for providing a key to gene-based treatments. Gene therapy aims to replace, augment or "repair" the mutated and improperly functioning genes with normal genes that can restore protein function when expressed in retinal cells.

Most gene-mediated therapeutic strategies developed today use viral vectors that enable efficient gene delivery and stable transgene expression. The adenoviral vectors were among the first to be tested for retinal transduction (Bennett et al. 1994). These vectors have a relatively large cloning capacity, ranging from 8 to ~40 kb. Subretinal injections of adeniviral vector lead to efficient transduction of the RPE but limited transduction of the photoreceptors. In addition, these vectors are proinflammatory and immunogenic (Hoffman et al. 1997). Lentiviral vectors derived from human immunodeficiency virus 1, almost completely devoid of viral coding sequences, have a cloning capacity in the range of 8–9 kb and are capable of transducing both dividing and nondividing cells (Naldini et al. 1996). In rodents, subretinal injection of lentiviral vector resulted in very effective targeting of the RPE, but targeting of retinal neurons appeared limited (Auricchio et al. 2001; Bemelmans et al. 2005). In addition, lentiviruses are RNAviruses, compared with adenoviruses and adeno-associated viruses (AAV), which are DNA viruses. Vectors in RNA viruses can potentially integrate at random positions in the genome, with potential subsequent carcinogenesis, whereas those from DNAviruses mainly remain episomal. This risk is limited in the eye, however, because subretinally injected viruses target postmitotic cells. AAV-derived vectors are currently the preferred vectors for ocular gene therapy because of several key properties. First, AAV vectors display low immunogenicity because their genome is completely devoid of viral coding sequences. Second, there are a variety of different AAV serotypes possessing distinct properties. For example, subretinal injection of serotype 4 specifically targets RPE cells, serotypes 7 and 8 are more specific for photoreceptors, and serotype 5 can target both layers with equivalent efficacy; intravitreal injection of AAV2 or 8 results in transduction of retinal ganglion cells (reviewed in Colella and Auricchio 2010). Finally, long-lasting transgene expression is achieved following AAV transduction—provided that the target cell survives and does not divide. In a majority of cases, this is an advantage, but it may also represent a disadvantage in cases that require cessation of treatment. Factors that determine the specificity or efficacy of retinal cell transduction include dose, administration route/site of delivery, disease state, animal model, and capsid (Vandenberghe and Auricchio 2012). Very efficient transduction of RPE (usually 100% transduction in the area of detachment) and variable transduction of photoreceptors (20%–80%, depending on the serotype and titer used) were reported for all subretinally administered AAV serotypes (Vandenberghe and Auricchio 2012). To date, subretinal administration is the most efficient method for targeting photoreceptors and RPE cells, but it is technically more challenging than intravitreal injection and could be associated with postsurgical complications. Use of a newly developed AAV variant (7m8) that mediates efficient panretinal delivery of the therapeutic gene from the vitreous has recently been reported in mice and nonhuman primates with X-linked retinoschisis and LCA (Dalkara et al. 2013). The 7m8 vector enabled noninvasive, long-term histological and functional rescue of these disease phenotypes across the entire retina, offering clinically relevant implications for further gene therapy development.

The therapeutic efficacy of the viral vectors has been shown in many experimental models of retinal disease, mainly those concerning monogenic recessive IRDs. In this case, a copy of the normal gene is introduced into an individual's target cells and tissues to prevent a disease, treat a disease, arrest disease progression, or slow down the degenerative process. Impressive rescue of retinal degeneration in animal models has been shown using adenovirus- (Bennett et al. 1996), AAV- (Ali et al. 2000), or lentivirus-based vector technology (Tschernutter et al. 2005). Today, *RPE65* gene-replacement is the most notable example of successful gene therapy for retinal degenerative disorders. Proof of concept for gene replacement therapy has been shown by the team of Jean Bennett (Acland et al. 2001) in the Swedish Briard dog, a model of human LCA. A single subretinal injection of AAV2.RPE65 restored visual function in this canine model of LCA in a safe, sustained, and long-term manner (Acland et al. 2005). On this basis, clinical trials of recombinant AAV (rAAV)-mediated gene therapy for patients with LCA have been implemented. Safety and efficacy of the gene transfer and stable rescue of visual function lasting for at least 3 yr have been shown (Bainbridge et al. 2008; Hauswirth et al. 2008; Maguire et al. 2008; Jacobson et al. 2012; Testa et al. 2013). Readministration of AAV has been studied using bilateral subretinal injections in mouse (Barker et al. 2009), dog (Annear et al. 2011), and monkey (Amado et al. 2010) models of IRDs. Readministration of *RPE65* gene-based treatment to the contralateral eye of adult patients with LCA was recently reported to evoke significantly greater responses in the second eye (Bennett et al. 2012), supporting the feasibility and benefits of repeated gene therapy in retinal degenerative diseases. Despite the improved vision after *RPE65* gene augmentation therapy, however, photoreceptor degeneration was shown to progress both in the canine model and in humans (Cideciyan et al. 2013). This report directs attention to the need for further studies to assess the long-term safety, morphological outcomes, and functional benefits of gene therapy in LCA and other forms of retinal degeneration, and to evaluate combination therapies to improve vision and slow retinal degeneration in the long term. Nevertheless, the relatively good safety profile of the *RPE65* gene replacement studies in humans has opened the path for other gene therapy studies.

Choroideremia, which is a recessive, monogenic retinal disorder without extraocular manifestations, could be considered an "ideal" target for gene augmentation therapy. As the *CHM* cDNA is <4.7 kb in length, it is suitable for packaging in rAAV (Vasireddy et al. 2013). Despite these favorable factors, the main challenge in developing gene therapy for choroideremia at present remains the lack of an animal model that accurately reflects the human condition. Recently, it has been reported that subretinal injections of a lentiviral CHM/REP1 cDNA transgene resulted in efficient transduction of the RPE, long-term expression for at least 6 mo and a rescued prenylation defect in the CHM mouse (Tolmachova et al. 2012). An open-label, dose-escalation phase 1 clinical trial is being undertaken in Oxford University to assess the safety and tolerability of the AAV2.REP1 vector administered at two different doses to the retina in 12 choroideremia patients (see http://ClinicalTrials.gov .identifier: NCT01461213, PI: Rob McLaren). This gene therapy is expected to restore REP1 activity in the RPE of choroideremia patients. So far, six patients have been included with no major safety issues (MacLaren et al. 2014).

Applying a similar approach, an open-label phase 1 study has been initiated by Dr. Alkuraya in Saudi Arabia, for gene replacement therapy of *MERTK* (rAAV2-VMD2-hMERTK) in patients with *MERTK*-associated retinal disease (see http://ClinicalTrials.gov. Identifier: NCT01482195). This study follows a proof-of-principle study in RCS rats (Conlon et al. 2013), a model of retinal degeneration. *MERTK* mutations are a rare cause of RP in humans and lead to retinal dystrophy in RCS rats.

Many preclinical studies using rAAVs are currently underway to prepare for future gene therapy trials. Targeted disorders include achromatopsia and X-linked retinoschisis. Canine *CNGB3* mutations have been identified in Alaskan malamute and German shorthaired pointer breeds, providing a valuable system for studying the disease mechanisms for achromatopsia and evaluating potential therapies (Sidjanin et al. 2002). A recent study in these naturally occurring canine models of a *CNGB3* defect showed rescue of cone photoreceptor function after a single subretinal injection of rAAV5-mediated gene replacement therapy using different forms of the human red cone opsin promoter (Komaromy et al. 2010). The rescued cone function was documented by cone-specific ERG, and recovery of day vision was sustained for >2 yr, suggesting that the correction is stable and probably permanent. Recent studies have also shown that AAV-mediated delivery (serotypes 2, 5, or 8) of the normal *RS1* gene can promote long-term rescue of retinal structure and function in a mouse model of X-linked retinoschisis (Zeng et al. 2004; Kjellstrom et al. 2007; Janssen et al. 2008; Park et al. 2009). Intravitreal administration of the 7m8 vector (7m8-RS1) in the *Rs1h* knockout mouse led to high-level, panretinal RS1 expression in photoreceptors and throughout all other retinal layers, to levels comparable to wild-type for this secreted protein. This treatment led to substantial and stable improvements in rod and cone photoreceptor-mediated visual function and synaptic transmission (Dalkara et al. 2013). These studies provide substantial evidence that gene replacement therapy can be considered as a potential treatment for X-linked retinoschisis.

The above-mentioned gene replacement studies targeted relatively small genes with relevant animal models for treatment validation through preclinical studies. Other diseases raise distinct challenges, including Stargardt disease and Usher syndrome, which have underlying genetic defects in large genes and lack animal models to obtain proof-of-principle validation of disease rescue. As mentioned above, the use of lentivirus vectors allows packaging of larger genes up to 9 kb and therefore offers a tool for delivery of genes that cannot be packaged in AAV. A better understanding of animal models that do not completely mimic human disease may allow identification of useful markers that are relevant in pathogenicity. Examples of such models include the $Abca^{-/-}$ mouse, which does not strictly develop the central photoreceptor degeneration observed in Stargardt disease, but does show progressive accumulation of A2E, a major component of the disease process in humans (Cideciyan et al. 2004). Similarly, the *shaker* mouse, which has mutations in *Myo7A* (also mutated in Usher syndrome type IB), shows abnormal rhodopsin trafficking within rod outer segments and abnormal melanosomes in RPE cells (Liu et al. 1998, 1999). These markers have been very useful for validating gene replacement therapy in the respective models. High transduction efficiency of both rod and cone photoreceptors was observed after subretinal injection of equine infectious anemia virus (EIAV)-derived lentiviral vectors expressing human *ABCA4* gene in a mouse model of Stargardt disease, and correction of the disease phenotype was shown (Kong et al. 2008). This opened the way for clinical evaluation of lentiviral gene therapy as potentially efficient tool for treating retinal diseases. Indeed, three clinical trials are currently underway to evaluate the safety of StarGen™ (NCT01367444) in patients with Stargardt macular degeneration, UshStat® (NCT01505062) in patients with Usher Syndrome Type IB and RetinoStat® (NCT01301443) in patients with age-related macular degeneration, with all three vectors designed and developed by Oxford BioMedica using the company's proprietary LentiVector® gene delivery technology.

The large number of genes involved in the pathogenesis of IRDs is a major challenge for gene augmentation therapy today. Gene therapy may also not be suitable for autosomal dominant diseases with a dominant negative effect as the pathogenic mechanism. In such cases, suppression of the mutated copy may be more relevant (Farrar et al. 2010). Other important factors that should be taken into account when considering gene therapy include availability of relevant animal models with suitable disease markers, prevalence of the disorder, knowledge of the disorder's natural history to determine a suitable window for treatment, function of the transgene product, and risks associated with overexpression of the transgene. Therapeutic strategies that are independent of the disease-causing mutation thus carry a great potential in IRDs.

Neuroprotection

A significant body of evidence has shown that neurotrophic factors such as brain-derived neurotrophic factor (BDNF), pigment epithelium-derived neurotrophic factor (PEDF), basic fibroblast growth factor (bFGF or FGF-2), and ciliary neurotrophic factor (CNTF) slow retinal degeneration in a number of animal models. A phase 1 trial performed in ten patients with advanced RP for a period of 6 mo indicated that CNTF delivered by intraocular encapsulated cell technology (NT-501 implant, Neurotech USA) is safe for the human retina even with severely compromised photoreceptors (Sieving et al. 2006). A recent study spanning four clinical trials confirmed consistent safety of intraocular delivery of CNTF by intraocular encapsulated cell technology (NT-501 implants) over a 2-yr period in patients with RP and geographic atrophy (Kauper et al. 2012). However, these studies have so far failed to show functional rescue as measured by best-corrected visual acuity and visual field sensitivity at 12 mo (Birch et al. 2013). A phase 1-2 clinical trial with an NT-501 intraocular implant releasing CNTF to the retina of patients affected with CNGB3 achromatopsia is currently underway (see http://ClinicalTrials.gov. Identifier: NCT01648452).

As previously emphasized, the initial loss of rods (owing to mutations in genes solely expressed in rods) is followed by degeneration of the cones, with loss of central vision and blindness. This is mechanistically puzzling, because the genetic lesion is present only in the rods. Preventing this secondary degeneration of cones may allow for treatment of a wide range of IRDs, as such therapy would be independent of the disease-causing mutation. Rod-derived cone viability factor (RdCVF) has been shown to induce cone survival and functional rescue in animal models of recessive and dominant RP (Leveillard et al. 2004; Yang et al. 2009) in a manner independent from either the mechanisms or extent of rod degeneration. RdCVF is now considered not only as an autocrine- and paracrine-acting neuroprotective agent but also as a physiological signal involved in the maintenance of photoreceptors, of importance during both aging and exposure to oxidative stress. It would be particularly well-suited for preventing the secondary degeneration of cones and for treating RP at a stage in which night blindness is associated with moderate central visual impairment (Leveillard and Sahel 2010).

Alternative Pharmacological Approaches

A variety of pharmacological strategies have shown some potential efficacy in treating retinal degeneration; these include retinoid replacement, valproic acid therapy, and treatment with calcium channel blockers. Mutations in *LRAT* and *RPE65* cause disruption in 11-*cis*-retinal regeneration and account for ~5% of all cases of LCA and RP (Thompson et al. 2001; Bereta et al. 2008). Pharmacological retinoid replacement therapy for 11-*cis*-retinal deficiency thus carries the potential for treatment of human disease. Indeed, administration of 9-*cis*-retinoid has been shown to bypass defects in the visual cycle, restore visual function and slow the progression of retinal degeneration in *Lrat*$^{-/-}$ and *Rpe65*$^{-/-}$ mice (Van Hooser et al. 2000; Maeda et al. 2009). Similarly, long-term treatment with the 9-*cis*-retinal analog QLT091001 was well-tolerated and able to maintain retinal thickness and morphology in *Lrat*$^{-/-}$, *Rpe65*$^{-/-}$ mice and *Gnat1*$^{-/-}$ mice (Maeda et al. 2013). Based on these encouraging preclinical results, a safety proof-of-concept study to evaluate the effects of oral QLT091001 in RP subjects with an autosomal dominant mutation in *RPE65* is currently underway (see http://ClinicalTrials.gov. Identifier: NCT01543906). The antiepileptic drug valproic acid has some properties (neuroprotective and anti-inflammatory effects) and was also shown to act as a chaperone molecule for proper folding of rhodopsin mutants allowing to hypothesize potential therapeutic value in retinal degenerative diseases. A preliminary study with valproic acid had suggested therapeutic benefit in some patients with RP (Clemson et al. 2011). However, the long-term follow-up of 31 RP patients revealed possible declines in visual acuity and field, suggesting caution in the use of this drug to treat pigmentary retinal dystrophies

(Bhalla et al. 2013). Efficacy and safety of oral valproic acid for RP is under clinical investigation (http://ClinicalTrials.gov. Identifier: NCT01399515). Some studies in animal models have shown that calcium channel blockers (e.g., diltiazem, nicardipine, nilvadipine, or nifedipine) inhibit photoreceptor degeneration (Frasson et al. 1999; Takano et al. 2004), and a 30-mo clinical trial recently reported that nilvadipine at 4 mg/d significantly retarded progression of central visual field defects in RP (Nakazawa et al. 2011).

Retinal Prosthetics

In IRDs, parts of the inner retina survive even after complete degeneration of the retinal photosensitive layer and remain responsive to electrical simulation even in late stages of the disease (Humayun et al. 1996). Visual neuroprosthetics use electrical stimulation to activate the remaining inner retinal network, allowing these cells to take over the function of the lost photoreceptors. Different groups worldwide are currently working on retinal implant devices. The longest and largest follow-up data at present were reported for the epiretinal implant Argus II, made by the U.S. company Second Sight Medical Products (Humayun et al. 2003). This device is positioned on the surface of the retina (between the surface of the vitreous and the retina). It communicates directly with the ganglion and bipolar cells, receiving light signals from an external camera system. Long-term safety results showed that 70% of patients with profound visual loss implanted with Argus II did not have any serious adverse events; most of them performed better on visual tasks, including object localization, motion- and oriented grating discrimination, identification of letters and words, and even reading short sentences (Humayun et al. 2012; da Cruz et al. 2013). Argus II can also simulate visual Braille as a sensory substitute for reading (Lauritzen et al. 2012). Argus II received the first-ever commercial use approval (Europe, 2011; the United States, 2013) for a retinal prosthesis device to treat adult patients with retinal degenerative diseases such as advanced RP.

Subretinal implants are positioned between the retina and the choroid to replace degenerated photoreceptors and receive light directly from the environment (Zrenner 2002). Because of the proximity to the surviving neurons in the visual pathway, this approach may offer better inherent mechanical stability and may possibly require less current for effective stimulation, but it remains challenging from a surgical point of view. Clinical trial data (NCT0102480) obtained with the subretinal device made by Retina Implant AG (the wirelessly powered subretinal implant alpha-IMS) in profoundly blind patients with RP showed stable visual percepts, restoration of useful vision in daily life, and even identification of objects and letters (Zrenner et al. 2011; Stingl et al. 2013). The subretinal implant technology of Retina Implant AG received CE marking in July 2013. In a novel prosthetic device, the photovoltaic subretinal prosthesis, video goggles deliver both power and visual information directly to each pixel through pulsed near-infrared illumination (Mathieson et al. 2012). The implant is thin and wireless, the surgical procedure appears simple, all pixels in it function independently, and the natural link between image perception and eye movement is preserved. Both epi- and subretinal implants require an intact optic nerve pathway to function. Despite the great technical progress, the quality of the images achieved with retinal prosthetic devices remains a challenge. New electrode designs and new materials aiming at improving visual resolution and safety profiles are currently under investigation.

Optogenetics

Optogenetics combines genetic strategies that target light-sensitive proteins within the cells and optical stimulation to activate these selectively targeted proteins. To restore useful vision in blind patients, optogenetics takes advantages of two facts: (i) Even after the occurrence of blindness caused by IRD, many cone photoreceptors survive and maintain their cell body for extended periods (Li et al. 1995, Lin et al. 2009); and (ii) the remarkable proteins channelrhodopsin-2 (ChR2) (Nagel et al. 2002; Boyden et al. 2005) and halorhodopsin (NpHR) (Zhang et al. 2007) function as light-gated ion channels. The key goal of optogenetic vision restoration is to convert strategically important retinal cell types into "artificial photoreceptors." Indeed, ChR2 has been targeted to ON bipolar cells of *rd1* mice, after which cells with morphological features of ON ganglion cells responded to increases in light intensity. Light-evoked activity was measured in the cortex, and visually evoked behavior was documented (Lagali et al. 2008). Recent studies have shown that NpHR introduced to surviving cone cell bodies in two mouse models of RP reactivated retinal ON and OFF pathways, as well as the retinal circuitry, and enabled RP mice to perform visually guided behaviors (Busskamp et al. 2010). Moreover, NpHR targeted to human postmortem photoreceptors with no measurable intrinsic rod- or cone-mediated photosensitivity restored light responses in photoreceptor cells, clearly showing that reactivation of the surviving retinal structures and phototransduction cascade required for vision is possible (Busskamp et al. 2010). These preclinical data hold promise that legally blind patients or severely visually impaired patients with no visual field but with a preserved layer of cone bodies (visible on OCT) could be eligible for optogenetic functional restoration of cones. Key advantages of optogenetics as a therapeutic approach for IRDs include: (i) It may provide artificially stimulated retinal activity that resembles the normal activity of retinal circuits, because these retinal cells are already connected to other retinal circuit elements in a biologically relevant way; and (ii) it is gene/mutation-independent. Different strategies for optogenetic vision restoration, including their advantages and possible combination with other methods to slow retinal degeneration and/or restore vision were recently reviewed in (Busskamp et al. 2011; Sahel and Roska 2013).

Cellular Therapy

Transplantation of retinal cells is another potential strategy to restore vision in patients with IRDs. Development of synaptic connections and functionality is of major importance, although efficacy and safety in implanting fetal retina with accompanying RPE in AMD and RP patients has already been reported (Radtke et al. 2008). Transplantation of photoreceptor precursor cells is an alternative approach. Indeed, initial data showed that transplanted progenitor or precursor cells isolated at the correct ontogenetic stage from the developing retina can integrate into the host retina and differentiate into rod photoreceptors (MacLaren et al. 2006). Recent findings confirmed the survival and differentiation of some photoreceptors derived from three-dimensional embryonic stem cell (ESC) cultures: ESC-derived photoreceptor cell precursors showed capability to integrate and mature, and to form outer segments and some synaptic connections after transplantation into the degenerate adult mouse retina, thus supporting the utility of ESC-derived cells for photoreceptor replacement therapy (whether similar integration can be achieved using human cells remains to be established as well as the functional improvement provided) (Gonzalez-Cordero et al. 2013). The main advantage of cell therapies as a source for regenerative therapy is that they are gene-independent and thus can be applicable to broader range of retinal diseases. Pluripotent stem cells like human embryonic stem cells (hESCs) or human induced pluripotent stem cells (hiPSCs) can be expanded indefinitely in culture and could be used as an unlimited source of retinal cells for treatment of IRDs (Zhao et al. 2002; Osakada et al. 2008; Hirami et al. 2009; Lamba et al. 2009; Lamba et al. 2010). The first-ever safety and tolerability prospective clinical trial to evaluate subretinal injection of hESC-derived RPE cells in patients with dry age-related macular degeneration and Stargardt macular dystrophy (see http://ClinicalTrials.gov. Identifier: NCT01345006) is currently underway, and very early results suggest no major safety concern (no signs of hyperproliferation, tumorigenicity, ectopic tissue formation, or apparent rejection after 4 mo) (Schwartz et al. 2012). As hiPSCs can be obtained directly from the patient, they have the advantage of being autologous and therefore less-immunogenic than hESCs (although hiPSCs vary in pluripotency and may differentiate less-efficiently than do ESCs). Retinal cells derived from hiPSCs have been generated by different laboratories worldwide, and some groups are currently setting up human clinical trials with hiPSC-derived RPE for treatment of age-related macular degeneration (e.g., pilot clinical study to assess the safety and feasibility of the transplantation of autologous iPSCs in patients with exudative age-related macular degeneration started in Japan in 2013) (see http://www.riken.jp/en/pr/press/2013/20130730_1). Advances in research into iPSC applications for treatment of retinal degeneration were recently reviewed in detail by Cramer and MacLaren (2013).

Sensory Substitution Devices

Technologies transforming auditory or tactile information into visual sensory information have recently been developed. Clinical studies currently assess the capacities of the visual-to-auditory sensory substitution device called "The vOICe." They showed that blind and blindfolded participants can locate and identify objects through images encoded by sound (Auvray et al. 2007; Merabet et al. 2009). Even congenitally fully blind adults could be taught to read and recognize complex images using "soundscapes," sounds topographically representing images (Striem-Amit et al. 2011, 2012a,b). Results of these studies clearly show the possibility of compensating for some effects of early and long-lasting or lifelong blindness or restore vision by providing visual-like experience via sensory substitution. BrainPort® is a device that translates information from a digital video camera to the tongue, because this organ has the capacity to act as a portal to convey somatosensory information to the visual cortex. The device uses a gentle electrical stimulation to create a tactile "image" that helps blind individuals to recognize high-contrast objects, their location and movement, and some aspects of perspective and depth (Sampaio et al. 2001; Chebat et al. 2007). As sensory substitution devices are noninvasive and cheap, although they require training in a scale of hours (Striem-Amit et al. 2012b), they represent an attractive alternative to other therapeutic approaches. They can serve as aids for the blind in daily visual tasks and can be used in combination with other therapeutic approaches for vision restoration.

APPROPRIATE PATIENT EVALUATION AND SELECTION

Identifying patients who can benefit from these innovative treatments is a crucial step in the process of assessing a patient's needs and selecting appropriate therapy. A key technology for this identification is in vivo, noninvasive imaging of the retina, which can provide objective clinical validation and may allow monitoring of both disease progression and treatment efficacy. Optical coherent tomography is particularly useful for examining retinal architecture and, more specifically, the outer retina structure, and photoreceptor inner/outer segment border. Adaptive optics fundus imaging is particularly suited for exploration of the healthy and dystrophic retinal structures, including photoreceptor detection and counting, and accurate documentation of RPE changes (Gocho et al. 2013). These high-resolution imaging techniques can help to select patients for clinical trials (e.g., to define the area of subretinal injection and diminish potential hazards resulting from injection) and may have important implications for establishing functional correlates and studying therapy outcomes. Functional studies (e.g., microperimetry) are also of crucial importance for establishing the benefit of these novel therapies, and they should be extended beyond testing visual field and visual acuity. Standardized mobility and task-related tests are needed both for assessment of the subjective visual handicap and for a reliable evaluation of the actual benefit for the patient. Development of new rehabilitation programs and devices, especially those that take advantage of visual plasticity (persisting even in old age) should be of paramount importance.

CONCLUDING REMARKS

An improved understanding of disease mechanisms is the first step in developing effective therapies for IRDs. To date, the advances in sequencing technologies have contributed to a rapid gain of knowledge and will certainly lead to discovery of new, as-yet unknown causative genes implicated in the pathophysiology of IRDs, with the ultimate goal of providing treatment for these incurable disorders. Indeed, a recent study using targeted RNA capture to perform large-scale validation of novel transcriptome features provided an unprecedented level of information regarding the human retinal transcriptome, identifying almost 30,000 novel exons and 116 putative novel genes (Farkas et al. 2013). Further studies will be required to uncover the function of these new genes in the retina. In addition to efficient and accurate genotyping, thorough clinical characterization of patients and families and genotype–phenotype association studies are the key toward improving diagnosis and allowing for appropriate genetic counseling with reliable predictions of disease course and prognosis. This knowledge will provide a foundation for development of preventive and/or therapeutic strategies, help to determine the risk/benefit profile of treatments and allow patients to make informed lifestyle decisions. The advent of several promising therapeutic approaches puts even more emphasis on genotype–phenotype correlations, extensive evaluation of disease markers during natural history, and analysis of treatment efficacy.

REFERENCES

Acland GM, Aguirre GD, Ray J, Zhang Q, Aleman TS, Cideciyan AV, Pearce-Kelling SE, Anand V, Zeng Y, Maguire AM, et al. 2001. Gene therapy restores vision in a canine model of childhood blindness. *Nat Genet* **28:** 92–95.

Acland GM, Aguirre GD, Bennett J, Aleman TS, Cideciyan AV, Bennicelli J, Dejneka NS, Pearce-Kelling SE, Maguire AM, Palczewski K, et al. 2005. Long-term restoration of rod and cone vision by single dose rAAV-mediated gene transfer to the retina in a canine model of childhood blindness. *Mol Ther* **12:** 1072–1082.

Adackapara CA, Sunness JS, Dibernardo CW, Melia BM, Dagnelie G. 2008. Prevalence of cystoid macular edema and stability in oct retinal thickness in eyes with retinitis pigmentosa during a 48-week lutein trial. *Retina* **28:** 103–110.

Aleman TS, Duncan JL, Bieber ML, de Castro E, Marks DA, Gardner LM, Steinberg JD, Cideciyan AV, Maguire MG, Jacobson SG. 2001. Macular pigment and lutein supplementation in retinitis pigmentosa and Usher syndrome. *Invest Ophthalmol Vis Sci* **42:** 1873–1881.

Ali RR, Sarra GM, Stephens C, Alwis MD, Bainbridge JW, Munro PM, Fauser S, Reichel MB, Kinnon C, Hunt DM, et al. 2000. Restoration of photoreceptor ultrastructure and function in retinal degeneration slow mice by gene therapy. *Nat Genet* **25:** 306–310.

Allikmets R, Singh N, Sun H, Shroyer NF, Hutchinson A, Chidambaram A, Gerrard B, Baird L, Stauffer D, Peiffer A, et al. 1997. A photoreceptor cell-specific ATP-binding transporter gene (*ABCR*) is mutated in recessive Stargardt macular dystrophy. *Nat Genet* **15:** 236–246.

Amado D, Mingozzi F, Hui D, Bennicelli JL, Wei Z, Chen Y, Bote E, Grant RL, Golden JA, Narfstrom K, et al. 2010. Safety and efficacy of subretinal readministration of a viral vector in large animals to treat congenital blindness. *Sci Transl Med* **2:** 21ra16.

Andreasson SO, Sandberg MA, Berson EL. 1988. Narrow-band filtering for monitoring low-amplitude cone electroretinograms in retinitis pigmentosa. *Am J Ophthalmol* **105:** 500–503.

Annear MJ, Bartoe JT, Barker SE, Smith AJ, Curran PG, Bainbridge JW, Ali RR, Petersen-Jones SM. 2011. Gene therapy in the second eye of RPE65-deficient dogs improves retinal function. *Gene Ther* **18:** 53–61.

Audo I, Robson AG, Holder GE, Moore AT. 2008. The negative ERG: Clinical phenotypes and disease mechanisms of inner retinal dysfunction. *Surv Ophthalmol* **53:** 16–40.

Auricchio A, Kobinger G, Anand V, Hildinger M, O'Connor E, Maguire AM, Wilson JM, Bennett J. 2001. Exchange of surface proteins impacts on viral vector cellular specificity and transduction characteristics: The retina as a model. *Hum Mol Genet* **10:** 3075–3081.

Auvray M, Hanneton S, O'Regan JK. 2007. Learning to perceive with a visuo-auditory substitution system: Localisation and object recognition with 'the vOICe'. *Perception* **36:** 416–430.

Ayuso C, Millan JM. 2010. Retinitis pigmentosa and allied conditions today: A paradigm of translational research. *Genome Med* **2:** 34.

Bahrami H, Melia M, Dagnelie G. 2006. Lutein supplementation in retinitis pigmentosa: PC-based vision assessment in a randomized double-masked placebo-controlled clinical trial [NCT00029289]. *BMC Ophthalmol* **6:** 23.

Bainbridge JW, Smith AJ, Barker SS, Robbie S, Henderson R, Balaggan K, Viswanathan A, Holder GE, Stockman A, Tyler N, et al. 2008. Effect of gene therapy on visual function in Leber's congenital amaurosis. *N Engl J Med* **358:** 2231–2239.

Barker SE, Broderick CA, Robbie SJ, Duran Y, Natkunarajah M, Buch P, Balaggan KS, MacLaren RE, Bainbridge JW, Smith AJ, et al. 2009. Subretinal delivery of adeno-associated virus serotype 2 results in minimal immune responses that allow repeat vector administration in immunocompetent mice. *J Gene Med* **11:** 486–497.

Bayyoud T, Bartz-Schmidt KU, Yoeruek E. 2013. Long-term clinical results after cataract surgery with and without capsular tension ring in patients with retinitis pigmentosa: A retrospective study. *BMJ Open* **26:** e002616.

Bemelmans AP, Bonnel S, Houhou L, Dufour N, Nandrot E, Helmlinger D, Sarkis C, Abitbol M, Mallet J. 2005. Retinal cell type expression specificity of HIV-1-derived gene transfer vectors upon subretinal injection in the adult rat: Influence of pseudotyping and promoter. *J Gene Med* **7:** 1367–1374.

Bennett J, Wilson J, Sun D, Forbes B, Maguire A. 1994. Adenovirus vector-mediated in vivo gene transfer into adult murine retina. *Invest Ophthalmol Vis Sci* **35:** 2535–2542.

Bennett J, Tanabe T, Sun D, Zeng Y, Kjeldbye H, Gouras P, Maguire AM. 1996. Photoreceptor cell rescue in retinal degeneration (*rd*) mice by in vivo gene therapy. *Nat Med* **2:** 649–654.

Bennett J, Ashtari M, Wellman J, Marshall KA, Cyckowski LL, Chung DC, McCague S, Pierce EA, Chen Y, Bennicelli JL, et al. 2012. AAV2 gene therapy readministration in three adults with congenital blindness. *Sci Transl Med* **4:** 120ra115.

Bereta G, Kiser PD, Golczak M, Sun W, Heon E, Saperstein DA, Palczewski K. 2008. Impact of retinal disease-associated *RPE65* mutations on retinoid isomerization. *Biochemistry* **47:** 9856–9865.

Berson EL, Rosner B, Sandberg MA, Hayes KC, Nicholson BW, Weigel-DiFranco C, Willett W. 1993. A randomized trial of vitamin A and vitamin E supplementation for retinitis pigmentosa. *Arch Ophthalmol* **111:** 761–772.

Berson EL, Rosner B, Sandberg MA, Weigel-DiFranco C, Moser A, Brockhurst RJ, Hayes KC, Johnson CA, Anderson EJ, Gaudio AR, et al. 2004. Further evaluation of docosahexaenoic acid in patients with retinitis pigmentosa receiving vitamin A treatment: Subgroup analyses. *Arch Ophthalmol* **122:** 1306–1314.

Berson EL, Rosner B, Sandberg MA, Weigel-DiFranco C, Brockhurst RJ, Hayes KC, Johnson EJ, Anderson EJ, Johnson CA, Gaudio AR, et al. 2010. Clinical trial of lutein in patients with retinitis pigmentosa receiving vitamin A. *Arch Ophthalmol* **128:** 403–411.

Bessant DA, Ali RR, Bhattacharya SS. 2001. Molecular genetics and prospects for therapy of the inherited retinal dystrophies. *Curr Opin Genet Dev* **11:** 307–316.

Bhalla S, Joshi D, Bhullar S, Kasuga D, Park Y, Kay CN. 2013. Long-term follow-up for efficacy and safety of treatment of retinitis pigmentosa with valproic acid. *Br J Ophthalmol* **97:** 895–899.

Birch DG, Sandberg MA. 1996. Submicrovolt full-field cone electroretinograms: Artifacts and reproducibility. *Doc Ophthalmol* **92:** 269–280.

Birch DG., Weleber RG, Duncan JL, Jaffe GJ., Tao W. 2013. Randomized trial of ciliary neurotrophic factor delivered by encapsulated cell intraocular implants for retinitis pigmentosa. *Am J Ophthalmol* **156:** 283–292.

Blacharski P. 1988. Fundus flavimaculatus. In *Retinal dystrophies and degenerations* (ed. Newsome DA), pp. 135–159. Raven, New York.

Boughman JA, Vernon M, Shaver KA. 1983. Usher syndrome: Definition and estimate of prevalence from two high-risk populations. *J Chronic Dis* **36:** 595–603.

Boyden ES, Zhang F, Bamberg E, Nagel G, Deisseroth K. 2005. Millisecond-timescale, genetically targeted optical control of neural activity. *Nat Neurosci* **8:** 1263–1268.

Bunker CH, Berson EL, Bromley WC, Hayes RP, Roderick TH. 1984. Prevalence of retinitis pigmentosa in Maine. *Am J Ophthalmol* **97:** 357–365.

Busskamp V, Duebel J, Balya D, Fradot M, Viney TJ, Siegert S, Groner AC, Cabuy E, Forster V, Seeliger M, et al. 2010. Genetic reactivation of cone photoreceptors restores visual responses in retinitis pigmentosa. *Science* **329:** 413–417.

Busskamp V, Picaud S, Sahel JA, Roska B. 2011. Optogenetic therapy for retinitis pigmentosa. *Gene Ther* **19:** 169–175.

Chebat DR, Rainville C, Kupers R, Ptito M. 2007. Tactile-'visual' acuity of the tongue in early blind individuals. *Neuroreport* **18:** 1901–1904.

Cideciyan AV, Aleman TS, Swider M, Schwartz SB, Steinberg JD, Brucker AJ, Maguire AM, Bennett J, Stone EM, Jacobson SG. 2004. Mutations in *ABCA4* result in accumulation of lipofuscin before slowing of the retinoid cycle: A reappraisal of the human disease sequence. *Hum Mol Genet* **13:** 525–534.

Cideciyan AV, Jacobson SG, Beltran WA, Sumaroka A, Swider M, Iwabe S, Roman AJ, Olivares MB, Schwartz SB, Komaromy AM, et al. 2013. Human retinal gene therapy for Leber congenital amaurosis shows advancing retinal degeneration despite enduring visual improvement. *Proc Natl Acad Sci* **110:** E517–E525.

Clemson CM, Tzekov R, Krebs M, Checchi JM, Bigelow C, Kaushal S. 2011. Therapeutic potential of valproic acid for retinitis pigmentosa. *Br J Ophthalmol* **95:** 89–93.

Colella P, Auricchio A. 2010. AAV-mediated gene supply for treatment of degenerative and neovascular retinal diseases. *Curr Gene Ther* **10:** 371–380.

Conlon TJ, Deng WT, Erger K, Cossette T, Pang JJ, Ryals R, Clement N, Cleaver B, McDoom I, Boye SE, et al. 2013. Preclinical potency and safety studies of an AAV2-mediated gene therapy vector for the treatment of MERTK associated retinitis pigmentosa. *Hum Gene Ther Clin Dev* **24:** 23–28.

Coppieters F, Lefever S, Leroy BP, De Baere E. 2010. *CEP290*, a gene with many faces: Mutation overview and presentation of CEP290*base*. *Hum Mutat* **31:** 1097–1108.

Cramer AO, MacLaren RE. 2013. Translating induced pluripotent stem cells from bench to bedside: Application to retinal diseases. *Curr Gene Ther* **13:** 139–151.

Cremers FP, van de Pol DJ, van Kerkhoff LP, Wieringa B, Ropers HH. 1990. Cloning of a gene that is rearranged in patients with choroideraemia. *Nature* **347:** 674–677.

Cremers FP, van de Pol DJ, van Driel M, den Hollander AI, van Haren FJ, Knoers NV, Tijmes N, Bergen AA, Rohrschneider K, Blankenagel A, et al. 1998. Autosomal recessive retinitis pigmentosa and cone-rod dystrophy caused by splice site mutations in the Stargardt's disease gene *ABCR*. *Hum Mol Genet* **7:** 355–362.

da Cruz L, Coley BF, Dorn J, Merlini F, Filley E, Christopher P, Chen FK, Wuyyuru V, Sahel J, Stanga P, et al. 2013. The Argus II epiretinal prosthesis system allows letter and word reading and long-term function in patients with profound vision loss. *Br J Ophthalmol* **97:** 632–636.

Daiger SP, Bowne SJ, Sullivan LS. 2007. Perspective on genes and mutations causing retinitis pigmentosa. *Arch Ophthalmol* **125:** 151–158.

Dalkara D, Byrne LC, Klimczak RR, Visel M, Yin L, Merigan WH, Flannery JG, Schaffer DV. 2013. In vivo-directed evolution of a new adeno-associated virus for therapeutic outer retinal gene delivery from the vitreous. *Sci Transl Med* **5:** p189ra176.

den Hollander AI, Roepman R, Koenekoop RK, Cremers FP. 2008. Leber congenital amaurosis: Genes, proteins and disease mechanisms. *Prog Retin Eye Res* **27:** 391–419.

Dikopf MS, Chow CC, Mieler WF, Tu EY. 2013. Cataract extraction outcomes and the prevalence of zonular insufficiency in retinitis pigmentosa. *Am J Ophthalmol* **156:** 82–88.

Drivas TG, Holzbaur EL, Bennett J. 2013. Disruption of CEP290 microtubule/membrane-binding domains causes retinal degeneration. *J Clin Invest* **123:** 4525–4539.

Dryja TP. 2000. Molecular genetics of Oguchi disease, fundus albipunctatus, and other forms of stationary night blindness: LVII Edward Jackson Memorial Lecture. *Am J Ophthalmol* **130:** 547–563.

Dryja TP, McGee TL, Reichel E, Hahn LB, Cowley GS, Yandell DW, Sandberg MA, Berson EL. 1990. A point mutation of the rhodopsin gene in one form of retinitis pigmentosa. *Nature* **343:** 364–366.

Dryja TP, Finn JT, Peng YW, McGee TL, Berson EL, Yau KW. 1995. Mutations in the gene encoding the α subunit of the rod cGMP-gated channel in autosomal recessive retinitis pigmentosa. *Proc Natl Acad Sci* **92:** 10177–10181.

Falk MJ, Zhang Q, Nakamaru-Ogiso E, Kannabiran C, Fonseca-Kelly Z, Chakarova C, Audo I, Mackay DS, Zeitz C, Borman AD, et al. 2012. *NMNAT1* mutations cause Leber congenital amaurosis. *Nat Genet* **44:** 1040–1045.

Farkas MH, Grant GR, White JA, Sousa ME, Consugar MB, Pierce EA. 2013. Transcriptome analyses of the human retina identify unprecedented transcript diversity and 3.5 Mb of novel transcribed sequence via significant alternative splicing and novel genes. *BMC Genomics* **14:** 486.

Farrar GJ, Palfi A, O'Reilly M. 2010. Gene therapeutic approaches for dominant retinopathies. *Curr Gene Ther* **10:** 381–388.

Fishman GA, Anderson RJ, Lourenco P. 1985. Prevalence of posterior subcapsular lens opacities in patients with retinitis pigmentosa. *Br J Ophthalmol* **69:** 263–266.

Fishman GA, Gilbert LD, Fiscella RG, Kimura AE, Jampol LM. 1989. Acetazolamide for treatment of chronic macular edema in retinitis pigmentosa. *Arch Ophthalmol* **107:** 1445–1452.

Forsythe E, Beales PL. 2012. Bardet-Biedl syndrome. *Eur J Hum Genet* **21:** 8–13.

Frasson M, Sahel JA, Fabre M, Simonutti M, Dreyfus H, Picaud S. 1999. Retinitis pigmentosa: Rod photoreceptor rescue by a calcium-channel blocker in the *rd* mouse. *Nat Med* **5:** 1183–1187.

Genead MA, Fishman GA, Rha J, Dubis AM, Bonci DM, Dubra A, Stone EM, Neitz M, Carroll J. 2011. Photoreceptor structure and function in patients with congenital achromatopsia. *Invest Ophthalmol Vis Sci* **52:** 7298–7308.

George ND, Yates JR, Moore AT. 1995. X linked retinoschisis. *Br J Ophthalmol* **79:** 697–702.

George ND, Yates JR, Moore AT. 1996. Clinical features in affected males with X-linked retinoschisis. *Arch Ophthalmol* **114:** 274–280.

Gerber S, Rozet JM, Bonneau D, Souied E, Camuzat A, Dufier JL, Amalric P, Weissenbach J, Munnich A, Kaplan J. 1995. A gene for late-onset fundus flavimaculatus with macular dystrophy maps to chromosome 1p13. *Am J Hum Genet* **56:** 396–399.

Gocho K, Sarda V, Falah S, Sahel JA, Sennlaub F, Benchaboune M, Ullern M, Paques M. 2013. Adaptive optics imaging of geographic atrophy. *Invest Ophthalmol Vis Sci* **54:** 3673–3680.

Goldberg NR, Greenberg JP, Laud K, Tsang S, Freund KB. 2013. Outer retinal tubulation in degenerative retinal disorders. *Retina* **33:** 1871–1876.

Gonzalez-Cordero A, West EL, Pearson RA, Duran Y, Carvalho LS, Chu CJ, Naeem A, Blackford SJ, Georgiadis A, Lakowski J, et al. 2013. Photoreceptor precursors derived from three-dimensional embryonic stem cell cultures integrate and mature within adult degenerate retina. *Nat Biotechnol* **31:** 741–747.

Grover S, Fishman GA, Fiscella RG, Adelman AE. 1997. Efficacy of dorzolamide hydrochloride in the management of chronic cystoid macular edema in patients with retinitis pigmentosa. *Retina* **17:** 222–231.

Hagiwara A, Yamamoto S, Ogata K, Sugawara T, Hiramatsu A, Shibata M, Mitamura Y. 2011. Macular abnormalities in patients with retinitis pigmentosa: Prevalence on OCT examination and outcomes of vitreoretinal surgery. *Acta Ophthalmol* **89:** e122–e125.

Haim M. 2002. Epidemiology of retinitis pigmentosa in Denmark. *Acta Ophthalmol Scand* **80**(S233): 1–34.

Hartong DT, Berson EL, Dryja TP. 2006. Retinitis pigmentosa. *Lancet* **368:** 1795–1809.

Hauswirth WW, Aleman TS, Kaushal S, Cideciyan AV, Schwartz SB, Wang L, Conlon TJ, Boye SL, Flotte TR, Byrne BJ, et al. 2008. Treatment of Leber congenital amaurosis due to *RPE65* mutations by ocular subretinal injection of adeno-associated virus gene vector: Short-term results of a phase I trial. *Hum Gene Ther* **19:** 979–990.

Heckenlively J. 1982. The frequency of posterior subcapsular cataract in the hereditary retinal degenerations. *Am J Ophthalmol* **93:** 733–738.

Heckenlively JR, Yoser SL, Friedman LH, Oversier JJ. 1988. Clinical findings and common symptoms in retinitis pigmentosa. *Am J Ophthalmol* **105:** 504–511.

Hirami Y, Osakada F, Takahashi K, Okita K, Yamanaka S, Ikeda H, Yoshimura N, Takahashi M. 2009. Generation of retinal cells from mouse and human induced pluripotent stem cells. *Neurosci Lett* **458:** 126–131.

Hoffman LM, Maguire AM, Bennett J. 1997. Cell-mediated immune response and stability of intraocular transgene expression after adenovirus-mediated delivery. *Invest Ophthalmol Vis Sci* **38:** 2224–2233.

Hoffman DR, Locke KG, Wheaton DH, Fish GE, Spencer R, Birch DG. 2004. A randomized, placebo-controlled clinical trial of docosahexaenoic acid supplementation for X-linked retinitis pigmentosa. *Am J Ophthalmol* **137:** 704–718.

Hood DC, Holopigian K, Greenstein V, Seiple W, Li J, Sutter EE, Carr RE. 1998. Assessment of local retinal function in patients with retinitis pigmentosa using the multi-focal ERG technique. *Vision Res* **38:** 163–179.

Humayun MS, de Juan E Jr, Dagnelie G, Greenberg RJ, Propst RH, Phillips DH. 1996. Visual perception elicited by electrical stimulation of retina in blind humans. *Arch Ophthalmol* **114:** 40–46.

Humayun MS, Weiland JD, Fujii GY, Greenberg R, Williamson R, Little J, Mech B, Cimmarusti V, Van Boemel G, Dagnelie G, et al. 2003. Visual perception in a blind subject with a chronic microelectronic retinal prosthesis. *Vision Res* **43:** 2573–2581.

Humayun MS, Dorn JD, da Cruz L, Dagnelie G, Sahel JA, Stanga PE, Cideciyan AV, Duncan JL, Eliott D, Filley E, et al. 2012. Interim results from the international trial of Second Sight's visual prosthesis. *Ophthalmology* **119:** 779–788.

Jackson H, Garway-Heath D, Rosen P, Bird AC, Tuft SJ. 2001. Outcome of cataract surgery in patients with retinitis pigmentosa. *Br J Ophthalmol* **85:** 936–938.

Jacobson SG, Cideciyan AV, Ratnakaram R, Heon E, Schwartz SB, Roman AJ, Peden MC, Aleman TS, Boye SL, Sumaroka A, et al. 2012. Gene therapy for Leber congenital amaurosis caused by *RPE65* mutations: Safety and efficacy in 15 children and adults followed up to 3 years. *Arch Ophthalmol* **130:** 9–24.

Janssen A, Min SH, Molday LL, Tanimoto N, Seeliger MW, Hauswirth WW, Molday RS, Weber BH. 2008. Effect of late-stage therapy on disease progression in AAV-mediated rescue of photoreceptor cells in the retinoschisin-deficient mouse. *Mol Ther* **16:** 1010–1017.

Jonas JB, Xu L, Wang YX. 2009. The Beijing Eye Study. *Acta Ophthalmol* **87:** 247–261.

Kamenarova K, Cherninkova S, Romero Duran M, Prescott D, Valdes Sanchez ML, Mitev V, Kremensky I, Kaneva R, Bhattacharya SS, Tournev I, et al. 2013. A novel locus for autosomal dominant cone-rod dystrophy maps to chromosome 10q. *Eur J Hum Genet* **21:** 338–342.

Kauper K, McGovern C, Sherman S, Heatherton P, Rapoza R, Stabila P, Dean B, Lee A, Borges S, Bouchard B, et al. 2012. Two-year intraocular delivery of ciliary neurotrophic factor by encapsulated cell technology implants in patients with chronic retinal degenerative diseases. *Invest Ophthalmol Vis Sci* **53:** 7484–7491.

Kjellstrom S, Bush RA, Zeng Y, Takada Y, Sieving PA. 2007. Retinoschisin gene therapy and natural history in the *Rs1h*-KO mouse: Long-term rescue from retinal degeneration. *Invest Ophthalmol Vis Sci* **48:** 3837–3845.

Koenekoop RK. 2004. An overview of Leber congenital amaurosis: A model to understand human retinal development. *Surv Ophthalmol* **49:** 379–398.

Koenekoop RK, Wang H, Majewski J, Wang X, Lopez I, Ren H, Chen Y, Li Y, Fishman GA, Genead M, et al. 2012. Mutations in *NMNAT1* cause Leber congenital amaurosis and identify a new disease pathway for retinal degeneration. *Nat Genet* **44:** 1035–1039.

Kohl S, Hamel C. 2013. Clinical utility gene card for: Achromatopsia–update 2013. *Eur J Hum Genet* **21.** http://www.nature.com/ejhg/journal/v21/n11/full/ejhg201344a.html

Kohl S, Coppieters F, Meire F, Schaich S, Roosing S, Brennenstuhl C, Bolz S, van Genderen MM, Riemslag FC, Lukowski R, et al. 2012. A nonsense mutation in *PDE6H* causes autosomal-recessive incomplete achromatopsia. *Am J Hum Genet* **91:** 527–532.

Koizumi H, Spaide RF, Fisher YL, Freund KB, Klancnik JM Jr, Yannuzzi LA. 2008. Three-dimensional evaluation of vitreomacular traction and epiretinal membrane using spectral-domain optical coherence tomography. *Am J Ophthalmol* **145:** 509–517.

Komaromy AM, Alexander JJ, Rowlan JS, Garcia MM, Chiodo VA, Kaya A, Tanaka JC, Acland GM, Hauswirth WW, Aguirre GD. 2010. Gene therapy rescues cone function in congenital achromatopsia. *Hum Mol Genet* **19:** 2581–2593.

Kong J, Kim SR, Binley K, Pata I, Doi K, Mannik J, Zernant-Rajang J, Kan O, Iqball S, Naylor S, et al. 2008. Correction of the disease phenotype in the mouse model of Stargardt disease by lentiviral gene therapy. *Gene Ther* **15:** 1311–1320.

Lagali PS, Balya D, Awatramani GB, Munch TA, Kim DS, Busskamp V, Cepko CL, Roska B. 2008. Light-activated channels targeted to ON bipolar cells restore visual function in retinal degeneration. *Nat Neurosci* **11:** 667–675.

Lamba DA, Gust J, Reh TA. 2009. Transplantation of human embryonic stem cell-derived photoreceptors restores some visual function in *Crx*-deficient mice. *Cell Stem Cell* **4:** 73–79.

Lamba DA, McUsic A, Hirata RK, Wang PR, Russell D, Reh TA. 2010. Generation, purification and transplantation of photoreceptors derived from human induced pluripotent stem cells. *PLoS ONE* **5:** e8763.

Lauritzen TZ, Harris J, Mohand-Said S, Sahel JA, Dorn JD, McClure K, Greenberg RJ. 2012. Reading visual braille with a retinal prosthesis. *Front Neurosci* **6:** 168.

Leveillard T, Sahel JA. 2010. Rod-derived cone viability factor for treating blinding diseases: From clinic to redox signaling. *Sci Transl Med* **2:** 26ps16.

Leveillard T, Mohand-Said S, Lorentz O, Hicks D, Fintz AC, Clerin E, Simonutti M, Forster V, Cavusoglu N, Chalmel F, et al. 2004. Identification and characterization of rod-derived cone viability factor. *Nat Genet* **36:** 755–759.

Li ZY, Kljavin IJ, Milam AH. 1995. Rod photoreceptor neurite sprouting in retinitis pigmentosa. *J Neurosci* **15:** 5429–5438.

Lin B, Masland RH, Strettoi E. 2009. Remodeling of cone photoreceptor cells after rod degeneration in *rd* mice. *Exp Eye Res* **88:** 589–599.

Liu X, Ondek B, Williams DS. 1998. Mutant myosin VIIa causes defective melanosome distribution in the RPE of shaker-1 mice. *Nat Genet* **19:** 117–118.

Liu X, Udovichenko IP, Brown SD, Steel KP, Williams DS. 1999. Myosin VIIa participates in opsin transport through the photoreceptor cilium. *J Neurosci* **19:** 6267–6274.

Lois N, Holder GE, Bunce C, Fitzke FW, Bird AC. 2001. Phenotypic subtypes of Stargardt macular dystrophy-fundus flavimaculatus. *Arch Ophthalmol* **119:** 359–369.

MacLaren RE, Pearson RA, MacNeil A, Douglas RH, Salt TE, Akimoto M, Swaroop A, Sowden JC, Ali RR. 2006. Retinal repair by transplantation of photoreceptor precursors. *Nature* **444:** 203–207.

MacLaren RE, Groppe M, Barnard AR, Cottriall CL, Tolmachova T, Seymour L, Clark KR, During MJ, Cremers FP,

Black GC, et al. 2014. Retinal gene therapy in patients with choroideremia: Initial findings from a phase 1/2 clinical trial. *Lancet* **383:** 1129–1137.

Maeda T, Cideciyan AV, Maeda A, Golczak M, Aleman TS, Jacobson SG, Palczewski K. 2009. Loss of cone photoreceptors caused by chromophore depletion is partially prevented by the artificial chromophore pro-drug, 9-cis-retinyl acetate. *Hum Mol Genet* **18:** 2277–2287.

Maeda T, Dong Z, Jin H, Sawada O, Gao S, Utkhede D, Monk W, Palczewska G, Palczewski K. 2013. QLT091001, a 9-cis-retinal analog, is well-tolerated by retinas of mice with impaired visual cycles. *Invest Ophthalmol Vis Sci* **54:** 455–466.

Maguire AM, Simonelli F, Pierce EA, Pugh EN Jr, Mingozzi F, Bennicelli J, Banfi S, Marshall KA, Testa F, Surace EM, et al. 2008. Safety and efficacy of gene transfer for Leber's congenital amaurosis. *N Engl J Med* **358:** 2240–2248.

Mathieson K, Loudin J, Goetz G, Huie P, Wang L, Kamins TI, Galambos L, Smith R, Harris JS, Sher A, et al. 2012. Photovoltaic retinal prosthesis with high pixel density. *Nat Photonics* **6:** 391–397.

McLaughlin ME, Sandberg MA, Berson EL, Dryja TP. 1993. Recessive mutations in the gene encoding the β-subunit of rod phosphodiesterase in patients with retinitis pigmentosa. *Nat Genet* **4:** 130–134.

Merabet LB, Battelli L, Obretenova S, Maguire S, Meijer P, Pascual-Leone A. 2009. Functional recruitment of visual cortex for sound encoded object identification in the blind. *Neuroreport* **20:** 132–138.

Michaelides M, Hunt DM, Moore AT. 2004. The cone dysfunction syndromes. *Br J Ophthalmol* **88:** 291–297.

Mitamura Y, Mitamura-Aizawa S, Nagasawa T, Katome T, Eguchi H, Naito T. 2012. Diagnostic imaging in patients with retinitis pigmentosa. *J Med Invest* **59:** 1–11.

Miyake Y, Yagasaki K, Horiguchi M, Kawase Y, Kanda T. 1986. Congenital stationary night blindness with negative electroretinogram. A new classification. *Arch Ophthalmol* **104:** 1013–1020.

Murakami T, Akimoto M, Ooto S, Suzuki T, Ikeda H, Kawagoe N, Takahashi M, Yoshimura N. 2008. Association between abnormal autofluorescence and photoreceptor disorganization in retinitis pigmentosa. *Am J Ophthalmol* **145:** 687–694.

Nagel G, Ollig D, Fuhrmann M, Kateriya S, Musti AM, Bamberg E, Hegemann P. 2002. Channelrhodopsin-1: A light-gated proton channel in green algae. *Science* **296:** 2395–2398.

Nakazawa M, Ohguro H, Takeuchi K, Miyagawa Y, Ito T, Metoki T. 2011. Effect of nilvadipine on central visual field in retinitis pigmentosa: A 30-month clinical trial. *Ophthalmologica* **225:** 120–126.

Naldini L, Blomer U, Gallay P, Ory D, Mulligan R, Gage FH, Verma IM, Trono D. 1996. In vivo gene delivery and stable transduction of nondividing cells by a lentiviral vector. *Science* **272:** 263–267.

Nangia V, Jonas JB, Khare A, Sinha A. 2012. Prevalence of retinitis pigmentosa in India: The Central India Eye and Medical Study. *Acta Ophthalmol* **90:** e649–e650.

Novarino G, Akizu N, Gleeson JG. 2011. Modeling human disease in humans: The ciliopathies. *Cell* **147:** 70–79.

Osakada F, Ikeda H, Mandai M, Wataya T, Watanabe K, Yoshimura N, Akaike A, Sasai Y, Takahashi M. 2008. Toward the generation of rod and cone photoreceptors from mouse, monkey and human embryonic stem cells. *Nat Biotechnol* **26:** 215–224.

Park TK, Wu Z, Kjellstrom S, Zeng Y, Bush RA, Sieving PA, Colosi P. 2009. Intravitreal delivery of AAV8 retinoschisin results in cell type-specific gene expression and retinal rescue in the *Rs1*-KO mouse. *Gene Ther* **16:** 916–926.

Petit C. 2001. Usher syndrome: From genetics to pathogenesis. *Annu Rev Genomics Hum Genet* **2:** 271–297.

Pimenides D, George ND, Yates JR, Bradshaw K, Roberts SA, Moore AT, Trump D. 2005. X-linked retinoschisis: Clinical phenotype and RS1 genotype in 86 UK patients. *J Med Genet* **42:** e35.

Potter MJ, Wong E, Szabo SM, McTaggart KE. 2004. Clinical findings in a carrier of a new mutation in the choroideremia gene. *Ophthalmology* **111:** 1905–1909.

Preising M, Ayuso C. 2004. Rab escort protein 1 (REP1) in intracellular traffic: A functional and pathophysiological overview. *Ophthalmic Genet* **25:** 101–110.

Prokisch H, Hartig M, Hellinger R, Meitinger T, Rosenberg T. 2007. A population-based epidemiological and genetic study of X-linked retinitis pigmentosa. *Invest Ophthalmol Vis Sci* **48:** 4012–4018.

Radtke ND, Aramant RB, Petry HM, Green PT, Pidwell DJ, Seiler MJ. 2008. Vision improvement in retinal degeneration patients by implantation of retina together with retinal pigment epithelium. *Am J Ophthalmol* **146:** 172–182.

Renner AB, Kellner U, Cropp E, Preising MN, MacDonald IM, van den Hurk JA, Cremers FP, Foerster MH. 2006. Choroideremia: Variability of clinical and electrophysiological characteristics and first report of a negative electroretinogram. *Ophthalmology* **113:** 2066.e1–e10.

The Retinoschisis Consortium. 1998. Functional implications of the spectrum of mutations found in 234 cases with X-linked juvenile retinoschisis (XLRS). *Hum Mol Genet* **7:** 1185–1192.

Robson AG, El-Amir A, Bailey C, Egan CA, Fitzke FW, Webster AR, Bird AC, Holder GE. 2003. Pattern ERG correlates of abnormal fundus autofluorescence in patients with retinitis pigmentosa and normal visual acuity. *Invest Ophthalmol Vis Sci* **44:** 3544–3550.

Robson AG, Tufail A, Fitzke F, Bird AC, Moore AT, Holder GE, Webster AR. 2011. Serial imaging and structure-function correlates of high-density rings of fundus autofluorescence in retinitis pigmentosa. *Retina* **31:** 1670–1679.

Roepman R, van Duijnhoven G, Rosenberg T, Pinckers AJ, Bleeker-Wagemakers LM, Bergen AA, Post J, Beck A, Reinhardt R, Ropers HH, et al. 1996. Positional cloning of the gene for X-linked retinitis pigmentosa 3: Homology with the guanine-nucleotide-exchange factor RCC1. *Hum Mol Genet* **5:** 1035–1041.

Romani M, Micalizzi A, Valente EM. 2013. Joubert syndrome: Congenital cerebellar ataxia with the molar tooth. *Lancet Neurol* **12:** 894–905.

Ronquillo CC, Bernstein PS, Baehr W. 2012. Senior-Loken syndrome: A syndromic form of retinal dystrophy associated with nephronophthisis. *Vision Res* **75:** 88–97.

Rosenfeld PJ, Cowley GS, McGee TL, Sandberg MA, Berson EL, Dryja TP. 1992. A null mutation in the rhodopsin gene causes rod photoreceptor dysfunction and autosomal recessive retinitis pigmentosa. *Nat Genet* **1:** 209–213.

Sahel JA, Roska B. 2013. Gene therapy for blindness. *Annu Rev Neurosci* **36:** 467–488.

Sampaio E, Maris S, Bach-y-Rita P. 2001. Brain plasticity: 'Visual' acuity of blind persons via the tongue. *Brain Res* **908:** 204–207.

Sauer CG, Gehrig A, Warneke-Wittstock R, Marquardt A, Ewing CC, Gibson A, Lorenz B, Jurklies B, Weber BH. 1997. Positional cloning of the gene associated with X-linked juvenile retinoschisis. *Nat Genet* **17:** 164–170.

Schwartz SD, Hubschman JP, Heilwell G, Franco-Cardenas V, Pan CK, Ostrick RM, Mickunas E, Gay R, Klimanskaya I, Lanza R. 2012. Embryonic stem cell trials for macular degeneration: A preliminary report. *Lancet* **379:** 713–720.

Sen P, Bhargava A, George R, Ve Ramesh S, Hemamalini A, Prema R, Kumaramanickavel G, Vijaya L. 2008. Prevalence of retinitis pigmentosa in South Indian population aged above 40 years. *Ophthalmic Epidemiol* **15:** 279–281.

Sidjanin DJ, Lowe JK, McElwee JL, Milne BS, Phippen TM, Sargan DR, Aguirre GD, Acland GM, Ostrander EA. 2002. Canine *CNGB3* mutations establish cone degeneration as orthologous to the human achromatopsia locus *ACHM3*. *Hum Mol Genet* **11:** 1823–1833.

Sieving PA, Arnold EB, Jamison J, Liepa A, Coats C. 1998. Submicrovolt flicker electroretinogram: Cycle-by-cycle recording of multiple harmonics with statistical estimation of measurement uncertainty. *Invest Ophthalmol Vis Sci* **39:** 1462–1469.

Sieving PA, Bingham EL, Kemp J, Richards J, Hiriyanna K. 1999. Juvenile X-linked retinoschisis from *XLRS1* Arg213Trp mutation with preservation of the electroretinogram scotopic b-wave. *Am J Ophthalmol* **128:** 179–184.

Sieving PA, Caruso RC, Tao W, Coleman HR, Thompson DJ, Fullmer KR, Bush RA. 2006. Ciliary neurotrophic factor (CNTF) for human retinal degeneration: Phase I trial of CNTF delivered by encapsulated cell intraocular implants. *Proc Natl Acad Sci* **103:** 3896–3901.

Stargardt K. 1909. Über familiäre, progressive degeneration under makulagegend des auges. *Albrecht von Graefes Arch Ophthalmol* **71:** 534–550.

Stingl K, Bartz-Schmidt KU, Besch D, Braun A, Bruckmann A, Gekeler F, Greppmaier U, Hipp S, Hortdorfer G, Kernstock C, et al. 2013. Artificial vision with wirelessly powered subretinal electronic implant α-IMS. *Proc Biol Sci* **280:** 20130077.

Striem-Amit E, Dakwar O, Reich L, Amedi A. 2011. The large-scale organization of "visual" streams emerges without visual experience. *Cereb Cortex* **22:** 1698–1709.

Striem-Amit E, Cohen L, Dehaene S, Amedi A. 2012a. Reading with sounds: Sensory substitution selectively activates the visual word form area in the blind. *Neuron* **76:** 640–652.

Striem-Amit E, Guendelman M, Amedi A. 2012b. 'Visual' acuity of the congenitally blind using visual-to-auditory sensory substitution. *PLoS ONE* **7:** e33136.

Sun H, Nathans J. 1997. Stargardt's ABCR is localized to the disc membrane of retinal rod outer segments. *Nat Genet* **17:** 15–16.

Takano Y, Ohguro H, Dezawa M, Ishikawa H, Yamazaki H, Ohguro I, Mamiya K, Metoki T, Ishikawa F, Nakazawa M. 2004. Study of drug effects of calcium channel blockers on retinal degeneration of *rd* mouse. *Biochem Biophys Res Commun* **313:** 1015–1022.

Talcott KE, Ratnam K, Sundquist SM, Lucero AS, Lujan BJ, Tao W, Porco TC, Roorda A, Duncan JL. 2011. Longitudinal study of cone photoreceptors during retinal degeneration and in response to ciliary neurotrophic factor treatment. *Invest Ophthalmol Vis Sci* **52:** 2219–2226.

Testa F, Maguire AM, Rossi S, Pierce EA, Melillo P, Marshall K, Banfi S, Surace EM, Sun J, Acerra C, et al. 2013. Three-year follow-up after unilateral subretinal delivery of adeno-associated virus in patients with Leber congenital amaurosis type 2. *Ophthalmology* **120:** 1283–1291.

Thompson DA, Li Y, McHenry CL, Carlson TJ, Ding X, Sieving PA, Apfelstedt-Sylla E, Gal A. 2001. Mutations in the gene encoding lecithin retinol acyltransferase are associated with early-onset severe retinal dystrophy. *Nat Genet* **28:** 123–124.

Tojo N, Nakamura T, Fuchizawa C, Oiwake T, Hayashi A. 2013. Adaptive optics fundus images of cone photoreceptors in the macula of patients with retinitis pigmentosa. *Clin Ophthalmol* **7:** 203–210.

Tolmachova T, Tolmachov OE, Wavre-Shapton ST, Tracey-White D, Futter CE, Seabra MC. 2012. *CHM/REP1* cDNA delivery by lentiviral vectors provides functional expression of the transgene in the retinal pigment epithelium of choroideremia mice. *J Gene Med* **14:** 158–168.

Tschernutter M, Schlichtenbrede FC, Howe S, Balaggan KS, Munro PM, Bainbridge JW, Thrasher AJ, Smith AJ, Ali RR. 2005. Long-term preservation of retinal function in the RCS rat model of retinitis pigmentosa following lentivirus-mediated gene therapy. *Gene Ther* **12:** 694–701.

Tsujikawa M, Wada Y, Sukegawa M, Sawa M, Gomi F, Nishida K, Tano Y. 2008. Age at onset curves of retinitis pigmentosa. *Arch Ophthalmol* **126:** 337–340.

Tsybovsky Y, Molday RS, Palczewski K. 2010. The ATP-binding cassette transporter ABCA4: Structural and functional properties and role in retinal disease. *Adv Exp Med Biol* **703:** 105–125.

Van Hooser JP, Aleman TS, He YG, Cideciyan AV, Kuksa V, Pittler SJ, Stone EM, Jacobson SG, Palczewski K. 2000. Rapid restoration of visual pigment and function with oral retinoid in a mouse model of childhood blindness. *Proc Natl Acad Sci* **97:** 8623–8628.

van Reeuwijk J, Arts HH, Roepman R. 2011. Scrutinizing ciliopathies by unraveling ciliary interaction networks. *Hum Mol Genet* **20:** R149–R157.

Vandenberghe LH, Auricchio A. 2012. Novel adeno-associated viral vectors for retinal gene therapy. *Gene Ther* **19:** 162–168.

Vasireddy V, Mills JA, Gaddameedi R, Basner-Tschakarjan E, Kohnke M, Black AD, Alexandrov K, Zhou S, Maguire AM, Chung DC, et al. 2013. AAV-mediated gene therapy for Choroideremia: Preclinical studies in personalized models. *PLoS ONE* **8:** e61396.

Waters AM, Beales PL. 2011. Ciliopathies: An expanding disease spectrum. *Pediatr Nephrol* **26:** 1039–1056.

Witkin AJ, Ko TH, Fujimoto JG, Chan A, Drexler W, Schuman JS, Reichel E, Duker JS. 2006. Ultra-high resolution optical coherence tomography assessment of photoreceptors in retinitis pigmentosa and related diseases. *Am J Ophthalmol* **142:** 945–952.

Yang Y, Mohand-Said S, Danan A, Simonutti M, Fontaine V, Clerin E, Picaud S, Leveillard T, Sahel JA. 2009. Functional cone rescue by RdCVF protein in a dominant model of retinitis pigmentosa. *Mol Ther* **17:** 787–795.

Yatsenko AN, Shroyer NF, Lewis RA, Lupski JR. 2001. Late-onset Stargardt disease is associated with missense mutations that map outside known functional regions of *ABCR* (*ABCA4*). *Hum Genet* **108:** 346–355.

You QS, Xu L, Wang YX, Liang QF, Cui TT, Yang XH, Wang S, Yang H, Jonas JB. 2013. Prevalence of retinitis pigmentosa in North China: The Beijing Eye Public Health Care Project. *Acta Ophthalmol* **91:** e499–e500.

Zeitz C, Jacobson SG, Hamel CP, Bujakowska K, Neuille M, Orhan E, Zanlonghi X, Lancelot ME, Michiels C, Schwartz SB, et al. 2013. Whole-exome sequencing identifies *LRIT3* mutations as a cause of autosomal-recessive complete congenital stationary night blindness. *Am J Hum Genet* **92:** 67–75.

Zeng Y, Takada Y, Kjellstrom S, Hiriyanna K, Tanikawa A, Wawrousek E, Smaoui N, Caruso R, Bush RA, Sieving PA. 2004. *RS-1* gene delivery to an adult *Rs1h* knockout mouse model restores ERG b-wave with reversal of the electronegative waveform of X-linked retinoschisis. *Invest Ophthalmol Vis Sci* **45:** 3279–3285.

Zhang K, Kniazeva M, Han M, Li W, Yu Z, Yang Z, Li Y, Metzker ML, Allikmets R, Zack DJ, et al. 2001. A 5-bp deletion in *ELOVL4* is associated with two related forms of autosomal dominant macular dystrophy. *Nat Genet* **27:** 89–93.

Zhang F, Wang LP, Brauner M, Liewald JF, Kay K, Watzke N, Wood PG, Bamberg E, Nagel G, Gottschalk A, et al. 2007. Multimodal fast optical interrogation of neural circuitry. *Nature* **446:** 633–639.

Zhao X, Liu J, Ahmad I. 2002. Differentiation of embryonic stem cells into retinal neurons. *Biochem Biophys Res Commun* **297:** 177–184.

Zrenner E. 2002. Will retinal implants restore vision? *Science* **295:** 1022–1025.

Zrenner E, Bartz-Schmidt KU, Benav H, Besch D, Bruckmann A, Gabel VP, Gekeler F, Greppmaier U, Harscher A, Kibbel S, et al. 2011. Subretinal electronic chips allow blind patients to read letters and combine them to words. *Proc Biol Sci* **278:** 1489–1497.

Genes and Mutations Causing Autosomal Dominant Retinitis Pigmentosa

Stephen P. Daiger, Sara J. Bowne, and Lori S. Sullivan

Human Genetics Center, School of Public Health, The University of Texas Health Science Center, Houston, Texas 77030

Correspondence: stephen.p.daiger@uth.tmc.edu

Retinitis pigmentosa (RP) has a prevalence of approximately one in 4000; 25%–30% of these cases are autosomal dominant retinitis pigmentosa (adRP). Like other forms of inherited retinal disease, adRP is exceptionally heterogeneous. Mutations in more than 25 genes are known to cause adRP, more than 1000 mutations have been reported in these genes, clinical findings are highly variable, and there is considerable overlap with other types of inherited disease. Currently, it is possible to detect disease-causing mutations in 50%–75% of adRP families in select populations. Genetic diagnosis of adRP has advantages over other forms of RP because segregation of disease in families is a useful tool for identifying and confirming potentially pathogenic variants, but there are disadvantages too. In addition to identifying the cause of disease in the remaining 25% of adRP families, a central challenge is reconciling clinical diagnosis, family history, and molecular findings in patients and families.

Retinitis pigmentosa (RP) is an inherited dystrophic or degenerative disease of the retina with a prevalence of roughly one in 4000 (Haim 2002; Daiger et al. 2007). Typically, the disease progresses from the midperiphery of the retina into the central retina and, in many cases, into the macula and fovea (Heckenlively and Daiger 2007; Fahim et al. 2013). Clinical features include night blindness starting in adolescence, followed by progressive loss of peripheral vision—referred to as "tunnel vision"—culminating in legal blindness or complete blindness in adulthood. Characteristic retinal findings on examination include bone-spicule formations and attenuated blood vessels, reduced visual fields, reduced and/or abnormal electroretinograms (ERGs), changes in structure imaged by optical coherence tomography (OCT), and subjective changes in visual function (Fishman et al. 2005). However, features and findings are highly variable among patients, even among patients within the same family.

RP is exceptionally heterogeneous at a genetic level. All modes of inheritance are encountered: dominant, recessive, autosomal, X-linked, and even mitochondrial (Berger et al. 2010). It is assumed that each patient has a monogenic form of disease (or digenic in rare cases) but many different genes account for disease in RP patients as a group. Currently, mutations in more than 66 genes are known to cause nonsyndromic RP and an additional 31 genes cause

Cite this article as *Cold Spring Harb Perspect Med* doi: 10.1101/cshperspect.a017129

syndromic forms such as Usher syndrome and Bardet–Biedl syndrome (Daiger et al. 2013; RetNet 2014). There are also many disease-causing mutations reported in these genes. More than 3100 mutations are listed in the Human Gene Mutation Database (HGMD) (HGMD 2014) in nonsyndromic RP genes alone (Daiger et al. 2013).

This review focuses on nonsyndromic autosomal dominant retinitis pigmentosa (adRP). This is partly to simplify the discussion but also because finding genes and mutations causing adRP entails unique opportunities and pitfalls. In addition, our laboratory has worked with adRP families for the past 25 years affording us insights into these issues. Despite the limited focus, many observations regarding genes and mutations causing adRP apply equally well to other forms of inherited retinopathy.

FINDING GENES AND MUTATIONS CAUSING adRP

The successes in finding adRP genes and disease-causing mutations over the past two decades are striking. Table 1 lists genes in which mutations are reported to cause adRP. References are in RetNet (RetNet 2014, see https://sph.uth.edu/retnet/). There are currently 25 reported adRP genes and an additional linked gene, RP63, which maps to human chromosome 6q23 (Kannabiran et al. 2012). The HGMD database (HGMD 2014) lists more than 1000 mutations in these genes, although not all are dominant-acting (and not all are pathogenic). To date, mutations in the known adRP genes account for 50%–75% of cases, depending on the tests performed and populations screened. Nonetheless, significant problems remain.

For example, it should be easy to name genes known to cause adRP, but it is not. In recent years, the simple idea that one gene leads to one disease has proven highly inaccurate, especially for inherited retinal diseases. A gene first identified as the cause of one form of disease, for example, recessive RP, may harbor mutations that cause another form of retinal disease or mutations with a different mode of inheritance for example, adRP. Table 1 lists alternate forms of disease associated with adRP genes. One consequence of this overlap is that any simple count of "RP genes" is often arbitrary.

Likewise, there are complications in detecting disease-causing mutations in adRP genes. For one, the initial diagnosis in a family may be misleading. That is, because of exceptional clinical variation, affected family members may have different clinical diagnoses, or the mode of inheritance may be misconstrued. For example, families with X-linked RP and affected carrier females may be mistaken as adRP (Churchill et al. 2013). Further, a significant fraction of RP patients present as isolated cases, with no known affected relatives, so the mode of inheritance is undetermined. Also, because different mutations in the same gene can produce different clinical consequences, the actual mutation may be in a known gene not commonly associated with adRP. Examples include rare adRP mutations in RPE65 (Bowne et al. 2011a) and RDH12 (Fingert et al. 2008), genes more likely to cause recessive RP or recessive Leber congenital amaurosis, respectively.

Beyond these complications, there is the general problem of variants of unknown significance (VUS), that is, rare, potentially pathogenic variants in known adRP genes for which the evidence is equivocal. This is a fundamental problem in medical genetics given the extensive background of rare and apparently damaging variants in the human population (Marth et al. 2011). Suggestions for scoring potentially pathogenic variants are discussed in the next section.

Finally, there are substantial difficulties in identifying novel adRP genes. Three advanced technologies using next-generation sequencing (NGS) are in use: targeted retinal-gene capture NGS (Simpson et al. 2011; Audo et al. 2012; Neveling et al. 2012; O'Sullivan et al. 2012; Chen et al. 2013; Eisenberger et al. 2013; Glockle et al. 2013; Wang et al. 2014), whole-exome NGS (Bowne et al. 2011a; Ozgul et al. 2011; Tucker et al. 2011; Zeitz et al. 2013; El Shamieh et al. 2014; Jin et al. 2014; Sergouniotis et al. 2014), and whole-genome NGS (Nishiguchi et al. 2013). Each has advantages and disadvantages.

Because targeted retinal-capture NGS examines only a small portion of the human

Table 1. Genes reported to cause autosomal dominant retinitis pigmentosa pigmentosa (in chromosomal order)

	Symbol	Gene/protein	Chromosome	Alternate diseases	Function
1	RPE65	Retinal pigment epithelium-specific 65 kD protein	1p31.2	Recessive retinitis pigmentosa; recessive Leber congenital amaurosis	Visual cycle
2	PRPF3	Pre-mRNA processing factor 3	1q21.2		RNA processing
3	SEMA4A	Semaphorin 4A	1q22	Dominant cone–rod dystrophy	Neuronal or immune response
4	SNRNP200	Small nuclear ribonucleoprotein 200 kDa (U5)	2q11.2		RNA processing
5	RHO	Rhodopsin	3q22.1	Dominant congenital stationary night blindness; recessive retinitis pigmentosa	Phototransduction, outer segment membrane structure
6	GUCA1B	Guanylate cyclase activating protein 1B	6p21.1	Dominant macular dystrophy	Phototransduction
7	PRPH2	Peripherin 2	6p21.1	Dominant macular dystrophy; digenic retinitis pigmentosa with ROM1; dominant adult vitelliform macular dystrophy; dominant cone–rod dystrophy; dominant central areolar choroidal dystrophy	Outer segment membrane structure
8	RP9	RP9 protein or PIM1-kinase associated protein 1	7p14.3		Unknown
9	KLHL7	Kelch-like 7 protein (*Drosophila*)	7p15.3		Ubiquitination pathway
10	IMPDH1	Inosine monophosphate dehydrogenase 1	7q32.1	Dominant Leber congenital amaurosis	Purine or amino acid synthesis
11	RP1	RP1 protein	8q12.1	Recessive retinitis pigmentosa	Ciliary structure/function
12	TOPORS	Topoisomerase I binding arginine/serine rich protein	9p21.1		Ciliary structure/function
13	PRPF4	Pre-mRNA processing factor 4	9q32		RNA processing
14	HK1	Hexokinase 1	10q22.1		Glucose metabolism
15	BEST1	Bestrophin 1	11q12.3	Dominant vitreoretinochoroidopathy; recessive bestrophinopathy; recessive retinitis pigmentosa; dominant macular dystrophy, Best type	Visual cycle and chloride channel

Continued

Table 1. *Continued*

	Symbol	Gene/protein	Chromosome	Alternate diseases	Function
16	ROM1	Retinal outer segment membrane protein 1	11q12.3	Digenic retinitis pigmentosa with PRPH2	Outer segment membrane structure
17	NRL	Neural retina lucine zipper	14q11.2	Recessive retinitis pigmentosa	Transcription factor
18	RDH12	Retinol dehydrogenase 12	14q24.1	Recessive Leber congenital amaurosis with severe childhood retinal dystrophy	Visual cycle
19	NR2E3	Nuclear receptor subfamily 2 group E3	15q23	Recessive retinitis pigmentosa in Portuguese Crypto Jews; recessive Goldmann–Favre syndrome; recessive enhanced S-cone syndrome (ESC); combined dominant and recessive retinopathy	Transcription factor
20	PRPF8	Pre-mRNA processing factor 8	17p13.3		RNA processing
21	CA4	Carbonic anhydrase IV	17q23.2		Retinal capillary structure/function
22	FSCN2	Retinal fascin homolog 2, actin bundling protein	17q25.3	Dominant macular dystrophy	Ciliary structure/ function
23	CRX	Cone–rod otx-like photoreceptor homeobox transcription factor	19q13.32	Recessive, dominant and de novo Leber congenital amaurosis; dominant cone–rod dystrophy	Transcription factor
24	PRPF31	Pre-mRNA processing factor 31	19q13.42		RNA processing
25	PRPF6	Pre-mRNA processing factor 6	20q13.33		RNA processing

References as in RetNet, https://sph.uth.edu/retnet/, and Sullivan et al. 2014 (HK1).

genome, that is, exons of known retinal genes and candidate genes, analysis of sequence data is simplified. Also, retinal capture panels are optimized for each exon and include retinal-specific splice variants. However, retinal-capture NGS is limited to known genes and detects a large number of VUS mutations (as do all NGS methods). In contrast, whole-exome sequencing is a powerful tool for identifying novel disease-causing genes but perforce is limited to exons, whereas whole genome NGS avoids this limitation but presents a very complex problem in data analysis. For autosomal dominant diseases, the problems are compounded by the need to detect a single, heterozygous mutation in a diploid organism, the proverbial needle-in-a-hay-stack.

Further, because NGS methods are based on short-read, paired-end, and shotgun sequencing, they are underpowered for detecting deletions, insertions, and variable-length repetitive elements. As examples, large deletions in the PRPF31 gene account for 2.5% of adRP cases (Sullivan et al. 2006b), but are generally not detectable by NGS, and the repetitive elements of the ORF15 region of the X-linked RP gene

RPGR are refractory to short-read sequencing (Churchill et al. 2013).

Fortunately, segregation testing and linkage analysis in adRP families address many of these problems. Segregation testing—determining if a putative disease-causing variant tracks with disease in a family—can support or exclude pathogenicity. Complications are the late onset of disease and nonpenetrance. That is, a clinically unaffected family member may carry a disease allele, either because the disease has not manifested yet or because the mutation is nonpenetrant in that individual. An example of the latter is mutations in PRPF31 for which nonpenetrance may be as high as 20% (McGee et al. 1997; Venturini et al. 2012). However, nonpenetrance is not common among other adRP genes. Conversely, absence of a putative mutation in an affected family member is usually strong evidence against pathogenicity.

Linkage analysis tests for cosegregation of polymorphic markers with disease in a family. Loosely, there are two contrasting approaches, linkage exclusion and linkage inclusion. Linkage exclusion is simply exclusion of a known adRP gene by recombination between polymorphic markers within or contiguous to the site. For example, small sets of highly variable STR (short-tandem repeat) polymorphisms can exclude many known adRP sites in families with five or more affected members available for testing (Sullivan et al. 2006b). In contrast, because of statistical issues, larger families are required for linkage inclusion, that is, mapping a disease gene by observing cosegregation of polymorphic markers. Since dominant retinal disease families may have many living, affected members, linkage mapping is an effective tool for localizing new adRP genes.

Contemporary marker sets for linkage mapping include hundreds of thousands of SNPs (single-nucleotide polymorphisms) such as markers in Affymetrix SNP Arrays (Friedman et al. 2009; Bowne et al. 2011a). Generally, in families with eight or more affected members available for testing, linkage mapping reduces the target region to one or a few chromosomal sites, each <10 Mb in length. This substantially reduces the "space" to search for novel adRP genes using NGS approaches. As an alternative to using SNP marker arrays, data from whole-exome NGS testing of multiple family members can be combined for linkage mapping in RP families based on regions identical-by-descent and shared rare variants (Koboldt et al. 2014).

Each approach is useful: Most adRP genes in Table 1 were first localized by linkage mapping; NGS methods were used to find most of the recently identified genes; and retinal capture NGS is a rapid, efficient approach to finding disease-causing mutations in known adRP genes. Taken together, advanced DNA sequencing and mapping methods have revolutionized gene discovery and mutation detection for adRP.

DETERMINING PATHOGENEITY OF adRP MUTATIONS

Determining which of the many rare variants in our genomes are pathogenic and which are benign, with all possibilities in between, is one of the fundamental problems in medical genetics (MacArthur et al. 2014). Dominant Mendelian diseases such as adRP offer the advantage of segregation testing to evaluate pathogenicity. However, this is only one of multiple steps in establishing causality. Although there is no fully accepted protocol, each of the NGS publications cited above follows similar strategies. Note that establishing pathogenicity overlaps with, but is distinct from, the "pipeline" for sequence assembly and detection of variants. Also, criteria for establishing pathogenicity of variants that may cause autosomal dominant diseases are distinct from criteria for recessive and X-linked diseases. With these caveats in mind, the following are reasonable steps for determining pathogenicity of potential adRP mutations (not necessarily in order), using retinal capture NGS as a model.

- Although the model assumes efficient retinal capture and a patient with autosomal inheritance, it is prudent to confirm coverage of the most common adRP genes, such as rhodopsin (RHO) and PRPH2, and to consider X-linked inheritance in the absence of male-to-male transmission.

- The filtering pipeline should flag all variants with an allele frequency of <0.1% in publically available databases such as 1000 Genomes, ESP, and dbSNP (Abecasis et al. 2012; Fernandez-Suarez et al. 2014; NCBI 2014). Note that some recessive RP mutations have population frequencies ≥0.1%, whereas all reported adRP mutations are more rare.
- Determine if any flagged variants are known, published disease-causing mutations. This requires searching, for example, relevant Leiden databases (Cremers et al. 2014), the HGMD database (HGMD 2014), and clinVAR (NCBI 2014). In-house databases should be consulted too, of course. Caution: Even though a variant is listed in a disease database, it may not be pathogenic. For uncertain variants, it is essential to confirm pathogenicity based on original publications.
- If there is no unequivocally pathogenic variant in a known adRP gene, consider deletion detection for PRPF31 (Sullivan et al. 2006b) and/or nested Sanger sequencing of ORF15 of RPGR (Churchill et al. 2013).
- In the remaining cases, rank variants by pathogenicity scores using publically available services such as PolyPhen, SIFT, NNSplice, and Mutation Taster (Schwarz et al. 2010; Knecht and Krawczak 2014). Published functional data on specific genes may be useful too.
- Confirm plausible mutations by conventional sequencing and test for segregation in available family members.
- Finally, *based on the totality of information available*, including all of the above, plus clinical information, family history, and the biology and clinical phenotypes of possible disease genes, score putative mutations (one or more) for the likelihood of causing disease in the patient and family tested. Several scoring systems have been suggested, largely ranging from "recognized cause of disorder," "expected cause of disorder," "may or may not cause disorder" (VUS), to "probably not causative" (Richards et al. 2008).

What do these NGS strategies miss? Mutations in known retinal disease genes outside of exons, mutations in novel genes, and mutations not detectable by shotgun sequencing (e.g., variable repeats), among others.

PREVALENCE OF DISEASE-CAUSING MUTATIONS IN adRP FAMILIES

Our research has focused principally on genetic studies of adRP patients and families. For purposes of tracking progress in gene discovery and mutation detection, we have established a cohort of well-characterized adRP families (Sohocki et al. 2001; Sullivan et al. 2006a; Bowne et al. 2008, 2013). Families in the cohort have a clinical diagnosis of adRP by a knowledgeable clinician, three or more affected generations with affected females, or two or more generations with male-to-male transmission (to bias against X-linked RP). Currently, there are 270 families in the cohort (Table 2). The families are largely Americans of European origin, 75% white, 5% African American, 5% Hispanic, 3% Asian, and the remainder other or unknown.

We have applied a variety of methods to detect disease-causing mutations in these families including linkage mapping (Sullivan et al. 1999; Bowne et al. 2002, 2011a), conventional Sanger sequencing (Bowne et al. 1999, 2006, 2008, 2013; Sullivan et al. 1999; Sohocki et al. 2001; Gire et al. 2007; Friedman et al. 2009), NGS (Bowne et al. 2011b; Wang et al. 2013), deletion detection (Sullivan et al. 2006b), and subclone sequencing of RPGR ORF15 (Churchill et al. 2013). Recently, we reported a novel adRP gene, hexokinase 1 (HK1), with a missense mutation in five independently ascertained families (Sullivan et al. 2014). This gene, too, was tested in the cohort.

Table 2 summarizes our findings. To date we have identified the disease-causing mutation in 78% of the families, leaving 22% in which the known dominant RP genes have been excluded. Figure 1 shows the fraction of cases caused by mutations in each gene.

Note that Table 2 includes mutations in two X-linked genes, RPGR and RP2, found in a total of 25 families (9%). Each of these families met

Cite this article as *Cold Spring Harb Perspect Med* doi: 10.1101/cshperspect.a017129

Table 2. Prevalence of disease-causing mutations in adRP families ($N = 270$), with number of mutation types

Gene	Families	Percent	Missense	Nonsense	Other
CRX	2	0.7	1	0	1
HK1	3	1.1	1	0	0
IMPDH1	10	3.7	2	0	0
KLHL7	3	1.1	3	0	0
NR2E3	6	2.2	1	0	1
NRL	2	0.7	2	0	0
PRPF3	4	1.5	2	0	0
PRPF31	24	8.9	4	3	17
PRPF8	7	2.6	4	0	1
RDH12	1	0.4	0	0	1
PRPH2	19	7.0	10	1	2
PRPH2+ROM1	1	0.4	1	0	1
RHO	83	30.7	30	2	1
RP1	13	4.8	0	3	1
RP2	3	1.1	1	0	2
RPE65	1	0.4	1	0	0
RPGR	22	8.1	4	2	13
SNRNP200	4	1.5	4	0	0
TOPORS	4	1.5	3	0	1
None	58	21.5			
Total	270	100			

reasonable criteria for inclusion in a cohort of "autosomal dominant" families, with multiple affected females and an initial diagnosis of adRP. On further review, most, but not all, affected females are more mildly affected than age-matched affected males (Wu et al. 2010; Churchill et al. 2013). Clinical symptoms are also more variable in carrier females, consistent with Lyonization or other factors modifying expression. This is an example of the power of molecular findings to dramatically change an initial diagnosis.

Based on the significant fraction of X-linked mutations among families with a diagnosis of adRP, mutations in RPGR are probably the most common cause of RP in the world. This is reinforced by the finding that RPGR mutations account for 13% of isolated RP in males (Branham et al. 2012).

The cohort families also have one instance of digenic inheritance of a PRPH2 Leu185Pro mutation combined with a ROM1 Leu114fs*131 mutation (Kajiwara et al. 1994; Sullivan et al. 2006a). Technically, the inheritance pattern deviates from classical adRP because an affected child must inherit both alleles from an affected parent, or one allele from an unaffected parent. This is a rare condition but other ROM1 (rod outer-membrane protein 1) mutations are known to cause digenic RP in combination with the PRPH2 Leu185Pro mutation (Dryja et al. 1997).

Table 2 also indicates the distribution of mutation types in three broad classes, missense, nonsense, and "other." From a functional prospective, missense mutations are likely to produce an abnormal protein and the mode of action is through partial loss-of-function, gain-of-function, dominant negative, or toxic effects. "Other" mutations most likely result in functional haploinsufficiency, that is, no protein or a nonfunctional protein. Nonsense mutations may or may not produce a protein depending on whether the premature stop is in the last exon, which escapes nonsense mediated decay, or earlier exons, which do not. Based on Table 2, most adRP mutations do not result in functional haploinsufficiency, except for PRPF31.

A substantial fraction of mutations detected in the cohort are "common," that is, they occur

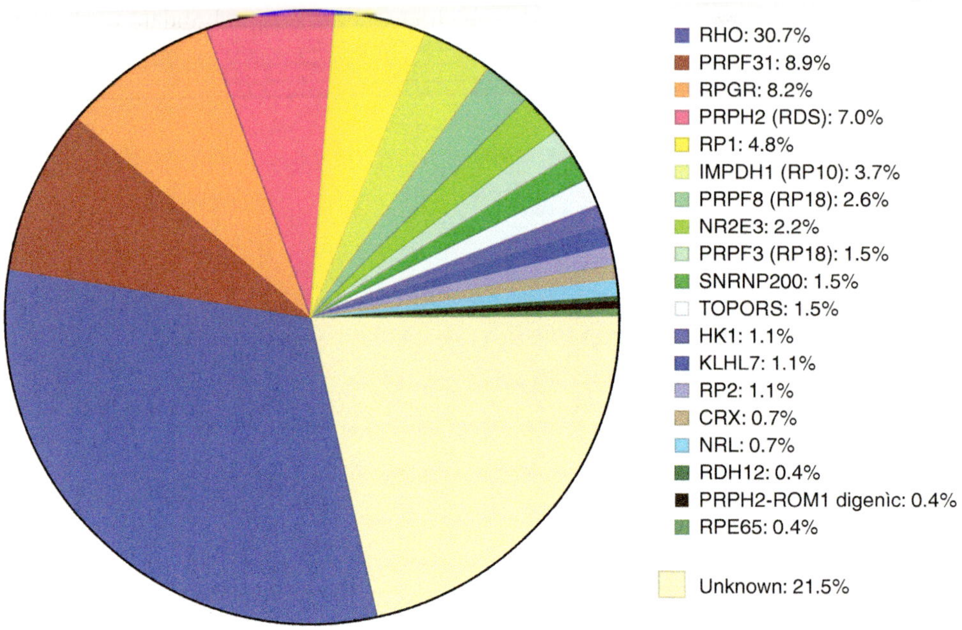

Figure 1. Fraction of mutations causing dominant RP in a cohort of 270 "adRP" families.

in three or more unrelated families. Table 3 lists the common mutations and the fraction of families with each. Twelve mutations in adRP genes account for nearly 30% of these families (i.e., excluding RPGR and RP2). Most of these mutations are ethnic-specific. Several arose by founder effect and have limited geographic distribution. That is, the mutation arose once only, increased in frequency by drift and population dynamics, and shares a distinct haplotype in *cis* to the mutation. For example, the rhodopsin Pro23His mutation (13%) and the peripherin 828+3A>T mutation (2%) arose by founder effect, are almost exclusive to the United States, and are found only in Americans of European origin (Dryja et al. 1990, 1991; Shankar et al. 2004). The hexokinase Glu847Lys mutation also arose from a common ancestor, but the mutation is found in North America and Europe (Sullivan et al. 2014). In contrast, the Asp226Asn mutation in the inosine monophosphate dehydrogenase 1 gene (IMPDH1) arose independently on multiple occasions (Sullivan et al. 2006a).

This is a general phenomenon for RP mutations: the prevalence of mutations in a given gene is often dominated by one or a few mutations that arose by founder effect. Thus, populations will have different prevalences as a result of founder mutations, even though the RP genes are universal and the fraction of new mutations is roughly the same worldwide. For example, rhodopsin mutations account for 30% of adRP cases among Americans of European origin but

Table 3. Common mutations in adRP genes and RPGR ($N = 270$)

Gene	Families	Mutation	Percent
HK1	3	Glu847Lys	1.1
IMPDH1	6	Asp226Asn	2.2
	4	Asp311Asn	1.5
NR2E3	5	Gly56Arg	1.9
PRPF3	3	Thr494Met	1.1
PRPH2	5	828+3A>T	1.9
	4	Pro216Ser	1.5
RHO	5	Arg135Leu	1.9
	5	Arg135Trp	1.9
	36	Pro23His	13.2
RP1	6	Arg677X	2.2
	4	Leu762Tyrfs*17	1.5
RPGR	3	Glu802Glyfs*32	1.1
Total			33.0

<10% in China, largely because the Pro23His mutation is absent from China (Li et al. 2010). In contrast, the prevalence of RPGR mutations, which are predominantly new mutations, is roughly the same worldwide (Bocquet et al. 2013; Xu et al. 2014).

DOMINANT-RECESSIVE ACTING adRP MUTATIONS

In most cases in which a gene in Table 1 has more than one disease association, this is the result of different mutations in the same gene causing different diseases. However, there are two instances in which the same mutation has different consequences depending on whether one or two copies are present, that is, whether the patient is heterozygous or homozygous. Technically, these mutations are dominant *and* recessive acting. In one large adRP family with the RP1 Arg677X mutation, two homozygous individuals are severely affected whereas heterozygous individuals are more mildly affected (Sullivan et al. 1999). In contrast, the consequences of this mutation are distinct from clinical expression of the several RP1 mutations, which are truly recessive, with unaffected carriers (Khaliq et al. 2005; Riazuddin et al. 2005). Similarly, in a large adRP family with the HK1 Glu847Lys mutation, a single homozygous individual is significantly more severely affected than heterozygotes (Sullivan et al. 2014). These cases may be rare, but because members of large, multigenerational adRP families occasionally live in the same community, this is more likely with adRP than with other dominant diseases.

NORMAL FUNCTION OF adRP GENES

Table 1 provides a brief phrase describing the functional class of each gene. Excellent, extensive reviews are also available (Berger et al. 2010; Wright et al. 2010). Even limiting discussion to genes that account for 1% or more of cases, genes causing adRP have diverse functional roles.

It is not surprising that mutations in genes coding for proteins that are abundant in rods or play fundamental roles in photoreceptor function may cause dominant RP. This includes rhodopsin, the most abundant rod protein; peripherin (PRPH2) and ROM1, which are essential structural components of rod outer membranes; and rod/cone expression factors such as CRX, NRL, and NR2E3. Mutations in these genes are frequent causes of adRP. On the other hand, the relationship between function and disease of other adRP genes is less clear.

For example, the protein products of four adRP genes, PRPF3, PRPF8, PRPF31, and SNRNP200, are essential components of the U4/U6-U5 tri-snRNP complex of the spliceosome involved in mRNA splicing (Liu and Zack 2013). The products of two less frequent causes of adRP, PRPF4 and PRPF6, are also components of this complex. These genes are expressed in all tissues and are highly conserved in all eukaryotes. Why mutations in these genes cause dominant RP, and only RP, is not known. However, genes coding for other proteins in this complex are attractive candidates for novel adRP genes.

The protein products of the remaining common adRP genes, HK1, IMPDH1, KLHL7, RP1, and TOPORS, are enzymes found in all cells (HK1 and IMPDH1), have a universal role in protein degradation (KLHL7), or are components of sensory cilia (RP1). That is, their roles are diverse and not obviously predictive of dominant, degenerative disease limited to the retina.

RECONCILING CLINICAL DIAGNOSIS, FAMILY HISTORY AND MOLECULAR FINDINGS

An emerging realization in inherited retinopathies is apparent discrepancies between clinical findings, inheritance pattern, and results of genetic testing. Clinical findings of retinitis pigmentosa and evidence from family history of dominant inheritance are consistent with a diagnosis of adRP. Fortunately, in most cases, a diagnosis of adRP is supported by the results of genetic testing. However, given the complex relationship between genes, mutations, and inherited retinopathies, there are opportunities for conflicts, for instance, when an apparent disease-causing mutation is in a gene not known to cause adRP, or the clinical phenotype in the family is more variable than just RP, or the apparent mode of inheritance is misleading or not determined. For these reasons, clinicians, counselors, and geneticists must work closely with each other to resolve these conflicts. In some cases, a reconsideration of the clinical, family, and molecular findings, taken together, may substantially alter the predicted mode of inheritance and prognosis. Thus, in addition to all the other benefits of genetic testing of patients with RP, molecular findings may substantially alter diagnosis, prognosis, counseling, and treatment.

CONCLUDING REMARKS

The long-term objective of research on genes and mutations causing inherited retinopathies is to enable effective genetic testing of patients and families, to incorporate this information into clinical care and counseling, and to develop treatments and cures based on a fundamental understanding of disease pathology. Currently, the success rate for finding the causative mutation in adRP patients is 50%–75%, but this fraction will increase rapidly with widespread adaptation of NGS testing and development of "third-generation" sequencing (Laszlo et al. 2014). Gene-specific and mutation-specific treatment trials have begun already. In time the limitation will not be genetic testing per se, but interpretation of variants, reconciling diagnosis and molecular findings, and providing meaningful information to clinicians and useful counseling to patients. The realization of these goals requires close integration of retinal specialists, genetic counselors, molecular geneticists, and bioinformaticists.

ACKNOWLEDGMENTS

Supported by Center and Individual Grants, and a Wynn-Gund TRAP Award, from the Foundation Fighting Blindness; by National Institutes of Health Grant EY007142; and by the Hermann Eye Fund.

REFERENCES

Abecasis GR, Auton A, Brooks LD, DePristo MA, Durbin RM, Handsaker RE, Kang HM, Marth GT, McVean GA. 2012. An integrated map of genetic variation from 1,092 human genomes. *Nature* **491:** 56–65.

Audo I, Bujakowska KM, Leveillard T, Mohand-Said S, Lancelot ME, Germain A, Antonio A, Michiels C, Saraiva JP, Letexier M, et al. 2012. Development and application of a next-generation-sequencing (NGS) approach to detect known and novel gene defects underlying retinal diseases. *Orphanet J Rare Dis* **7:** 8.

Berger W, Kloeckener-Gruissem B, Neidhardt J. 2010. The molecular basis of human retinal and vitreoretinal diseases. *Prog Retin Eye Res* **29:** 335–375.

Bocquet B, Lacroux A, Surget MO, Baudoin C, Marquette V, Manes G, Hebrard M, Senechal A, Delettre C, Roux AF, et al. 2013. Relative frequencies of inherited retinal dystrophies and optic neuropathies in Southern France: Assessment of 21-year data management. *Ophthalmic Epidemiol* **20:** 13–25.

Bowne SJ, Daiger SP, Hims MM, Sohocki MM, Malone KA, McKie AB, Heckenlively JR, Birch DG, Inglehearn CF, Bhattacharya SS, et al. 1999. Mutations in the *RP1* gene causing autosomal dominant retinitis pigmentosa. *Hum Mol Genet* **8:** 2121–2128.

Bowne SJ, Sullivan LS, Blanton SH, Cepko CL, Blackshaw S, Birch DG, Hughbanks-Wheaton D, Heckenlively JR, Daiger SP. 2002. Mutations in the inosine monophosphate dehydrogenase 1 gene (IMPDH1) cause the RP10 form of autosomal dominant retinitis pigmentosa. *Hum Mol Genet* **11:** 559–568.

Bowne SJ, Sullivan LS, Mortimer SE, Hedstrom L, Zhu J, Spellicy CJ, Gire AI, Hughbanks-Wheaton D, Birch DG, Lewis RA, et al. 2006. Spectrum and frequency of mutations in IMPDH1 associated with autosomal dominant retinitis pigmentosa and Leber congenital amaurosis. *Invest Ophthalmol Vis Sci* **47:** 34–42.

Bowne SJ, Sullivan LS, Gire AI, Birch DG, Hughbanks-Wheaton D, Heckenlively JR, Daiger SP. 2008. Mutations in the *TOPORS* gene cause 1% of autosomal dominant retinitis pigmentosa. *Mol Vis* **14:** 922–927.

Bowne SJ, Humphries MM, Sullivan LS, Kenna PF, Tam LCS, Kiang AS, Campbell M, Weinstock GM, Koboldt DC, Ding L, et al. 2011a. A dominant mutation in *RPE65* identified by whole-exome sequencing causes retinitis pigmentosa with choroidal involvement. *Euro J Hum Genet* **19:** 1074–1081.

Bowne SJ, Sullivan LS, Koboldt DC, Ding L, Fulton R, Abbott RM, Sodergren EJ, Birch DG, Wheaton DH, Heckenlively JR, et al. 2011b. Identification of disease-causing mutations in autosomal dominant retinitis pigmentosa (adRP) using next-generation DNA sequencing. *Invest Ophthalmol Vis Sci* **52:** 494–503.

Bowne SJ, Sullivan LS, Avery CE, Sasser EM, Roorda A, Duncan JL, Wheaton DH, Birch DG, Branham KE, Heckenlively JR, et al. 2013. Mutations in the *SNRNP200* gene cause 1.6% of autosomal dominant retinitis pigmentosa. *Mol Vis.* **19:** 2407–2417.

Branham K, Othman M, Brumm M, Karoukis AJ, Atmaca-Sonmez P, Yashar BM, Schwartz SB, Stover NB, Trzupek K, Wheaton D, et al. 2012. Mutations in *RPGR* and *RP2* account for 15% of males with simplex retinal degenerative disease. *Invest Ophthalmol Vis Sci* **53:** 8232–8237.

Chen X, Zhao K, Sheng X, Li Y, Gao X, Zhang X, Kang X, Pan X, Liu Y, Jiang C, et al. 2013. Targeted sequencing of 179 genes associated with hereditary retinal dystrophies and 10 candidate genes identifies novel and known mutations in patients with various retinal diseases. *Invest Ophthalmol Vis Sci* **54:** 2186–2197.

Churchill JD, Bowne SJ, Sullivan LS, Lewis RA, Wheaton DK, Birch DG, Branham KE, Heckenlively JR, Daiger SP. 2013. Mutations in the X-linked retinitis pigmentosa genes *RPGR* and *RP2* found in 8.5% of families with a provisional diagnosis of autosomal dominant retinitis pigmentosa. *Invest Ophthalmol Vis Sci* **54:** 1411–1416.

Cremers FP, den Dunnen JT, Ajmal M, Hussain A, Preising MN, Daiger SP, Qamar R. 2014. Comprehensive registration of DNA sequence variants associated with inherited retinal diseases in Leiden Open Variation Databases. *Hum Mutat* **35:** 147–148.

Daiger SP, Bowne SJ, Sullivan LS. 2007. Perspective on genes and mutations causing retinitis pigmentosa. *Arch Ophthalmol* **125:** 151–158.

Daiger SP, Sullivan LS, Bowne SJ. 2013. Genes and mutations causing retinitis pigmentosa. *Clin Genet* **84:** 132–141.

Dryja TP, McGee TL, Hahn LB, Cowley GS, Olsson JE, Reichel E, Sandberg MA, Berson EL. 1990. Mutations within the rhodopsin gene in patients with autosomal dominant retinitis pigmentosa. *N Engl J Med* **323:** 1302–1307.

Dryja TP, Hahn LB, Cowley GS, McGee TL, Berson EL. 1991. Mutation spectrum of the rhodopsin gene among patients with autosomal dominant retinitis pigmentosa. *Proc Natl Acad Sci* **88:** 9370–9374.

Dryja TP, Hahn LB, Kajiwara K, Berson EL. 1997. Dominant and digenic mutations in the *peripherin/RDS* and *ROM1* genes in retinitis pigmentosa. *Invest Ophthalmol Vis Sci* **38:** 1972–1982.

Eisenberger T, Neuhaus C, Khan AO, Decker C, Preising MN, Friedburg C, Bieg A, Gliem M, Charbel Issa P, Holz FG, et al. 2013. Increasing the yield in targeted next-generation sequencing by implicating CNV analysis, non-coding exons and the overall variant load: The example of retinal dystrophies. *PLoS ONE* **8:** e78496.

El Shamieh S, Neuille M, Terray A, Orhan E, Condroyer C, Demontant V, Michiels C, Antonio A, Boyard F, Lancelot ME, et al. 2014. Whole-exome sequencing identifies *KIZ* as a ciliary gene associated with autosomal-recessive rod-cone dystrophy. *Am J Hum Genet* **94:** 625–633.

Fahim AT, Daiger SP, Weleber RG. 2013. Retinitis pigmentosa overview. In *GeneReviews* (ed. Pagon RA, Adam MP, Bird TD, Dolan CR, Fong CT, Stephens K), University of Washington, Seattle.

Fernandez-Suarez XM, Rigden DJ, Galperin MY. 2014. The 2014 Nucleic Acids Research Database Issue and an updated NAR online Molecular Biology Database Collection. *Nucleic Acids Res* **42:** D1–D6.

Fingert JH, Oh K, Chung M, Scheetz TE, Andorf JL, Johnson RM, Sheffield VC, Stone EM. 2008. Association of a novel mutation in the retinol dehydrogenase 12 (*RDH12*) gene with autosomal dominant retinitis pigmentosa. *Arch Ophthalmol* **126:** 1301–1307.

Fishman GA, Jacobson SG, Alexander KR, Cideciyan AV, Birch DG, Weleber RG, Hood DC. 2005. Outcome measures and their application in clinical trials for retinal degenerative diseases: Outline, review, and perspective. *Retina* **25:** 772–777.

Friedman JS, Ray JW, Waseem N, Johnson K, Brooks MJ, Hugosson T, Breuer D, Branham KE, Krauth DS, Bowne SJ, et al. 2009. Mutations in a BTB-Kelch protein, KLHL7, cause autosomal-dominant retinitis pigmentosa. *Am J Hum Genet* **84:** 792–800.

Gire AI, Sullivan LS, Bowne SJ, Birch DG, Hughbanks-Wheaton D, Heckenlively JR, Daiger SP. 2007. The Gly56Arg mutation in NR2E3 accounts for 1–2% of autosomal dominant retinitis pigmentosa. *Mol Vis* **13:** 1970–1975.

Glockle N, Kohl S, Mohr J, Scheurenbrand T, Sprecher A, Weisschuh N, Bernd A, Rudolph G, Schubach M, Poloschek C, et al. 2013. Panel-based next generation sequencing as a reliable and efficient technique to detect mutations in unselected patients with retinal dystrophies. *Eur J Hum Genet.* **22:** 99–104.

Haim M. 2002. Epidemiology of retinitis pigmentosa in Denmark. *Acta Ophthalmol Scand Suppl* **233:** 1–34.

Heckenlively JR, Daiger SP. 2007. Hereditary retinal and choroidal degenerations. In *Emery and Rimoin's principles and practice of medical genetics*, Chap. 147, pp. 3197–3227, Churchill Livingston, London.

HGMD. 2014. Human Gene Mutation Database, http://www.hgmd.cf.ac.uk/. Biobase Biological Databases.

Jin ZB, Huang XF, Lv JN, Xiang L, Li DQ, Chen J, Huang C, Wu J, Lu F, Qu J. 2014. *SLC7A14* linked to autosomal recessive retinitis pigmentosa. *Nat Commun* **5:** 3517.

Kajiwara K, Berson EL, Dryja TP. 1994. Digenic retinitis pigmentosa due to mutations at the unlinked peripherin/RDS and ROM1 loci. *Science* **264:** 1604–1608.

Kannabiran C, Singh HP, Jalali S. 2012. Mapping of locus for autosomal dominant retinitis pigmentosa on chromosome 6q23. *Hum Genet* **131:** 717–723.

Khaliq S, Abid A, Ismail M, Hameed A, Mohyuddin A, Lall P, Aziz A, Anwar K, Mehdi SQ. 2005. Novel association of *RP1* gene mutations with autosomal recessive retinitis pigmentosa. *J Med Genet* **42:** 436–438.

Knecht C, Krawczak M. 2014. Molecular genetic epidemiology of human diseases: From patterns to predictions. *Hum Genet* **133:** 425–430.

Koboldt DC, Larson DE, Sullivan LS, Bowne SJ, Steinberg KM, Churchill JD, Buhr AC, Nutter N, Pierce EA, Blanton SH, et al. 2014. Exome-based mapping and variant prioritization for inherited Mendelian disorders. *Am J Hum Genet* **94:** 373–384.

Laszlo AH, Derrington IM, Ross BC, Brinkerhoff H, Adey A, Nova IC, Craig JM, Langford KW, Samson JM, Daza R, et al. 2014. Decoding long nanopore sequencing reads of natural DNA. *Nat Biotechnol* **32:** 829–833.

Li S, Xiao X, Wang P, Guo X, Zhang Q. 2010. Mutation spectrum and frequency of the *RHO* gene in 248 Chinese families with retinitis pigmentosa. *Biochem Biophys Res Commun* **401:** 42–47.

Liu MM, Zack DJ. 2013. Alternative splicing and retinal degeneration. *Clin Genet* **84:** 142–149.

MacArthur DG, Manolio TA, Dimmock DP, Rehm HL, Shendure J, Abecasis GR, Adams DR, Altman RB, Antonarakis SE, Ashley EA, et al. 2014. Guidelines for investigating causality of sequence variants in human disease. *Nature* **508:** 469–476.

Marth GT, Yu F, Indap AR, Garimella K, Gravel S, Leong WF, Tyler-Smith C, Bainbridge M, Blackwell T, Zheng-Bradley X, et al. 2011. The functional spectrum of low-frequency coding variation. *Genome Biol* **12:** R84.

McGee TL, Devoto M, Ott J, Berson EL, Dryja TP. 1997. Evidence that the penetrance of mutations at the RP11 locus causing dominant retinitis pigmentosa is influenced by a gene linked to the homologous RP11 allele. *Am J Hum Genet* **61:** 1059–1066.

NCBI. 2014. Database resources of the National Center for Biotechnology Information. *Nucleic Acids Res* **42:** D7–D17.

Neveling K, Collin RW, Gilissen C, van Huet RA, Visser L, Kwint MP, Gijsen SJ, Zonneveld MN, Wieskamp N, de Ligt J, et al. 2012. Next-generation genetic testing for retinitis pigmentosa. *Hum Mutat* **33:** 963–972.

Nishiguchi KM, Tearle RG, Liu YP, Oh EC, Miyake N, Benaglio P, Harper S, Koskiniemi-Kuendig H, Venturini G, Sharon D, et al. 2013. Whole genome sequencing in patients with retinitis pigmentosa reveals pathogenic DNA structural changes and *NEK2* as a new disease gene. *Proc Natl Acad Sci* **110:** 16139–16144.

O'Sullivan J, Mullaney BG, Bhaskar SS, Dickerson JE, Hall G, O'Grady A, Webster A, Ramsden SC, Black GC. 2012. A paradigm shift in the delivery of services for diagnosis of inherited retinal disease. *J Med Genet* **49:** 322–326.

Ozgul RK, Siemiatkowska AM, Yucel D, Myers CA, Collin RW, Zonneveld MN, Beryozkin A, Banin E, Hoyng CB, van den Born LI, et al. 2011. Exome sequencing and cis-regulatory mapping identify mutations in *MAK*, a gene encoding a regulator of ciliary length, as a cause of retinitis pigmentosa. *Am J Hum Genet* **89:** 253–264.

RetNet. 2014. The Retinal Information Network, http://www.sph.uth.edu/RetNet/. Stephen P. Daiger, Ph.D., Administrator, The University of Texas Health Science Center at Houston.

Riazuddin SA, Zulfiqar F, Zhang Q, Sergeev YV, Qazi ZA, Husnain T, Caruso R, Riazuddin S, Sieving PA, Hejtmancik JF. 2005. Autosomal recessive retinitis pigmentosa is associated with mutations in *RP1* in three consanguineous Pakistani families. *Invest Ophthalmol Vis Sci* **46:** 2264–2670.

Richards CS, Bale S, Bellissimo DB, Das S, Grody WW, Hegde MR, Lyon E, Ward BE. 2008. ACMG recommendations for standards for interpretation and reporting of sequence variations: Revisions 2007. *Genet Med* **10:** 294–300.

Schwarz JM, Rodelsperger C, Schuelke M, Seelow D. 2010. MutationTaster evaluates disease-causing potential of sequence alterations. *Nat Methods* **7:** 575–576.

Sergouniotis PI, Chakarova C, Murphy C, Becker M, Lenassi E, Arno G, Lek M, MacArthur DG, Bhattacharya SS, Moore AT, et al. 2014. Biallelic variants in *TTLL5*, encoding a tubulin glutamylase, cause retinal dystrophy. *Am J Hum Genet* **94:** 760–769.

Shankar SP, Kozma P, Birch DG, Hughbanks-Wheaton D, Locke KG, Ruiz RS, Sullivan LS, Bowne SJ, Stone EM, Daiger SP. 2004. Analysis of protein haplotypes in *trans* as factors modifying phenotypic variation of retinal dystrophies caused by a splice site mutation in the *peripherin/RDS* gene. *Invest Ophthalmol Vis Sci* **45:** 3719.

Simpson DA, Clark GR, Alexander S, Silvestri G, Willoughby CE. 2011. Molecular diagnosis for heterogeneous genetic diseases with targeted high-throughput DNA sequencing applied to retinitis pigmentosa. *J Med Genet* **48:** 145–151.

Sohocki MM, Daiger SP, Bowne SJ, Rodriquez JA, Northrup H, Heckenlively JR, Birch DG, Mintz-Hittner H, Ruiz RS, Lewis RA, et al. 2001. Prevalence of mutations causing retinitis pigmentosa and other inherited retinopathies. *Hum Mutat* **17:** 42–51.

Sullivan LS, Heckenlively JR, Bowne SJ, Zuo J, Hide WA, Gal A, Denton M, Inglehearn CF, Blanton SH, Daiger SP. 1999. Mutations in a novel retina-specific gene cause autosomal dominant retinitis pigmentosa. *Nat Genet* **22:** 255–259.

Sullivan LS, Bowne SJ, Birch DG, Hughbanks-Wheaton D, Heckenlively JR, Lewis RA, Garcia CA, Ruiz RS, Blanton SH, Northrup H, et al. 2006a. Prevalence of disease-causing mutations in families with autosomal dominant retinitis pigmentosa: A screen of known genes in 200 families. *Invest Ophthalmol Vis Sci* **47:** 3052–3064.

Sullivan LS, Bowne SJ, Seaman CR, Blanton SH, Lewis RA, Heckenlively JR, Birch DG, Hughbanks-Wheaton D, Daiger SP. 2006b. Genomic rearrangements of the *PRPF31* gene account for 2.5% of autosomal dominant retinitis pigmentosa. *Invest Ophthalmol Vis Sci* **47:** 4579–4588.

Sullivan LS, Koboldt DC, Bowne SJ, Lang S, Blanton SH, Cadena EL, Avery CE, Lewis RA, Webb-Jones K, Wheaton DK, et al. 2014. A dominant mutation in hexokinase 1 (HK1) causes retinitis pigmentosa. *Invest Ophthalmol Vis Sci* doi: 10.1167/iovs.14-15419.

Tucker BA, Scheetz TE, Mullins RF, DeLuca AP, Hoffmann JM, Johnston RM, Jacobson SG, Sheffield VC, Stone EM. 2011. Exome sequencing and analysis of induced pluripotent stem cells identify the cilia-related gene *male germ cell-associated kinase* (*MAK*) as a cause of retinitis pigmentosa. *Proc Natl Acad Sci* **108:** E569–576.

Venturini G, Rose AM, Shah AZ, Bhattacharya SS, Rivolta C. 2012. *CNOT3* is a modifier of *PRPF31* mutations in retinitis pigmentosa with incomplete penetrance. *PLoS Genet* **8:** e1003040.

Wang F, Wang H, Tuan HF, Nguyen DH, Sun V, Keser V, Bowne SJ, Sullivan LS, Luo H, Zhao L, et al. 2013. Next generation sequencing-based molecular diagnosis of retinitis pigmentosa: Identification of a novel genotype-phenotype correlation and clinical refinements. *Hum Genet* **133:** 331–345.

Wang J, Zhang VW, Feng Y, Tian X, Li FY, Truong C, Wang G, Chiang PW, Lewis RA, Wong LJ. 2014. Dependable and efficient clinical utility of target capture based deep sequencing in molecular diagnosis of retinitis pigmentosa. *Invest Ophthalmol Vis Sci.* doi: 10.1167/iovs.14-14936.

Wright AF, Chakarova CF, Abd El-Aziz MM, Bhattacharya SS. 2010. Photoreceptor degeneration: Genetic and mechanistic dissection of a complex trait. *Nat Rev Genet* **11:** 273–284.

Wu DM, Khanna H, Atmaca-Sonmez P, Sieving PA, Branham K, Othman M, Swaroop A, Daiger SP, Heckenlively JR. 2010. Long-term follow-up of a family with dominant X-linked retinitis pigmentosa. *Eye* **24:** 764–774.

Xu Y, Guan L, Shen T, Zhang J, Xiao X, Jiang H, Li S, Yang J, Jia X, Yin Y, et al. 2014. Mutations of 60 known causative genes in 157 families with retinitis pigmentosa based on exome sequencing. *Hum Genet.* doi: 10.1007/s00439-014-1460-2.

Zeitz C, Jacobson SG, Hamel CP, Bujakowska K, Neuille M, Orhan E, Zanlonghi X, Lancelot ME, Michiels C, Schwartz SB, et al. 2013. Whole-exome sequencing identifies *LRIT3* mutations as a cause of autosomal-recessive complete congenital stationary night blindness. *Am J Hum Genet* **92:** 67–75.

Genomic Approaches for the Discovery of Genes Mutated in Inherited Retinal Degeneration

Anna M. Siemiatkowska[1,2], Rob W.J. Collin[1,2], Anneke I. den Hollander[1,2,3], and Frans P.M. Cremers[1,2]

[1]Department of Human Genetics, Radboud University Medical Center, Nijmegen, The Netherlands

[2]Radboud Institute for Molecular Life Sciences, Radboud University Medical Center, Nijmegen, The Netherlands

[3]Department of Ophthalmology, Radboud University Medical Center, Nijmegen, The Netherlands

Correspondence: Frans.Cremers@radboudumc.nl

In view of their high degree of genetic heterogeneity, inherited retinal diseases (IRDs) pose a significant challenge for identifying novel genetic causes. Thus far, more than 200 genes have been found to be mutated in IRDs, which together contain causal variants in >80% of the cases. Accurate genetic diagnostics is particularly important for isolated cases, in which X-linked and de novo autosomal dominant variants are not uncommon. In addition, new gene- or mutation-specific therapies are emerging, underlining the importance of identifying causative mutations in each individual. Sanger sequencing of selected genes followed by cost-effective targeted next-generation sequencing (NGS) can identify defects in known IRD-associated genes in the majority of the cases. Exome NGS in combination with genetic linkage or homozygosity mapping studies can aid the identification of the remaining causal genes. As these are thought to be mutated in <1% of the cases, validation through functional modeling in, for example, zebrafish and/or replication through the genotyping of large patient cohorts is required. In the near future, whole genome NGS in combination with transcriptome NGS may reveal mutations that are currently hidden in the noncoding regions of the human genome.

Inherited retinal dystrophies are degenerative disorders of the retina characterized by photoreceptor cell death, which may lead to complete blindness. In general, they display significant clinical and genetic heterogeneity (Berger et al. 2010; den Hollander et al. 2010). These disorders may be subdivided into two groups, either primarily affecting rod photoreceptor cells (e.g., retinitis pigmentosa, RP; congenital stationary night blindness, CSNB) or mainly affecting cone photoreceptors (e.g., cone dystrophy [CD], cone-rod dystrophy [CRD], achromatopsia [ACHM]). In the case of Leber congenital amaurosis (LCA), both types of photoreceptors or the retinal pigment epithelium can be affected, resulting in severe visual impairment in the first year of life. The majority of retinal dystrophies show a progressive degen-

Cite this article as *Cold Spring Harb Perspect Med* doi: 10.1101/cshperspect.a017137

eration, but some are thought not to progress with age, such as CSNB and ACHM. Because some of these diseases have common characteristics (Fig. 1), the differential diagnosis may be problematic. Additionally, with 200 genes known to be involved in various inherited retinal diseases (RetNet, see https://sph.uth.edu/RetNet/sum-dis.htm#A-genes), the genetic diagnostics can be challenging.

Within this group of disorders, two major types can be distinguished: retinal dystrophies that are part of a syndrome and nonsyndromic disorders affecting solely the retina. Most inherited retinal dystrophies are monogenic, displaying all patterns of Mendelian inheritance. However, there is growing evidence of additional contribution of alleles in other genes to the disease outcome in certain IRDs (see Katsanis 2014).

In this review we outline the state of the art genomic approaches to identify defects underlying nonsyndromic IRDs that show a moderate or high degree of genetic heterogeneity, that is, ACHM, CD, CRD, LCA, and RP. We present examples of studies that illustrate the approaches we deem most effective at this moment, taking the associated costs into consideration. As the majority of IRD-associated genes have been identified, we discuss how mutations in known IRD genes can be excluded (e.g., by Sanger sequencing of frequently mutated genes or targeted NGS of sets of genes) before exome NGS is applied to identify defects in novel disease genes. Finally, we provide a future outlook on how the remaining genetic causes can be identified using whole genome NGS and transcriptomics.

GENETIC ANALYSIS OF HOMOGENOUS MONOGENIC DISEASES

Presently, 200 genes are known to be involved in the pathogenesis of IRDs. The most common retinal dystrophy, RP, is particularly heterogeneous, with 61 causative genes described so far. On the other side of the spectrum lie the diseases where most of the cases are explained by mutations in a single gene, such as ornithine amino transferase (*OAT*) in gyrate atrophy, *CHM* in choroideremia, or *ABCA4* in Stargardt disease. Further details of such diseases are provided in Daiger et al. (2015). These homogeneous diseases are relatively undemanding in terms of genetic diagnostics. The preferred method of choice in these cases is Sanger se-

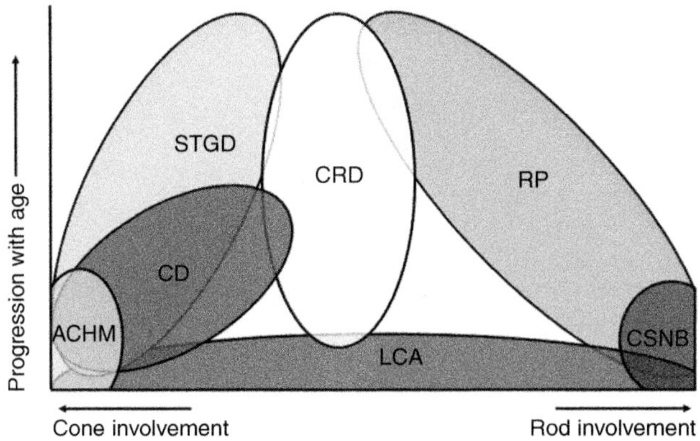

Figure 1. Photoreceptor involvement and progression with age showing clinical overlap between autosomal recessive retinal diseases. (From den Hollander et al. 2010; adapted, with permission.) Leber congenital amaurosis (LCA), as the most severe disorder, is rapidly progressing, reaching blindness at an early age. Retinitis pigmentosa (RP), cone dystrophy (CD), cone-rod dystrophy (CRD), and Stargardt disease (STGD) have a broad spectrum of ages of onset and do not always lead to complete vision loss. Stationary disorders (achromatopsia, ACHM; congenital stationary night blindness, CSNB) are on the edges of the graph, displaying sole cone and rod involvement, respectively.

 Cite this article as *Cold Spring Harb Perspect Med* doi: 10.1101/cshperspect.a017137

quencing, which is cost-effective for genes spanning no more than 50 amplicons. For autosomal recessive inheritance both alleles must be affected. If only one of the two alleles harbors a clear-cut mutation, looking for exonic deletions or duplications using the multiplex ligation probe amplification technique may be applied. For the genes expressed at detectable levels in peripheral blood lymphocytes, for instance in choroideremia, X-linked CSNB, or retinoschisis, RNA analysis may rather be considered. Reverse transcription and subsequent direct cDNA sequencing enables the discovery of splicing abnormalities such as the insertion of cryptic exons (den Hollander et al. 2006), or the deletion of coding exons (van den Hurk et al. 2003). This technique is particularly valuable because it also enables detection of mutation events that abolish transcription from one allele. This approach can be applied when a mutation is found in a heterozygous state in genomic DNA. In some of these cases, cDNA analysis may reveal the presence of only the mutated allele, indicating that the other allele either is not transcribed or is degraded via nonsense-mediated decay (Ozgul et al, 2011). Unfortunately, many genes are not expressed at sufficient levels in peripheral blood lymphocytes, and in these instances other approaches are necessary to uncover the causative alteration (see below).

GENOMIC APPROACHES FOR HETEROGENEOUS MONOGENIC DISEASES

Prescreening for Genes/Variants Responsible for a Significant Proportion of the Cases

For the majority of monogenic retinal dystrophies, mutations in multiple genes can be responsible for the phenotype. These genetically heterogeneous retinal dystrophies, such as CD, CRD, LCA, and RP, present a challenge, as mutations can be expected in any of 8–61 genes. However, in some subtypes, only one or a few genes or mutations explain a significant proportion of cases, rendering a specific prescreening for these genes or variants a cost-effective diagnostic method. In Figure 2, screening procedures for these types of retinal diseases are proposed. The majority of mutations responsible for ACHM are found in *CNGB3* (50%–87%), followed by *CNGA3* (5%–20%) (Wissinger et al. 2001; Thiadens et al. 2009; Kohl et al. 2005). Although autosomal dominant RP can be caused by mutations in 23 genes, alterations in rhodopsin (*RHO*) account for 20%–30% of

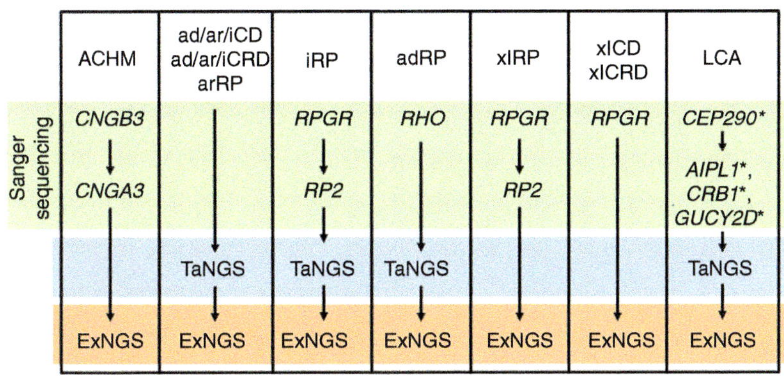

Figure 2. Genotyping strategy for genetically heterogeneous retinal dystrophies. ACHM, achromatopsia; ad, autosomal dominant; ar, autosomal recessive; CD, cone dystrophy; CRD, cone-rod dystrophy; ExNGS, exome next-generation sequencing; i, isolated; LCA, Leber congenital amaurosis; RP, retinitis pigmentosa; TaNGS, targeted next-generation sequencing. *In many Western countries, Sanger sequencing of the intronic *CEP290* variant (c.2991+1655A>G) solves ~15% of the cases. Sequence analysis of *AIPL1* exon 6 (p.W278*), *CRB1* exons 7 and 9, and *GUCY2D* exon 12 (p.R768W) reveals at least one variant in another 20% of the cases. For ExNGS, if multiple affected cases are available, at least two should be analyzed to minimize the number of putative causal variants.

the cases (Daiger et al. 2008). *RPGR* is mutated in ~70% of X-linked RP families (Vervoort and Wright 2002; Bader et al. 2003; Sharon et al. 2003), as well as in ~15% of isolated male RP cases (Branham et al. 2012). The most common LCA-causing mutation in the Caucasian population (*CEP290*, c.2991+1655A>G), is responsible for ~15% of all cases (den Hollander et al. 2006; Perrault et al. 2007; Coppieters et al. 2010). In addition, the *AIPL1* variant p.W278* in exon 6, the *GUCY2D* p.R768W variant in exon 12, as well as *CRB1* variants in exons 7 and 9 together explain another 20% of LCA alleles (Yzer et al. 2006; Testa et al. 2011; Bujakowska et al. 2012). Sequence analysis of these four exons is therefore proposed by the authors as a second prescreening step in LCA. Possibly, in specific populations, other genetic variants are so frequent that their prescreening may be cost-effective. In such cases, a balance between Sanger sequencing costs and expected mutation yield should be assessed on an individual basis.

Targeted NGS

NGS encompasses many different massive parallel sequencing strategies. At least eight NGS methods are currently available, and many others are under development. Older NGS sequencing strategies were originally designed to sequence entire genomes in a high-throughput manner, but have not been tailored to analyze smaller sets of genes. Many NGS methods have been shown to be reasonably sensitive, identifying genetic defects in 40%–50% of persons with autosomal recessive/isolated RP (Booij et al. 2011; Neveling et al. 2012; O'Sullivan et al. 2012; Schorderet et al. 2013; Shanks et al. 2013). However, most of the techniques have two major shortcomings. First, analysis of protein coding sequences of selected genes requires an enrichment step, which invariably leads to underrepresentation or noncoverage of up to 15% of exons. In most cases this is caused by high GC-content, in particular at 5′ ends of genes. Nonenrichment can also be caused by the repetitive nature of targeted sequences, as in *RPGR* ORF15. Second, material costs for target enrichment and sequencing are substantial (~€1000/sample), which limits their use in routine diagnostics.

Two of the targeted NGS approaches can be performed for less than €200 per sample, assuming sequence analysis of a maximum of 100 IRD genes, parallel analysis of at least 100 patient samples and use of the Illumina HiSeq 2000 or a comparable platform. With the first approach, fragment enrichment of protein coding exons or other relevant sequences is achieved by hybridization, either in solution (Agilent SureSelect Target Enrichment System, NimbleGen SeqCap EZ) or on an array (NimbleGen, Bodi et al. 2013). With the second approach, the enrichment utilizes highly multiplexed PCR with molecular inversion probes designed to amplify the fragments of interest (Absalan and Ronaghi 2007; Jacob et al. 2007; Turner et al. 2009; Igartua et al. 2010; Teer et al. 2010; O'Roak et al. 2012).

A key advantage of targeted NGS is that it represents an unbiased approach. The analysis of the entire set of ~100 genes associated with nonsyndromic CD, CRD, LCA, and RP provides flexibility regarding the clinical diagnosis, which can be difficult at early and late stages of disease (see Fig. 1). This is also important for isolated cases with RP, which is often caused by de novo mutations. Indeed, de novo mutations were identified in 4 of 28 cases of isolated RP, with the mutations in both autosomal dominant and autosomal recessive genes (Neveling et al. 2012).

Exome NGS

When prescreening of specific IRD genes or targeted NGS of a larger set of IRD genes does not reveal causative variants, exome NGS is currently the method of choice to reveal defects in "novel" IRD genes.

The following two data sets illustrate typical yields of gene mutations for genetically heterogeneous diseases. Abu-Safieh et al. (2013) employed genome-wide homozygosity mapping and exome NGS to identify the underlying mutations in 78 unrelated consanguineous families with RP or allied dystrophies. This yielded variants in previously identified IRD genes in 78%

of the cases, variants in possible novel IRD genes in 8% of the cases, and no result in 14% of the cases. Similar studies in 41 Pakistani families yielded causal variants in known IRD genes in 32 (78%) of the families (Khan et al. 2014; MI Khan and M Ajmal, unpubl.).

As the majority of genes associated with genetically heterogeneous IRDs has most likely been identified, alterations are expected to be found in genes mutated at low frequency (1% or less). If multiple affected persons are available in a family, at least two affected individuals should be analyzed in parallel. This is particularly important in the case of autosomal dominant diseases, as the number of novel heterozygous variants identified in each individual by exome sequencing (~500) can be daunting. By analyzing affected persons that are remote relatives, the expected number of shared sequence variants decreases significantly. Below, we outline additional techniques and novel approaches to identify the culprit mutation(s).

GENETIC LINKAGE STUDIES AND COPY NUMBER VARIANT DETECTION

Throughout the years, molecular diagnostics of genetically heterogeneous diseases like IRDs have been performed using different techniques. Genetic linkage studies have been employed to narrow down the critical genomic regions for all Mendelian inheritance types of IRDs and are still valuable in this era of high-throughput sequencing technologies. For example, two novel genes underlying autosomal dominant exudative vitreoretinopathy, *TSPAN12* and *ZNF408*, were identified by combining linkage mapping and targeted (to a 40 Mb genomic region) or exome NGS, respectively (Nikopoulos et al. 2010; Collin et al. 2013). Homozygosity mapping combined with exome sequencing identified several other novel IRD genes (for example *MAK*, *DHDDS*, and *RAB28*) (Ozgul et al. 2011; Tucker et al. 2011; Zelinger et al. 2011; Zuchner et al. 2011; Roosing et al. 2013).

In the past, identity-by-descent (IBD) mapping was the method of choice for narrowing down the critical regions in families with an autosomal recessive inheritance pattern. Half of the genes underlying autosomal recessive RP have been identified using this approach, both in consanguineous (Bareil et al. 2001; den Hollander et al. 2009; Bandah-Rozenfeld et al. 2010a,b; Collin et al. 2010), and in nonconsanguineous families (den Hollander et al. 2007; Collin et al. 2008). In brief, a microarray hybridization technique is used to genotype single nucleotide polymorphisms (SNPs) equally spread across the genome. Subsequently, runs of homozygosity shared between the affected individuals can be determined using freely available software for genome-wide SNP analysis such as PLINK (Purcell et al. 2007) or Homozygosity Mapper (Seelow et al. 2009). Theoretically, the IBD regions in an affected person of which the parents are first-cousins on average span 33 Mb (Woods et al. 2006), and in several studies the causal variant in >90% of the cases was found in the largest or second largest homozygous region (Littink et al. 2010; Collin et al. 2011; Siemiatkowska et al. 2011). In nonconsanguineous families, however, the size of IBD regions can vary between ~1.0 Mb and 30 Mb. Because small homozygous regions in the genome are numerous and are less likely to contain the causative mutation, the initial cutoff should be set to 2 Mb. Exome data may also be used to determine the location, number, and length of homozygous regions (Pippucci et al. 2011).

Homozygous mutations are frequently present in populations where consanguineous unions are culturally established, such as in Indonesia, Pakistan, or Saudi Arabia (Siemiatkowska et al. 2011; Khan et al. 2012; Abu-Safieh et al. 2013). In Western populations, homozygous IBD regions within one family are smaller, because more generations have passed since the original founder. A significant proportion (~70%) of recessive inheritance in these populations is attributable to compound heterozygous alterations. Linkage analysis using SNP arrays may be more suitable for this type of data. Recently, a software tool, Haplobot, has been developed to extract stretches of common haplotypes between affected individuals within one family (A Henkes and RWJ Collin, unpubl.). Based on the same principle as PLINK (Purcell et al. 2007), it analyzes common haplotypes within a given window with variable parameters (mismatches and no-calls between individuals per window and size threshold). After listing the common haplotype regions, the program automatically filters out variants from the exome data file that reside in unshared regions. Hence, it enables narrowing down the list of probable causative variants identified by exome NGS. This approach recently aided the identification of causative mutations in *MVK* in an autosomal recessive RP family (Siemiatkowska et al. 2013). Exome data can also be filtered against existing linkage data for a given family, including previously obtained linkage loci.

High density SNP arrays also enable the detection of copy number variations, which may still explain an underrated part of the undiscovered heritability. At the moment, the highest probe density of 2.7 M is provided by CytoScan HD (Affymetrix); among those, 700,000 SNPs have a high minor allele frequency, which is very informative for linkage and homozygosity mapping, or for the detection of uniparental isodisomy (Roosing et al. 2013). Two million probes on the array are quantitatively assessed to detect deletions, duplications, and amplifications larger than 20 kb. Changes smaller in size, e.g., encompassing several exons of a given gene, were previously analyzed by multiplex ligation probe amplification. However, because this method requires custom designed probes for every gene, quantitative assessment of exome NGS data may replace this strategy. In the near future, with sufficient read depth, it is expected that exome NGS will allow a reliable detection of homo- and heterozygous deletions and duplications.

Mutations in Genes Causing Syndromic and Nonsyndromic IRDs

As illustrated by the abovementioned *MVK* case, novel genotype–phenotype correlations are constantly emerging. In the past, such associations were identified for many genes that were initially described as causative of syndromic forms of retinal dystrophies. Examples include *OFD1*, a Joubert syndrome gene recently found to be mutated in nonsyndromic X-linked RP (Coene et al. 2009; Webb et al. 2012) and *CEP290*, a gene that was initially found to be mutated in Joubert syndrome and later turned out to be frequently involved in LCA (den Hollander et al. 2006; Sayer et al. 2006; Valente et al. 2006). *IQCB1*, a gene known for many years to be mutated in Senior-Løken syndrome, was found to be involved in LCA (Otto et al. 2005; Estrada-Cuzcano et al. 2011), and finally the *Bardet-Biedl Syndrome 1 (BBS1)* gene was discovered to be involved in the pathogenesis of wide spectrum of syndromic and nonsyndromic retinal dystrophies (Mykytyn et al. 2002; Estrada-Cuzcano et al. 2012). The recent implementation of whole-exome sequencing has facilitated the discovery of many of such novel associations. Mutations found in *ALMS1*, *CNGA3*, and *MYO7A*, involved in either syndromic or other nonsyndromic forms of IRD, were discovered in LCA families (Wang et al. 2011). In some cases, mutations reside in exons that are only present in retina specific transcripts, e.g., in *BBS8* and *OFD1* (Riazuddin et al. 2010; Webb et al. 2012).

In many instances, autosomal recessive mutations show varying degrees of severity, and the allelic combinations determine the final clinical outcome. For example, missense mutations in the Usher syndrome type 3A gene *CLRN1* were found in nonsyndromic RP (Khan et al. 2011); the hypomorphic *CEP290* c.2991 + 1655A>G variant was found predominantly in persons with LCA, but not in Joubert and Meckel-Gruber syndrome (den Hollander et al. 2006); and the *USH2A* variant p.C759F was found at higher frequency in persons with RP without hearing loss (Eudy et al. 1998; Rivolta et al. 2000). As a consequence, the panels for targeted NGS should ideally contain genes involved in diseases that display retinal dystrophy as one of the symptoms of a multiorgan disorder, although this may double the analysis costs. However, in some instances, the exact same mutation can cause either a syndromic or a nonsyndromic form of IRD, and different models have been proposed to explain this phenomenon among which are modifier loci and digenic/oligogenic inheritance (Katsanis 2004; Estrada-Cuzcano et al. 2012). The novel approaches that are emerging to identify such modifier loci are described in Katsanis (2014).

 Cite this article as *Cold Spring Harb Perspect Med* doi: 10.1101/cshperspect.a017137

WHOLE GENOME SEQUENCING AND TRANSCRIPTOME ANALYSIS

Whole Genome Sequencing

For nonsyndromic RP, recent publications describe the percentage of readily "solved" exome sequencing samples to be approximately 80% (Abu-Safieh et al. 2013). Because exome sequencing does not detect deep intronic variants, which may cause aberrant splicing events, or variants in regulatory sequences that may cause a decrease or imbalance in transcript levels, next-generation sequencing of the whole genome may be the next method to analyze "unsolved" samples. With the costs of whole genome sequencing constantly decreasing, this method is now becoming available for a broader group of laboratories. However, the analysis of whole genome data is still very difficult. First, a very large number of variants ($\sim$3 million in each individual) is obtained and the filtering of potentially causative variants may prove challenging. Second, the effects of regulatory and intronic mutations are not certain, even with the use of contemporary prediction software. An additional cDNA analysis can provide crucial evidence regarding the functional significance of a variant at the RNA level. In the near future, a combination of whole genome sequencing and transcriptome sequencing may effectively decrease the number of candidate variants that require follow-up.

Transcriptome Analysis of Retinal Cells Derived from Induced Pluripotent Stem Cells

The term "transcriptome" refers to all mRNA transcripts that are synthesized in a particular cell type or tissue. Whole transcriptome sequencing provides the most complete analysis possible at the cDNA level (see Farkas et al. 2015). Many described alterations can be detected by examining their consequences at the mRNA level: small insertions and deletions in exons, exon inversions, erroneous splicing events, transcript-level variations (e.g., a mutation is heterozygous in the genomic DNA, but the transcript is not produced from the second allele), exonic and intronic splice site enhancer/silencer changes as well as nonsense mediated exon skipping (Flanigan et al. 2011). Some of these variants are detectable only at the transcript level; the genomic DNA alterations are not visible and require additional Sanger sequencing. In the case of regulatory sequences, identification of these mutations may be problematic.

An additional challenge regarding cDNA analysis in IRDs is the low level of gene transcription. Many genes involved in IRDs are expressed solely, or at least predominantly, in the retina and have very low expression levels in peripheral blood leukocytes or fibroblasts. Recently, an interesting option arose to overcome this difficulty. Transcriptomes may now be derived from photoreceptor-like cells that have been differentiated from induced pluripotent stem cells derived from somatic cells of affected persons. mRNA libraries derived from such cells will not exactly match transcription levels or patterns in the retina, but they do provide the best use of cells currently available (see Tucker et al. 2011; Wiley et al. 2015). Furthermore, transcriptome analysis requires a reference sequence created for the appropriate tissue. This sequence, targeted to human retina and other ocular tissues, was assembled by several different groups (Farkas et al. 2013; Peng et al. 2013; Wagner et al. 2013). Shortly, the transcript library from photoreceptor-like cells derived from induced pluripotent stem cells will also become available. However, because transcriptome analysis is a novel tool, confirmation and comparison from other laboratories will be necessary to ensure high quality of this analysis.

DISEASE VARIANT INTERPRETATION

Allele Frequency Analysis in Control Cohorts

With the increasing possibilities of mutation detection via NGS methods, there is an unprecedented need for additional measures to assess the pathogenicity of the variants. Typically, exome NGS for a single patient using the SOLiD technique yields around 30,000 variations. Because the reference sequence was obtained via Sanger sequencing by the Human Genome Project (International Human Genome Sequencing 2004) and Celera Genomics (Istrail et al. 2004), which involved a small number of anonymous donors, it is not always accurate. Some nucleotides present in the reference are in fact rare variants or sequencing artifacts, and, therefore, these loci will appear as "mutated" in almost every analyzed sample. An improved reference genome, based on novel genomic sequences involving a large number of studied individuals and, as a result, more reliable frequencies, is being assembled. Before it becomes available, the only method of eliminating these variants from exome data is filtering against variant frequencies. Depending on the software used for analysis, SNP frequency from the dbSNP database may be available (see http://www.ncbi.nlm.nih.gov/projects/SNP/). The newest build of this database (138) also contains data from the NHLBI Exome Variant Server (see http://evs.gs.washington.edu/EVS/), 1000 genomes (see http://www.1000genomes.org), and the HapMap project (see http://hapmap.ncbi.nlm.nih.gov/). It is crucial to also incorporate in-house exome variant frequency data in order to eliminate population specific frequent variants or systematic equipment errors, which may not be present in the dbSNP database. After eliminating the polymorphic alterations and common false positives, further frequency filtering depends on prevalence of the disease. Keeping in mind that most novel genes will be mutated rarely in IRD, the allele frequency cutoff for autosomal recessive IRD may be set to 0.5%. All variants below this threshold have a higher probability of being causative; however, there are exceptions to this rule. For instance, a disease may be caused by a null allele combined with a SNP or a mild allele, such as *ABCA4* c.2588G>C, which occurs heterozygously in 3% of healthy individuals in the Netherlands (Maugeri et al. 1999). Obviously, establishing such associations may be challenging. Because of the extremely high heterogeneity of IRDs, it is estimated that one in five individuals bears a null allele in an autosomal recessive IRD-associated gene with proven causality (Nishiguchi and Rivolta 2012). In general, recessive IRDs mainly involve mutations that result in a loss-of-function. In contrast, a dominant inheritance pattern can be caused by null or regulatory mutations (haploinsufficiency) or by missense mutations that cause a gain-of-function or exert a dominant-negative effect on the wild-type protein. Because of incomplete penetrance, which is occasionally observed in dominant IRDs, or recessive hypomorphic alleles, the frequency threshold may need to be set as high as 1%.

Variant Prioritization

In the analysis of autosomal recessive diseases, null alleles should receive utmost priority. Insertion/deletion variants, nonsense variants, and canonical splice site variants, which may lead to the introduction of a premature termination codon, should be examined first. Subsequently, missense alleles and in-frame deletions/insertions should be analyzed. Last, intronic sequence changes and synonymous variants should be given attention. There are several in silico prediction programs and tools that may be helpful in the analysis and prioritization of the variants. For missense mutations, one such tool is PhyloP, which is a nucleotide conservation score derived from 46 vertebrate species (available for all genomic positions at http://genome.ucsc.edu/cgi-bin/hgTables). Most causative mutations have been shown to have a high PhyloP score (>2.5) (Booij et al. 2011). Therefore, filtering out variants with lower PhyloP scores may facilitate identification of the causative mutation. A complementary value in assessing mutation pathogenicity is the Grantham score, which is a measure of physicochemical differences between amino acids that takes features such as size, charge, and polarity into consideration (Grantham 1974). The higher the value, the more different the properties of the amino acids are, and the more likely it is that the missense change will affect protein structure or function. In addition, pathogenicity prediction software, such as Sorting Intolerant From Tolerant (SIFT) (Ng and Henikoff 2003), PolyPhen2 (Adzhubei et al. 2010), and Mutation Assessor (MASS) (Reva et al. 2011) take various features such as evolutionary conservation and Grantham scores into account and predict a variant to be benign or pathogenic. One should bear in mind, however, that false negative results may arise from such an analysis and a "neutral" score does not necessarily mean that the alteration is not causative.

Extreme caution must be exercised in pathogenicity evaluation. As stated above, rare clear-cut null recessive mutations within autosomal recessive IRD genes may be present heterozygously in about one in five individuals (Nishiguchi and Rivolta 2012). Coding sequence length of a given gene also plays a major role in the number of discovered missense alterations. In *RP1L1* and *HMCN1* the rate of such variants reaches 4%, and many of these changes are indicated as deleterious by prediction software (Strom and Gorin 2013).

Canonical splice site mutations (affecting donor and acceptor nucleotides −1, −2, +1, and +2) are usually considered clear splice site abolishing mutations and are expected to significantly diminish the percentage of the normal transcript. The flanking regions of splice sites, including noncanonical sequences, may be evaluated with splice site prediction programs, such as NNSPLICE, Human Splicing Finder, Gene Splicer, SpliceSiteFinder-like, MaxEntScan, or AlaMut, which is a software package containing all of the above. For the purpose of identifying mutations abrogating exonic splice enhancers and silencers, SKIPPY, an online analysis tool, may be applied (Woolfe et al. 2010) (see http://research.nhgri.nih.gov/skippy/input.shtml). Intronic splice enhancers and silencers are more complicated in their nature, and a program enabling their analysis has not yet been devised, although it is known that these modifiers are enriched near alternatively spliced exons (Yeo et al. 2007).

Candidate genes obtained by exome sequencing data may be further prioritized using existing databases of animal model phenotypes, such as Mouse Genome Informatics (MGI) (see http://www.informatics.jax.org/searches/allele_form.shtml) or Zebrafish International Resource Center (ZFIN) (see http://zfin.org/). Other helpful tools involve binding data for retina-specific transcription factors necessary for photoreceptor development and maintenance (e.g., CRX, NRL) (Corbo et al. 2010; Hao et al. 2012). Such data have already facilitated the identification of two retinal dystrophy-associated genes, namely *MAK* and *FAM161A* (Langmann et al. 2010; Ozgul et al. 2011). Because many IRD-associated genes are involved in the development and maintenance of the photoreceptor connecting cilium, the database containing ciliary proteins (see http://www.sfu.ca/~leroux/ciliome_database.htm) may be used to prioritize candidate IRD genes from exome data.

Allele-Specific Control and Large Patient Cohort Analyses

Mutations that are classified as likely responsible for a phenotype must undergo further scrutiny. A population-specific polymorphism that is not present in available SNP databases can be excluded using ethnically matched control panel analysis. This may be achieved even by indirect allele assessment methods such as the amplification-refractory mutation system (ARMS) or, in case of some amplicons, restriction fragment length polymorphism (RFLP) analysis. Alternatively, especially when working with large patient numbers, Taqman/Kaspar assays can be used.

To exclude the possibility that rare variants represent benign polymorphisms, DNA samples of ethnically matched, healthy individuals must be analyzed. Assuming a variant allele frequency of 1%, to achieve 80% power of significance at least 210 chromosomes must be analyzed; for 95% power 340 chromosomes should be analyzed (Collins and Schwartz 2002). However, one should bear in mind that relatively common alleles may still exert a negative effect on the protein (Maugeri et al. 1999). Subsequently, allele-specific analysis can be performed on a large cohort of IRD patients with no identified disease cause. This may reveal other patients with the same mutation, either in homozygous or heterozygous state. In the latter case, Sanger sequencing of the remaining exons may enable the identification of the second hit in the same gene. For the same purpose, if genome-wide SNP genotyping data are available and a homozygous stretch encompasses the respective gene, one can directly sequence all of its exons in other individuals with the same phenotype and overlapping homozygous regions. Both of these methods, however, require significant numbers of patient samples. As such, it is essential to have access to large patient cohorts, which unequivocally addresses the need for multicenter collaborations, especially for rare diseases.

Functional Assessment of Mutation Pathogenicity

Although null alleles, such as frameshift deletions/insertions, canonical splice site alterations, and nonsense mutations are usually considered to result in no protein function, this is not always the case. A mechanism discovered two decades ago, nonsense-mediated exon skipping, may restore the reading frame. Briefly, a nonsense codon introduced within an exon (with the exception of a premature termination codon in the last exon) causes the spliceosome machinery to exclude this exon from the mRNA transcript. Provided that the nucleotide number of the excised exon is divisible by three, the reading frame is preserved. If the portion of the protein encoded by the exon in question does not significantly influence its structure and it is not crucial for the protein function, such an allele may be relatively mild. This mechanism was found for *CEP290*, in which a protein-truncating mutation in exon 7 (c.451C>T, p.Arg151*) resulted in the skipping of exon 7, or exons 7 and 8, and an in-frame deletion (Littink et al. 2010). Persons carrying this *CEP290* variant showed a relatively mild retinal dystrophy. Therefore, transcript analysis is highly advised, even for variants that are expected to result in null alleles.

Recent advances in morpholino-induced gene knockdown enabled the accurate and relatively fast evaluation of missense variants in genes that have zebrafish orthologues. In particular, genes acting in cilia were positively evaluated: the rescue of the morpholino-induced phenotype was obtained using human wild-type RNA (Zaghloul and Katsanis 2011). Because ~70% of human genes have zebrafish counterparts (Santoriello and Zon 2012), this assay is an important tool in functional assessment of potentially pathogenic mutations. Further details are described in Katsanis (2014). If available, functional analysis is best performed in a mammalian model, such as knockout mice or appropriate murine cell lines. Other experiments to consider, which are relatively simple, are subcellular localization studies. Immunostaining of the desired protein in appropriate cell type (e.g., ciliated cell when studying a ciliary protein) may give a clue about the pathogenicity of the variant. Such studies may also be performed in induced pluripotent stem cells differentiated into photoreceptor-like cells.

CONCLUDING REMARKS

Over the recent years, we have witnessed a dramatic change in the methods of gene identification. Contemporary techniques enable faster detection of genetic defects, even in large patient cohorts. Nevertheless, pathogenicity evaluation of the identified variants remains a challenging endeavor. The abundance of known pathogenic mutations in the heterozygous state, observed also in healthy individuals, confers further difficulty in identifying the causative alleles. Adding to the complexity, variants in other genes may contribute to the phenotype. With rapidly decreasing costs of the newest next-generation sequencing techniques, exome sequencing is already becoming a standard in diagnostics of retinal dystrophies. Transcriptome analysis of photoreceptor cells derived from induced pluripotent stem cells and whole-genome sequencing may soon become the next advancements widely used in this field. Many of the IRD genes that have been identified to date, and those that remain to be identified, are mutated in only a small proportion of affected individuals. Therefore, there is an emerging need for worldwide networks of patients that can contribute to studies aiming at future therapeutic trials.

REFERENCES

Reference is also in this subject collection.

Absalan F, Ronaghi M. 2007. Molecular inversion probe assay. *Methods Mol Biol* **396:** 315–330.

Abu-Safieh L, Alrashed M, Anazi S, Alkuraya H, Khan AO, Al-Owain M, Al-Zahrani J, Al-Abdi L, Hashem M, Al-Tarimi S, et al. 2013. Autozygome-guided exome sequencing in retinal dystrophy patients reveals pathogenetic mutations and novel candidate disease genes. *Genome Res* **23:** 236–247.

Adzhubei IA, Schmidt S, Peshkin L, Ramensky VE, Gerasimova A, Bork P, Kondrashov AS, Sunyaev SR. 2010. A method and server for predicting damaging missense mutations. *Nat Methods* **7:** 248–249.

Bader I, Brandau O, Achatz H, Apfelstedt-Sylla E, Hergersberg M, Lorenz B, Wissinger B, Wittwer B, Rudolph G, Meindl A, et al. 2003. X-linked retinitis pigmentosa: *RPGR* mutations in most families with definite X linkage and clustering of mutations in a short sequence stretch of exon ORF15. *Invest Ophthalmol Vis Sci* **44:** 1458–1463.

Bandah-Rozenfeld D, Collin RWJ, Banin E, van den Born LI, Coene KLM, Siemiatkowska AM, Zelinger L, Khan MI, Lefeber DJ, Erdinest I, et al. 2010a. Mutations in *IMPG2*, encoding interphotoreceptor matrix proteoglycan 2, cause autosomal-recessive retinitis pigmentosa. *Am J Hum Genet* **87:** 199–208.

Bandah-Rozenfeld D, Mizrahi-Meissonnier L, Farhy C, Obolensky A, Chowers I, Pe'er J, Merin S, Ben-Yosef T, Ashery-Padan R, Banin E, et al. 2010b. Homozygosity mapping reveals null mutations in *FAM161A* as a cause of autosomal-recessive retinitis pigmentosa. *Am J Hum Genet* **87:** 382–391.

Bareil C, Hamel CP, Delague V, Arnaud B, Demaille J, Claustres M. 2001. Segregation of a mutation in *CNGB1* encoding the β-subunit of the rod cGMP-gated channel in a family with autosomal recessive retinitis pigmentosa. *Hum Genet* **108:** 328–334.

Berger W, Kloeckener-Gruissem B, Neidhardt J. 2010. The molecular basis of human retinal and vitreoretinal diseases. *Prog Retin Eye Res* **29:** 335–375.

Bodi K, Perera AG, Adams PS, Bintzler D, Dewar K, Grove DS, Kieleczawa J, Lyons RH, Neubert TA, Noll AC, et al. 2013. Comparison of commercially available target enrichment methods for next-generation sequencing. *J Biomol Tech* **24:** 73–86.

Booij JC, Bakker A, Kulumbetova J, Moutaoukil Y, Smeets B, Verheij J, Kroes HY, Klaver CCW, van Schooneveld MJ, Bergen AAB, et al. 2011. Simultaneous mutation detection in 90 retinal disease genes in multiple patients using a custom-designed 300-kb retinal resequencing chip. *Ophthalmology* **118:** 160–167 e161–163.

Branham KE, Othman M, Brumm M, Karoukis AJ, Atmaca-Sonmez P, Yashar BM, Schwartz SB, Stover NB, Trzupek K, Wheaton D, et al. 2012. Mutations in *RPGR* and *RP2* account for 15% of males with simplex retinal degenerative disease. *Invest Ophthalmol Vis Sci* **53:** 8232–8237.

Bujakowska K, Audo I, Mohand-Said S, Lancelot ME, Antonio A, Germain A, Leveillard T, Letexier M, Saraiva JP, Lonjou C, et al. 2012. *CRB1* mutations in inherited retinal dystrophies. *Hum Mutat* **33:** 306–315.

Coene KLM, Roepman R, Doherty D, Afroze B, Kroes HY, Letteboer SJF, Ngu LH, Budny B, van Wijk E, Gorden NT, et al. 2009. OFD1 is mutated in X-linked Joubert syndrome and interacts with *LCA5*-encoded lebercilin. *Am J Hum Genet* **85:** 465–481.

Collin RWJ, Littink KW, Klevering BJ, van den Born LI, Koenekoop RK, Zonneveld-Vrieling MN, Blokland EAW, Strom TM, Hoyng CB, den Hollander AI, et al. 2008. Identification of a 2 Mb human ortholog of *Drosophila eyes shut/spacemaker* that is mutated in patients with retinitis pigmentosa. *Am J Hum Genet* **83:** 594–603.

Collin RWJ, Safieh C, Littink KW, Shalev SA, Garzozi HJ, Rizel L, Abbasi AH, Cremers FPM, den Hollander AI, Klevering BJ, et al. 2010. Mutations in *C2ORF71* cause autosomal-recessive retinitis pigmentosa. *Am J Hum Genet* **86:** 783–788.

Collin RWJ, Van den Born LI, Klevering BJ, De Castro Miro M, Littink KW, Arimadyo K, Azam M, Yazar V, Zonneveld-Vrieling MN, Paun CC, et al. 2011. High-resolution homozygosity mapping is a powerful tool to detect novel mutations causative of autosomal recessive RP in the Dutch population. *Invest Ophthalmol Vis Sci* **52:** 2227–2239.

Collin RWJ, Nikopoulos K, Dona M, Gilissen C, Hoischen A, Boonstra FN, Poulter JA, Kondo H, Berger W, Toomes C, et al. 2013. *ZNF408* is mutated in familial exudative vitreoretinopathy and is crucial for the development of zebrafish retinal vasculature. *Proc Natl Acad Sci* **110:** 9856–9861.

Collins JS, Schwartz CE. 2002. Detecting polymorphisms and mutations in candidate genes. *Am J Hum Genet* **71:** 1251–1252.

Coppieters F, Casteels I, Meire F, De Jaegere S, Hooghe S, van Regemorter N, Van Esch H, Matuleviciene A, Nunes L, Meersschaut V, et al. 2010. Genetic screening of LCA in Belgium: Predominance of *CEP290* and identification of potential modifier alleles in *AHI1* of *CEP290*-related phenotypes. *Hum Mutat* **31:** E1709–1766.

Corbo JC, Lawrence KA, Karlstetter M, Myers CA, Abdelaziz M, Dirkes W, Weigelt K, Seifert M, Benes V, Fritsche LG, et al. 2010. CRX ChIP-seq reveals the *cis*-regulatory architecture of mouse photoreceptors. *Genome Res* **20:** 1512–1525.

Daiger SP, Sullivan LS, Gire AI, Birch DG, Heckenlively JR, Bowne SJ. 2008. Mutations in known genes account for 58% of autosomal dominant retinitis pigmentosa (adRP). *Adv Exp Med Biol* **613:** 203–209.

* Daiger SP, Bowne SJ, Sullivan LS. 2015. Genes and mutations causing autosomal dominant retinitis pigmentosa. *Cold Spring Harb Perspect Med* doi: 10.1101/cshperspect.a017129.

den Hollander AI, Koenekoop RK, Yzer S, Lopez I, Arends ML, Voesenek KEJ, Zonneveld-Vrieling MN, Strom TM, Meitinger T, Brunner HG, et al. 2006. Mutations in the *CEP290* (*NPHP6*) gene are a frequent cause of Leber congenital amaurosis. *Am J Hum Genet* **79:** 556–561.

den Hollander AI, Koenekoop RK, Mohamed MD, Arts HH, Boldt K, Towns KV, Sedmak T, Beer M, Nagel-Wolfrum K, McKibbin M, et al. 2007. Mutations in *LCA5*, encoding the ciliary protein lebercilin, cause Leber congenital amaurosis. *Nat Genet* **39:** 889–895.

den Hollander AI, McGee TL, Ziviello C, Banfi S, Dryja TP, Gonzalez-Fernandez F, Ghosh D, Berson EL. 2009. A homozygous missense mutation in the *IRBP* gene (*RBP3*) associated with autosomal recessive retinitis pigmentosa. *Invest Ophthalmol Vis Sci* **50:** 1864–1872.

den Hollander AI, Black A, Bennett J, Cremers FPM. 2010. Lighting a candle in the dark: Advances in genetics and gene therapy of recessive retinal dystrophies. *J Clin Invest* **120:** 3042–3053.

Estrada-Cuzcano A, Koenekoop RK, Coppieters F, Kohl S, Lopez I, Collin RWJ, De Baere EBW, Roeleveld D, Marek J, Bernd A, et al. 2011. *IQCB1* mutations in patients with leber congenital amaurosis. *Invest Ophthalmol Vis Sci* **52:** 834–839.

Estrada-Cuzcano A, Koenekoop RK, Senechal A, De Baere EBW, de Ravel T, Banfi S, Kohl S, Ayuso C, Sharon D, Hoyng CB, et al. 2012. *BBS1* mutations in a wide spectrum of phenotypes ranging from nonsyndromic retinitis pigmentosa to Bardet-Biedl syndrome. *Arch Ophthalmol* **130:** 1425–1432.

Eudy JD, Weston MD, Yao S, Hoover DM, Rehm HL, Ma-Edmonds M, Yan D, Ahmad I, Cheng JJ, Ayuso C, et al. 1998. Mutation of a gene encoding a protein with extracellular matrix motifs in Usher syndrome type IIa. *Science* **280:** 1753–1757.

Farkas MH, Grant GR, White JA, Sousa ME, Consugar MB, Pierce EA. 2013. Transcriptome analyses of the human retina identify unprecedented transcript diversity and 3.5 Mb of novel transcribed sequence via significant alternative splicing and novel genes. *BMC Genomics* **14:** 486.

* Farkas MH, Du EA, Sousa ME, Pierce EA. 2015. RNA-seq: Improving our understanding of retinal biology and disease. *Cold Spring Harb Perspect Med* doi: 10.1101/cshperspect.a017152.

Flanigan KM, Dunn D, Larsen CA, Medne L, Bonnemann CB, Weiss RB. 2011. Becker muscular dystrophy due to an inversion of exons 23 and 24 of the *DMD* gene. *Muscle Nerve* **44:** 822–825.

Grantham R. 1974. Amino acid difference formula to help explain protein evolution. *Science* **185:** 862–864.

Hao H, Kim DS, Klocke B, Johnson KR, Cui K, Gotoh N, Zang C, Gregorski J, Gieser L, Peng W, et al. 2012. Transcriptional regulation of rod photoreceptor homeostasis revealed by *in vivo* NRL targetome analysis. *PLoS Genet* **8:** e1002649.

Igartua C, Turner EH, Ng SB, Hodges E, Hannon GJ, Bhattacharjee A, Rieder MJ, Nickerson DA, Shendure J. 2010. Targeted enrichment of specific regions in the human genome by array hybridization. *Curr Protoc Hum Genet* Chapter 18: Unit 18 13.

International Human Genome Sequencing C. 2004. Finishing the euchromatic sequence of the human genome. *Nature* **431:** 931–945.

Istrail S, Sutton GG, Florea L, Halpern AL, Mobarry CM, Lippert R, Walenz B, Shatkay H, Dew I, Miller JR, et al. 2004. Whole-genome shotgun assembly and comparison of human genome assemblies. *Proc Natl Acad Sci* **101:** 1916–1921.

Jacob CO, Reiff A, Armstrong DL, Myones BL, Silverman E, Klein-Gitelman M, McCurdy D, Wagner-Weiner L, Nocton JJ, Solomon A, et al. 2007. Identification of novel susceptibility genes in childhood-onset systemic lupus erythematosus using a uniquely designed candidate gene pathway platform. *Arthritis Rheum* **56:** 4164–4173.

Katsanis N. 2004. The oligogenic properties of Bardet-Biedl syndrome. *Hum Mol Genet* **13:** R65–71.

* Katsanis N. 2014. *Cold Spring Harb Perspect Med* doi: 10.1101/cshperspect.a017145.

Khan MI, Kersten FFJ, Azam M, Collin RWJ, Hussain A, Shah ST, Keunen JEE, Kremer H, Cremers FPM, Qamar R, et al. 2011. *CLRN1* mutations cause nonsyndromic retinitis pigmentosa. *Ophthalmology* **118:** 1444–1448.

Khan MI, Ajmal M, Micheal S, Azam M, Hussain A, Shahzad A, Venselaar H, Bokhari H, de Wijs I, Hoefsloot LH, et al. 2012. Homozygosity mapping identifies genetic defects in four consanguineous families with retinal dystrophy from Pakistan. *Clin Genet* **84:** 290–293.

Khan MI, Azam M, Ajmal M, Collin RWJ, den Hollander AI, Cremers FPM, Qamar R. 2014. The molecular basis of retinal dystrophies in Pakistan. *Genes (Basel)* **5:** 176–195.

Kohl S, Varsanyi B, Antunes GA, Baumann B, Hoyng CB, Jagle H, Rosenberg T, Kellner U, Lorenz B, Salati R, et al. 2005. *CNGB3* mutations account for 50% of all cases with autosomal recessive achromatopsia. *Eur J Hum Genet* **13:** 302–308.

Langmann T, Di Gioia SA, Rau I, Stohr H, Maksimovic NS, Corbo JC, Renner AB, Zrenner E, Kumaramanickavel G, Karlstetter M, et al. 2010. Nonsense mutations in *FAM161A* cause *RP28*-associated recessive retinitis pigmentosa. *Am J Hum Genet* **87:** 376–381.

Littink KW, Koenekoop RK, van den Born LI, Collin RWJ, Moruz L, Veltman JA, Roosing S, Zonneveld-Vrieling MN, Omar A, Darvish M, et al. 2010. Homozygosity mapping in patients with cone-rod dystrophy: Novel mutations and clinical characterizations. *Invest Ophthalmol Vis Sci* **51:** 5943–5951.

Maugeri A, van Driel MA, van de Pol DJ, Klevering BJ, van Haren FJ, Tijmes N, Bergen AAB, Rohrschneider K, Blankenagel A, Pinckers AJ, et al. 1999. The 2588G-->C mutation in the *ABCR* gene is a mild freq5uent founder mutation in the Western European population and allows the classification of *ABCR* mutations in patients with Stargardt disease. *Am J Hum Genet* **64:** 1024–1035.

Mykytyn K, Nishimura DY, Searby CC, Shastri M, Yen HJ, Beck JS, Braun T, Streb LM, Cornier AS, Cox GF, et al. 2002. Identification of the gene (*BBS1*) most commonly involved in Bardet-Biedl syndrome, a complex human obesity syndrome. *Nat Genet* **31:** 435–438.

Neveling K, Collin RWJ, Gilissen C, van Huet RAC, Visser L, Kwint MP, Gijsen SJ, Zonneveld-Vrieling MN, Wieskamp N, de Ligt J, et al. 2012. Next-generation genetic testing for retinitis pigmentosa. *Hum Mutat* **33:** 963–972.

Ng PC, Henikoff S. 2003. SIFT: Predicting amino acid changes that affect protein function. *Nucleic Acids Res* **31:** 3812–3814.

Nikopoulos K, Gilissen C, Hoischen A, van Nouhuys CE, Boonstra FN, Blokland EAW, Arts P, Wieskamp N, Strom TM, Ayuso C, et al. 2010. Next-generation sequencing of a 40 Mb linkage interval reveals *TSPAN12* mutations in patients with familial exudative vitreoretinopathy. *Am J Hum Genet* **86:** 240–247.

Nishiguchi KM, Rivolta C. 2012. Genes associated with retinitis pigmentosa and allied diseases are frequently mutated in the general population. *PLoS ONE* **7:** e41902.

O'Roak BJ, Vives L, Fu W, Egertson JD, Stanaway IB, Phelps IG, Carvill G, Kumar A, Lee C, Ankenman K, et al. 2012. Multiplex targeted sequencing identifies recurrently mutated genes in autism spectrum disorders. *Science* **338:** 1619–1622.

O'Sullivan J, Mullaney BG, Bhaskar SS, Dickerson JE, Hall G, O'Grady A, Webster AR, Ramsden SC, Black GC. 2012. A paradigm shift in the delivery of services for diagnosis of inherited retinal disease. *J Med Genet* **49:** 322–326.

Otto EA, Loeys B, Khanna H, Hellemans J, Sudbrak R, Fan S, Muerb U, O'Toole JF, Helou J, Attanasio M, et al. 2005. Nephrocystin-5, a ciliary IQ domain protein, is mutated in Senior-Loken syndrome and interacts with RPGR and calmodulin. *Nat Genet* **37:** 282–288.

Ozgul RK, Siemiatkowska AM, Yucel D, Myers CA, Collin RWJ, Zonneveld-Vrieling MN, Beryozkin A, Banin E, Hoyng CB, van den Born LI, et al. 2011. Exome sequencing and *cis*-regulatory mapping identify mutations in *MAK*, a gene encoding a regulator of ciliary length, as a cause of retinitis pigmentosa. *Am J Hum Genet* **89:** 253–264.

Peng SM, Gan GL, Qiu CH, Zhong M, An HY, Adelman RA, Rizzolo LJ. 2013. Engineering a blood-retinal barrier with human embryonic stem cell-derived retinal pigment epithelium: Transcriptome and functional analysis. *Stem Cell Transl Med* **2:** 534–544.

Perrault I, Delphin N, Hanein S, Gerber S, Dufier JL, Roche O, Defoort-Dhellemmes S, Dollfus H, Fazzi E, Munnich A, et al. 2007. Spectrum of *NPHP6/CEP290* mutations in Leber congenital amaurosis and delineation of the associated phenotype. *Hum Mutat* **28:** 416.

Pippucci T, Benelli M, Magi A, Martelli PL, Magini P, Torricelli F, Casadio R, Seri M, Romeo G. 2011. EX-HOM (EXome HOMozygosity): A proof of principle. *Hum Hered* **72:** 45–53.

Purcell S, Neale B, Todd-Brown K, Thomas L, Ferreira MA, Bender D, Maller J, Sklar P, de Bakker PI, Daly MJ, et al. 2007. PLINK: A tool set for whole-genome association and population-based linkage analyses. *Am J Hum Genet* **81:** 559–575.

Reva B, Antipin Y, Sander C. 2011. Predicting the functional impact of protein mutations: Application to cancer genomics. *Nucleic Acids Res* **39:** e118.

Riazuddin SA, Iqbal M, Wang Y, Masuda T, Chen Y, Bowne S, Sullivan LS, Waseem NH, Bhattacharya SS, Daiger SP, et al. 2010. A splice-site mutation in a retina-specific exon of *BBS8* causes nonsyndromic retinitis pigmentosa. *Am J Hum Genet* **86:** 805–812.

Rivolta C, Sweklo EA, Berson EL, Dryja TP. 2000. Missense mutation in the *USH2A* gene: Association with recessive retinitis pigmentosa without hearing loss. *Am J Hum Genet* **66:** 1975–1978.

Roosing S, Rohrschneider K, Beryozkin A, Sharon D, Weisschuh N, Staller J, Kohl S, Zelinger L, Peters TA, Neveling K, et al. 2013. Mutations in *RAB28*, encoding a farnesylated small GTPase, are associated with autosomal-recessive cone-rod dystrophy. *Am J Hum Genet* **93:** 110–117.

Santoriello C, Zon LI. 2012. Hooked! Modeling human disease in zebrafish. *J Clin Invest* **122:** 2337–2343.

Sayer JA, Otto EA, O'Toole JF, Nurnberg G, Kennedy MA, Becker C, Hennies HC, Helou J, Attanasio M, Fausett BV, et al. 2006. The centrosomal protein nephrocystin-6 is mutated in Joubert syndrome and activates transcription factor ATF4. *Nat Genet* **38:** 674–681.

Schorderet DF, Iouranova A, Favez T, Tiab L, Escher P. 2013. IROme, a new high-throughput molecular tool for the diagnosis of inherited retinal dystrophies. *Biomed Res Int* **2013:** 198089.

Seelow D, Schuelke M, Hildebrandt F, Nurnberg P. 2009. HomozygosityMapper—an interactive approach to homozygosity mapping. *Nucleic Acids Res* **37:** W593–599.

Shanks ME, Downes SM, Copley RR, Lise S, Broxholme J, Hudspith KA, Kwasniewska A, Davies WI, Hankins MW, Packham ER, et al. 2013. Next-generation sequencing (NGS) as a diagnostic tool for retinal degeneration reveals a much higher detection rate in early-onset disease. *Eur J Hum Genet* **21:** 274–280.

Sharon D, Sandberg MA, Rabe VW, Stillberger M, Dryja TP, Berson EL. 2003. *RP2* and *RPGR* mutations and clinical correlations in patients with X-linked retinitis pigmentosa. *Am J Hum Genet* **73:** 1131–1146.

Siemiatkowska AM, Arimadyo K, Moruz LM, Astuti GD, de Castro-Miro M, Zonneveld-Vrieling MN, Strom TM, de Wijs IJ, Hoefsloot LH, Faradz SM, et al. 2011. Molecular genetic analysis of retinitis pigmentosa in Indonesia using genome-wide homozygosity mapping. *Mol Vis* **17:** 3013–3024.

Siemiatkowska AM, van den Born LI, van Hagen PM, Stoffels M, Neveling K, Henkes A, Kipping-Geertsema M, Hoefsloot LH, Hoyng CB, Simon A, et al. 2013. Mutations in the mevalonate kinase (*MVK*) gene cause nonsyndromic retinitis pigmentosa. *Ophthalmology* **120:** 2697–2679.

Strom SP, Gorin MB. 2013. Evaluation of autosomal dominant retinal dystrophy genes in an unaffected cohort suggests rare or private missense variants may often be benign. *Mol Vis* **19:** 980–985.

Teer JK, Bonnycastle LL, Chines PS, Hansen NF, Aoyama N, Swift AJ, Abaan HO, Albert TJ, Program NCS, Margulies EH, et al. 2010. Systematic comparison of three genomic enrichment methods for massively parallel DNA sequencing. *Genome Res* **20:** 1420–1431.

Testa F, Surace EM, Rossi S, Marrocco E, Gargiulo A, Di Iorio V, Ziviello C, Nesti A, Fecarotta S, Bacci ML, et al. 2011. Evaluation of Italian patients with leber congenital amaurosis due to *AIPL1* mutations highlights the potential applicability of gene therapy. *Invest Ophthalmol Vis Sci* **52:** 5618–5624.

Thiadens AAHJ, Slingerland NW, Roosing S, van Schooneveld MJ, van Lith-Verhoeven JJC, van Moll-Ramirez NG, van den Born LI, Hoyng CB, Cremers FPM, Klaver CC. 2009. Genetic etiology and clinical consequences of complete and incomplete achromatopsia. *Ophthalmology* **116:** 1984–1989 e1981.

Tucker BA, Scheetz TE, Mullins RF, DeLuca AP, Hoffmann JM, Johnston RM, Jacobson SG, Sheffield VC, Stone EM. 2011. Exome sequencing and analysis of induced pluripotent stem cells identify the cilia-related gene *male germ cell-associated kinase* (*MAK*) as a cause of retinitis pigmentosa. *Proc Natl Acad Sci* **108:** E569–576.

Turner EH, Lee C, Ng SB, Nickerson DA, Shendure J. 2009. Massively parallel exon capture and library-free resequencing across 16 genomes. *Nat Methods* **6:** 315–316.

Valente EM, Silhavy JL, Brancati F, Barrano G, Krishnaswami SR, Castori M, Lancaster MA, Boltshauser E, Boccone L, Al-Gazali L, et al. 2006. Mutations in *CEP290*, which encodes a centrosomal protein, cause pleiotropic forms of Joubert syndrome. *Nat Genet* **38:** 623–625.

van den Hurk JAJM, van de Pol DJ, Wissinger B, van Driel MA, Hoefsloot LH, de Wijs I, van den Born LI, Heckenlively JR, Brunner HG, Zrenner E, et al. 2003. Novel types of mutation in the choroideremia (*CHM*) gene: A full-length L1 insertion and an intronic mutation activating a cryptic exon. *Hum Genet* **113:** 268–275.

Vervoort R, Wright AF. 2002. Mutations of *RPGR* in X-linked retinitis pigmentosa (RP3). *Hum Mutat* **19:** 486–500.

Wagner AH, Anand VN, Wang WH, Chatterton JE, Sun D, Shepard AR, Jacobson N, Pang IH, DeLuca AP, Casavant TL, et al. 2013. Exon-level expression profiling of ocular tissues. *Exp Eye Res* **111:** 105–111.

Wang X, Wang H, Cao M, Li Z, Chen X, Patenia C, Gore A, Abboud EB, Al-Rajhi AA, Lewis RA, et al. 2011. Whole-exome sequencing identifies *ALMS1*, *IQCB1*, *CNGA3*, and *MYO7A* mutations in patients with Leber congenital amaurosis. *Hum Mutat* **32:** 1450–1459.

Webb TR, Parfitt DA, Gardner JC, Martinez A, Bevilacqua D, Davidson AE, Zito I, Thiselton DL, Ressa JH, Apergi M, et al. 2012. Deep intronic mutation in *OFD1*, identified by targeted genomic next-generation sequencing, causes a severe form of X-linked retinitis pigmentosa (RP23). *Hum Mol Genet* **21:** 3647–3654.

* Wiley LA, Burnight EA, Mullins RF, Stone EM, Tucker BA. 2015. Stem cells as tools for studying the genetics of inherited retinal degenerations. *Cold Spring Harb Perspect Med* doi: 10.1101/cshperspect.a017160.

Wissinger B, Gamer D, Jagle H, Giorda R, Marx T, Mayer S, Tippmann S, Broghammer M, Jurklies B, Rosenberg T, et al. 2001. *CNGA3* mutations in hereditary cone photoreceptor disorders. *Am J Hum Genet* **69:** 722–737.

Woods CG, Cox J, Springell K, Hampshire DJ, Mohamed MD, McKibbin M, Stern R, Raymond FL, Sandford R, Malik SS, et al. 2006. Quantification of homozygosity in consanguineous individuals with autosomal recessive disease. *Am J Hum Genet* **78:** 889–896.

Woolfe A, Mullikin JC, Elnitski L. 2010. Genomic features defining exonic variants that modulate splicing. *Genome Biol* **11:** pR20.

Yeo GW, Van Nostrand EL, Liang TY. 2007. Discovery and analysis of evolutionarily conserved intronic splicing regulatory elements. *PLoS Genet* **3:** e85.

Yzer S, Leroy BP, De Baere EBW, de Ravel TJ, Zonneveld-Vrieling MN, Voesenek KEJ, Kellner U, Ciriano JP, de Faber JT, Rohrschneider K, et al. 2006. Microarray-based mutation detection and phenotypic characterization of patients with Leber congenital amaurosis. *Invest Ophthalmol Vis Sci* **47:** 1167–1176.

Zaghloul NA, Katsanis N. 2011. Zebrafish assays of ciliopathies. *Methods Cell Biol* **105:** 257–272.

Zelinger L, Banin E, Obolensky A, Mizrahi-Meissonnier L, Beryozkin A, Bandah-Rozenfeld D, Frenkel S, Ben-Yosef T, Merin S, Schwartz SB, et al. 2011. A missense mutation in *DHDDS*, encoding dehydrodolichyl diphosphate synthase, is associated with autosomal-recessive retinitis pigmentosa in Ashkenazi Jews. *Am J Hum Genet* **88:** 207–215.

Zuchner S, Dallman J, Wen R, Beecham G, Naj A, Farooq A, Kohli MA, Whitehead PL, Hulme W, Konidari I, et al. 2011. Whole-exome sequencing links a variant in *DHDDS* to retinitis pigmentosa. *Am J Hum Genet* **88:** 201–206.

Genetic Modifiers and Oligogenic Inheritance

Maria Kousi and Nicholas Katsanis

Center for Human Disease Modeling, Duke University, Durham, North Carolina 27710

Correspondence: katsanis@cellbio.duke.edu

Despite remarkable progress in the identification of mutations that drive genetic disorders, progress in understanding the effect of genetic background on the penetrance and expressivity of causal alleles has been modest, in part because of the methodological challenges in identifying genetic modifiers. Nonetheless, the progressive discovery of modifier alleles has improved both our interpretative ability and our analytical tools to dissect such phenomena. In this review, we analyze the genetic properties and behaviors of modifiers as derived from studies in patient populations and model organisms and we highlight conceptual and technological tools used to overcome some of the challenges inherent in modifier mapping and cloning. Finally, we discuss how the identification of these modifiers has facilitated the elucidation of biological pathways and holds the potential to improve the clinical predictive value of primary causal mutations and to develop novel drug targets.

Since the mapping of the first locus for autosomal dominant retinitis pigmentosa (RP) on the long arm of chromosome 3 (McWilliam et al. 1989) and the subsequent identification of rhodopsin (*RHO*) as the causal transcript (Dryja et al. 1990), the genetic dissection of disorders in which retinal degeneration comprises a core phenotypic component has accelerated rapidly, leading to the report of more than 250 loci and genes cataloged in RetNet (as of May 2014; see https://sph.uth.edu/retnet/disease.htm). These advances have had a clear contribution to both our understanding of photoreceptor biology and in providing genetic diagnoses to families. At the same time, however, post hoc knowledge of disease-causing genes and mutations had a modest impact on the predictive ability of prognosis with regard to key aspects of disease expressivity, such as age-of-onset, rate of progression, severity, and manifestation of other comorbidities. Numerous reports exist in the literature in which patients with the same primary mutation show stark differences in phenotypic expressivity, with the more striking examples coming from nonidentical twin studies in which patients that grow under a shared environment and carry the same primary mutation display distinct phenotypes, most likely because of genetic determinants that act as modifiers (Walia et al. 2008). The example above is not an isolated oddity. Accumulating clinical and genetic evidence now suggests that, even for classically monogenic disorders, the view that the expressivity of the phenotype is exclusively the property of dominant or recessive mutations at a single locus

Cite this article as *Cold Spring Harb Perspect Med* doi: 10.1101/cshperspect.a017145

might be an oversimplification of the biological phenomena (Dipple and McCabe 2000; Badano and Katsanis 2002; Schäffer 2013).

The concept of modifier genes and alleles is not new (Haldane 1941). Nonetheless, the field of retinal degeneration disorders has been in a unique position to lead the efforts to understand genetic architecture, causality, and variable expressivity. This is in part because of (1) large and well-phenotyped multiethnic cohorts; (2) a substantial (and growing) mutational target of almost 300 genes, each known to be necessary for retinal biogenesis, homeostasis, and/or function; and (3) the availability of in vitro and in vivo tools to model genetic interaction phenomena. Here we will discuss the concepts of modifier genes and alleles, including their evolving terminology; we will highlight examples that illustrate the still episodic, yet significant, advances in dissecting the genetic basis of modification of penetrance and expressivity; and we will discuss possible avenues toward improving our interpretative ability of such events.

PROPERTIES OF GENETIC MODIFIERS

A critical step in understanding genetic modification phenomena consists of providing a clear definition for the term itself. Phenomena described by terms such as epistasis, oligogenic inheritance, or genetic interaction/modification, are all effective synonyms of the same process, namely, the effect of one gene/allele on the phenotypic outcome of a second gene/locus. A distinction that can aid better defining these genetic phenomena consists in establishing whether the primary locus is both necessary and sufficient to cause disease. If yes, then the presence of allele(s) at a second locus/gene exerts purely a modifying role on the severity of the phenotype as defined by the rate of disease progression; the severity of the phenotype with regard to its pleiotropy; or in the manifestation of endophenotypes that necessitate genetic interactions; if not, then the requirement of an allele in a second gene to manifest pathology defines a case of digenic or oligogenic inheritance (Fig. 1). In general, in the context of dissecting modifier phenomena, four major parameters play a prominent role:

1. *Allelic heterogeneity.* Phenotypic variability can stem from mutations in different genes that contribute to disease endophenotypes. However, simpler models of genetic heterogeneity and their influence on phenotypic expressivity should first be considered. Locus and allelic heterogeneity are highlighted in Leber congenital amaurosis (LCA), a disorder for which at least 11 causative genes have been reported under a recessive paradigm (reviewed in Davis and Katsanis 2012). In addition to genetic heterogeneity, LCA is also an example of allelic heterogeneity. For example, nonsense and frameshift, as well as missense mutations in *CEP290* drive disorders ranging between nonsyndromic LCA to Joubert syndrome (JBTS) to the more severe Meckel Gruber syndrome (MKS) phenotype. These observations have reasonably suggested that modifier genetic factors account for this marked variance in clinical presentation (den Hollander et al. 2006, 2008; Sayer et al. 2006; Valente et al. 2006; Baala et al. 2007; Frank et al. 2007; Perrault et al. 2007). However, a discrete intronic mutation (c.2991+1655A>G) in *CEP290* that creates a strong splice-donor site and inserts a cryptic exon in the *CEP290* mRNA resulting in an aberrantly spliced transcript, appears to be sufficient to cause LCA (den Hollander et al. 2006, 2008; Sayer et al. 2006; Valente et al. 2006; Baala et al. 2007; Frank et al. 2007; Perrault et al. 2007). These data argue that, at least in some instances, this mutational event alone is sufficient to explain the disease without necessarily evoking the action of additional alleles. In this example, recurrence of the specific mutation has facilitated that argument. However, typically bereft of such data, dissecting phenotype–genotype correlations within a primary causal locus from modifier effects can be challenging, especially because most such correlations are made on the basis of a few mutations.

2. *Multiple interactions and gene/allele-specific interactions.* The effect of genetic modifiers

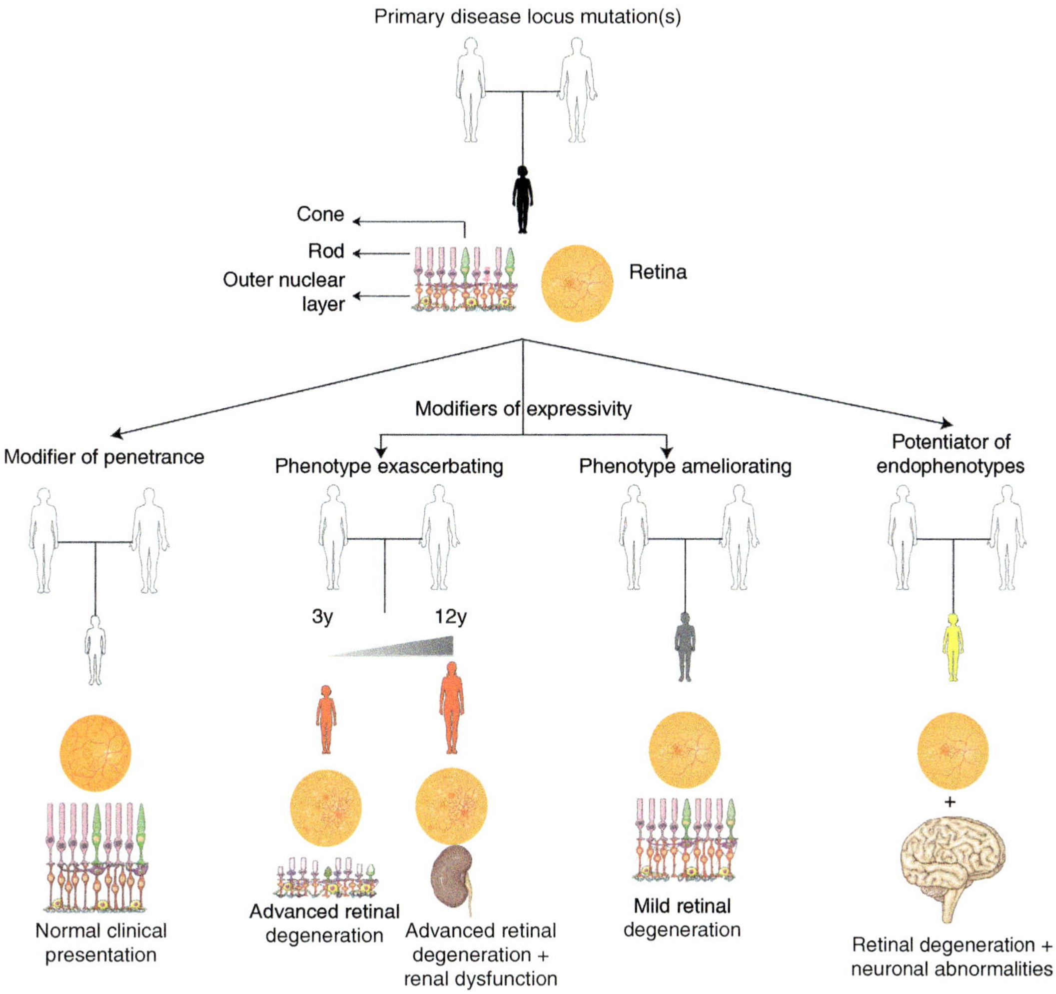

Figure 1. Schematic of the effects of modifiers on causal mutations. A genetic modifier can exert its effect on the phenotype established by mutation(s) at the primary locus in a number of ways. Depending on the nature of the modifier, this interaction can result in reduced penetrance of specific endophenotype(s) and/or disorders; in variable expressivity with the modifying locus resulting in either exacerbated phenotypes (i.e., earlier age of onset and faster progression of the disease); in a milder clinical presentation (i.e., later age of onset, attenuated disease progression, and absence/protection from specific endophenotypes); and modifiers that potentiate the manifestation of specific endophenotypes resulting in what is described as novel forms of disease. This figure was prepared using Servier Medical Art (http://www.servier.com/Powerpoint-image-bank).

on penetrance and/or expressivity can vary from a "monogenic" model of modification, in which one modifier can account for most of the observed variability, to a more complex model in which more than one genetic determinant interacts with the primary disease locus. Although identification of major or "panmodifiers" is feasible, the dissection of more than one gene modulating the phenotype caused by the primary locus is challenging, due primarily to lack of genetic power. An example illustrating the mapping of a "panmodifier" was described in a Bardet-Biedl syndrome (BBS) cohort of 226 patients not preselected for mutations at any specific locus. Within this group, an allele in *CCDC28B* was associated with a more severe BBS phenotype, a discovery based on association analysis and transmission disequilibrium testing (TDT) and dissected further by biochemical studies (Badano et al. 2006). Had the modifying effect of *CCDC28B* been specific to a particular BBS locus, unmasking of such a genetic interaction would have been difficult. In contrast to "panmodifiers," the interplay of multiple modifiers, each of which has a variable strength of effect on the final disease expression is probably common, but the most challenging to unravel. A good example is cystic fibrosis, a life-shortening recessive disorder in which 90% of the affected patients die because of obstructive pulmonary disease (Cutting 2010). Despite the majority of patients carrying identical genotypes (homozygosity for *CFTR* F508del), striking differences in lung function have been described (Kerem et al. 1990). Candidate modifier studies reported that functional variants in *MBL2* and alleles in the promoter and first exon of *TGFb1* were associated with lower lung function measures (Garred et al. 1999; Drumm et al. 2005; Darrah et al. 2010). More recently, genome-wide association studies revealed additional modifiers of lung function; *IL-8*, *IFRD1* and *ENDRA* associated with neutrophil function (Vanscoy et al. 2007; Hillian et al. 2008). Taken together, the aforementioned genetic modifiers are believed to alter lung disease severity by affecting the ability of the host to tolerate infection, which can be further modified by nongenetic determinants such as air pollutants, secondhand smoking, or even access to medical care and treatment (Rubin 1990; Goss et al. 2004). Under such a model, each modifier explains only a small portion of the variability, similar to the genetic risk factors involved in complex traits.

3. *Modifiers in the same locus/region with the disease driver.* Genetic modifiers in *cis* with the disease driver gene might be considered to be variants tagging and being transmitted in linkage disequilibrium with the primary mutation. An example of a modifier in *cis* comes from several studies showing that variants within *FTO* were reported to confer susceptibility to developing obesity (Dina et al. 2007; Frayling et al. 2007; Scuteri et al. 2007; Church et al. 2010). Although *FTO* was shown to regulate body mass, the variants identified appeared to have no effect on the expression and stability of the protein (Klöting et al. 2008; Grunnet et al. 2009). Instead, the variants within the *FTO* region are regulating the expression of a transcription factor located in *cis*, *IRX3* that is now thought to potentially act as the primary susceptibility gene for developing obesity (Smemo et al. 2014). An example of *trans* modification within the same locus was described in a pedigree diagnosed with erythropoietic protoporphyria (EPP), in which the patients carry a splice donor site deletion resulting in skipping of exon 10 (Δex10) of ferrochelatase (*FECH*). When this change is accompanied by an in *trans* intragenic variant (IVS3-48C), the phenotype is aggravated with the levels of ferrochelatase in those patients being significantly lower than in asymptomatic carriers (Gouya et al. 1996, 2006). The mechanism underlying this phenomenon consists in IVS3-48C modulating the use of a constitutive aberrant acceptor splice site on *FECH* resulting in an aberrantly spliced mRNA that is subject to nonsense-mediated decay and therefore leading to *FECH* deficiency (Gouya et al. 2002).

4. *Frequency of the modifying variants in the general population.* Assuming that a modifier allele alone is not sufficient to induce pathology, it might be relatively common in the general population, thus complicating the dissection of phenotypically relevant versus benign variants. In the study that identified an allele that confers susceptibility to Hirschsprung disease (HSCR), the causal variant had a minor allele frequency (MAF) of 0.45 in Asia, 0.25 in Europe and was virtually absent (0.01) in the African population (Emison et al. 2005). Unmasking such common variants may require the use of multiple methods; in this case the combinatorial use of careful phenotyping combined with human genetic, comparative genomic, functional, and population genetic analyses

(Emison et al. 2005). At a second tier, there are alleles of intermediate frequency in the general population. An example of this is the p.A229T allele in *RPGRIP1L* which aggravates the retinal phenotype in ciliopathy patients, present in 3% of Northern Europeans (Khanna et al. 2009). Finally, rare variants that are enriched in patients compared with controls can have a modifying effect on disease expressivity and penetrance. In age-related macular degeneration (AMD), in which most primary driver variants are common, rare alleles (MAF<1%) within the complement pathway can alter the disease phenotype. The first example described the rare p.R1210C mutation in *CFH* as a penetrant allele that confers high risk to AMD and was followed by the discovery of an additional five risk and 15 protective variants through a study that evaluated components of the complement pathway (Raychaudhuri et al. 2011; Seddon et al. 2013). Although it is easier to establish the relevance of a rare variant to disease causality or predisposition, the same is not true for common variants that are overrepresented in the control population. In the context of genetic modification the true debate is not how common or rare a variant is, but rather how those variants work together and what is their cumulative effect (Gibson 2012).

CHALLENGES IN IDENTIFYING MODIFIER GENES/ALLELES

In contrast to the remarkable progress in identification of disease causing genes, the dissection of oligogenic and epistatic phenomena is lagging, in part because of the reduced power of traditional genetic analyses to uncover such phenomena. Beyond methodological limitations, there are additional challenges to consider:

1. *Availability of accurate clinical evaluation and longitudinal studies.* The identification of genetic modifying phenomena relies heavily on the detailed characterization of the aspect(s) of the phenotype under modification. It is thus imperative to have detailed clinical longitudinal information. Historically, cohorts have been characterized qualitatively for the presence/absence of a trait (i.e., RP or macular degeneration), with since-point proxies used as an imperfect means of expressing disease progression; these have included age of onset of a specific phenotype (Badano et al. 2006), thickness of the outer nuclear layer (ONL) (Danciger et al. 2008), or number of photoreceptors (Haider et al. 2008). The literature however, is populated by incomplete phenotypic information on the cases presented, often focusing on specific aspects of disease. In BBS, a multisystemic disorder characterized by rod–cone dystrophy, central obesity, polydactyly, and retinal degeneration, a cardinal symptom of the disorder, renal dysfunction had been overlooked (Brattgard 1949; Landau et al. 1949). A reason for this could have been that, although renal structural abnormalities might be present, only a small fraction of the patients develop symptoms consistent with kidney functional impairment that would prompt clinical evaluation (Magro and Peres 1970; Labrune et al. 1974; Gershoni-Baruch et al. 1992; Beales et al. 1999). In the case of *RPGRIP1L*, thorough description of the retinal phenotype across a cohort of patients with syndromic disorders falling under the umbrella of the ciliopathies, led to the dissection of the p.A229T allele as a variant associated with increased loss of photoreceptors, whereas absence of this change was proposed to have a potential protective effect from RP (Khanna et al. 2009).

2. *Nongenetic factors.* The effect of nongenetic factors poses a major confounder. In humans, one way to determine whether the phenotypic variability observed is caused by genetic modifiers or environmental factors is to compare inter- and intrafamilial variability. A second approach is that of comparing the phenotype in monozygotic (MZ) and dizygotic (DZ) twins that share the same environmental influence. One of the best characterized examples of nongenet-

ic determinants leading to disease manifestation comes from studies linking pregnancies complicated by fetal neural tube defects (NTDs) with folate insufficiency, and the evidence that periconceptional folate supplementation can reduce the risk of NTDs and other congenital abnormalities (Laurence et al. 1980; Tolarova 1982; Czeizel and Dudás 1992; Wald et al. 2001).

STRATEGIES FOR CLONING GENETIC MODIFIERS

The examples of disease modifier identification existing in the literature have used a plethora of techniques and approaches (Fig. 2), typically combining several lines of investigation:

1. *Linkage analyses.* If nuclear families with individuals carrying the same primary locus mutation and displaying discordant phenotypes are available, linkage analyses to identify alleles identical by descent (IBD) in individuals sharing a specific trait or endophenotype can be performed. The same can be applied in sib pairs concordant or discordant for a given phenotype. Knowing the primary disease causing mutation, linkage analysis for the detection of modifier loci can be performed by evaluating the sample set for qualitative phenotypes (mutation carriers with the phenotype, mutation carriers without the phenotype, and mutation carriers with more severe disease form), or for quantitative phenotypes (i.e., age of onset). One of the reasons that could account for the inability to map modifiers is that, especially in human studies, large pedigrees are often necessary to map the regions harboring the genes of interest. This is exemplified in Fuchs corneal dystrophy (FCD), in which genome-wide linkage in a large multigenerational pedigree carrying the *TCF8* p.Q840P allele that drives disease, revealed a second locus on 9p that, when combined with *TCF8* p.Q840P, results in a more severe form of disease (Riazuddin et al. 2010). Even when large pedigrees are available, variable intrafamilial phenotypic expression, in association with the difficulty to identify families with uniform phenotypes, can complicate mapping of modifiers. To address this, screening pedigrees from genetic isolates can prove beneficial. Such a study was performed on the Menonite genetic isolate to identify genes underlying HSCR (Carrasquillo et al. 2002). Using a genome-wide association study coupled with multipoint-linkage disequilibrium analysis, which searches for association arising from common mutation ancestry, linkage over known HSCR loci was detected. However, this signal was insufficient to explain disease manifestation (Carrasquillo et al. 2002). Instead, it was an epistatic interaction between the receptor tyrosine kinase (*RET*) and the endothelin receptor type B (*EDNRB*) that was necessary for disease manifestation (Carrasquillo et al. 2002).

2. *Candidate locus association studies.* The advantage of this approach consists mainly in that data from singletons can be compared with other unrelated patients with similar phenotypes. A limitation of this approach is that once association is established, it is difficult to discern whether it is truly owing to the polymorphism/marker identified, to a variant that is in linkage disequilibrium (LD) with the marker used, or to an unknown confounding factor that might not even be genetic (Génin et al. 2008). An alternative is family-based association and TDT, in which the preferential transmission of alleles from parent to affected offspring is evaluated (Speilman et al. 1993). In HSCR, linkage of modifiers has been shown consistently to the *RET* locus, harboring the main HSCR driver, *RET*, although in most of these studies no coding mutations could be identified (Bolk et al. 2000; Borrego et al. 2000; Gabriel et al. 2002; Garcia-Barceló et al. 2003; Sancandi et al. 2003). In these studies, it was hypothesized that the genetic determinant conferring increased susceptibility to HSCR when combined with mutations in other loci, would lie within the *RET* locus (Emison et al. 2005). As such, a combination of human ge-

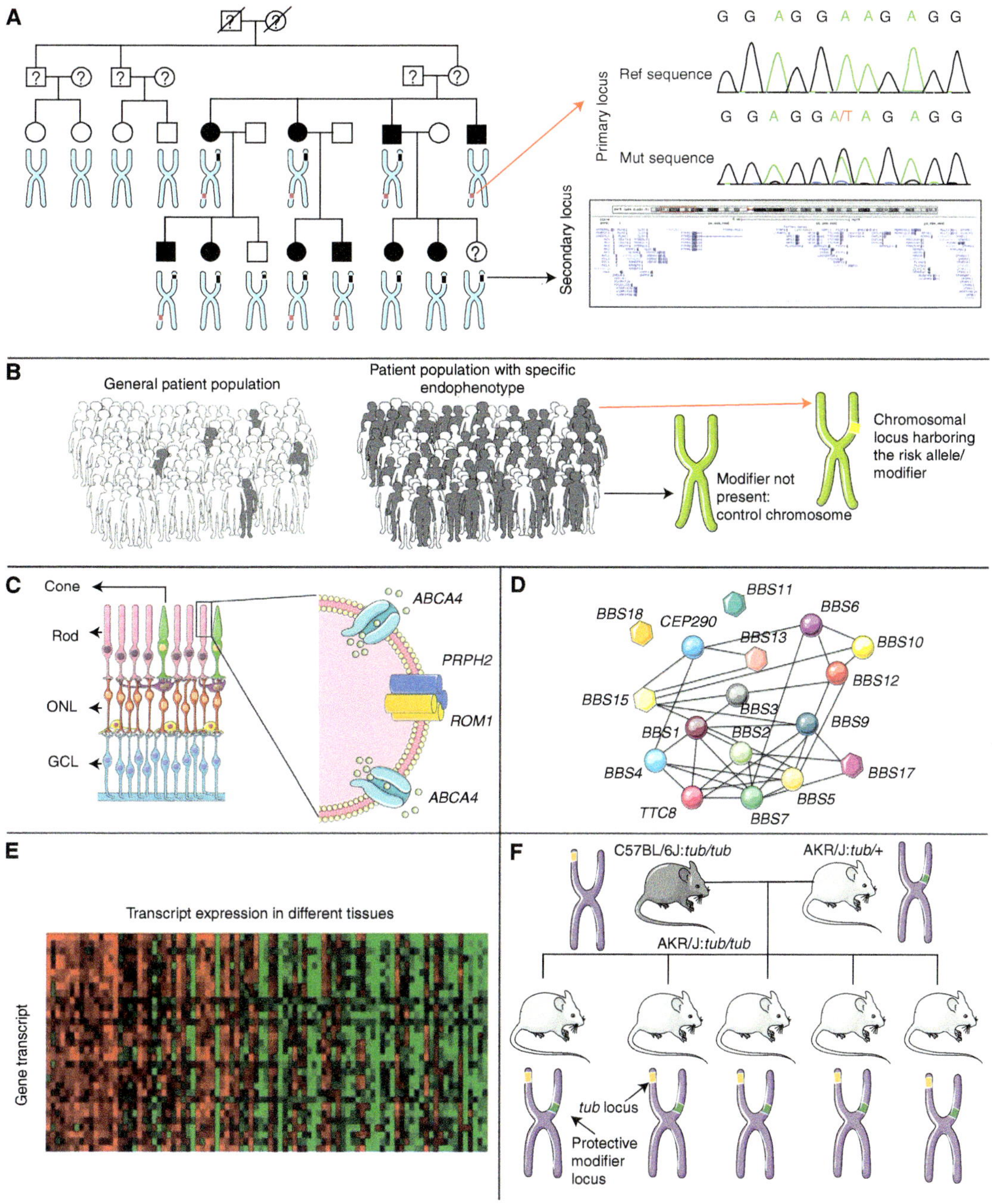

Figure 2. Examples of strategies for cloning modifiers. *A*. Linkage analysis, with the affected family members manifesting specific endophenotypes or differential disease severity. By evaluating the sample set for the endophenotype or trait of interest, the candidate modifier loci can be mapped. The snapshot of chromosome 9 in panel *A* is from the UCSC browser (http://genome.ucsc.edu/). *B*. Association studies compare patient cohorts with (gray figures) or without (white figures) a modifier of disease severity/expressivity, to obtain a signal for the locus/position that harbors the modifying allele(s). *C*. The candidate gene approach evaluates whether genes whose products operate within the same pathway can exert a modifying effect on each other. The example illustrated comes from the observation that mutations in *PRPH2* and *ABCA4* can aggravate disease severity when combined with primary disease mutations in *ROM1*. *D*. The system-based hypothesis evaluates the likelihood of specific genes to physically interact or manifest similar expression profile changes in control versus affected individuals to build genetic networks that drive disease pathogenesis. Such network interactions among genes that cause the same or similar disorders is exemplified by BBS, in which the responsible genes are shown to operate and interact together. *E*. In transcriptome analyses, heatmaps compare changes in expression levels of genes, between healthy and affected individuals. *F*. The use of mouse congenic strains to map modifiers in a more simplified genetic background. This figure was prepared using Servier Medical Art (http://www.servier.com/Powerpoint-image-bank).

netic, comparative genomic, functional and population genetic analyses were undertaken to show that the variant sought was an intronic change within a conserved enhancer sequence in intron 1 of *RET* (Emison et al. 2005). A similar approach was used to show the overtransmission of the *CCDC28B* modifier in BBS (Badano et al. 2006).

3. *Candidate gene approach.* One strategy to identify genetic modifiers is by applying a hypothesis-based candidate gene approach through the screening of genes that operate within the same biological pathways/processes as the primary disease driver gene(s). Such hypotheses can be formulated either through current experimental or in silico knowledge of gene networks or from evidence from model organisms. Using this approach, Poloschek and colleagues screened 15 family members for mutations in genes known to cause retinal degeneration. They identified heterozygous mutations in *PRPH2*, *ABCA4*, and *ROM1*; family members carrying the p.R172W mutation in *PRPH2* were severely affected, patients carrying heterozygous alterations in only one of those genes displayed a milder phenotype and patients with heterozygous mutations in all three genes evaluated, show an even more severe form of disease (Poloschek et al. 2010). Another example based on the candidate gene approach involved the identification of the genetic interaction between *NPHP1* and *AHI1*, with *NPHP1* accounting for the nephronopthisis phenotype and the *AHI1* p.R830W allele being the major determinant driving the retinal phenotype in the NPHP cohort (Louie et al. 2010).

4. *System-based candidates.* This approach requires a priori knowledge of the specific genes driving the pathogenesis of the trait of interest. In the human disease network hypothesis, genes associated with similar disorders show higher likelihood of physical interactions and higher expression profiling similarity between their products (Goh et al. 2007). Such an interaction network was constructed for 54 proteins involved in 23 distinct types of human inherited ataxias (Lim et al. 2006). Within this network, different ataxia-causing proteins showed physical interactions and revealed common cellular pathways potentially relevant to disease (Lim et al. 2006). To test the robustness of this approach, the ataxia network was evaluated for its ability to unravel both modifiers and disease drivers. Two major modifiers of spinocerebellar ataxia type 1 (SCA1), ataxin-2 (ATXN2) and RNA binding protein with multiple splicing (RBPMS) were present on the "ataxia-genome" map as nodes that shared strong physical interactions with ataxin-1 (ATXN1) (Lim et al. 2006). BBS represents another example of this approach, with more than 20 causative genes participating in the function of the cilium and thus showing that they are related to each other at a higher level of cellular and organismal organization (Davis and Katsanis 2012). As such, other proteins localizing and operating within the cilium emerge as candidates to either drive disease pathology or modulate phenotypic expressivity. Starting with the bona fide genes that can cause BBS under a recessive paradigm in some families, and thus representing de facto contributors to the molecular etiology of BBS, an excess of pathogenic heterozygous BBS alleles were found in families with recessive mutations in other BBS loci (Katsanis et al. 2001; Badano et al. 2003; Beales et al. 2003; Stoetzel et al. 2006, 2007; Leitch et al. 2008). These phenomena were not restricted to genes mutated in BBS under a recessive paradigm; the BBS modifier *CCDC28B* was screened based on its interaction and colocalization with multiple BBS proteins, in addition to the fact that it was belonging to the ciliary proteome and hence operating in the same system as the other BBS proteins (Li et al. 2004; Badano et al. 2006; Gherman et al. 2006).

5. *Transcriptome analyses.* Methodologies that evaluate the expression of proteins such as microarrays and RNA-seq present powerful tools for studying the transcriptional landscape of a given cell or tissue. Transcrip-

tome analyses compare the expression levels of proteins between different phenotypic groups, such as control versus disease organism. The comparison can be applied to the whole transcriptome of the tissue of interest, or it can be combined with other methodologies such as linkage analyses, to identify only the genes that have altered expression within the locus of interest. Whole transcriptome comparison was performed between four siblings (two of which were asymptomatic) and two unrelated patients affected by spinal muscular atrophy (SMA), all of which carried identical *SMN1/SMN2* genotypes (Oprea et al. 2008). One transcript showing statistically significant differential expression between the individuals with discordant phenotypes was plastin 3 (*PLS3*), a protein that elevates the F actin levels and promotes axonogenesis, comprising the first protective modifier in SMA reported (Oprea et al. 2008). The protective effect of *PLS3* was illustrated further in a conditional mouse model overexpressing *PLS3* into an SMA background (SMA_{PLS3}), with the motor neurons of the SMA_{PLS3} mice showing restored actin dynamics, increased size of the somata, increased quantal content of the neuromuscular junctions, axon stabilization, increase in the size of innervated muscle fibers, and overall prolonged survival (Ackermann et al. 2013; Lyon et al. 2014).

6. *Considering whole-exome data in toto.* A more unbiased approach to screen for genetic modifiers is through interrogation of the whole exome. Advances in massively parallel sequencing over the past years have made such analyses feasible. The caveat in using such large-scale screens lies in the small sample size available to screen for modifiers, the failure to correct for multiple hypotheses testing when several variants and genetic markers are examined, as well as the effects of population stratification (Gusella and MacDonald 2009). Nonetheless, the advantage of using these technologies consists mainly in the fact that they provide an unbiased approach. This is illustrated by recent studies in Gordon Holmes syndrome (GHS), a rare form of cerebellar ataxia associated with hypogonadotropic hypogonadism. Analysis of whole-exome sequencing (WES) identified rare alleles in a large consanguineous pedigree and when the genetic findings were coupled to functional studies concluded that, in that family GHS was hypomorphic caused by combinatorial mutations in two independent genes (*RNF216* and *OTUD4*), both of which participate in the ubiquitin proteasome pathway (Margolin et al. 2013). There are several conclusions that can be drawn by this study: (1) if significant linkage was obtained over the locus of one or both of the genes identified, it would have most probably led to the mapping of the one of the genes of this interaction, leaving the second locus unexplored; (2) if the epistatic interaction in GHS had not been underlay by homozygous hits in both genes, but rather was mediated by a homozygous hit in the primary locus and a heterozygous hit in the second or epistatic locus, it would have likely been missed by "typical" WES allele filtering; (3) without the use of the in vivo functional model uncovering the functional synergy of the two genes, *RNF216* would have been proposed as the gene underlying GHS because of identification of mutations in this gene in unrelated patients, leading to the false conclusion that *OTUD4* is not relevant to disease.

7. *Modifiers in inbred and mutation-induced mouse strains.* The most successful approach to map genetic modifiers are mouse models that show phenotypic divergence caused by their different genetic background. A study illustrating the power of this approach to identify genetic modifiers consisted of crossing C57BL/6J-*tub/tub* mice that display retinal and cochlear degeneration (Heckenlively et al. 1995; Ohlemiller et al. 1997) with AKR/J$^{-/+}$ animals. In the F2 generation, the C57BL/6J:AKR/J-*tub/tub* mice were protected from retinal degeneration, having an almost normal ONL thickness and number of photoreceptors when compared with the C57BL/6J-*tub/tub* littermates (Ikeda

et al. 2002a). Subsequent analysis identified significant linkage over the *motr1* locus on chromosome 11 and yielded suggestive evidence for linkage at two loci on chromosomes 2 and 8, respectively (Ikeda et al. 2002a).

GENETIC MODIFIERS OF RETINAL DEGENERATION IN HUMANS

The report of a nuclear family with a 3 bp deletion in peripherin (*RDS*) presenting with three distinct clinical phenotypes (RP, pattern macular dystrophy, and fundus flavimaculatus; Table 1), provided the first example of complex inheritance in retinal degeneration (Weleber et al. 1993). The identification of additional families with *RDS* mutations and significant inter- and intrafamilial variability ensued (Apfelstedt-Sylla et al. 1995). Kajiwara and colleagues then chose three clinically variable families carrying the heterozygous *RDS* p.L185P allele; the investigators undertook a candidate gene approach and screened for mutations in the gene encoding the retinal outer segment membrane protein 1 (*ROM1*), whose homodimer protein products complex with those encoded by *RDS* (Goldberg and Molday 1996). This study revealed that only family members that were double heterozygotes for the *RDS* p.L185P alleles and the *ROM1* p.114fsX developed RP, whereas individuals that were heterozygous for either one of these mutations did not (Kajiwara et al. 1994; Rivolta et al. 2002). The mechanism through which such a genetic interaction can affect the clinical phenotype has also been elucidated, revealing that RDS mutant subunits fail to homodimerize and that the formation of functional complexes is further decreased by the frameshifting mutation in ROM1, thus leading to the ultimate degeneration of photoreceptors in the retina (Goldberg and Molday 1996; Loewen et al. 2001). The effect of *ROM1* as a modifier of phenotype was highlighted further in a study in which cases with heterozygous *ROM1* mutations (p.R172W or p.R229H) combined with mutations in *RDS* result in a more severe phenotype, with pronounced loss in rod but not cone function (Poloschek et al. 2010). In the same study, a subset of patients with mutations in yet a third gene (*ABCA4*: p.R172W, p.R229H or p.V2050L) were present together with *ROM1* and *RDS* mutations; the phenotype was even more severe, with advanced macular degeneration, nyctalopia, and severe rod and cone function decline (Poloschek et al. 2010).

A second modifier of retinal degeneration identified through the candidate gene approach was *AHI1* in a study evaluating patients with nephronophthisis (NPHP), a hereditary kidney disease (Louie et al. 2010; Table 1). More specifically, within a pedigree with three NPHP diagnosed patients, one brother was also carrying the heterozygous *AHI1* p.R830W mutation (Louie et al. 2010). This variant was shown to be associated with retinal degeneration both in this familial case but also among sporadic NPHP patients (Louie et al. 2010), thus attributing a retinal degeneration modifying effect role to *AHI1*. In addition to the NPHP cohort, *AHI1* was also screened for mutations and reported as a genetic modifier in a Belgian cohort of eight *CEP290* mutation positive patients affected by LCA and mental retardation (Coppieters et al. 2010). The patients most severely affected were carriers of *AHI1* p.N811K and p.H758P, leading to the conclusion that *CEP290* and *AHI1* are likely to be operating in the same pathway and that within this cohort *AHI1* serves as a modifier of the neurological phenotype (Coppieters et al. 2010).

A third example came from the screening of *RPGRIP1L*, a gene known to cause MKS and JBTS (Arts et al. 2007; Delous et al. 2007), for a cohort of patients with various ciliary disorder diagnoses (Khanna et al. 2009). Among the 10 novel nonsynonymous changes identified in *RPGRIP1L*, one allele (p.A229T) was enriched significantly in patients with ciliary disease coupled by retinal degeneration (Khanna et al. 2009; Table 1). The effect of the modifier allele was established in a zebrafish model in which it scored as pathogenic, and in a yeast two-hybrid screen in which the mutant RPGRIP1L was exerting a significantly lower affinity to form complexes with the retinitis pigmentosa GTPase regulator protein (RPGR), with which it interacts (Khanna et al. 2009). It is thought that the observed photoreceptor degeneration in patients with the modifying *RPGRIP1L* p.A229T allele are because of the attenuation of the RPGRIP1L–RPGR interaction (Khanna et al. 2009). The observation that *RPGRIP1L* contributes modifying alleles was shown further in X-linked RP caused by mutations in *RPGR* (Fahim et al. 2011). Affected males from 56 families with *RPGR* mutations were genotyped for common alleles in each of *RPGRIP1*, *RPGRIP1L*, *CEP290*, and *IQCB1* based on the fact that they all interact with RPGR as determined by coimmunoprecipitation experiments (Boylan and Wright 2000; Otto et al. 2005; Chang et al. 2006; Khanna et al. 2009). Two alleles, the *IQCB1* p.I393N and the common *RPGRIP1L* p.R744Q, showed significant association with disease severity, with the minor allele in *IQCB1* and the common allele in *RPGRIP1L* being associated with more severe disease (Fahim et al. 2011).

In Usher syndrome, a genetically heterogeneous recessive disease characterized by hearing loss and RP, a genetic modifier of the retinal phenotype was identified by blasting for homologous proteins to harmonin causing Usher syndrome subtype 1C (USH1C) and whirlin underlying USH2D that cross-link other Usher proteins to form a multimolecular complex in the photoreceptors and hearing cells (Kremer et al. 2006; Ebermann et al. 2007). *PDZD7* was identified and screened for mutations in patients with an Usher syndrome diagnosis (Ebermann et al. 2010; Table 1). Although no changes in *PDZD7* were identified in Usher patients with any molecular diagnosis, in familial cases with mutations in known Usher genes, *PDZD7* seemed to be contributing to a digenic mode of inheritance and to also be contributing modifying alleles (Ebermann et al. 2010). For example, in a family with two *USH2A* (p.C1447QfsX29) affected sisters, the one that also carried a heterozygous frameshift mutation in *PDZD7* (p.R56PfsX24) displayed an earlier age of onset and more severe progression of RP, whereas in a distinct case of a family with two affected offspring, only the individual with a heterozygous *USH2C* (*GPR98* p.A5713LfsX3) mutation and a second heterozygous hit in *PDZD7* is affected, suggesting that *GPR98* and *PDZD7* seem to be participating in a digenic mode of inheritance (Ebermann et al. 2010). Similar to the study identifying *RPGRIP1L* as a genetic modifier, the direction of effect of the *PDZD7* alleles as pathogenic and the digenic inheritance of *GPR98* and *PDZD7* were confirmed in a zebrafish in vivo model for RP (Ebermann et al. 2010).

BBS has contributed substantially to understanding the contribution of genetic modifiers to disease (Katsanis et al. 2001; Badano et al. 2006; Table 1). The disorder is genetically and clinically heterogeneous, with well-documented examples of inter- and intrafamilial phenotypic variability (Carmi et al. 1995; Riise et al. 1997). Although initially reported to follow an autosomal recessive mode of inheritance, BBS was the first disorder to follow a "triallelic" model of disease transmission with three alleles at two independent loci being required for disease manifestation (Katsanis et al. 2001). More specifically, in a nuclear family with one affected and two unaffected siblings, compound heterozygosity in *BBS2* for the nonsense alleles p.Y24X and p.Q59X was not sufficient to cause the phenotype, but required the presence of a third allele at a second BBS locus, *BBS6* p.Q147X, which acts essentially as a modifier of penetrance (Katsanis et al. 2001). A second example of genetic modification coming from the study of BBS samples is the identification of *CCDC28B* p.C430T as a modifier affecting RP; the patients that carried p.C430T displayed an earlier onset of RP and accelerated disease progression (Badano et al. 2006). In addition to contributing modifying alleles, *CCDC28B* has also been postulated to represent an example of complex inheritance because it seems to be required for disease manifestation in a family with *BBS1* p.M390R homozygous siblings and also asymptomatic father. It is therefore hypothesized that the third allele (p.C430T) located in *CCDC28B* might be required for disease manifestation or be acting as a modifier of penetrance similar to the *BBS6* and *BBS2* epistatic interaction (Beales et al. 2003; Badano et al. 2006).

GENETIC MODIFIERS OF RETINAL DEGENERATION IN MICE

The cloning of modifiers in human genetic disorders is confounded by genetic and allelic heterogeneity. Some of these challenges can be overcome in model organisms. Laboratory mice in particular, have been successfully used to map modifier genes and alleles in a wide range of genetic disorders (Table 2). Although in most successful studies the modification of the primary phenotype is because of the effects of a single locus, independent from the primary locus (Danciger et al. 2000; Ikeda et al. 2002a), mapping of modifiers can be complicated when the modification results from the combined effects of several genes at discrete loci (Table 2) (Ikeda et al. 2002a).

The first report of a genetic modifier of retinal degeneration in mice was the identification of protective alleles in the *rd5* or tubby mouse for both the hearing and retinal degeneration phenotypes (Danciger et al. 2000; Ikeda et al. 2002a,b). The tubby mouse has been proposed as animal model for Usher syndrome 1, BBS and Alström syndrome because of the phenotypic convergence of the clinical phenotypes of retinal and cochlear degeneration, and maturity onset insulin-resistant obesity (Coleman and Eicher 1990; Heckenlively et al. 1995). Originally, the profound hearing loss in B6-*tub*/*tub* mice was fully rescued in F2 *tub*/*tub* homozygotes crossed with AKR/J, 129P2/OlaHsd and CAST/Ei mice, suggesting the presence of a protective allele (Ikeda et al. 2002a). Linkage analysis and subsequent sequencing identified 10 amino acid substitutions and an Ala-Pro repeat length difference in the microtubule-associated protein 1A (*Mtap1a*) residing within the modifier of *tubby* hearing 1 (*moth1*) locus on chromosome 2, between the B6-*tub*/*tub* and the *tub*/*tub* homozygotes in protective strains (Ikeda et al. 1999, 2002a). *Mtap1a* was suggested to play a role in vesicular trafficking of proteins to the neuronal synaptic junctions and further work demonstrating differential binding affinities of *Mtap1a* with the postsynaptic marker PSD95 support a role of the *Mtap1a* modifier gene in synaptic maintenance and architecture (Brenman et al. 1998; Halpain and Dehmelt 2006). The second modifier hunt in the tubby strain consisted in the identification of the protective allele for the retinal degeneration phenotype of this model (Ikeda et al. 2002a). The degree of retinal degeneration was quantitatively assessed by measuring the thickness of the ONL and the number of photoreceptors in a defined area of the ONL between C57BL/6J-*tub*/*tub* mice and *tub*/*tub* homozygotes in the protective AKR/J strain (Ikeda et al. 2002a). Linkage analysis comparing the two strains identified a significant signal on chromosome 11, a locus termed modifier of *tubby* retinal degeneration 1 (*motr1*) whereby a recessive mode of inheritance was assumed for the mapping of the protective allele and two suggestive signals on chromosomes 2 and 8, where dominant protective alleles were likely to segregate (Ikeda et al. 2002a). Interestingly, the locus on chromosome 2 identified in the study for the retinal degeneration modifier, maps to the same locus as *moth1* harboring the *Mtap1a* hearing modifier (Ikeda et al. 2002a,b). Subsequent screening of *Mtap1a* revealed nonsynonymous sequence alterations between the C57BL/6J-*tub*/*tub* and AKR/J-*tub*/*tub* mice, suggesting that the same gene contributes protective alleles that account for the amelioration of both the hearing and retinal degeneration phenotypes of the *tubby* mouse (Maddox et al. 2012).

The use of ONL thickness as a quantitative trait that reflects retinal damage to perform linkage analysis led to the successful identification of a protective modifier in the *Rpe65* mouse model for light-induced photoreceptor damage, corresponding to human LCA (Akhmedov et al. 2000). The two strains compared were C57BL/6J-c(2J) (c2J) albino mice that showed less damage to their photoreceptors after exposure to prolonged light than BALB/c mice and other albino strains, suggesting that the c2J strain was contributing protective allele(s) (Danciger et al. 2000). The strongest linkage signal was on chromosome 3; subsequent analyses let to the mapping of *Rpe65*, in which p.Leu450 was present on the BALB/c strain and was associated with light-induced photoreceptor damage, although the c2J strain carried the

Table 1. Genetic modifiers in retinal degeneration from studies in humans

Disorder	Primary disease driver	Second-site modifier	Clinical aspect affected by modifier	Reference(s)
BBS	*BBS2* (p.Y24X, p.Q59X)	*BBS6* (p.Q147X)	Disease penetrance; digenic inheritance	Katsanis et al. 2001
BBS		*MGC1203* (p.C430T)	Earlier onset of RP; accelerated disease progression	Badano et al. 2006
BBS	*BBS1* (p.M390R)	*MGC1203* (p.C430T)	Disease penetrance; digenic inheritance	Badano et al. 2006
Ciliopathies		*RPGRIP1L* (p.A229T)	Retinal degeneration	Khanna et al. 2009
Dominant cone or cone–rod dystrophy (COD3)	*GUCA1A* (p.P50 L)	Unknown	Disease severity	Downes et al. 2001
LCA	*CEP290*	*AHI1* (p.N811K and p.H758P)	Neurological phenotype; disease severity	Coppieters et al. 2010
LCA	*AIPL1* (p.Q163X)	*CRX* (p.T273L)	Earlier disease onset; disease severity	Zernant et al. 2005
LCA	*AIPL1* (p.R302 L)	*CRB1* (p.R1331H)	Accelerated disease progression	Zernant et al. 2005
LCA	*RPE65* (p.E102X)	*GUCY2D* (p.I573V)	Disease severity	Zernant et al. 2005
LCA	*GUCY2D* (p.S448X)	*CRX* (p.A158T)	Development of macular coloboma in both eyes	Zernant et al. 2005
Macular dystrophy	*PRPH2*	*ROM1* (p.R172 W or p.R229H)	Disease severity; loss of rod function	Poloschek et al. 2010
Macular dystrophy	*PRPH2*	*ABCA4* (p.R172 W, p.R229H or p.V2050L)	Aggravated disease course; loss of cone and rod function	Poloschek et al. 2010
Nephronopthisis	*NPHP1*	*AHI1* (p.R830 W)	Retinal degeneration	Louie et al. 2010
Oguchi's disease/ autosomal recessive RP	*SAG* (p.383fsX)	Unknown	Development of macular degeneration and golden-yellow fundus reflex	Nakazawa et al. 1998
Retinoschisis (X-linked)	*XLRS1* (p.125fsX)	Unknown	Disease severity and progression	Tantri et al. 2003
RP, pattern macular dystrophy, fundus flavimaculatus	*RDS* (p.L185P)	*ROM1* (p.114fsx)	Development of RP	Kajiwara et al. 1993; Weleber et al. 1993
RP (X-linked)	*RPGR*	*RPGRIP1L* (p.R744Q)	Disease severity	Fahim et al. 2011
RP (X-linked)	*RPGR*	*IQCB1* (p.I393N)	Disease severity	Fahim et al. 2011
RP (autosomal dominant)	*PRPF31*	*CNOT3*	Disease penetrance through transcriptional repression	Venturini et al. 2012

Continued

Table 1. *Continued*

Disorder	Primary disease driver	Second-site modifier	Clinical aspect affected by modifier	Reference(s)
RP (autosomal dominant)	*PRPF31*	Unknown (linkage on 14q21-23)	Disease penetrance	Frio et al. 2008
RP1	*RP1* (p.R677X)	Unknown	Disease severity	Jacobson et al. 2000
RP9	*PAP-1* (p.H137 L)	Unknown	Disease severity	Keen et al. 2002; Kim et al. 1995
RP48	*GUCA1B* (p.G157R)	Unknown	Disease severity	Sato et al. 2005
Stargardt type 3	*ELOVL4* (5 bp deletion)	ABCA4	Disease severity ranging from Stargardt-like macular dystrophy to pattern dystrophy	Zhang et al. 1999; Bernstein et al. 2001
Sorby fundus dystrophy (SFD)	*TIMP3* (S181C)	Unknown	Pathological findings ranging from absence of fundus spots to yellow deposits associated with macular degeneration	Hamilton et al. 1989; Weber et al. 1994; Wijesuriya et al. 1996; Felbor et al. 1997
Usher syndrome	*USH2A* (p. C1447QfsX29)	*PDZD7* (p.R56PfsX24)	Earlier disease onset; aggravation of RP severity	Ebermann et al. 2010
Usher syndrome	*USH2C* (*GPR98* p.A5713LfsX3)	*PDZD7*	Disease penetrance; digenic inheritance	Ebermann et al. 2010
Usher syndrome	*USH1D* (p.R1746Q)	Unknown	Severity and progression of RP	Bolz et al. 2001; Astuto et al. 2002
Usher syndrome	*USH3A* (p.N48 K)	Unknown	Progression of RP	Ness et al. 2003
Vitelliform macular dystrophy type 2	*VMD2*	Unknown	Disease severity and penetrance; development of macular degeneration	Nordström and Thorburn 1980

p.Met450 that appeared to be driving the protection against light-induced damage (Danciger et al. 2000). The protective effect of *Rpe65* p.Met450 was also confirmed in other forms of retinal degeneration (Samardzija et al. 2006) and was supported further by introducing the allele in a *c-Fos*$^{-/-}$ mouse (Wenzel et al. 2003). *C-Fos* is essential for light-induced photoreceptor apoptosis because of a sustained increase in the DNA-binding activity of AP-1 (Hafezi et al. 1997; Wenzel et al. 2000) and as a result *c-Fos*$^{-/-}$ mice appear resistant to light-induced damage (Wenzel et al. 2000). When the endogenous *Rpe65* gene (carrying p.Met450) in *c-Fos*$^{-/-}$ mice is substituted by *Rpe65* p.Leu450, *Rpe65* p.Leu450 resulted in an increase in the levels of rhodopsin and therefore led to light-induced photoreceptor loss despite the protective role of *c-Fos* deficiency (Wenzel et al. 2003).

A third successful application of linkage analysis for the mapping of a quantitative trait locus (QTL) was performed in *Rs1* mouse model for X-linked retinoschisis (XLRS) (George et al. 1995; Johnson et al. 2010). XLRS is a form of juvenile-onset macular degeneration, whereby there is splitting of the retina (schisis) and loss of synaptic transmission (George et al. 1995; Johnson et al. 2010). When C57BL/6J *Rs1*^{tmgc1} mice were backcrossed into the AKR/J background, a recessive modifier seemed to be protecting *Rs1*^{tmgc1} mice from retinoschisis

 Cite this article as *Cold Spring Harb Perspect Med* doi: 10.1101/cshperspect.a017145

Table 2. Genetic modifiers in retinal degeneration from studies in mice

Disorder	Primary disease driver/ mouse model	Second-site modifier	Phenotypic aspect affected by modifier	Strains involved	Reference(s)
Fibrous retrolental tissue	*p53*	Not identified	Disease penetrance	C57BL/6J, 129/SvJ	Ikeda et al. 1999
Glaucoma	*BMP4*	Not identified	Disease severity	C57BL/6J, BliA, CAST/Ei, C3H, AKR/J, BALB/C, 129/SvEvTac	Hong et al. 1999
Iris atrophy/ Glaucoma	*Ipd*	*Isa* (*Tyrp1*)	Disease manifestation	C57BL/6J, DBA/2J	Chang et al. 1999
Iris digment dispersion	*Ipd*	Not identified	Disease penetrance	AKXD-28/Ty	Anderson et al. 2001
Iris stromal atrophy	*Isa*	Not identified	Disease severity; increased cell death	AKXD-28/Ty	Anderson et al. 2001
LCA	*Rd16*	*Bbs6*	Variability in photoreceptor degeneration	C57BL/6J, 129/Sv, C57BL/6	Rachel et al. 2012
Light-induced retinal degeneration	*Rpe65*	*Rpe65* p.Leu450, *Rpe65* p.Met450	Disease penetrance	BALB/c2J	Danciger et al. 2000; Wenzel et al. 2003
Ocular retardation	*Chx10*	Not identified	Disease penetrance	CASA/Rk	Bone-Larson et al. 2000
Oguchi disease (stationary night blindness)	*Arrestin*$^{-/-}$	*Arrestin*$^{P365/P365}$	Light-damage susceptibility	C57BL/6, 129/SvJ	Chen et al. 1999
Light-induced RP	*Rho*$^{-/-}$	*Rho* p.V20G, *Rho* p.P23H, *Rho* p.P27L	Disease penetrance	C57BL/6, FVB	Naash et al. 1996; Wang et al. 1997
Retinoschisis	*Rs1*	*Tyr* (*Mor1*)	Disease penetrance	C57BL/6J, AKR/J	Johnson et al. 2010
RP (recessive)	*Pde6a*	Not identified	Disease severity; photoreceptor loss rate	G3 A.B6-*Tyr*$^{+}$/J	Sakamoto et al. 2009
RP1	*Rp1h*	Not identified	Disease severity	(N6) B6.129S, DBA.129S(B6), A.129S(B6)	Liu et al. 2009
RP	*Tub or Rd5*	*Mtap1a* (*motr1*)	RP penetrance; disease progression	B6.Cg-*rd5*/*rd5*, AKR/J	Ikeda et al. 2002b; Maddox et al. 2012
Retinal degeneration	*Rd3*	Not identified	Onset and progression of photoreceptor degeneration	RBF/Dn, Meta-In(1)Rk, Rb(11.13)4Bnr, In-30	Heckenlively et al. 1993

Continued

Table 2. *Continued*

Disorder	Primary disease driver/ mouse model	Second-site modifier	Phenotypic aspect affected by modifier	Strains involved	Reference(s)
Retinal degeneration	*Rd7*	Chr 8 and 19 (CAST/EiJ), Chr 7 and 11 (AKR/J)	Suppression of retinal spotting	B6.Cg-*rd7/rd7*, CAST/EiJ, AKR/J, NOD.NON-*H2*^{nb1}	Akhmedov et al. 2000; Haider et al. 2008
Retinal degeneration	*Rho*$^{-/-}$	Not identified	Variability in photoreceptor degeneration	129/SV, C57BL/6	Humphries et al. 2001
Retinal degeneration	*Rd16*	*Bbs4*	Variability in photoreceptor degeneration	129/SV, BXD24	Zhang et al. 2014

(George et al. 1995; Johnson et al. 2010). Linkage analysis identified the modifier for *Rs1* (*Mor1*) locus on chromosome 7 (Johnson et al. 2010). Within the critical interval mapped in AKR/J *Rs1*^{tmgc1} mice, a recessive mutation in tyrosinase (*Tyr*$^{c\text{-}2J}$) was identified as the *Mor1* gene responsible for protection from the development of the schisis phenotype (George et al. 1995; Johnson et al. 2010).

CONCLUSIONS AND FUTURE PERSPECTIVES

Knowledge of the primary disease-causing mutation is rarely coupled by accurate prognosis. In many instances, the clinical phenotype of a patient with an identified driver mutation can either be ameliorated on the presence of protective alleles or exacerbated when disease-promoting alleles are present in the genome. Despite the numerous reports supporting the presence and importance of genetic modifiers, this field has not progressed as rapidly compared with the identification of primary disease drivers. One of the reasons for this difference, is our inability to recognize interactions among alleles and variants (Eichler et al. 2010). This is true not only for disorders considered to be monogenic but also for complex traits, in which "missing heritability," the fraction of the genetic contribution not explained/explainable by single-locus analysis for rare or common alleles, has been attributed, in part, to the presence of locus interactions and modifiers (Marchini et al. 2005; Zuk et al. 2012). It is possible to consider epistasis and genetic modification to uncover additional genetic contributions; in a study of ankylosing spondylitis, a common form of inflammatory arthritis, nonancestral *ERAP1* alleles have been shown to interact with disease predisposition alleles in *HLA-B27* to confer protection from disease manifestation (Evans et al. 2011). The protective role of *ERAP1* was validated further in a second multifactorial disorder, psoriasis, uncovering the interaction of this gene with *HLA-Cw6*, one of the major psoriasis susceptibility genes (Genetic Analysis of Psoriasis Consortium & the Wellcome Trust Case Control Consortium 2, 2010). Despite the advances in the sequencing technologies, the number of successful genetic modifier identification studies remains small to date owing to many reasons such as the limited disease population sizes, genetic heterogeneity, the low frequency at which any particular combination of alleles is present in the population, and incomplete clinical descriptions (Flint and Mackay 2009). Animal models have provided a powerful tool for the identification of genetic modifiers. Congenic mouse strains have facilitated the mapping of protective and disease-aggravating alleles in a number of cases, some of which have been illustrated here. Zebrafish in vivo assays have aided in the functional annotation and direction of effect of candidate alleles arising by such screens.

The most efficient method to unravel phenomena of genetic modification and oligogenic or complex inheritance, is to interrogate the identified candidate alleles starting from a discrete number of likely interacting loci. Higher throughput technologies provide a unique opportunity toward this goal; a complete genetic profile of cohorts or even specific cell types such as photoreceptors in retinal disorders can be generated through whole-exome or whole-genome sequencing providing the opportunity to mind the same data set multiple times to dissect specific and discrete endophenotypes associated with a genetic condition and its progression, and the development of induced pluripotent stem (iPS) cell technology offers the promise to provide differentiated products from individual human subjects. Although each of these methodologies appear promising, the majority of successful genetic modifier identification reports have relied on the combinatorial use of such tools. Shedding light into the field of genetic modifiers will lead to a more insightful comprehension of the affected pathways and cellular processes. Understanding the basis of disease is the only way toward designing new and more efficient therapeutic paradigms, improve prognosis and even prevent disease manifestation by attempting to mimic the effect of modifiers that affect disease penetrance.

REFERENCES

Ackermann B, Kröber S, Torres-Benito L, Borgmann A, Peters M, Hosseini Barkooie SM, Tejero R, Jakubik M, Schreml J, Milbradt J, et al. 2013. Plastin 3 ameliorates spinal muscular atrophy via delayed axon pruning and improves neuromuscular junction functionality. *Hum Mol Genet* **22:** 1328–1347.

Akhmedov NB, Piriev NI, Chang B, Rapoport AL, Hawes NL, Nishina PM, Nusinowitz S, Heckenlively JR, Roderick TH, Kozak CA, et al. 2000. A deletion in a photoreceptor-specific nuclear receptor mRNA causes retinal degeneration in the *rd7* mouse. *Proc Natl Acad Sci* **97:** 5551–5556.

Anderson M, Smith R, Savinova O, Hawes N, Chang B, Zabaleta A, Wilpan R, Heckenlively J, Davisson M, John S. 2001. Genetic modification of glaucoma associated phenotypes between AKXD-28/Ty and DBA/2J mice. *BMC Genet* **2:** 1.

Apfelstedt-Sylla E, Theischen M, Rüther K, Wedemann H, Gal A, Zrenner E. 1995. Extensive intrafamilial and interfamilial phenotypic variation among patients with autosomal dominant retinal dystrophy and mutations in the human RDS/peripherin gene. *Br J Ophthalmol* **79:** 28–34.

Arts HH, Doherty D, van Beersum SEC, Parisi MA, Letteboer SJF, Gorden NT, Peters TA, Marker T, Voesenek K, Kartono A, et al. 2007. Mutations in the gene encoding the basal body protein RPGRIP1L, a nephrocystin-4 interactor, cause Joubert syndrome. *Nat Genet* **39:** 882–888.

Astuto LM, Bork JM, Weston MD, Askew JW, Fields RR, Orten DJ, Ohliger SJ, Riazuddin S, Morell RJ, Khan S, et al. 2002. *CDH23* mutation and phenotype heterogeneity: A profile of 107 diverse families with Usher Syndrome and nonsyndromic deafness. *Am J Hum Genet* **71:** 262–275.

Baala L, Audollent S, Martinovic J, Ozilou C, Babron M-C, Sivanandamoorthy S, Saunier S, Salomon R, Gonzales M, Rattenberry E, et al. 2007. Pleiotropic effects of *CEP290* (*NPHP6*) mutations extend to Meckel syndrome. *Am J Hum Genet* **81:** 170–179.

Badano JL, Katsanis N. 2002. Beyond Mendel: An evolving view of human genetic disease transmission. *Nat Rev Genet* **3:** 779–789.

Badano JL, Kim JC, Hoskins BE, Lewis RA, Ansley SJ, Cutler DJ, Castellan C, Beales PL, Leroux MR, Katsanis N. 2003. Heterozygous mutations in *BBS1*, *BBS2* and *BBS6* have a potential epistatic effect on Bardet–Biedl patients with two mutations at a second BBS locus. *Hum Mol Genet* **12:** 1651–1659.

Badano JL, Mitsuma N, Beales PL, Katsanis N. 2006. The ciliopathies: An emerging class of human genetic disorders. Annu Rev Genomics Hum Genet. **7:** 125–148.

Beales PL, Elcioglu N, Woolf AS, Parker D, Flinter FA. 1999. New criteria for improved diagnosis of Bardet-Biedl syndrome: Results of a population survey. *J Med Genet* **36:** 437–446.

Beales PL, Badano JL, Ross AJ, Ansley SJ, Hoskins BE, Kirsten B, Mein CA, Froguel P, Scambler PJ, Lewis RA, et al. 2003. Genetic interaction of *BBS1* mutations with alleles at other *BBS* loci can result in non-Mendelian Bardet-Biedl syndrome. *Am J Hum Genet* **72:** 1187–1199.

Bernstein PS, Tammur J, Singh N, Hutchinson A, Dixon M, Pappas CM, Zabriskie NA, Zhang K, Petrukhin K, Leppert M, et al. 2001. Diverse macular dystrophy phenotype caused by a novel complex mutation in the *ELOVL4* gene. *Invest Ophthalmol Vis Sci* **42:** 3331–3336.

Bolk S, Pelet A, Hofstra RMW, Angrist M, Salomon R, Croaker D, Buys CHCM, Lyonnet S, Chakravarti A. 2000. A human model for multigenic inheritance: Phenotypic expression in Hirschsprung disease requires both the *RET* gene and a new 9q31 locus. *Proc Natl Acad Sci* **97:** 268–273.

Bolz H, von Brederlow B, Ramirez A, Bryda EC, Kutsche K, Nothwang HG, Seeliger M, Cabrera MdCS, Vila MC, Molina OP, et al. 2001. Mutation of *CDH23*, encoding a new member of the cadherin gene family, causes Usher syndrome type 1D. *Nat Genet* **27:** 108–112.

Bone-Larson C, Basu S, Radel JD, Liang M, Perozek T, Kapousta-Bruneau N, Green DG, Burmeister M, Hankin

MH. 2000. Partial rescue of the ocular retardation phenotype by genetic modifiers. *J Neurobiol* **42:** 232–247.

Borrego S, Ruiz A, Saez ME, Gimm O, Gao X, López-Alonso M, Hernández A, Wright FA, Antiñolo G, Eng C. 2000. *RET* genotypes comprising specific haplotypes of polymorphic variants predispose to isolated Hirschsprung disease. *J Med Genet* **37:** 572–578.

Boylan JP, Wright AF. 2000. Identification of a novel protein interacting with RPGR. *Hum Mol Genet* **9:** 2085–2093.

Brattgard S. 1949. The pathology of the Laurence-Moon-Biedl syndrome. *Acta Path Microbiol Scand* **26:** 525–537.

Brenman JE, Topinka JR, Cooper EC, McGee AW, Rosen J, Milroy T, Ralston HJ, Bredt DS. 1998. Localization of postsynaptic density-93 to dendritic microtubules and interaction with microtubule-associated protein 1A. *J Neurosci* **18:** 8805–8813.

Carmi R, Elbedour K, Stone EM, Sheffield VC. 1995. Phenotypic differences among patients with Bardet-Biedl syndrome linked to three different chromosome loci. *Am J Med Genet* **59:** 199–203.

Carrasquillo MM, McCallion AS, Puffenberger EG, Kashuk CS, Nouri N, Chakravarti A. 2002. Genome-wide association study and mouse model identify interaction between RET and EDNRB pathways in Hirschsprung disease. *Nat Genet* **32:** 237–244.

Chang B, Smith RS, Hawes NL, Anderson MG, Zabaleta A, Savinova O, Roderick TH, Heckenlively JR, Davisson MT, John SWM. 1999. Interacting loci cause severe iris atrophy and glaucoma in DBA/2J mice. *Nat Genet* **21:** 405–409.

Chang B, Khanna H, Hawes N, Jimeno D, He S, Lillo C, Parapuram SK, Cheng H, Scott A, Hurd RE, et al. 2006. In-frame deletion in a novel centrosomal/ciliary protein CEP290/NPHP6 perturbs its interaction with RPGR and results in early-onset retinal degeneration in the *rd16* mouse. *Hum Mol Genet* **15:** 1847–1857.

Chen J, Simon MI, Matthes MT, Yasumura D, LaVail MM. 1999. Increased susceptibility to light damage in an arrestin knockout mouse model of Oguchi disease (stationary night blindness). *Invest Ophthalmol Vis Sci* **40:** 2978–2982.

Church C, Moir L, McMurray F, Girard C, Banks GT, Teboul L, Wells S, Bruning JC, Nolan PM, Ashcroft FM, et al. 2010. Overexpression of *Fto* leads to increased food intake and results in obesity. *Nat Genet* **42:** 1086–1092.

Coleman DL, Eicher EM. 1990. Fat (*fat*) and tubby (*tub*): Two autosomal recessive mutations causing obesity syndromes in the mouse. *J Hered* **81:** 424–427.

Coppieters F, Casteels I, Meire F, De Jaegere S, Hooghe S, van Regemorter N, Van Esch H, Matulevičienė A, Nunes L, Meersschaut V, et al. 2010. Genetic screening of LCA in Belgium: Predominance of *CEP290* and identification of potential modifier alleles in *AHI1* of *CEP290*-related phenotypes. *Hum Mutat* **31:** E1709–E1766.

Cutting GR. 2010. Modifier genes in Mendelian disorders: The example of cystic fibrosis. *Ann NY Acad Sci* **1214:** 57–69.

Czeizel AE, Dudás I. 1992. Prevention of the first occurrence of neural-tube defects by periconceptional vitamin supplementation. *N Engl J Med* **327:** 1832–1835.

Danciger M, Matthes MT, Yasamura D, Akhmedov NB, Rickabaugh T, Gentleman S, Redmond TM, La Vail MM, Farber DB. 2000. A QTL on distal Chromosome 3 that influences the severity of light-induced damage to mouse photoreceptors. *Mamm Genome* **11:** 422–427.

Danciger M, Ogando D, Yang H, Matthes MT, Yu N, Ahern K, Yasumura D, Williams RW, LaVail MM. 2008. Genetic modifiers of retinal degeneration in the *rd3* mouse. *Invest Ophthalmol Vis Sci* **49:** 2863–2869.

Darrah R, McKone E, O'Connor C, Rodgers C, Genatossio A, McNamara S, Gibson R, Stuart Elborn J, Ennis M, et al. 2010. *EDNRA* variants associate with smooth muscle mRNA levels, cell proliferation rates, and cystic fibrosis pulmonary disease severity. *Physiol Genomics* **41:** 71–77.

Davis EE, Katsanis N. 2012. The ciliopathies: A transitional model into systems biology of human genetic disease. *Curr Opin Genet Dev* **22:** 290–303.

Delous M, Baala L, Salomon R, Laclef C, Vierkotten J, Tory K, Golzio C, Lacoste T, Besse L, Ozilou C, et al. 2007. The ciliary gene *RPGRIP1L* is mutated in cerebello-oculo-renal syndrome (Joubert syndrome type B) and Meckel syndrome. *Nat Genet* **39:** 875–881.

den Hollander AI, Koenekoop RK, Yzer S, Lopez I, Arends ML, Voesenek KEJ, Zonneveld MN, Strom TM, Meitinger T, Brunner HG, et al. 2006. Mutations in the *CEP290* (*NPHP6*) gene are a frequent cause of Leber congenital amaurosis. *Am J Hum Genet* **79:** 556–561.

den Hollander AI, Roepman R, Koenekoop RK, Cremers FPM. 2008. Leber congenital amaurosis: Genes, proteins and disease mechanisms. *Prog Retin Eye Res* **27:** 391–419.

Dina C, Meyre D, Gallina S, Durand E, Korner A, Jacobson P, Carlsson LMS, Kiess W, Vatin V, Lecoeur C, et al. 2007. Variation in *FTO* contributes to childhood obesity and severe adult obesity. *Nat Genet* **39:** 724–726.

Dipple KM, McCabe ERB. 2000. Phenotypes of patients with "simple" Mendelian disorders are complex traits: Thresholds, modifiers, and systems dynamics. *Am J Hum Genet* **66:** 1729–1735.

Downes SM, Holder GE, Fitzke FW, et al. 2001. Autosomal dominant cone and cone–rod dystrophy with mutations in the guanylate cyclase activator 1a gene-encoding guanylate cyclase activating protein-1. *Arch Ophthalmol* **119:** 96–105.

Drumm ML, Konstan MW, Schluchter MD, Handler A, Pace R, Zou F, Zariwala M, Fargo D, Xu A, Dunn JM, et al. 2005. Genetic modifiers of lung disease in cystic fibrosis. *N Engl J Med* **353:** 1443–1453.

Dryja TP, McGee TL, Hahn LB, Cowley GS, Olsson JE, Reichel E, Sandberg MA, Berson EL. 1990. Mutations within the rhodopsin gene in patients with autosomal dominant retinitis pigmentosa. *N Engl J Med* **323:** 1302–1307.

Ebermann I, Scholl HN, Charbel Issa P, Becirovic E, Lamprecht J, Jurklies B, Millán J, Aller E, Mitter D, Bolz H. 2007. A novel gene for Usher syndrome type 2: Mutations in the long isoform of whirlin are associated with retinitis pigmentosa and sensorineural hearing loss. *Hum Genet* **121:** 203–211.

Ebermann I, Phillips JB, Liebau MC, Koenekoop RK, Schermer B, Lopez I, Schaefer E, Roux A-F, et al. 2010. *PDZD7* is a modifier of retinal disease and a contributor to digenic Usher syndrome. *J Clin Invest* **120:** 1812–1823.

Eichler EE, Flint J, Gibson G, Kong A, Leal SM, Moore JH, Nadeau JH. 2010. Missing heritability and strategies for finding the underlying causes of complex disease. *Nat Rev Genet* **11:** 446–450.

Emison ES, McCallion AS, Kashuk CS, Bush RT, Grice E, Lin S, Portnoy ME, Cutler DJ, Green ED, Chakravarti A. 2005. A common sex-dependent mutation in a *RET* enhancer underlies Hirschsprung disease risk. *Nature* **434:** 857–863.

Evans DM, Spencer CCA, Pointon JJ, Su Z, Harvey D, Kochan G, Oppermann U, Dilthey A, Pirinen M, Stone MA, et al. 2011. Interaction between *ERAP1* and HLA-B27 in ankylosing spondylitis implicates peptide handling in the mechanism for HLA-B27 in disease susceptibility. *Nat Genet* **43:** 761–767.

Fahim AT, Bowne SJ, Sullivan LS, Webb KD, Williams JT, Wheaton DK, Birch DG, Daiger SP. 2011. Allelic heterogeneity and genetic modifier loci contribute to clinical variation in males with X-linked retinitis pigmentosa due to *RPGR* mutations. *PLoS ONE* **6:** e23021.

Felbor U, Benkwitz C, Klein ML, Greenberg J, Gregory CY, Weber BF. 1997. Sorsby fundus dystrophy: Reevaluation of variable expressivity in patients carrying a *TIMP3* founder mutation. *Arch Ophthalmol* **115:** 1569–1571.

Flint J, Mackay TFC. 2009. Genetic architecture of quantitative traits in mice, flies, and humans. *Genome Res* **19:** 723–733.

Frank V, Ortiz Brüchle N, Mager S, Frints SGM, Bohring A, du Bois G, Debatin I, Seidel H, Senderek J, Besbas N, et al. 2007. Aberrant splicing is a common mutational mechanism in *MKS1*, a key player in Meckel-Gruber syndrome. *Hum Mutat* **28:** 638–639.

Frayling TM, Timpson NJ, Weedon MN, Zeggini E, Freathy RM, Lindgren CM, Perry JRB, Elliott KS, Lango H, Rayner NW, et al. 2007. A common variant in the *FTO* gene is associated with body mass index and predisposes to childhood and adult obesity. *Science* **316:** 889–894.

Frio TR, Civic N, Ransijn A, Beckmann JS, Rivolta C. 2008. Two trans-acting eQTLs modulate the penetrance of *PRPF31* mutations. *Hum Mol Genet* **17:** 3154–3165.

Gabriel SB, Salomon R, Pelet A, Angrist M, Amiel J, Fornage M, Attie-Bitach T, Olson JM, Hofstra R, Buys C, et al. 2002. Segregation at three loci explains familial and population risk in Hirschsprung disease. *Nat Genet* **31:** 89–93.

Garcia-Barceló M-M, Sham M-H, Lui VC-H, Chen BL-S, Song Y-Q, Lee W-S, Yung S-K, Romeo G, Tam PK-H. 2003. Chinese patients with sporadic Hirschsprung's disease are predominantly represented by a single *RET* haplotype. *J Med Genet* **40:** e122.

Garred P, Pressler T, Madsen HO, Frederiksen B, Svejgaard A, Fiby N, Schwartz M, Koch C. 1999. Association of mannose-binding lectin gene heterogeneity with severity of lung disease and survival in cystic fibrosis. *J Clin Invest* **104:** 431–437.

Genetic Analysis of Psoriasis Consortium & the Wellcome Trust Case Control Consortium 2, Strange A, Capon F, Spencer CC, Knight J, Weale ME, Allen MH, Barton A, Band G, Bellenguez C, et al. 2010. A genome-wide association study identifies new psoriasis susceptibility loci and an interaction between *HLA-C* and *ERAP1*. *Nat Genet* **42:** 985–990.

Génin E, Feingold J, Clerget-Darpoux F. 2008. Identifying modifier genes of monogenic disease: Strategies and difficulties. *Hum Genet* **124:** 357–368.

George ND, Yates JR, Moore AT. 1995. X linked retinoschisis. *Br J Ophthalmol* **79:** 697–702.

Gershoni-Baruch R, Nachlieli T, Leibo R, Degani S, Weissman I. 1992. Cystic kidney dysplasia and polydactyly in 3 sibs with Bardet-Biedl syndrome. *Am J Med Genet* **44:** 269–273.

Gherman A, Davis EE, Katsanis N. 2006. The ciliary proteome database: An integrated community resource for the genetic and functional dissection of cilia. *Nat Genet* **38:** 961–962.

Gibson G. 2012. Rare and common variants: Twenty arguments. *Nat Rev Genet* **13:** 135–145.

Goh K-I, Cusick ME, Valle D, Childs B, Vidal M, Barabási A-L. 2007. The human disease network. *Proc Natl Acad Sci* **104:** 8685–8690.

Goldberg AFX, Molday RS. 1996. Defective subunit assembly underlies a digenic form of retinitis pigmentosa linked to mutations in peripherin/rds and rom-1. *Proc Natl Acad Sci* **93:** 13726–13730.

Goss CH, Newsom SA, Schildcrout JS, Sheppard L, Kaufman JD. 2004. Effect of ambient air pollution on pulmonary exacerbations and lung function in cystic fibrosis. *Am J Respir Crit Care Med* **169:** 816–821.

Gouya LDJ, Lamoril J, Da Silva V, Beaumont C, Grandchamp B, Nordmann Y. 1996. Modulation of the phenotype in dominant erythropoietic protoporphyria by a low expression of the normal ferrochelatase allele. *Am J Hum Genet* **58:** 292–299.

Gouya L, Puy H, Robreau A-M, Bourgeois M, Lamoril J, Da Silva V, Grandchamp B, Deybach J-C. 2002. The penetrance of dominant erythropoietic protoporphyria is modulated by expression of wildtype *FECH*. *Nat Genet* **30:** 27–28.

Gouya L, Martin-Schmitt C, Robreau A-M, Austerlitz F, Da Silva V, Brun P, Simonin S, Lyoumi S, Grandchamp B, Beaumont C, et al. 2006. Contribution of a common single-nucleotide polymorphism to the genetic predisposition for erythropoietic protoporphyria. *Am J Hum Genet* **78:** 2–14.

Grunnet LG, Brøns C, Jacobsen S, Nilsson E, Astrup A, Hansen T, Pedersen O, Poulsen P, Quistorff B, Vaag A. 2009. Increased recovery rates of phosphocreatine and inorganic phosphate after isometric contraction in oxidative muscle fibers and elevated hepatic insulin resistance in homozygous carriers of the A-allele of *FTO* rs9939609. *J Clin Endocrinol Metab* **94:** 596–602.

Gusella J, MacDonald M. 2009. Huntington's disease: The case for genetic modifiers. *Genome Med* **1:** 80.

Hafezi F, Steinbach JP, Marti A, Munz K, Wang ZQ, Wagner EF, Aguzzi A, Remé CE. 1997. The absence of *c-fos* prevents light-induced apoptotic cell death of photoreceptors in retinal degeneration in vivo. *Nat Med* **3:** 346–349.

Haider N, Zhang W, Hurd R, Ikeda A, Nystuen A, Naggert J, Nishina P. 2008. Mapping of genetic modifiers of $Nr2e3^{rd7/rd7}$ that suppress retinal degeneration and restore blue cone cells to normal quantity. *Mamm Genome* **19:** 145–154.

Haldane J. 1941. The relative importance of principal and modifying genes in determining some human diseases. *J Genet* **41:** 149–157.

Halpain S, Dehmelt L. 2006. The MAP1 family of microtubule-associated proteins. *Genome Biol* **7:** 224.

Hamilton WK, Ewing CC, Ives EJ, Carruthers JD. 1989. Sorsby's Fundus Dystrophy. *Ophthalmology* **96:** 1755–1762.

Heckenlively JR, Chang B, Peng C, Hawes NL, Roderick TH. 1993. Variable expressivity of rd-3 retinal degeneration dependent on background strain. In *Retinal degeneration* (ed. Hollyfield JG, Anderson RE, LaVail MM), pp. 273–280. Plenum, New York.

Heckenlively JR, Chang B, Erway LC, Peng C, Hawes NL, Hageman GS, Roderick TH. 1995. Mouse model for Usher syndrome: Linkage mapping suggests homology to Usher type I reported at human chromosome 11p15. *Proc Natl Acad Sci* **92:** 11100–11104.

Hillian AD, Londono D, Dunn JM, Goddard KAB, Pace RG, Knowles MR, Drumm ML. 2008. Modulation of cystic fibrosis lung disease by variants in interleukin-8. *Genes Immun* **9:** 501–508.

Hong H-K, Lass JH, Chakravarti A. 1999. Pleiotropic skeletal and ocular phenotypes of the mouse mutation congenital hydrocephalus (*ch/Mf1*) arise from a winged helix/forkhead transcription factor gene. *Hum Mol Genet* **8:** 625–637.

Humphries MM, Kiang S, McNally N, Donovan MA, Sieving PA, Bush RA, Machida S, Cotter T, Hobson A, Farrar J, et al. 2001. Comparative structural and functional analysis of photoreceptor neurons of *Rho*$^{-/-}$ mice reveal increased survival on C57BL/6J in comparison to 129Sv genetic background. *Vis Neurosci* **18:** 437–443.

Ikeda A, Yin Zheng Q, Rosenstiel P, Maddatu T, Zuberi AR, Roopenian DC, North MA, Naggert JK, Johnson KR, Nishina PM. 1999. Genetic modification of hearing in tubby mice: Evidence for the existence of a major gene (*moth1*) which protects tubby mice from hearing loss. *Hum Mol Genet* **8:** 1761–1767.

Ikeda A, Naggert JK, Nishina PM. 2002a. Genetic modification of retinal degeneration in tubby mice. *Exp Eye Res* **74:** 455–461.

Ikeda A, Zheng QY, Zuberi AR, Johnson KR, Naggert JK, Nishina PM. 2002b. Microtubule-associated protein 1A is a modifier of tubby hearing (*moth1*). *Nat Genet* **30:** 401–405.

Jacobson SG, Cideciyan AV, Iannaccone A, Weleber RG, Fishman GA, Maguire AM, Affatigato LM, Bennett J, Pierce EA, Danciger M, et al. 2000. Disease expression of RP1 mutations causing autosomal dominant retinitis pigmentosa. *Invest Opthalmol Vis Sci* **41:** 1898–1908.

Johnson BA, Cole BS, Geisert EE, Ikeda S, Ikeda A. 2010. Tyrosinase is the modifier of retinoschisis in mice. *Genetics* **186:** 1337–1344.

Kajiwara K, Sandberg MA, Berson EL, Dryja TP. 1993. A *null* mutation in the human peripherin/RDS gene in a family with autosomal dominant retinitis punctata albescens. *Nat Genet* **3:** 208–212.

Kajiwara K, Berson E, Dryja T. 1994. Digenic retinitis pigmentosa due to mutations at the unlinked peripherin/*RDS* and *ROM1* loci. *Science* **264:** 1604–1608.

Katsanis N, Ansley SJ, Badano JL, Eichers ER, Lewis RA, Hoskins BE, Scambler PJ, Davidson WS, Beales PL, Lupski JR. 2001. Triallelic inheritance in Bardet-Biedl syndrome, a Mendelian recessive disorder. *Science* **293:** 2256–2259.

Keen TJ, Himms MM, McKie AB, Moore AT, Doran RM, Mackey DA, Mansfield DC, Mueller RF, Bhattacharya SS, Bird AC, et al. 2002. Mutations in a protein target of the Pim-1 kinase associated with the RP9 form of autosomal dominant retinitis pigmentosa. *Eur J Hum Genet* **10:** 245–249.

Kerem BS, Zielenski J, Markiewicz D, Bozon D, Gazit E, Yahav J, Kennedy D, Riordan JR, Collins FS, Rommens JM. 1990. Identification of mutations in regions corresponding to the two putative nucleotide (ATP)-binding folds of the cystic fibrosis gene. *Proc Natl Acad Sci* **87:** 8447–8451.

Khanna H, Davis EE, Murga-Zamalloa CA, Estrada-Cuzcano A, Lopez I, den Hollander AI, Zonneveld MN, Othman MI, Waseem N, Chakarova CF, et al. 2009. A common allele in *RPGRIP1L* is a modifier of retinal degeneration in ciliopathies. *Nat Genet* **41:** 739–745.

Kim RY, Fitzke FW, Moore AT, Jay M, Inglehearn C, Arden GB, Bhattacharya SS, Bird AC. 1995. Autosomal dominant retinitis pigmentosa mapping to chromosome 7p exhibits variable expression. *Br J Ophthalmol* **79:** 23–27.

Klöting N, Schleinitz D, Ruschke K, Berndt J, Fasshauer M, Tönjes A, Schön MR, Kovacs P, Stumvoll M, Blüher M. 2008. Inverse relationship between obesity and *FTO* gene expression in visceral adipose tissue in humans. *Diabetologia* **51:** 641–647.

Kremer H, van Wijk E, Märker T, Wolfrum U, Roepman R. 2006. Usher syndrome: Molecular links of pathogenesis, proteins and pathways. *Hum Mol Genet* **15:** R262–R270.

Labrune M, Gaux JC, Brault B. 1974. The Laurence-Moon-Bardet-Biedl syndrome. Urographic signs. *Ann Radiol* **17:** 385–389.

Landau J, Bromberg Y, Schorr J. 1949. Laurence-Moon-Biedl syndrome with mulitple congenital malformations of the urinary tract. *Acta Med Orient* **8:** 205–210.

Laurence KM, James N, Miller M, Campbell H. 1980. Increased risk of recurrence of pregnancies complicated by fetal neural tube defects in mothers receiving poor diets, and possible benefit of dietary counselling. *BMJ* **281:** 1592–1594.

Leitch CC, Zaghloul NA, Davis EE, Stoetzel C, Diaz-Font A, Rix S, Alfadhel M, Lewis RA, Eyaid W, Banin E, et al. 2008. Hypomorphic mutations in syndromic encephalocele genes are associated with Bardet-Biedl syndrome. *Nat Genet* **40:** 443–448.

Li JB, Gerdes JM, Haycraft CJ, Fan Y, Teslovich TM, May-Simera H, Li H, Blacque OE, Li L, Leitch CC, et al. 2004. Comparative genomics identifies a flagellar and basal body proteome that includes the *BBS5* human disease gene. *Cell* **117:** 541–552.

Lim J, Hao T, Shaw C, Patel AJ, Szabó G, Rual J-F, Fisk CJ, Li N, Smolyar A, Hill DE, et al. 2006. A protein–protein interaction network for human inherited ataxias and disorders of Purkinje cell degeneration. *Cell* **125:** 801–814.

Liu Q, Saveliev A, Pierce EA. 2009. The severity of retinal degeneration in *Rp1h* gene-targeted mice is dependent on genetic background. *Invest Ophthalmol Vis Sci* **50:** 1566–1574.

Loewen CJR, Moritz OL, Molday RS. 2001. Molecular characterization of peripherin-2 and rom-1 mutants responsible for digenic retinitis pigmentosa. *J Biol Chem* **276:** 22388–22396.

Louie CM, Caridi G, Lopes VS, Brancati F, Kispert A, Lancaster MA, Schlossman AM, Otto EA, Leitges M, Grone H-J, et al. 2010. *AHI1* is required for photoreceptor outer segment development and is a modifier for retinal degeneration in nephronophthisis. *Nat Genet* **42:** 175–180.

Lyon AN, Pineda RH, Hao lT, Kudryashova E, Kudryashov DS, Beattie CE. 2014. Calcium binding is essential for plastin 3 function in Smn-deficient motoneurons. *Hum Mol Genet* **23:** 1990–2004.

Maddox DM, Ikeda S, Ikeda A, Zhang W, Krebs MP, Nishina PM, Naggert JK. 2012. An allele of microtubule-associated protein 1A (*Mtap1a*) reduces photoreceptor degeneration in *Tulp1* and *Tub* mutant mice. *Invest Ophthalmol Vis Sci* **53:** 1663–1669.

Magro F, Peres E. 1970. Nefropathia do sindrome do Laurence–Moon–Bardet–Biedl. *Revista Iberica de Endocrinologia* **17:** 243–253.

Marchini J, Donnelly P, Cardon LR. 2005. Genome-wide strategies for detecting multiple loci that influence complex diseases. *Nat Genet* **37:** 413–417.

Margolin DH, Kousi M, Chan Y-M, Lim ET, Schmahmann JD, Hadjivassiliou M, Hall JE, Adam I, Dwyer A, Plummer L, et al. 2013. Ataxia, dementia, and hypogonadotropism caused by disordered ubiquitination. *N Engl J Med* **368:** 1992–2003.

McWilliam P, Farrar GJ, Kenna P, Bradley DG, Humphries MM, Sharp EM, McConnell DJ, Lawler M, Sheils D, Ryan C, et al. 1989. Autosomal dominant retinitis pigmentosa (ADRP): Localization of an ADRP gene to the long arm of chromosome 3. *Genomics* **5:** 619–622.

Naash ML, Peachey NS, Li ZY, Gryczan CC, Goto Y, Blanks J, Milam AH, Ripps H. 1996. Light-induced acceleration of photoreceptor degeneration in transgenic mice expressing mutant rhodopsin. *Invest Ophthalmol Vis Sci* **37:** 775–782.

Nakazawa M, Wada Y, Tamai M. 1998. Arrestin gene mutations in autosomal recessive retinitis pigmentosa. *Arch Ophthalmol* **116:** 498–501.

Ness SL, Ben-Yosef T, Bar-Lev A, Madeo AC, Brewer CC, Avraham KB, Kornreich R, Desnick RJ, Willner JP, Friedman TB, et al. 2003. Genetic homogeneity and phenotypic variability among Ashkenazi Jews with Usher syndrome type III. *J Med Genet* **40:** 767–772.

Nordström S, Thorburn W. 1980. Dominantly inherited macular degeneration (Best's disease) in a homozygous father with 11 children. *Clin Genet* **18:** 211–216.

Ohlemiller KK, Hughes RM, Lett JM, Ogilvie JM, Speck JD, Wright JS, Faddis BT. 1997. Progression of cochlear and retinal degeneration in the *tubby* (*rd5*) mouse. *Audiol Neurootol* **2:** 175–185.

Oprea GE, Kröber S, McWhorter ML, Rossoll W, Müller S, Krawczak M, Bassell GJ, Beattie CE, Wirth B. 2008. Plastin 3 is a protective modifier of autosomal recessive spinal muscular atrophy. *Science* **320:** 524–527.

Otto EA, Loeys B, Khanna H, Hellemans J, Sudbrak R, Fan S, Muerb U, O'Toole JF, Helou J, Attanasio M, et al. 2005. Nephrocystin-5, a ciliary IQ domain protein, is mutated in Senior-Loken syndrome and interacts with RPGR and calmodulin. *Nat Genet* **37:** 282–288.

Perrault I, Delphin N, Hanein S, Gerber S, Dufier J-L, Roche O, Defoort-Dhellemmes S, Dollfus H, Fazzi E, Munnich A, et al. 2007. Spectrum of NPHP6/CEP290 mutations in Leber congenital amaurosis and delineation of the associated phenotype. *Hum Mutat* **28:** 416–416.

Poloschek CM, Bach M, Lagrèze WA, Glaus E, Lemke JR, Berger W, Neidhardt J. 2010. *ABCA4* and *ROM1*: Implications for modification of the *PRPH2*-associated macular dystrophy phenotype. *Invest Ophthalmol Vis Sci* **51:** 4253–4265.

Rachel RA, May-Simera HL, Veleri S, Gotoh N, Choi BY, Murga-Zamalloa C, McIntyre JC, Marek J, Lopez I, Hackett AN, et al. 2012. Combining Cep290 and Mkks ciliopathy alleles in mice rescues sensory defects and restores ciliogenesis. *J Clin Ivest* **122:** 1233–1245.

Raychaudhuri S, Iartchouk O, Chin K, Tan PL, Tai AK, Ripke S, Gowrisankar S, Vemuri S, Montgomery K, Yu Y, et al. 2011. A rare penetrant mutation in *CFH* confers high risk of age-related macular degeneration. *Nat Genet* **43:** 1232–1236.

Riazuddin SA, Shahzadi A, Zeitz C, Ahmed ZM, Ayyagari R, Chavali VRM, Ponferrada VG, Audo I, Michiels C, Lancelot M-E, et al. 2010. A mutation in *SLC24A1* implicated in autosomal-recessive congenital stationary night blindness. *Am J Hum Genet* **87:** 523–531.

Riise R, Andréasson S, Borgström MK, Wright AF, Tommerup N, Rosenberg T, Tornqvist K. 1997. Intrafamilial variation of the phenotype in Bardet–Biedl syndrome. *Br J Ophthalmol* **81:** 378–385.

Rivolta C, Sharon D, DeAngelis MM, Dryja TP. 2002. Retinitis pigmentosa and allied diseases: Numerous diseases, genes, and inheritance patterns. *Hum Mol Genet* **11:** 1219–1227.

Rubin BK. 1990. Exposure of children with cystic fibrosis to environmental tobacco smoke. *N Engl J Med* **323:** 782–788.

Sakamoto K, McCluskey M, Wensel TG, Naggert JK, Nishina PM. 2009. New mouse models for recessive retinitis pigmentosa caused by mutations in the *Pde6a* gene. *Hum Mol Genet* **18:** 178–192.

Samardzija M, Wenzel A, Naash M, Remé CE, Grimm C. 2006. *Rpe65* as a modifier gene for inherited retinal degeneration. *Eur J Neurosci* **23:** 1028–1034.

Sancandi M, Griseri P, Pesce B, Patrone G, Puppo F, Lerone M, Martucciello G, Romeo G, Ravazzolo R, Devoto M, et al. 2003. Single nucleotide polymorphic alleles in the 5′ region of the *RET* proto-oncogene define a risk haplotype in Hirschsprung's disease. *J Med Genet* **40:** 714–718.

Sato M, Nakazawa M, Usui T, Tanimoto N, Abe H, Ohguro H. 2005. Mutations in the gene coding for guanylate cyclase-activating protein 2 (*GUCA1B* gene) in patients with autosomal dominant retinal dystrophies. *Graefes Arch Clin Exp Ophthalmol* **243:** 235–242.

Sayer JA, Otto EA, O'Toole JF, Nurnberg G, Kennedy MA, Becker C, Hennies HC, Helou J, Attanasio M, Fausett BV, et al. 2006. The centrosomal protein nephrocystin-6 is mutated in Joubert syndrome and activates transcription factor ATF4. *Nat Genet* **38:** 674–681.

Schäffer AA. 2013. Digenic inheritance in medical genetics. *J Med Genet* **50:** 641–652.

Scuteri A, Sanna S, Chen W-M, Uda M, Albai G, Strait J, Najjar S, Nagaraja R, Orrú M, Usala G, et al. 2007. Genome-wide association scan shows genetic variants in the *FTO* gene are associated with obesity-related traits. *PLoS Genet* **3:** e115.

Seddon JM, Yu Y, Miller EC, Reynolds R, Tan PL, Gowrisankar S, Goldstein JI, Triebwasser M, Anderson HE, Zerbib J, et al. 2013. Rare variants in *CFI, C3* and *C9* are associated with high risk of advanced age-related macular degeneration. *Nat Genet* **45:** 1366–1370.

Smemo S, Tena JJ, Kim K-H, Gamazon ER, Sakabe NJ, Gomez-Marin C, Aneas I, Credidio FL, Sobreira DR, Wasserman NF, et al. 2014. Obesity-associated variants within *FTO* form long-range functional connections with *IRX3*. *Nature* **507:** 371–375.

Speilman RS, McGinnis RE, Ewens WJ. 1993. Transmission test for linkage disequilibrium: The insulin gene region and insulin-dependent diabetes mellitus (IDDM). *Am J Hum Genet* **52:** 506–516.

Stoetzel C, Laurier V, Davis EE, Muller J, Rix S, Badano JL, Leitch CC, Salem N, Chouery E, Corbani S, et al. 2006. *BBS10* encodes a vertebrate-specific chaperonin-like protein and is a major BBS locus. *Nat Genet* **38:** 521–524.

Stoetzel C, Muller J, Laurier V, Davis EE, Zaghloul NA, Vicaire S, Jacquelin C, Plewniak F, Leitch CC, Sarda P, et al. 2007. Identification of a novel BBS gene (*BBS12*) highlights the major role of a vertebrate-specific branch of chaperonin-related proteins in Bardet-Biedl syndrome. *Am J Hum Genet* **80:** 1–11.

Tantri A, Vrabec TR, Cu-Unjieng A, Frost A, Annesley WH Jr, Donoso LA. 2003. X-linked retinoschisis: Report of a family with a rare deletion in the xLRS1 gene. *Am J Ophthalmol* **136:** 547–549.

Tolarova M. 1982. Periconceptional supplementation with vitamins and folic acid to prevent recurrence of cleft lip. *Lancet* **320:** 217.

Valente EM, Silhavy JL, Brancati F, Barrano G, Krishnaswami SR, Castori M, Lancaster MA, Boltshauser E, Boccone L, Al-Gazali L, et al. 2006. Mutations in *CEP290*, which encodes a centrosomal protein, cause pleiotropic forms of Joubert syndrome. *Nat Genet* **38:** 623–625.

Vanscoy LL, Blackman SM, Collaco JM, Bowers A, Lai T, Naughton K, Algire M, McWilliams R, Beck S, Hoover-Fong J, et al. 2007. Heritability of lung disease severity in cystic fibrosis. *Am J Respir Crit Care Med* **175:** 1036–1043.

Venturini G, Rose AM, Shah AZ, Bhattacharya SS, Rivolta C. 2012. *CNOT3* is a modifier of *PRPF31* mutations in retinitis pigmentosa with incomplete penetrance. *PLoS Genet* **8:** e1003040.

Wald NJ, Law MR, Morris JK, Wald DS. 2001. Quantifying the effect of folic acid. *Lancet* **358:** 2069–2073.

Walia S, Fishman GA, Swaroop A, Branham KEH, Lindemena M, Othman M, Weleber RG. 2008. Discordant phenotypes in fraternal twins having an identical mutation in exon ORF15 of the *RPGR* gene. *Arch Ophthalmol* **126:** 379–384.

Wang M, Lam TT, Tso MOM, Naash MI. 1997. Expression of a mutant opsin gene increases the susceptibility of the retina to light damage. *Vis Neurosci* **14:** 55–62.

Weber BHF, Vogt G, Pruett RC, Stohr H, Felbor U. 1994. Mutations in the tissue inhibitor of metalloproteinases-3 (*TIMP3*) in patients with Sorsby's fundus dystrophy. *Nat Genet* **8:** 352–356.

Weleber RG, Carr RE, Murphey WH, Sheffield VC, Stone EM. 1993. Phenotypic variation including retinitis pigmentosa, pattern dystrophy, and fundus flavimaculatus in a single family with a deletion of codon 153 or 154 of the peripherin/*RDS* gene. *Arch Ophthalmol* **111:** 1531–1542.

Wenzel A, Grimm C, Marti A, Kueng-Hitz N, Hafezi F, Niemeyer G, Remé CE. 2000. *c-fos* controls the "private pathway" of light-induced apoptosis of retinal photoreceptors. *J Neurosci* **20:** 81–88.

Wenzel A, Grimm C, Samardzija M, Remé CE. 2003. The genetic modifier $Rpe65Leu_{450}$: Effect on light damage susceptibility in *c-Fos*-deficient mice. *Invest Ophthalmol Vis Sci* **44:** 2798–2802.

Wijesuriya SD, Evans K, Jay MR, Davison C, Weber BH, Bird AC, Bhattacharya SS, Gregory CY. 1996. Sorsby's fundus dystrophy in the British Isles: Demonstration of a striking founder effect by microsatellite-generated haplotypes. *Genome Res* **6:** 92–101.

Zernant J, Külm M, Dharmaraj S, den Hollander AI, Perrault I, Preising MN, Lorenz B, Kaplan J, Cremers FPM, Maumenee I, et al. 2005. Genotyping microarray (disease chip) for Leber congenital amaurosis: Detection of modifier alleles. *Invest Ophthalmolo Vis Sci* **46:** 3052–3059.

Zhang K, Kniazeva M, Hutchinson A, Han M, Dean M, Allikmets R. 1999. The *ABCR* gene in recessive and dominant Stargardt diseases: A genetic pathway in macular degeneration. *Genomics* **60:** 234–237.

Zhang Y, Seo S, Bhattarai S, Bugge K, Searby CC, Zhang Q, Drack AV, Stone EM, Sheffield VC. 2014. BBS mutations modify phenotypic expression of CEP290-related ciliopathies. *Hum Mol Genet* **23:** 40–51.

Zuk O, Hechter E, Sunyaev SR, Lander ES. 2012. The mystery of missing heritability: Genetic interactions create phantom heritability. *Proc Natl Acad Sci* **109:** 1193–1198.

RNA-Seq: Improving Our Understanding of Retinal Biology and Disease

Michael H. Farkas, Elizabeth D. Au, Maria E. Sousa, and Eric A. Pierce

Ocular Genomics Institute, Department of Ophthalmology, Massachusetts Eye and Ear Infirmary, Harvard Medical School, Boston, Massachusetts 02114

Correspondence: eric_pierce@meei.harvard.edu

Over the past several years, rapid technological advances have allowed for a dramatic increase in our knowledge and understanding of the transcriptional landscape, because of the ability to study gene expression in greater depth and with more detail than previously possible. To this end, RNA-Seq has quickly become one of the most widely used methods for studying transcriptomes of tissues and individual cells. Unlike previously favored analysis methods, RNA-Seq is extremely high-throughput, and is not dependent on an annotated transcriptome, laying the foundation for novel genetic discovery. Additionally, RNA-Seq derived transcriptomes provide a basis for widening the scope of research to identify potential targets in the treatment of retinal disease.

The study of whole transcriptome gene expression in disease research is not a novel concept. Early methods of gene expression analysis, such as the use of expressed sequence tags (EST) and serial analysis of gene expression (SAGE), have been in use since the early 1990s. In the late 1990s, microarrays quickly became the method of choice for the study of gene expression, owing to their higher throughput nature. These methods allowed scientists to study transcriptomes in great detail and in less time, giving rise to large amounts of information more quickly than previously thought possible.

Early gene expression studies using EST analysis were first published by Adams et al. (1991), and quickly gained popularity as a means to identify novel alternate splice sites and examine differential expression in data sets. This technique involves sequencing a cloned cDNA and mapping the sequence (100–800 bp) to a genome of interest. In 1999, 83 EST clusters were identified as potential retinal specific genes, with 14 further classified as potential disease genes (Malone et al. 1999). By 2000, the first analysis of the retinal transcriptome was published (Bortoluzzi et al. 2000). Nearly 5000 known retinal genes were studied, levels of expression were estimated, and several genes were noted to be potentially associated with disease. Although EST studies laid the groundwork for analysis of the retinal transcriptome, they are extremely low-throughput, making whole transcriptome analyses time consuming and difficult.

The use of SAGE analysis was first published in 1995 as a means to study differences in gene expression in patients with cancer (Velculescu

Cite this article as *Cold Spring Harb Perspect Med* doi: 10.1101/cshperspect.a017152

et al. 1995). SAGE studies produce a list of short (10–20 bp) sequences, which can then be mapped back to a genome of interest, whereas EST studies are based on the sequencing of one longer sequence. In 2002, SAGE libraries constructed from two eye tissue samples were studied, identifying 26,355 retinal transcripts, and 10,404 RPE (retinal pigment epithelium) transcripts (Sharon et al. 2002). SAGE studies, although an improvement on ESTs, are still low-throughput, and the analysis of an entire transcriptome is both time-consuming and expensive, necessitating the use of more high-throughput analysis methods to comprehensively study the retinal transcriptome (Swaroop and Zack 2002).

DNA microarrays were an answer to the call for higher throughput methods of expression analysis, and were first used to study a "complete" genome in 1997 (Lashkari et al. 1997). Microarrays evolved from the technique of Southern blotting. Complementary sequence that aligns uniquely to each gene of interest are mapped on an array, and used to determine the relative levels of expression of each gene in a given sample. In 2010, microarray analysis identified 154 "signature RPE genes," in which expression in the RPE was at least 10-fold higher than published expression levels in other tissues (Strunnikova et al. 2010). The high-throughput nature of microarrays makes this method preferable to EST and SAGE for whole transcriptome analyses. However, microarrays only allow for relative quantitation of transcripts compared with all other transcripts on the array. Additionally, microarrays are reliant on a properly annotated genome. It is only possible to study previously identified transcripts, without the ability to identify alternate splice sites or novel exons.

RNA-Seq is the newest and most widely used method for transcriptome analyses, combining the qualitative nature of EST and SAGE studies with the high-throughput and quantitative abilities of microarrays. Importantly, RNA-Seq experiments are extremely cost-effective considering the large amount of data produced, and allow for the identification of novel exons, splice sites, and transcripts. Whereas EST and SAGE sequencing studies required the researcher to clone a small section of a genome at a time, RNA-Seq allows for the sequencing of an entire transcriptome (we define the transcriptome as all expressed RNAs, both coding and noncoding). This greatly enhances the possibility of finding novel transcripts, and offers increased insight into the transcriptional dynamics of a particular cell.

Next generation sequencing (NGS) has become a ubiquitous research tool in all fields of science, and has greatly enhanced the field of ophthalmology. The rise of NGS was possible because of the many advantages it offered over previously preferred techniques. Now, with only nanogram levels of starting material, the current NGS technologies can create more than one hundred million paired-end reads, covering a large portion of the genome, or transcriptome, while maintaining sensitivity and specificity (Mardis 2008; Morozova 2008; Shendure 2008; Reis-Filho 2009). The data generated is useful in a variety of applications because of its dual qualitative and quantitative nature (Reis-Filho 2009). This enables individual investigators to pursue projects previously accessible only to larger consortia, particularly because of its cost effectiveness over Sanger sequencing (Schuster 2007; Morozova 2008; Shendure 2008).

One of the most prominent challenges of RNA-Seq has been the bioinformatic analysis of such large data sets. The massive amount of data generated by each sequencing run has created a high demand for pipelines capable of accurately analyzing the data in a timely manner (Shendure 2008). In addition, as RNA-Seq studies continue to produce more and more data, it becomes increasingly difficult to sift through the results to discover pertinent biological insights (Reis-Filho 2009).

NEXT GENERATION SEQUENCING IN OPHTHALMOLOGY

Since its commercial availability in 2004, NGS has been used in a variety of cases within ophthalmology (Mardis 2008). Whole exome sequencing has identified both novel and known mutations in DHDDS, SNRNP200, MAK,

NMNAT1, and RPE65, in patients with Leber congenital amuarosa (LCA) and retinitis pigmentosa (RP) (Benaglio 2011; Bowne 2011; Özgül 2011; Tucker 2011; Wang 2012). Similarly, NGS has been used to search for mutations in other ocular conditions. In 2010, mutations were discovered in TSPAN12, in patients who exhibited familial exudative vitreoretinopathy (Nikopoulos 2010). NGS has also been used to investigate variants in ABCA4, which is associated with a number of retinal dystrophies including Stargardt disease, cone–rod dystrophy and RP (Zernant 2011). Furthermore, this technology has aided in the discovery of mutations in GPR179 and ATOH7, which are associated with autosomal-recessive complete congenital stationary night blindness and global eye defects, respectively (Khan 2012).

Increasingly, NGS has been used in a clinical setting for diagnostic purposes within ophthalmology. This method has the ability to aid in the diagnosis of diseases such as RP, which has dozens of causative genes associated with it (Audo 2012; Neveling 2012; Schrader 2011). NGS has the ability to continue to shape both the future of diagnostics and ophthalmology research as a whole.

RNA-SEQUENCING

RNA-Seq is a powerful NGS method that allows for the study of transcriptomes in great detail and with a high degree of accuracy, providing unprecedented resolution of gene expression at the level of the transcript down to a single base (Chepelev et al. 2009; Costa et al. 2010; Marguerat and Bahler 2010). This affords the ability to study RNA editing, alternative splicing, and isoform quantification (Costa et al. 2010; Ozsolak and Milos 2011; Rosenberg et al. 2011; Djebali et al. 2012). Further, the relatively unbiased nature of the technology captures novel transcriptome events including novel isoforms and novel gene expression (Chen et al. 2011; Halvardson et al. 2013; Kim et al. 2012; Mercer et al. 2012). RNA-Seq studies provide a vast wealth of information, and hence require sophisticated methodologies and bioinformatic algorithms for data analysis. As NGS technology continues to improve, the RNA-Seq library preparation techniques and analysis packages are quickly evolving as well. These innovations, along with the development of appropriate models, allow for RNA-Seq to be applied to vision research.

NEXT GENERATION LIBRARY PREPARATION

Initially, RNA-Seq was limited by the relatively large amount (1–10 μg) of total RNA required for library preparation (Farkas et al. 2012; Grant et al. 2011). This amount of RNA was needed because of long protocols with many inefficient purification steps that lead to significant loss of product. Even with such large starting amounts of RNA, the loss of sample at each step required PCR amplification to have enough final product for sequencing. It is important to note that over-amplification has the potential to lead to amplification bias and PCR artifacts (Wang et al. 2009; Costa et al. 2010, 2012). These initial preparations were labor-intensive, relatively low-throughput, multi-day protocols.

Lower input, higher-throughput methods have since been developed, which allow for starting total RNA concentrations as low as 100 ng (Brooks et al. 2011, 2012). An initial concern with using minimal starting material was that samples would be underrepresented when compared with data produced using the earlier, high-input protocols. Brooks et al. (2012), however, showed in mouse retina that the two methods are comparable (Brooks et al. 2011). Although an improvement on the first library preparation protocols, these methods are still subject to PCR bias because of necessary amplification before sequencing, and require multiple days to complete.

A newer innovation involves transposon-mediated fragmentation and adaptor ligation, processes originally designed for DNA sequencing that can be adapted for RNA-Seq library preparation (Syed 2010; Gertz et al. 2012). Unlike previous RNA-Seq preparation methods, in which polyadenylated RNA (polyA RNA) was selected and fragmented, then converted to double-stranded cDNA (ds cDNA), the new method involves a polyA RNA selection step during first-strand cDNA synthesis followed by transposon-based fragmentation of ds cDNA. This offers significant improvements to the process, eliminating purification steps and minimizing loss of product. Further, because there are fewer purification steps in this process, the number of amplification cycles is reduced to only five, and PCR bias is minimized. Finally, this newest method is higher throughput and can be performed in hours rather than days.

BIOINFORMATIC ANALYSIS—ALIGNMENT OF RNA-Seq DATA

One of the most critical steps in any RNA-Seq experiment is the alignment of reads to a reference genome and/or transcriptome. This is also one of the most challenging steps because of splicing of exons to form transcripts. RNA-Seq aligners are continually being developed, and improved, to overcome this challenge. Many of the currently available alignment algorithms have been comprehensively characterized and reviewed (Fonseca et al. 2012; Lindner and Friedel 2012). The most important factors to consider when choosing an RNA-Seq aligner are its ability to: 1) accurately align reads; 2) maximize the number of reads aligned (sensitivity); 3) detect splice junctions (both annotated and novel); and 4) efficiently align reads (i.e., speed of alignment with minimal compute resources).

Currently, no RNA-Seq alignment algorithm is able to outperform the others in all four categories. In choosing which algorithm is most suitable for a particular RNA-Seq experiment, it is important to weigh the benefits of each. For example, of the most popular aligners, RUM (RNA-Seq unified mapper) and GSNAP (Genomic Short-Read Nucleotide Alignment Program) are the most accurate, sensitive, and capable of detecting splice junctions (Grant et al. 2011; Dobin et al. 2013). However, they are only able to achieve this by being compute-intensive and having slower alignment speeds, relative to other programs. The most recently developed algorithm, STAR, is an ultrafast aligner that uses fewer compute resources relative to RUM and GSNAP, but does so at the cost of sensitivity and accuracy (Dobin et al. 2013). Even so, STAR outperforms some of the most popular alignment algorithms such as TopHat and MapSplice.

Although alignment speed is certainly important, with such large data sets being produced by NGS studies, it may be the least important factor, taking into account the amount of data needed to fully cover a transcriptome. We have reported that 100 million reads are necessary to fully cover both the human and mouse neural retina transcriptome (Grant et al. 2011; Farkas et al. 2012, 2013). Because transcriptome complexity varies between tissues and organisms, it is necessary to independently determine the appropriate depth of coverage for each RNA-Seq study (Wang et al. 2008; Barbosa-Morais et al. 2012; Gonzalez-Porta et al. 2012). With the amount of relatively inexpensive resources available on the cloud, if a read depth of 100 million read is considered sufficient, aligner speed becomes less important than accuracy, sensitivity, and junction detection (Karlsson et al. 2012; Kienzler et al. 2012; Morgan et al. 2012; Nekrutenko and Taylor 2012; Zhang et al. 2012).

BIOINFORMATIC ANALYSIS—DIFFERENTIAL EXPRESSION

Although an important part of the analysis process, sequence alignment is only the first step in the bioinformatic processing of RNA-Seq data. Downstream analysis algorithms are necessary to obtain more useful information, and can address a range of issues, from basic tasks such as quantification of differential gene expression, to more challenging projects such as determining alternative splicing and RNA-editing (Peng et al. 2012). Unfortunately, as with the alignment algorithms, development of algorithms to perform such downstream analyses have lagged behind the advances in sequencing technology, and there is limited consensus as to which perform optimally.

Often, one of the first postalignment questions regarding sequencing data is the determination of differential expression (DE) between conditions. This is not a new concept; analysis of transcriptome data for DE features has been performed since the first experiments utilizing SAGE (Lorenz and Dean 2002; Baggerly et al. 2003; Lu et al. 2005). Microarrays soon replaced SAGE as the method of choice to study transcriptomes, and a new set of DE algorithms were developed (Cui and Churchill 2003; Smyth 2004). When RNA-Seq was developed, it was assumed that the statistical models developed for microarrays could be adapted for RNA-Seq DE analyses. Indeed, some RNA-Seq DE algorithms borrow statistical assumptions from microarray packages (Oshlack et al. 2010). However, microarray quantification is based on a continuous intensity distribution, whereas RNA-Seq quantification is the result of a discrete measurement (i.e., number of reads mapped to a feature). The differences in data distribution and the biases associated with each method suggest that DE algorithms would not be compatible between the two. Microarray data is modeled using a normal distribution, although a Poisson distribution was initially determined to be the most appropriate for modeling RNA-Seq data (Marioni et al. 2008; Bullard et al. 2010). In fact, analysis of RNA-Seq experiments in which the same sample was run over multiple lanes of a flowcell showed that RNA-Seq data was Poisson distributed (Marioni et al. 2008). Poisson modeling of biological replicates, however, does not account for biological variability, and is prone to high false positive rates (Anders and Huber 2010). Interestingly, the analysis method that most appropriately fits RNA-Seq data was first developed for SAGE analyses. Because these two methods are relatively similar and mainly differ in the amount of data generated from a single experiment, a negative binomial distribution has been considered the most appropriate for DE analysis of RNA-Seq data (Robinson and Smyth 2008; Anders and Huber 2010; Hardcastle 2010; Robinson et al. 2010). Two of the most popular DE algorithms, DESeq and EdgeR, incorporate the negative binomial statistical approach, but differ in their normalization methods (Anders and Huber 2010; Robinson et al. 2010). Multiple studies comparing the two methods have been published with the consensus being that DESeq is more conservative and better limits the false positive rate, although EdgeR is able to call more truly DE genes, but at the expense of a higher false positive rate (Rapaport et al. 2013; Soneson and Delorenzi 2013). Ultimately, the best algorithm will be the one that best fits the research design of the end user.

In addition to quantification of gene expression, RNA-Seq can be used to study RNA splicing. Detecting splice junctions is not a trivial task, as it requires mapping reads to multiple locations in the genome, separated by anywhere from a few bases to as many as a few hundred thousand bases. The ability to perform such mapping functions are built into alignment algorithms, but are performed differently by each. RUM, for example, identifies annotated splice junctions by using a concatenated transcriptome index, which does not include introns or intergenic regions (Grant et al. 2011). This allows RUM to quickly align reads to annotated junctions without the need for gapped alignment. Novel splice junction detection by RUM is more compute intensive because it is performed using the BLAST-Like Alignment Tool (BLAT) (Kent 2002). BLAT uses an "anchor-extension" strategy, in which a portion of the read is aligned to the genome, and is considered to "anchor" the alignment. The remaining read is then aligned to another region in the genome. In contrast, TopHat uses an alternative method for detecting splice junctions, which relies on the aligner Bowtie, assembly algorithm Maq, and canonical splice site information to map reads crossing splice junctions (Li et al. 2008; Trapnell et al. 2009). TopHat splice junction mapping differs from the "anchor-extension" method in that it maps reads to build "islands" that represent exons, using the canonical splice site information to find the exon/intron boundaries.

The "anchor-extension" strategy is acknowledged to be an excellent method for novel splice junction determination. Notably, using RUM, we have identified thousands of novel splicing events in the mouse neural retina, including exon skipping, novel exons, and alternate 3′ and 5′ splicing (Grant et al. 2011). Several new algorithms use statistical modeling methods as an alternative approach. Most recently, Fine-

Splice, PASTA, and TrueSight have been developed to use regression modeling to identify splice junctions, and claim to enhance sensitivity and specificity over traditional splice junction detection methods, but have not been independently verified (Li et al. 2013; Tang and Riva 2013; Gatto et al. 2014).

RNA-Seq STUDIES IN THE RETINA

The rapid development of bioinformatic tools has enabled a complete genomic characterization of the retina, which is necessary to properly study the basic biological mechanisms that drive cellular physiology, morphology, and development, as well as disease. To date, only a few RNA-Seq studies have set out to characterize the transcriptome of the normal or diseased retina. Original characterizations of the retina using SAGE and microarray technology, although useful, are antiquated and inadequate for fully sampling the transcriptome (Mortazavi et al. 2008; Wang et al. 2009; Li et al. 2010). Microarrays can comprehensively sample the annotated transcriptome, but are limited to providing information about known features (exons, genes, etc.), and are unable to aid in the discovery of novel features. In contrast, SAGE analyses are able to detect novel features, but are limited by minimal data output (Oshlack et al. 2010). Although RNA-Seq does have its own biases, such as problems caused by PCR amplification, it addresses many issues of the earlier technologies and allows for a much more comprehensive transcriptome analysis (Costa et al. 2012).

Given the importance of mouse models for vision research, and the difficulty in obtaining high quality human retinal samples, it is no surprise that the first RNA-Seq retinal transcriptome articles to be published examine the mouse retina. These studies have found between 16,000–34,000 transcripts expressed in the mouse retina, which is in line with prior SAGE analyses of human retina, where 26,000 transcripts were found to be expressed (Swaroop and Zack 2002; Brooks et al. 2011). Analyses regarding the overlap of transcript expression in the retina between the two species, including isoform abundance, has not yet been performed, but would be particularly useful for studying retinal dystrophies in mouse models.

More comprehensive RNA-Seq studies of the mouse retina have shed light onto the overall expression and alternative splicing of known retinal disease genes. For example, Gamsiz et al. (2012) noted that many of these genes are among the most highly expressed in the retina, with rhodopsin being at the top of the list (Gamsiz et al. 2012). The investigators also point out that these genes are among the largest, and are susceptible to more alternative splicing events. This is interesting, and confirms previous observations that the number of alternative splicing events a transcript undergoes is proportional to the number of exons in the transcript (Pickrell et al. 2010).

Although new RNA-Seq studies are continuously increasing our knowledge of the mouse retina, alternative splicing has not yet been fully characterized, and, in particular, novel alternative splicing events remain to be fully investigated. Grant et al. (2011) set out to identify and validate novel alternative splicing events, including exon skipping, alternate 3′/5′ splice sites, and novel exons, concluding that tens of thousands of novel alternative splicing events occur in the mouse retina (Grant et al. 2011). A majority of the novel features identified were seen in lower abundance than their annotated counterparts, however, there are also novel features with expression levels suggesting they may in fact be the major isoform of a given gene. Further research is required to determine the biological function of these novel features. Additionally, the fact that the highly expressed novel features have not yet been discovered in other tissues raises the question of their specific importance in the retina.

MODELS FOR STUDYING DISEASE

RNA-Seq captures a snapshot of the transcriptome at a given point in time (Wang et al. 2009; Costa et al. 2010; Marguerat and Bahler 2010). This fact complicates studying disease in humans. In the case of inherited retinal dystrophies (IRDs), for example, high quality human retinal tissue is particularly hard to obtain. In

 Cite this article as *Cold Spring Harb Perspect Med* doi: 10.1101/cshperspect.a017152

addition, transcriptome changes occur because of degeneration of the retina and extended postmortem times to RNA isolation, further complicating the issue (Koppelkamm et al. 2011). To appropriately study the pathogenesis of an IRD, one would need to view the transcriptome before degeneration. In light of these inherent difficulties, mouse models have been studied as an alternative, although these models are still not a perfect solution.

Mouse models are clearly the method of choice for studying visual dystrophies (Buch et al. 2008; Liu et al. 2010; Jaillard et al. 2012). From a disease standpoint, they have played a major role in elucidating the mechanisms of pathogenesis for many types of blindness (Won et al. 2011). Mouse models have helped identify the role of oxidative damage, lipid metabolism, inflammation, and immune response in the development of age-related macular degeneration (AMD) (Hollyfield and Kuttner-Kondo 2010; Pennesi et al. 2012). In this last case, however, there are obvious deficiencies in using mice as a model for AMD. Most notably, mice lack a macula, and hence true AMD has not been recapitulated. Another issue arises in terms of RNA-Seq data itself. Expression levels of gene isoforms in the transcriptomes of mice vary relative to those expressed in humans (Matlin et al. 2005; Meena Kishore et al. 2005; Pan et al. 2005; Konopka et al. 2009; Stahl and Wainszelbaum 2009; Nilsen and Graveley 2010). This can be caused by variation in alternative splicing between the two species, as well as differences in the degree of expression of each isoform in the tissue. It is well known that splicing is not well conserved between species, especially between human and mouse. It is currently not well understood how these variations affect normal tissue function, and it is unknown how they may affect disease models. Despite this issue, mouse and zebrafish models have commonly been considered the best alternative for disease research, since obtaining retinal samples is not always possible. In cases in which disease genes are conserved between species, these models have proven effective. In other instances, such as the study of mutations in the RNA splicing factors, which cause RP, animal models may not be the best choice, because aberrant splicing is hypothesized to underlie disease pathogenesis (Ivings et al. 2008; Graziotto et al. 2011; Farkas et al. 2012; Cvačková et al. 2014).

One possible alternative to animal models is the use of induced pluripotent stem cells (iPS); with iPS, it is possible to derive RPE and photoreceptor-like cells from human, or animal, fibroblast cells or blood (Takahashi et al. 2007; Aoi et al. 2008; Okamoto and Takahashi 2011; Phillips et al. 2012). This technology offers a lot of promise from a research standpoint, as expression profiles closely match those found in human tissue samples, providing a more accurate disease model. Specifically, in cases in which differences in splicing patterns present complications, iPS cells from patients affected with RNA splicing factor RP may provide a better alternative to understanding disease onset. Further, since the discovery, and practicality, of genome editing, affected patient samples are no longer necessary because mutations can be readily introduced into iPS cells. Additionally, the use of iPS cells offers clinical promise, as functional iPS-derived retina cells have the potential for therapeutic use (Carr et al. 2009; Carr 2011; Schmeer et al. 2012). Before clinical use, a thorough characterization is warranted and necessary, because iPS-dervived RPE have been shown to have a short lifespan after transplantation in the rat eye (Carr et al. 2009). Currently, it is unknown why iPS-derived RPE do not survive in vivo, especially since functional characterization suggests the RPE are indeed functional (Kokkinaki et al. 2011; Westenskow et al. 2012).

RNA-Seq STUDIES TO UNDERSTAND DISEASE MECHANISMS

To date, many mouse models of human visual dystrophies have been developed, but only a few have been studied using RNA-Seq. Age-related retinal degeneration (ARD) is the most common cause of vision loss (Mustafi et al. 2012). It is defined as likely being caused by a myriad of factors that are both genetic and environmental (Donoso et al. 2010; Hong et al. 2011; Pennesi et al. 2012; Sui et al. 2012). Little is known about the genetic factors underlying the disease, which makes it an ideal candidate for RNA-Seq studies. In mice, genetic background plays a role in the development of ARD. Mice on the A/J background are more susceptible to retinal degeneration than are BALB/c or B6 mice (Mustafi et al. 2012). In A/J mice, transcriptome analysis of the whole eye, rather than a specific retinal tissue, revealed an increase in proinflammatory factors and a decrease in protective factors such as those involved in the oxidative stress response. These differentially expressed genes were ultimately localized to the RPE, suggesting a role for the RPE in ARD development.

Diabetic retinopathy is another leading cause of vision loss worldwide (Klein et al. 2009; Visser 2010). The pattern of gene expression changes in mouse models of diabetic retinopathy as the disease progresses, are notable (Kandpal et al. 2012). Inflammation has been shown to be critical to the pathogenesis of diabetic retinopathy. RNA-Seq studies have found that the degree of up-regulation of inflammation related genes actually decreases over time as disease severity progresses, while at the same time other genes, such as those involved in the Wnt signaling pathway, crystallins, and various transcription factors are newly up-regulated (Li et al. 2009; Tang and Kern 2011; Kandpal et al. 2012). Further, these RNA-Seq studies note that disease-specific alternative splicing events, which were previously found to occur in the disease state, in fact accumulate as disease progresses. Interestingly, potential inhibitors known to slow the progression of diabetic retinopathy by targeting specific metabolic pathways were shown to regulate the expression of some of the over expressed genes, most notably the crystallins, in the disease models. Additionally, these inhibitors reversed the levels of the disease-specific alternative splicing events implicated in disease progression.

Although RNA-Seq-based transcriptome analyses of the eye are still in their infancy, it is clear the tremendous potential this technology provides the field. RNA-Seq will likely play an important role in uncovering everything from the eye's basic transcriptional landscape to providing unprecedented insight into the mechanisms underlying disease.

CONCLUDING REMARKS

RNA-Seq has proven to be a powerful, albeit underutilized, tool for studying disease in the eye. Studying the transcriptome of patients with retinal disease is difficult and largely dependent on mouse models. Because the transcriptomes of humans and mice differ quite significantly, these models are not always sufficient for RNA-Seq studies. With the advancement of iPS technology, and the ability to derive RPE and photoreceptor progenitor cells, the technology necessary to perform suitable human studies will now be readily available. These studies will be essential for furthering both genetic and clinical studies to help bring therapies to patients.

The increase in demand for a genetic diagnosis by patients with ocular disease is rising because of the recent advances in gene therapy. In addition, the fact that many ocular diseases present with a similar phenotype caused by a heterogeneous group of genes (e.g., RP) necessitates the need to have a genetic diagnosis before treatment is possible. Whole-exome sequencing (WES) provides the quickest and most practical technology available for screening and providing a genetic diagnosis to patients with mutations in protein coding genes. However, it has become evident that we do not have a complete understanding of many diseases, as many patients with an obvious Mendelian disease cannot be diagnosed using current methods. Although this might be attributed to our incomplete understanding of the exome, it is highly likely that noncoding RNAs and other unexplored regions of the genome contribute to disease. RNA-Seq is both more affordable and powerful to explore these regions, compared with other NGS technologies. Future advances in whole exome sequencing technology, RNA-Seq, analysis, bioinformatics, and functional models should provide clinicians with powerful tools to diagnose and treat ocular disease.

REFERENCES

Adams MD, Kelley JM, Gocayne JD, Dubnick M, Polymeropoulos MH, Xiao H, Merril CR, Wu A, Olde B, Moreno RF. 1991. Complementary DNA sequencing: Expressed sequence tags and human genome project. *Science* **252:** 1651–1656.

Anders S, Huber W. 2010. Differential expression analysis for sequence count data. *Genome Biol* **11:** R106.

Aoi T, Yae K, Nakagawa M, Ichisaka T, Okita K, Takahashi K, Chiba T, Yamanaka S. 2008. Generation of pluripotent stem cells from adult mouse liver and stomach cells. *Science* **321:** 699–702.

Audo I, Bujakowska K, Mohand-Said S, Lancelot M-E, Moskova-Doumanova V, Waseem N, Antonio A, Sahel J-A, Bhattacharya S, Zeitz C. 2010. Prevalence and novelty of PRPF31 mutations in French autosomal dominant rod-cone dystrophy patients and a review of published reports. *BMC Med Genet* **11:** 145.

Baggerly KA, Deng L, Morris JS, Aldaz CM. 2003. Differential expression in SAGE: Accounting for normal between-library variation. *Bioinformatics* **19:** 1477–1483.

Barbosa-Morais NL, Irimia M, Pan Q, Xiong HY, Gueroussov S, Lee LJ, Slobodeniuc V, Kutter C, Watt S, Sáolak R. 2012. The evolutionary landscape of alternative splicing in vertebrate species. *Science* **338:** 1587–1593.

Benaglio P, McGee TL, Capelli LP, Harper S, Berson EL, Rivolta C. 2011. Next generation sequencing of pooled samples reveals new SNRNP200 mutations associated with retinitis pigmentosa. *Hum Mutat* **32:** E2246–E2258.

Bortoluzzi S, d'Alessi F, Danieli GA. 2000. A novel resource for the study of genes expressed in the adult human retina. *Invest Ophthalmol Vis Sci* **41:** 3305–3308.

Bowne SJ, Humphries MM, Sullivan LS, Kenna PF, Tam LCS, Kiang AS, Campbell M, Weinstock GM, Koboldt DC, Ding L. 2011. A dominant mutation in RPE65 identified by whole-exome sequencing causes retinitis pigmentosa with choroidal involvement. *Eur J Hum Genet* **19:** 1074–1081.

Brooks MJ, Rajasimha HK, Roger JE, Swaroop A. 2011. Next-generation sequencing facilitates quantitative analysis of wild-type and Nrl$^{-/-}$ retinal transcriptomes. *Mol Vis* **17:** 3034–3054.

Brooks MJ, Rajasimha HK, Swaroop A. 2012. Retinal transcriptome profiling by directional next-generation sequencing using 100 ng of total RNA. *Methods Mol Biol* **884:** 319–334.

Buch P, Bainbridge J, Ali R. 2008. AAV-mediated gene therapy for retinal disorders: From mouse to man. *Gene Ther* **15:** 849–857.

Bullard JH, Purdom E, Hansen KD, Dudoit S. 2010. Evaluation of statistical methods for normalization and differential expression in mRNA-Seq experiments. *BMC Bioinformatics* **11:** 94.

Carr A. 2011. iPS cells—An alternative source of RPE? *Acta Ophthalmol* doi: 10.1111/j.1755-3768.2011.2231.x

Carr AJ, Vugler AA, Hikita ST, Lawrence JM, Gias C, Chen LL, Buchholz DE, Ahmado A, Smart MJK, Hasan S. 2009. Protective effects of human iPS-derived retinal pigment epithelium cell transplantation in the retinal dystrophic rat. *PLoS ONE* **4:** e8152.

Chen G, Li R, Shi L, Qi J, Hu P, Luo J, Liu M, Shi T. 2011. Revealing the missing expressed genes beyond the human reference genome by RNA-Seq. *BMC Genomics* **12:** 590.

Chepelev I, Wei G, Tang Q, Zhao K. 2009. Detection of single nucleotide variations in expressed exons of the human genome using RNA-Seq. *Nucleic Acids Res* **37:** e106.

Costa V, Angelini C, De Feis I, Ciccodicola A. 2010. Uncovering the complexity of transcriptomes with RNA-Seq. *J Biomed Biotechnology* **2010:** 853916.

Costa V, Aprile M, Esposito R, Ciccodicola A. 2012. RNA-Seq and human complex diseases: Recent accomplishments and future perspectives. *Eur J Hum Genet* **21:** 134–142.

Cui X, Churchill GA. 2003. Statistical tests for differential expression in cDNA microarray experiments. *Genome Biol* **4:** 210.

Cvačková Z, Matějů D, Staněk D. 2014. Retinitis pigmentosa mutations of *SNRNP200* enhance cryptic splice-site recognition. *Hum Mutat* **35:** 308–317.

Djebali S, Davis CA, Merkel A, Dobin A, Lassmann T, Mortazavi A, Tanzer A, Lagarde J, Lin W, Schlesinger F, et al. 2012. Landscape of transcription in human cells. *Nature* **489:** 101–108.

Dobin A, Davis CA, Schlesinger F, Drenkow J, Zaleski C, Jha S, Batut P, Chaisson M, Gingeras TR. 2013. STAR: Ultrafast universal RNA-Seq aligner. *Bioinformatics* **29:** 15–21.

Donoso LA, Vrabec T, Kuivaniemi H. 2010. The role of complement factor H in age-related macular degeneration: A review. *Surv Ophthalmol* **55:** 227–246.

Farkas MH, Grant GR, Pierce EA. 2012. Transcriptome analyses to investigate the pathogenesis of RNA splicing factor retinitis pigmentosa retinal degenerative diseases. (ed. LaVail MM, Ash JD, Anderson RE, Hollyfield JG, Grimm C), pp. 519–525. Springer, New York.

Farkas MH, Grant GR, White JA, Sousa ME, Consugar MB, Pierce EA. 2013. Transcriptome analyses of the human retina identify unprecedented transcript diversity and 3.5 Mb of novel transcribed sequence via significant alternative splicing and novel genes. *BMC Genomics* **14:** 486.

Fonseca NA, Rung J, Brazma A, Marioni JC. 2012. Tools for mapping high-throughput sequencing data. *Bioinformatics* **28:** 3169–3177.

Gamsiz ED, Ouyang Q, Schmidt M, Nagpal S, Morrow EM. 2012. Genome-wide transcriptome analysis in murine neural retina using high-throughput RNA sequencing. *Genomics* **99:** 44–51.

Gatto A, Torroja-Fungairino C, Mazzarotto F, Cook SA, Barton PJ, Sanchez-Cabo F, Lara-Pezzi E. 2014. FineSplice, enhanced splice junction detection and quantification: A novel pipeline based on the assessment of diverse RNA-Seq alignment solutions. *Nucleic Acids Res* **42:** e71.

Gertz J, Varley KE, Davis NS, Baas BJ, Goryshin IY, Vaidyanathan R, Kuersten S, Myers RM. 2012. Transposase mediated construction of RNA-Seq libraries. *Genome Res* **22:** 134–141.

Gonzalez-Porta M, Calvo M, Sammeth M, Guigo R. 2012. Estimation of alternative splicing variability in human populations. *Genome Res* **22:** 528–538.

Grant GR, Farkas MH, Pizarro AD, Lahens NF, Schug J, Brunk BP, Stoeckert CJ, Hogenesch JB, Pierce EA. 2011. Comparative analysis of RNA-Seq alignment algorithms and the RNA-Seq unified mapper (RUM). *Bioinformatics* **27:** 2518–2528.

Graziotto JJ, Farkas MH, Bujakowska K, Deramaudt BM, Zhang Q, Nandrot EF, Inglehearn CF, Bhattacharya SS, Pierce EA. 2011. Three gene-targeted mouse models of RNA splicing factor RP show late-onset RPE and retinal degeneration. *Invest Ophthalmol Vis Sci* **52:** 190–198.

Halvardson J, Zaghlool A, Feuk L. 2013. Exome RNA sequencing reveals rare and novel alternative transcripts. *Nucleic Acids Res* doi: 10.1093/nar/gks816.

Hardcastle TJ. 2010. baySeq: Empirical Bayesian analysis of patterns of differential expression in count data. *BMC Bioinformatics* **11:** 442.

Hollyfield JG, Kuttner-Kondo L. 2010. Animal models for age-related macular degeneration. In Animal models for retinal diseases (ed. Pang IH, Clark AF), pp. 81–98. Springer, New York.

Hong T, Tan AG, Mitchell P, Wang JJ. 2011. A review and meta-analysis of the association between C-reactive protein and age-related macular degeneration. *Surv Ophthalmol* **56:** 184–194.

Ivings L, Towns KV, Matin M, Taylor C, Ponchel F, Grainger RJ, Ramesar RS, Mackey DA, Inglehearn CF. 2008. Evaluation of splicing efficiency in lymphoblastoid cell lines from patients with splicing-factor retinitis pigmentosa. *Mol Vis* **14:** 2357.

Jaillard C, Mouret A, Niepon ML, Clerin E, Yang Y, Lee-Rivera I, Ait-Ali N, Millet-Puel G, Cronin T, Sedmak T. 2012. *Nxnl2* splicing results in dual functions in neuronal cell survival and maintenance of cell integrity. *Hum Mol Genet* **21:** 2298–2311.

Kandpal RP, Rajasimha HK, Brooks MJ, Nellissery J, Wan J, Qian J, Kern TS, Swaroop A. 2012. Transcriptome analysis using next generation sequencing reveals molecular signatures of diabetic retinopathy and efficacy of candidate drugs. *Mol Vis* **18:** 1123–1146.

Karlsson J, Torreno O, Ramet D, Klambauer G, Cano M, Trelles O. 2012. Enabling large-scale bioinformatics data analysis with cloud computing. In *Parallel and Distributed Processing with Applications (ISPA), 2012 IEEE 10th International Symposium*, pp. 640–645. IEEE.

Kent WJ. 2002. BLAT: The BLAST-like alignment tool. *Genome Res* **12:** 656–664.

Khan K, Logan CV, McKibbin M, Sheridan E, Elçioglu NH, Yenice O, Parry DA, Fernandez-Fuentes N, Abdelhamed ZIA, Al-Maskari A. 2012. Next generation sequencing identifies mutations in Atonal homolog 7 (ATOH7) in families with global eye developmental defects. *Hum Mol Genet* **21:** 776–783.

Kienzler R, Bruggmann R, Ranganathan A, Tatbul N. 2012. Large-Scale DNA sequence analysis in the cloud: A stream-based approach. In *Euro-Par 2011: Parallel Processing Workshops*, pp. 467–476. Springer, New York.

Kim J, Zhao K, Jiang P, Lu Z-X, Wang J, Murray J, Xing Y. 2012. Transcriptome landscape of the human placenta. *BMC Genomics* **13:** 115.

Klein R, Klein BEK, Moss SE. 2009. The Wisconsin epidemiological study of diabetic retinopathy: A review. *Diabetes Metab Rev* **5:** 559–570.

Kokkinaki M, Sahibzada N, Golestaneh N. 2011. Human induced pluripotent stem-derived retinal pigment epithelium (RPE) cells exhibit ion transport, membrane potential, polarized vascular endothelial growth factor secretion, and gene expression pattern similar to native RPE. *Stem Cells* **29:** 825–835.

Konopka G, Bomar JM, Winden K, Coppola G, Jonsson ZO, Gao F, Peng S, Preuss TM, Wohlschlegel JA, Geschwind DH. 2009. Human-specific transcriptional regulation of CNS development genes by FOXP2. *Nature* **462:** 213–217.

Koppelkamm A, Vennemann B, Lutz-Bonengel S, Fracasso T, Vennemann M. 2011. RNA integrity in post-mortem samples: Influencing parameters and implications on RT-qPCR assays. *Int J Legal Med* **125:** 1–8.

Lashkari DA, DeRisi JL, McCusker JH, Namath AF, Gentile C, Hwang SY, Brown PO, Davis RW. 1997. Yeast microarrays for genome wide parallel genetic and gene expression analysis. *Proc Natl Acad Sci* **94:** 13057–13062.

Li H, Ruan J, Durbin R. 2008. Mapping short DNA sequencing reads and calling variants using mapping quality scores. *Genome Res* **18:** 1851–1858.

Li J, Wang JJ, Yu Q, Wang M, Zhang SX. 2009. Endoplasmic reticulum stress is implicated in retinal inflammation and diabetic retinopathy. *FEBS Lett* **583:** 1521–1527.

Li B, Ruotti V, Stewart RM, Thomson JA, Dewey CN. 2010. RNA-Seq gene expression estimation with read mapping uncertainty. *Bioinformatics* **26:** 493–500.

Li Y, Li-Byarlay H, Burns P, Borodovsky M, Robinson GE, Ma J. 2013. TrueSight: A new algorithm for splice junction detection using RNA-seq. *Nucleic Acids Res* **41:** e51.

Lindner R, Friedel CC. 2012. A comprehensive evaluation of alignment algorithms in the context of RNA-Seq. *PloS ONE* **7:** e52403.

Liu Q, Zhang Q, Pierce EA. 2010. Photoreceptor sensory cilia and inherited retinal degeneration. *Adv Exp Med Biol* **664:** 223–232.

Lorenz WW, Dean JFD. 2002. SAGE profiling and demonstration of differential gene expression along the axial developmental gradient of lignifying xylem in loblolly pine (*Pinus taeda*). *Tree Physiol* **22:** 301–310.

Lu J, Tomfohr J, Kepler T. 2005. Identifying differential expression in multiple SAGE libraries: An overdispersed log-linear model approach. *BMC Bioinformatics* **6:** 165.

Malone K, Sohocki MM, Sullivan LS, Daiger SP. 1999. Identifying and mapping novel retinal-expressed ESTs from humans. *Mol Vis* **5:** 5.

Mardis ER. 2008. Next-generation DNA sequencing methods. *Annu Rev Genomics Hum Genet* **9:** 387–402.

Marguerat S, Bahler J. 2010. RNA-Seq: From technology to biology. *Cell Mol Life Sci* **67:** 569–579.

Marioni JC, Mason CE, Mane SM, Stephens M, Gilad Y. 2008. RNA-Seq: An assessment of technical reproducibility and comparison with gene expression arrays. *Genome Res* **18:** 1509–1517.

Matlin AJ, Clark F, Smith CWJ. 2005. Understanding alternative splicing: Towards a cellular code. *Nat Rev Mol Cell Biol* **6:** 386–398.

Meena Kishore S, Bagavathi SP, Yun Ping L, Lee Pern C, Yiting Y, Pandjassarame K. 2005. Alternatively spliced human genes by exon skipping—A database (ASHESdb). *In Silico Biol* **5:** 221–225.

Mercer TR, Gerhardt DJ, Dinger ME, Crawford J, Trapnell C, Jeddeloh JA, Mattick JS, Rinn JL. 2012. Targeted RNA sequencing reveals the deep complexity of the human transcriptome. *Nat Biotech* **30:** 99–104.

Morgan JC, Chapman RW, Anderson PE. 2012. A next generation sequence processing and analysis platform with integrated cloud-storage and high performance computing resources. In *Proceedings of the ACM Conference on Bioinformatics, Computational Biology and Biomedicine*, pp. 594–594. ACM.

Morozova O, Marra MA. 2008. Applications of next-generation sequencing technologies in functional genomics. *Genomics* **92:** 255–264.

Mortazavi A, Williams BA, McCue K, Schaeffer L, Wold B. 2008. Mapping and quantifying mammalian transcriptomes by RNA-Seq. *Nat Meth* **5:** 621–628.

Mustafi D, Maeda T, Kohno H, Nadeau JH, Palczewski K. 2012. Inflammatory priming predisposes mice to age-related retinal degeneration. *J Clin Invest* **122:** 2989–3001.

Nekrutenko A, Taylor J. 2012. Next-generation sequencing data interpretation: Enhancing reproducibility and accessibility. *Nat Rev Genet* **13:** 667–672.

Neveling K, Collin RWJ, Gilissen C, van Huet RAC, Visser L, Kwint MP, Gijsen SJ, Zonneveld MN, Wieskamp N, de Ligt J. 2012. Next-generation genetic testing for retinitis pigmentosa. *Hum Mutat* **33:** 963–972.

Nikopoulos K, Gilissen C, Hoischen A, Erik van Nouhuys C, Boonstra FN, Blokland EAW, Arts P, Wieskamp N, Strom TM, Ayuso C. 2010. Next-generation sequencing of a 40 Mb linkage interval reveals *TSPAN12* mutations in patients with familial exudative vitreoretinopathy. *Am J Hum Genet* **86:** 240–247.

Nilsen TW, Graveley BR. 2010. Expansion of the eukaryotic proteome by alternative splicing. *Nature* **463:** 457–463.

Okamoto S, Takahashi M. 2011. Induction of retinal pigment epithelial cells from monkey iPS cells. *Invest Ophthalmol Vis Sci* **52:** 8785–8790.

Oshlack A, Robinson MD, Young MD. 2010. From RNA-Seq reads to differential expression results. *Genome Biol* **11:** 220.

Özgül RK, Siemiatkowska AM, Yücel D, Myers CA, Collin RWJ, Zonneveld MN, Beryozkin A, Banin E, Hoyng CB, van den Born LI. 2011. Exome sequencing and *cis*-regulatory mapping identify mutations in *MAK*, a gene encoding a regulator of ciliary length, as a cause of retinitis pigmentosa. *Am J Hum Genet* **89:** 253–264.

Ozsolak F, Milos PM. 2011. RNA sequencing: Advances, challenges and opportunities. *Nat Rev Genet* **12:** 87–98.

Pan Q, Bakowski MA, Morris Q, Zhang W, Frey BJ, Hughes TR, Blencowe BJ. 2005. Alternative splicing of conserved exons is frequently species-specific in human and mouse. *Trends Genet* **21:** 73–77.

Peng Z, Cheng Y, Tan BC-M, Kang L, Tian Z, Zhu Y, Zhang W, Liang Y, Hu X, Tan X. 2012. Comprehensive analysis of RNA-Seq data reveals extensive RNA editing in a human transcriptome. *Nat Biotechnol* **30:** 253–260.

Pennesi ME, Neuringer M, Courtney RJ. 2012. Animal models of age related macular degeneration. *Mol Aspects Med* **33:** 487–509.

Phillips MJ, Wallace KA, Dickerson SJ, Miller MJ, Verhoeven AD, Martin JM, Wright LS, Shen W, Capowski EE, Percin EF. 2012. Blood-derived human iPS cells generate optic vesicle-like structures with the capacity to form retinal laminae and develop synapses. *Invest Ophthalmol Vis Sci* **53:** 2007–2019.

Pickrell JK, Pai AA, Gilad Y, Pritchard JK. 2010. Noisy splicing drives mRNA isoform diversity in human cells. *PLoS Genet* **6:** e1001236.

Rapaport F, Khanin R, Liang Y, Pirun M, Krek A, Zumbo P, Mason CE, Socci ND, Betel D. 2013. Comprehensive evaluation of differential gene expression analysis methods for RNA-Seq data. *Genome Biol* **14:** R95.

Reis-Filho JS. 2009. Next-generation sequencing. *Breast Cancer Res* **11:** S12.

Robinson MD, Smyth GK. 2008. Small-sample estimation of negative binomial dispersion, with applications to SAGE data. *Biostatistics* **9:** 321–332.

Robinson MD, McCarthy DJ, Smyth GK. 2010. edgeR: A Bioconductor package for differential expression analysis of digital gene expression data. *Bioinformatics* **26:** 139–140.

Rosenberg BR, Hamilton CE, Mwangi MM, Dewell S, Papavasiliou FN. 2011. Transcriptome-wide sequencing reveals numerous APOBEC1 mRNA-editing targets in transcript 3′ UTRs. *Nat Struct Mol Biol* **18:** 230–236.

Schmeer CW, Wohl SG, Isenmann S. 2012. Cell-replacement therapy and neural repair in the retina. *Cell Tissue Res* 1–12.

Schrader KA, Heravi-Moussavi A, Waters PJ, Senz J, Whelan J, Ha G, Eydoux P, Nielsen T, Gallagher B, Oloumi A. 2011. Using next-generation sequencing for the diagnosis of rare disorders: A family with retinitis pigmentosa and skeletal abnormalities. *J Pathol* **225:** 12–18.

Schuster SC. 2008. Next-generation sequencing transforms today's biology. *Nat Methods* **5:** 16–18.

Sharon D, Blackshaw S, Cepko CL, Dryja TP. 2002. Profile of the genes expressed in the human peripheral retina, macula, and retinal pigment epithelium determined through serial analysis of gene expression (SAGE). *Proc Natl Acad Sci* **99:** 315–320.

Shendure J, Ji H. 2008. Next-generation DNA sequencing. *Nat Biotechnol* **26:** 1135–1145.

Smyth GK. 2004. Linear models and empirical Bayes methods for assessing differential expression in microarray experiments. *Stat Appl Genet Mol Biol* **3:** 1544–6115.

Soneson C, Delorenzi M. 2013. A comparison of methods for differential expression analysis of RNA-Seq data. *BMC Bioinformatics* **14:** 91.

Stahl PD, Wainszelbaum MJ. 2009. Human-specific genes may offer a unique window into human cell signaling. *Sci Signal* **2:** pe59.

Strunnikova N, Maminishkis A, Barb J, Wang F, Zhi C, Sergeev Y, Chen W, Edwards A, Stambolian D, Abecasis G. 2010. Transcriptome analysis and molecular signature of human retinal pigment epithelium. *Hum Mol Genet* **19:** 2468–2486.

Sui GY, Liu GC, Liu GY, Gao YY, Deng Y, Wang WY, Tong SH, Wang L. 2012. Is sunlight exposure a risk factor for age-related macular degeneration? A systematic review and meta-analysis. *Br J Ophthalmol* **97:** 389–394.

Swaroop A, Zack D. 2002. Transcriptome analysis of the retina. *Genome Biol* **3:** reviews1022.1021–reviews1022.1024.

Syed F. 2010. Application of Nextera technology to RNA-seq library preparation. *Nature Methods* **7:** an2–an3.

Takahashi K, Tanabe K, Ohnuki M, Narita M, Ichisaka T, Tomoda K, Yamanaka S. 2007. Induction of pluripotent stem cells from adult human fibroblasts by defined factors. *Cell* **131:** 861–872.

Tang J, Kern TS. 2011. Inflammation in diabetic retinopathy. *Prog Retin Eye Res* **30:** 343–358.

Tang S, Riva A. 2013. PASTA: Splice junction identification from RNA-Sequencing data. *BMC Bioinformatics* **14:** 116.

Trapnell C, Pachter L, Salzberg SL. 2009. TopHat: Discovering splice junctions with RNA-Seq. *Bioinformatics* **25:** 1105–1111.

Tucker BA, Scheetz TE, Mullins RF, DeLuca AP, Hoffmann JM, Johnston RM, Jacobson SG, Sheffield VC, Stone EM. 2011. Exome sequencing and analysis of induced pluripotent stem cells identify the cilia-related gene male germ cell-associated kinase (MAK) as a cause of retinitis pigmentosa. *Proc Nat Acad Sci* **108:** E569–E576.

Velculescu VE, Zhang L, Vogelstein B, Kinzler KW. 1995. Serial analysis of gene expression. *Science* **270:** 484–487.

Visser L. 2010. What's new in diabetic retinopathy?: Review. *S African J Diabetes Vasc Disease* **7:** 93–98.

Wang ET, Sandberg R, Luo S, Khrebtukova I, Zhang L, Mayr C, Kingsmore SF, Schroth GP, Burge CB. 2008. Alternative isoform regulation in human tissue transcriptomes. *Nature* **456:** 470–476.

Wang Z, Gerstein M, Snyder M. 2009. RNA-Seq: A revolutionary tool for transcriptomics. *Nat Rev Genet* **10:** 57–63.

Wang Y, Guo L, Cai SP, Dai M, Yang Q, Yu W, Yan N, Zhou X, Fu J, Guo X. 2012. Exome sequencing identifies compound heterozygous mutations in CYP4V2 in a pedigree with retinitis pigmentosa. *PLoS ONE* **7:** e33673.

Westenskow PD, Moreno SK, Krohne TU, Kurihara T, Zhu S, Zhang Z, Zhao T, Xu Y, Ding S, Friedlander M. 2012. Using flow cytometry to compare the dynamics of photoreceptor outer segment phagocytosis in iPS-derived RPE cells. *Invest Ophthalmol Vis Sci* **53:** 6282–6290.

Won J, Shi LY, Hicks W, Wang J, Hurd R, Naggert JK, Chang B, Nishina PM. 2011. Mouse model resources for vision research. *J Ophthalmol* doi: 10.1155/2011/391384

Zernant J, Schubert C, Im KM, Burke T, Brown CM, Fishman GA, Tsang SH, Gouras P, Dean M, Allikmets R. 2011. Analysis of the ABCA4 gene by next-generation sequencing. *Invest Ophthalmol Vis Sci* **52:** 8479–8487.

Zhang Y, Erdmann J, Chilton J, Onsongo G, Bower M, Beckman K, Thyagarajan B, Silverstein K, Lamblin AF. 2012. CLIA-certified next-generation sequencing analysis in the cloud. In *BMC Proceedings*, p. P54. BioMed Central Ltd.

Stem Cells as Tools for Studying the Genetics of Inherited Retinal Degenerations

Luke A. Wiley[1], Erin R. Burnight[1], Robert F. Mullins[1], Edwin M. Stone[1,2], and Budd A. Tucker[1]

[1]Stephen A. Wynn Institute for Vision Research, Department of Ophthalmology and Visual Sciences, University of Iowa, Iowa City, Iowa 52242

[2]Howard Hughes Medical Institute, University of Iowa, Iowa City, Iowa 52242

Correspondence: budd-tucker@uiowa.edu

The ability to provide early clinical intervention for inherited disorders is heavily dependent on knowledge of a patient's disease-causing mutations and the resultant pathophysiologic mechanism(s). Without knowing a patient's disease-causing gene, and how gene mutations alter the health and functionality of affected cells, it would be difficult to develop and deliver patient-specific molecular or small molecule therapies. Many believe that the field of stem cell biology holds the keys to the future development of disease-, patient-, and cell-specific therapies. In the case of the eye, which is susceptible to an extremely common late-onset degenerative disease known as age-related macular degeneration, stem cell-based therapies could increase the quality of life for millions of patients worldwide. Furthermore, autologous, patient-specific induced pluripotent stem cells could be a viable source to treat rare Mendelian retinal degenerative diseases such as retinitis pigmentosa, Stargardt disease, and Best disease, to name a few.

The retina is a complex tissue that is responsible for converting light energy into changes in neuronal membrane potential that are then relayed to the brain as trains of action potentials and processed to yield a picture of the surrounding visual environment. Many of the diseases that impair vision occur in the outermost layers of the retina, namely, the photoreceptor layer and the underlying supportive retinal pigment epithelium (RPE). Many of the diseases that will be discussed in this review occur within the area highlighted by the red bracket shown in Figure 1. Although the ability to identify disease-causing genetic mutations has dramatically improved in recent years, it is still challenging to investigate the pathophysiologic mechanisms associated with these mutations because of the inability to obtain samples of diseased tissue from living patients.

Despite this difficulty, the retina is a good candidate for gene and cell replacement therapies for a number of reasons. Compared with other components of the central nervous system, the posterior retina is very accessible to therapeutic delivery via subretinal injection, a procedure that can be performed by most vitre-

Cite this article as *Cold Spring Harb Perspect Med* doi: 10.1101/cshperspect.a017160

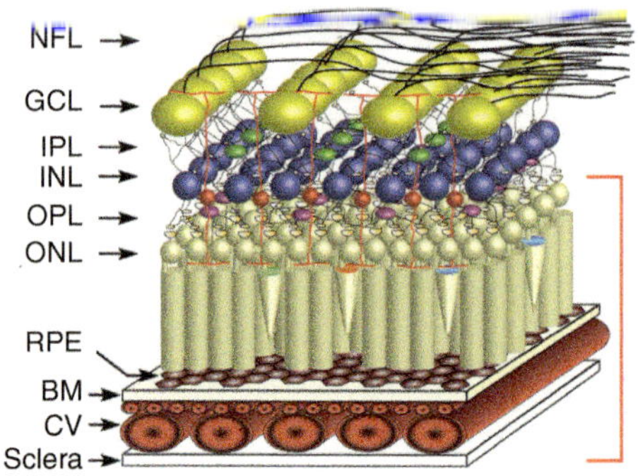

Figure 1. Schematic of the human retina. The major layers of the retina are shown schematically: NFL, nerve fiber layer; GCL, ganglion cell layer; IPL, inner plexiform layer; INL, inner nuclear layer; OPL, outer plexiform layer; ONL, outer nuclear layer; RPE, retinal pigment epithelium; BM, Bruch's membrane; and CV, choroidal vasculature. The photoreceptors, retinal pigment epithelium, and choroidal vasculature (indicated by red bracket on *right* of schematic) are the cell types that are most commonly affected by inherited retinal diseases.

oretinal surgeons. Clinical diagnosis and post-intervention monitoring of the retina are also easier than other parts of the CNS because of transparency of the cornea, lens, and intraocular media.

The cells that comprise the outer retina are highly specified to perform visual processing. Cone and rod photoreceptor cells consist of a cell body and an extremely metabolically active outer segment that is responsible for converting light energy into hyperpolarization of the cell membrane. This phototransduction involves the isomerization of retinoids and the subsequent activation of other signaling molecules in an amplifying cascade (Tang et al. 2013). Hyperpolarization of the photoreceptor cells results in a graded stimulation of bipolar cells, which then cause ganglion cells to send trains of action potentials via their axons in the optic nerves and tracts to the lateral geniculate nuclei in the brain. Photoreceptor outer segments are shed in a diurnal rhythm and then phagocytized, degraded, and recycled by the RPE. The RPE is a polarized monolayer of neuroepithelial origin that is tasked with this phagocytic activity as well as the reisomerization of all-*trans*-retinol to the light sensitive 11-*cis* isomer needed for photon capture in the photoreceptors (Ramsden et al. 2013). Rod photoreceptors cannot survive long without close proximity to healthy, functional RPE. The RPE also provides some nutrients to the photoreceptors and contains pigment that limits light scattering (Ramsden et al. 2013). Both photoreceptor cells and RPE cells are highly metabolic and consume large amounts of oxygen, which is supplied by the lobular, fenestrated capillary bed, the choriocapillaris. The physiological interdependence of photoreceptors, RPE cells, and the choriocapillaris results in the injury of all three of these cell types in most inherited retinal degenerative disorders.

Retinal degenerative disorders are the leading cause of irreversible blindness worldwide (McClements and MacLaren 2013). Some well-studied diseases within this large and heterogenous group are age-related macular degeneration (AMD), retinitis pigmentosa, Stargardt disease, Leber congenital amaurosis, and Best disease, to name just a few. AMD is a complex disorder of older individuals that results from the interaction among a number of genetic loci and the environment (Swaroop et al. 2007; Ryu et al. 2010; Priya et al. 2012). In contrast, retinitis pigmentosa and the other degenerative disorders listed above are Mendelian retinal dystrophies, each caused primarily by the absence or dysfunction of a single gene product. The commonality between AMD and the single gene disorders is that they each are associated with damage to the photoreceptors, RPE, and underlying choroidal vessels. An additional complexity to the single gene disorders is that some of them selectively injure the macula (the cone photoreceptor-rich central area of retina that is responsible for visual acuity), whereas others selectively injure the rod photoreceptor-rich mid-peripheral retina.

For the development of some types of disease-specific therapies, it is first necessary to understand the underlying disease mechanisms and the natural history of the disease in some detail. There are large clinical differences among the diseases listed above, but in addition, there are often significant differences among individ-

 Cite this article as *Cold Spring Harb Perspect Med* doi: 10.1101/cshperspect.a017160

uals affected with the same disease that are traceable to differences in severity of their mutations and the presence or absence of modifying alleles. These factors will cause the ideal therapeutic options to vary from patient to patient, as will the point in the patient's disease course that therapy is being contemplated.

Figure 2 depicts the relationships between various treatment options and the time course and mechanistic understanding of a given patient's disease. When knowledge of disease mechanism is abundant, such as knowing that a person harbors a well-characterized disease allele of high penetrance, preventative measures such as preimplantation genetic testing can be taken. If the disease is already clinically manifest and there is some knowledge of the mechanism of cell loss, drug therapy specifically targeted against mediators of a specific pathway may be applied. Similarly, when specific disease-causing mutations have been identified and there are still viable retinal cells remaining to rescue, gene therapy can be used to replace the mutated gene and restore normal gene function thereby arresting or slowing the progress of the disease. When the disease has progressed to the point that extensive cellular loss has occurred, cell replacement therapy using stem cell technology will be needed to restore useful vision. If autologous induced pluripotent stem cells (iPSCs) were used for such transplantation, the patient's disease-causing mutations would still be present and would be expected to injure the transplanted cells at the same or a faster rate as they did before treatment. However, if the disease-causing gene is first corrected with viral-mediated gene replacement or genome editing, one can take advantage of the near-perfect immunologic match of an autologous transplant without suffering the disadvantage of the disease-causing genotype. Recent advances in genome editing using RNA-mediated clustered regularly interspaced short palindromic repeats (CRISPRs) allow the delivery of corrected, fully functioning cells into diseased tissues (Cong et al. 2013; Joung and Sander 2013). Last, when knowledge of disease mechanism is sparse or in the cases of individuals that have had disease for an extended period of time and undergone near or total loss of photoreceptor cells, RPE, and/or choriocapillaris, optogenetic strategies, or a retinal prosthesis could be viable therapeu-

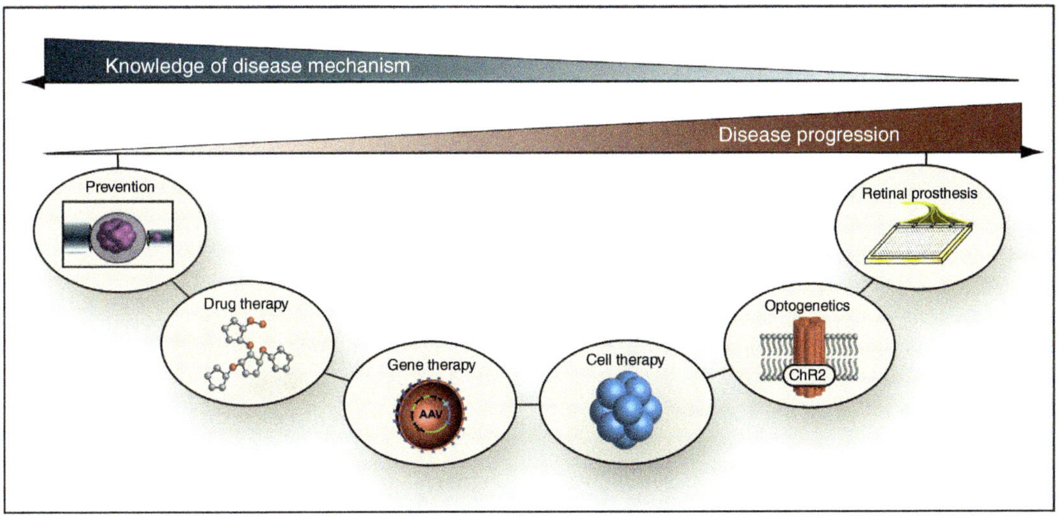

Figure 2. Relationship between knowledge of disease mechanism and disease progression on therapeutic options. Some therapeutic options are more suitable for earlier stages of disease than others. Similarly, some require a precise understanding of the cause and/or mechanism of the disease, whereas others are more generally usable.

tic options to restore some visual function. Optogenetics uses light to trigger responses in genetically targeted groups of cells. In contrast to traditional gene therapy approaches whose goal is to correct a mutated gene and restore normal protein function, optogenetics introduces novel light sensitive proteins into neurons like bipolar cells and ganglion cells to cause them to function as photoreceptors to restore some visual function (Garg and Federman 2013; Packer et al. 2013; Yonehara et al. 2013). Retinal prostheses typically consist of arrays of photodiodes that are surgically implanted beneath or above the retina to electrically stimulate the remaining inner retinal cells (Loudin et al. 2007; Zrenner et al. 2011). Another strategy that is being pursued for patients with very advanced disease is a three-dimensional transplants consisting of stem-cell-derived sheets of photoreceptors and RPE cells grown on a biocompatible polymer scaffold (Zhang et al. 2007; Yao et al. 2011; Tucker et al. 2011a; Shepherd et al. 2013).

USING STEM CELLS TO INTERROGATE PATHOPHYSIOLOGY OF DISEASE

Stem cells, which can be isolated from various tissues during different points in development, have the ability to continually self-propagate and differentiate into multiple cell types. Embryonic stem cells (ESCs), harvested from the inner cell mass of the blastocyst of preimplantation embryos, are classified as pluripotent. That is, they are capable of forming tissues of all three embryonic germ layers: endoderm, mesoderm, and ectoderm. Fetal stem cells are isolated from fetal tissue and are multipotent. They can differentiate into a limited number of cell types depending on their individual degree of differentiation at the time of isolation. Adult stem cells (ASCs) are present in small numbers in most major organs and also display multipotency. For example, ASCs can be found in bone marrow, intestinal crypts, and the eye, near the limbal region posterior to the cornea (Davanger and Evensen 1971; Jiang et al. 2002; Snippert et al. 2010).

Induced iPSCs were originally generated via retroviral transduction of mouse dermal fibroblasts with the transcription factors Oct4, Sox2, Klf4, and c-myc (Yamanaka and Takahashi 2006). They have since been derived from a variety of different tissues and species. Like ESCs, iPSCs have both an unlimited capacity for self-renewal and are pluripotent. They are therefore suitable for tissue-specific cell generation. Our laboratory and others have become proficient in generating retinal progenitor cells (RPCs) from iPSCs and further differentiating them into RPE and photoreceptor cells (Wang et al. 2008; Meyer et al. 2011; Tucker et al. 2011b, 2013a,b). Using these protocols we have recently been able to show that following transplantation into the subretinal space of retinal degenerative hosts, iPSC-derived photoreceptor precursor cells aid in the restoration of retinal structure and function (Tucker et al. 2011b).

Apart from being a promising cell source for autologous transplantation, a major advantage of the iPSC technology is that it provides the ability to model and study human disease in vitro. In particular, iPSCs are a useful tool for confirmation of newly identified disease-causing mutations and interrogation of disease pathophysiology in relatively inaccessible tissues such as the retina that cannot be routinely subjected to molecular analysis in living patients. As shown in Figure 2, the ability to develop an in-depth understanding of disease mechanism will increase the number of therapeutic options available to a physician. The following paragraphs provide an overview of the ways in which iPSCs have been used to model Mendelian diseases such as retinitis pigmentosa and Best disease, as well as complex disorders such as AMD.

MODELING OF MENDELIAN RETINAL DEGENERATIONS

Most inherited retinal diseases are caused by mutations in a single gene. For instance, mutations in the gene *ABCA4* (ATP-binding cassette, subfamily A, member 4), cause a wide spectrum of recessive photoreceptor cell-specific retinal phenotypes including Stargardt disease, cone–rod dystrophy, and even retinitis pigmentosa (RP). ABCA4 is a flippase that facilitates the movement of the visual cycle intermediate, *N*-retinylidene-phosphatidylethanolamine (NR-PE), from the intradiscal leaflet of photoreceptor disc membranes to the cytoplasmic leaflet (Quazi et al. 2012). Once translocated, NR-PE is reduced to vitamin A, transferred to the RPE and reisomerized into 11-*cis*-retinal. When *ABCA4* is mutated, the flippase function of the protein is lost, leading to the formation and accumulation of the insoluble bisretinoid *N*-retinylidene-*N*-retinyl-ethanolamine (A2E). A2E acts similarly to a detergent and is toxic to the RPE and photoreceptors (Schindler et al. 2010; Sheffield and Stone 2011; Braun et al. 2013). Stargardt disease typically presents with reduced visual acuity and a gradually enlarging central scotoma that is associated with the progressive accumulation of autofluorescent deposits of A2E-containing lipofuscin. The age of onset for Stargardt disease can vary from early childhood to adulthood (Schindler et al. 2010). Within the phenotypic spectrum of Stargardt disease, some patients have very severe degeneration, including near complete loss of RPE and cone and rod photoreceptors (resembling retinitis pigmentosa), whereas other individuals have much milder disease in which the foveal photoreceptors are relatively spared and the visual acuity remains quite good for many years. A comprehensive understanding of the function of *ABCA4* and its gene product have facilitated current gene therapy trials designed to deliver wild-type *ABCA4* to patients with this disease (Al-Saikhan 2013; Boye et al. 2013). As indicated above, for patients with extensive photoreceptor cell loss, cell replacement therapy to provide new functional photoreceptor and RPE cells will likely be required. For Mendelian disorders like Stargardt disease, an autologous iPSC-based approach would likely require correction of the disease-causing genetic mutation before cellular transplantation. If left uncorrected, the deleterious effect of the genetic mutation would likely reduce the longevity of the newly transplanted cells. This would likely be especially true for early onset diseases. Although undesirable for cell replacement purposes, as indicated above, one could take advantage of the presence of the mutant alleles in the iPSCs to interrogate disease pathophysiology and develop new treatment strategies.

Unlike *ABCA4*-associated disease, which is relatively well understood mechanistically, a large number of patients' disease-causing genes are either currently unknown or the function of these genes is poorly understood. By using iPSC-derived photoreceptor precursor cells generated from patients with retinal degenerative disease, we were recently able to show that a homozygous Alu insertion, identified in exon 9 of the gene male germ cell-associated kinase (*MAK*), results in loss of the transcript and an inability to produce normal MAK protein (Tucker et al. 2011b). Loss of MAK was found to disrupt normal photoreceptor cell structure leading to cell death and irreversible blindness. In addition to allowing us to confirm pathogenicity of the *MAK* mutation, we were also able to identify and confirm the involvement of a unique *MAK*-specific retinal transcript in disease pathophysiology. This transcript contains an extra 75-bp exon (exon 12), which is phylogenetically conserved. It only exists in transcripts that also contain *MAK* exon 9. Collectively these findings have enabled the development of gene-based interventions for *MAK*-associated RP in which patient-specific iPSC-derived photoreceptor cells are being used to confirm therapeutic efficacy.

In a similar study, iPSC-derived photoreceptor precursor cells were used to confirm the pathogenicity of two *USH2A* mutations in an adult patient with autosomal recessive RP (Tucker et al. 2013b). In this study, keratinocyte-derived iPSCs were differentiated into multilayer eyecup-like structures with an outer-pigmented layer of RPE and an inner layer containing photoreceptor precursor cells. The latter cells expressed photoreceptor-specific markers and showed axonemes and basal bodies structurally characteristic of outer segments. Analysis of the identified *USH2A* transcripts in these cells revealed that one of the patient's mutations causes exonification of intron 40, a translation frameshift and a premature stop codon. Upregulation of the proteins GRP78 and GRP94 suggested that the patient's other *USH2A* variant (a single point mutation resulting in an

Arginine to Histidine transition at position 4192) causes disease through protein misfolding and endoplasmic reticulum (ER) stress. To further support the idea that this disease is ER stress-related rather than a developmental defect, photoreceptor precursor cells were transplanted into 4-d-old immunodeficient *Crb1*$^{-/-}$ mice. Newly integrated patient-derived cells formed morphologically and immunohistochemically recognizable photoreceptor cells, suggesting that the mutations in this patient cause degeneration of developmentally normal photoreceptors. The role of ER stress in RP-associated photoreceptor cell death is consistent with previous findings in other disease causing mutations. For instance, in a similar study, Jin and colleagues were able to show that iPSC-derived rod photoreceptor precursor cells generated from a patient with autosomal dominant rhodopsin-associated RP have elevated levels of ER stress-related proteins and subsequently succumb to apoptic cell death in vitro (Jin et al. 2011).

Unlike RP, which is usually caused by mutations in genes expressed in photoreceptor cells, Best disease results from mutations in the RPE-specific gene, *BEST1*. Best disease selectively affects the region of the human retina within one disk diameter of the fovea and predisposes affected individuals to vision threatening choroidal neovascular membrane formation. Late stages of Best disease are often marked by geographic loss of the RPE underlying the macula. Although *BEST1* mutations have been known to cause this disease for quite some time, the mechanism by which these mutations cause Best disease remain unclear. In an elegant study recently published by Singh et al. (2013), human iPSC-derived RPE were generated from patients and unaffected siblings and used to examine the cellular and molecular processes underlying Best disease. The investigators found that RPE derived from patients with Best disease displayed disrupted fluid flux and increased accumulation of autofluorescent material after long-term feeding of photoreceptor outer segments (Singh et al. 2013). Furthermore, following chronic photoreceptor outer segment feeding, rhodopsin degradation was found to be delayed, cellular responses to calcium were up-regulated, and oxidative stress levels were altered (Abramoff et al. 2013; Singh et al. 2013). Collectively, these findings suggest that *BEST1* plays an important role in photoreceptor outer segment turnover and implicates disruption of this pathway in the pathogenesis of Best disease.

MODELING OF COMPLEX RETINAL DEGENERATIVE DISEASE

AMD is a genetically heterogeneous and complex disease with more than 50 different genetic risk loci identified to date (Gorin 2012; Liu et al. 2012), 19 of which meet genome wide significance (Fritsche et al. 2013). Early AMD typically presents in the sixth decade of life with the formation of lipid-like deposits, commonly referred to as drusen, which can accumulate within and beneath the RPE layer (Curcio et al. 2013). A subset of patients with early AMD later develop geographic atrophy of the retinal pigment epithelium and underlying choriocapillaris, and the loss of these tissues results in the loss of the overlying photoreceptor cells. Other patients with early AMD develop a complication sometimes referred to as "wet AMD" in which the underlying choroidal vasculature grows into the sub-RPE and/or subretinal space forming fenestrated, leaky vascular networks known as choroidal neovascular membranes (CNVs) (Jager et al. 2008). For AMD, all of the therapeutic interventions shown in Figure 2 could eventually come into play. Drug therapy using the antivascular endothelial growth factor (VEGF) agents Avastin and Lucentis have proven very efficacious in ameliorating CNVs and slowing vision loss in wet AMD (Agosta et al. 2012; Scott and Bressler 2013). Because of the fact that AMD is genetically heterogenous, traditional gene augmentation approaches seem less promising than for Mendelian disease. However, cell replacement therapy for patients with loss of photoreceptor, RPE, and choroidal (choriocapillaris) endothelial cells is being pursued by a number of groups and, if successful, would be extremely beneficial for thousands of patients. In very late stage disease, in which significant cell death has occurred, optogenetic and retinal prosthetic approaches may eventually be viable options, although the resolution of the latter devices will need to be improved if they are to offer AMD patients a significant improvement in visual acuity.

The greatest opportunity for AMD treatment lies in understanding the genetic causes and pathogenic mechanisms well enough to be able to identify those who will develop the disease and prevent it from happening through early and efficacious intervention. Although the notion that AMD has a strong genetic component was advocated as early as the 1970s (Gass 1973), our understanding of the biological mechanisms through which specific genetic loci contribute to the development and progression of AMD is still rather poorly understood. Genome wide association studies of AMD identified two loci on chromosomes 1 and 10 that are highly associated with disease risk (Edwards et al. 2005; Haines et al. 2005; Jakobsdottir et al. 2005; Klein et al. 2005; Rivera et al. 2005; Zareparsi et al. 2005; Schwartz et al. 2012). The risk associated with the chromosome 1q locus is predominantly because of a haplotype that harbors a missense mutation in the complement factor H (*CFH*) gene (Tyr402His) (Hageman et al. 2006; Zhang et al. 2008). The complement cascade was implicated in the pathogenesis of AMD before the association of *CFH* variants with the disease (Johnson et al. 2000, 2001; Mullins et al. 2000, 2001; Bora et al. 2005), and thus the involvement of this inhibitor in AMD fits into a mechanistic framework of impaired complement regulation and bystander cell injury (Mullins et al. 2011). In contrast, the mechanism by which the chromosome 10q locus increases AMD risk has been—and remains—controversial. The most common high-risk haplotype contains two genes (*ARMS2* and *HTRA1*) with plausible disease-causing variants. The variants include a nonconservative polymorphism in the *ARMS2* gene (Ala69Ser), a complex 144 bp deletion and a 54 bp insertion in the 3′ untranslated region of the *ARMS2* transcript, and a promoter polymorphism in the *HTRA1* gene (Fig. 3) (Fritsche et al. 2008).

These variants are in strong linkage disequilibrium such that only a few percent of 10q alleles harboring *ARMS2* Ala69Ser lack the *HTRA1* promoter variant and vice versa. This, coupled with the overall genetic complexity of AMD (and the nonspecificity of the AMD phenotype recorded in written clinical records) have made it difficult to determine which, if either, of these two genes is responsible for conferring the AMD risk associated with this locus. Recently, Yang and colleagues (2014) used an unbiased proteome screen of A2E-aged patient-specific iPSC-derived RPE cell lines derived from patients with high and low risk 10q26 loci. They found that cells from patients who were homozygous for the high-risk haplotype had a reduction in superoxide dismutase 2 (SOD2)-mediated antioxidative defense. The investigators concluded that the *ARMS2/HTRA1* risk alleles decrease SOD2 defense, making RPE more susceptible to oxidative damage and thereby contributing to AMD pathogenesis. By elucidating the disease mechanism(s) associated with this locus, new targets for therapeutic intervention have potentially been identified.

CONCLUSION

For genetically heterogeneous retinal diseases like RP, a large number of disease-causing genes and mutations have yet to be identified. Each of these remaining genes is likely to be responsible for a small fraction of patients affected with the

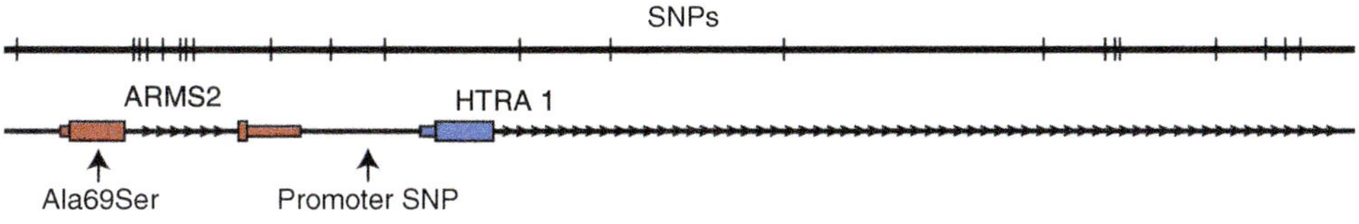

Figure 3. Schematic depiction of the 10q26 risk haplotype and associated mutations.

disease. The *MAK* gene for instance, although enriched in people of Ashkenazi Jewish ancestry, is responsible for only 1% of all cases of RP. To develop treatments for disorders like these, inexpensive model systems that faithfully recapitulate key disease phenotypes are very useful. iPSCs can provide attractive alternatives to animal models. There are now many examples in which patient-specific iPSCs have been found to accurately recapitulate a disease phenotype in a dish. One can use such systems to rapidly interrogate disease pathophysiology and test the efficacy of a variety of different drug- and gene-based therapies.

ACKNOWLEDGMENTS

The authors acknowledge grant support from National Institutes of Health (NIH) Directors New Innovator Award 1-DP2-OD007483-01, NEI EY017451, F32 EY022834, Howard Hughes Medical Institute, Foundation Fighting Blindness, Stephen A. Wynn Foundation, Grousbeck Family Foundation, Leo, Jacques & Marion Hauser Family Vision Restoration Fund.

REFERENCES

Abramoff MD, Mullins RF, Lee K, Hoffmann JM, Sonka M, Critser DB, Stasheff SF, Stone EM. 2013. Human photoreceptor outer segments shorten during light adaptation. *Invest Ophthalmol Vis Sci* **54:** 3721–3728.

Agosta E, Lazzeri S, Orlandi P, Figus M, Fioravanti A, Di Desidero T, Sartini MS, Nardi M, Danesi R, Bocci G. 2012. Pharmacogenetics of antiangiogenic and antineovascular therapies of age-related macular degeneration. *Pharmacogenomics* **13:** 1037–1053.

Al-Saikhan FI. 2013. The gene therapy revolution in ophthalmology. *Saudi J Ophthalmol* **27:** 107–111.

Bora PS, Sohn J-H, Cruz JMC, Jha P, Nishihori H, Wang Y, Kaliappan S, Kaplan HJ, Bora NS. 2005. Role of complement and complement membrane attack complex in laser-induced choroidal neovascularization. *J Immunol* **174:** 491–497.

Boye SE, Boye SL, Lewin AS, Hauswirth WW. 2013. A comprehensive review of retinal gene therapy. *Mol Ther* **21:** 509–519.

Braun TA, Mullins RF, Wagner AH, Andorf JL, Johnston RM, Bakall BB, DeLuca AP, Fishman GA, Lam BL, Weleber RG, et al. 2013. Non-exomic and synonymous variants in *ABCA4* are an important cause of Stargardt disease. *Hum Mol Genet* **22:** 5136–5145.

Cong L, Ran FA, Cox D, Lin S, Barretto R, Habib N, Hsu PD, Wu X, Jiang W, Marraffini LA, et al. 2013. Multiplex genome engineering using CRISPR/Cas systems. *Science* **339:** 819–823.

Curcio CA, Messinger JD, Sloan KR, McGwin G, Medeiros NE, Spaide RF. 2013. Subretinal drusenoid deposits in non-neovascular age-related macular degeneration: Morphology, prevalence, topography, and biogenesis model. *Retina* **33:** 265–276.

Davanger M, Evensen A. 1971. Role of the pericorneal papillary structure in renewal of corneal epithelium. *Nature* **229:** 560–561.

Edwards AO, Ritter R, Abel KJ, Manning A, Panhuysen C, Farrer LA. 2005. Complement factor H polymorphism and age-related macular degeneration. *Science* **308:** 421–424.

Fritsche LG, Loenhardt T, Janssen A, Fisher SA, Rivera A, Keilhauer CN, Weber BHF. 2008. Age-related macular degeneration is associated with an unstable *ARMS2* (*LOC387715*) mRNA. *Nat Genet* **40:** 892–896.

Fritsche LG, Chen W, Schu M, Yaspan BL, Yu Y, Thorleifsson G, Zack DJ, Arakawa S, Cipriani V, Ripke S, et al. 2013. Seven new loci associated with age-related macular degeneration. *Nat Genet* **45:** 433-9–439e1-2.

Garg SJ, Federman J. 2013. Optogenetics, visual prosthesis and electrostimulation for retinal dystrophies. *Curr Opin Ophthalmol* **24:** 407–414.

Gass JD. 1973. Drusen and disciform macular detachment and degeneration. *Arch Ophthalmol* **90:** 206–217.

Gorin MB. 2012. Genetic insights into age-related macular degeneration: Controversies addressing risk, causality, and therapeutics. *Mol Aspects Med* **33:** 467–486.

Hageman GS, Hancox LS, Taiber AJ, Gehrs KM, Anderson DH, Johnson LV, Radeke MJ, Kavanagh D, Richards A, Atkinson J, et al. 2006. Extended haplotypes in the complement factor H (*CFH*) and CFH-related (*CFHR*) family of genes protect against age-related macular degeneration: Characterization, ethnic distribution and evolutionary implications. *Ann Med* **38:** 592–604.

Haines JL, Hauser MA, Schmidt S, Scott WK, Olson LM, Gallins P, Spencer KL, Kwan SY, Noureddine M, Gilbert JR, et al. 2005. Complement factor H variant increases the risk of age-related macular degeneration. *Science* **308:** 419–421.

Jager RD, Mieler WF, Miller JW. 2008. Age-related macular degeneration. *N Engl J Med* **358:** 2606–2617.

Jakobsdottir J, Conley YP, Weeks DE, Mah TS, Ferrell RE, Gorin MB. 2005. Susceptibility genes for age-related maculopathy on chromosome 10q26. *Am J Hum Genet* **77:** 389–407.

Jiang Y, Jahagirdar BN, Reinhardt RL, Schwartz RE, Keene CD, Ortiz-Gonzalez XR, Reyes M, Lenvik T, Lund T, Blackstad M, et al. 2002. Pluripotency of mesenchymal stem cells derived from adult marrow. *Nature* **418:** 41–49.

Jin Z-B, Okamoto S, Osakada F, Homma K, Assawachananont J, Hirami Y, Iwata T, Takahashi M. 2011. Modeling retinal degeneration using patient-specific induced pluripotent stem cells. *PLoS ONE* **6:** e17084.

Johnson LV, Ozaki S, Staples MK, Erickson PA, Anderson DH. 2000. A potential role for immune complex pathogenesis in drusen formation. *Exp Eye Res* **70:** 441–449.

Johnson LV, Leitner WP, Staples MK, Anderson DH. 2001. Complement activation and inflammatory processes in drusen formation and age related macular degeneration. *Exp Eye Res* **73:** 887–896.

Joung JK, Sander JD. 2013. TALENs: A widely applicable technology for targeted genome editing. *Nat Rev Mol Cell Biol* **14:** 49–55.

Klein RJ, Zeiss C, Chew EY, Tsai J-Y, Sackler RS, Haynes C, Henning AK, SanGiovanni JP, Mane SM, Mayne ST, et al. 2005. Complement factor H polymorphism in age-related macular degeneration. *Science* **308:** 385–389.

Liu MM, Chan C-C, Tuo J. 2012. Genetic mechanisms and age-related macular degeneration: Common variants, rare variants, copy number variations, epigenetics, and mitochondrial genetics. *Hum Genomics* **6:** 13.

Loudin JD, Simanovskii DM, Vijayraghavan K, Sramek CK, Butterwick AF, Huie P, McLean GY, Palanker DV. 2007. Optoelectronic retinal prosthesis: System design and performance. *J Neural Eng* **4:** S72–S84.

McClements ME, MacLaren RE. 2013. Gene therapy for retinal disease. *Transl Res* **161:** 241–254.

Meyer JS, Howden SE, Wallace KA, Verhoeven AD, Wright LS, Capowski EE, Pinilla I, Martin JM, Tian S, Stewart R, et al. 2011. Optic vesicle-like structures derived from human pluripotent stem cells facilitate a customized approach to retinal disease treatment. *Stem Cells* **29:** 1206–1218.

Mullins RF, Russell SR, Anderson DH, Hageman GS. 2000. Drusen associated with aging and age-related macular degeneration contain proteins common to extracellular deposits associated with atherosclerosis, elastosis, amyloidosis, and dense deposit disease. *FASEB J* **14:** 835–846.

Mullins RF, Aptsiauri N, Hageman GS. 2001. Structure and composition of drusen associated with glomerulonephritis: Implications for the role of complement activation in drusen biogenesis. *Eye (Lond)* **15:** 390–395.

Mullins RF, Dewald AD, Streb LM, Wang K, Kuehn MH, Stone EM. 2011. Elevated membrane attack complex in human choroid with high risk complement factor H genotypes. *Exp Eye Res* **93:** 565–567.

Packer AM, Roska B, Häusser M. 2013. Targeting neurons and photons for optogenetics. *Nat Neurosci* **16:** 805–815.

Priya RR, Chew EY, Swaroop A. 2012. Genetic studies of age-related macular degeneration: Lessons, challenges, and opportunities for disease management. *Ophthalmology* **119:** 2526–2536.

Quazi F, Lenevich S, Molday RS. 2012. ABCA4 is an *N*-retinylidene-phosphatidylethanolamine and phosphatidylethanolamine importer. *Nat Commun* **3:** 925.

Ramsden CM, Powner MB, Carr A-JF, Smart MJK, da Cruz L, Coffey PJ. 2013. Stem cells in retinal regeneration: Past, present and future. *Development* **140:** 2576–2585.

Rivera A, Fisher SA, Fritsche LG, Keilhauer CN, Lichtner P, Meitinger T, Weber BHF. 2005. Hypothetical *LOC387715* is a second major susceptibility gene for age-related macular degeneration, contributing independently of complement factor H to disease risk. *Hum Mol Genet* **14:** 3227–3236.

Ryu E, Fridley BL, Tosakulwong N, Bailey KR, Edwards AO. 2010. Genome-wide association analyses of genetic, phenotypic, and environmental risks in the age-related eye disease study. *Mol Vis* **16:** 2811–2821.

Schindler EI, Nylen EL, Ko AC, Affatigato LM, Heggen AC, Wang K, Sheffield VC, Stone EM. 2010. Deducing the pathogenic contribution of recessive *ABCA4* alleles in an outbred population. *Hum Mol Genet* **19:** 3693–3701.

Schwartz SG, Agarwal A, Kovach JL, Gallins PJ, Cade W, Postel EA, Wang G, Ayala-Haedo J, Spencer KM, Haines JL, et al. 2012. The *ARMS2* A69S variant and bilateral advanced age-related macular degeneration. *Retina* **32:** 1486–1491.

Scott AW, Bressler SB. 2013. Long-term follow-up of vascular endothelial growth factor inhibitor therapy for neovascular age-related macular degeneration. *Curr Opin Ophthalmol* **24:** 190–196.

Sheffield VC, Stone EM. 2011. Genomics and the eye. *N Engl J Med* **364:** 1932–1942.

Shepherd RK, Shivdasani MN, Nayagam DAX, Williams CE, Blamey PJ. 2013. Visual prostheses for the blind. *Trends Biotechnol* **10:** 562–571.

Singh R, Shen W, Kuai D, Martin JM, Guo X, Smith MA, Perez ET, Phillips MJ, Simonett JM, Wallace KA, et al. 2013. iPS cell modeling of Best disease: Insights into the pathophysiology of an inherited macular degeneration. *Hum Mol Genet* **22:** 593–607.

Snippert HJ, van der Flier LG, Sato T, van Es JH, van den Born M, Kroon-Veenboer C, Barker N, Klein AM, van Rheenen J, Simons BD, et al. 2010. Intestinal crypt homeostasis results from neutral competition between symmetrically dividing Lgr5 stem cells. *Cell* **143:** 134–144.

Swaroop A, Branham KE, Chen W, Abecasis G. 2007. Genetic susceptibility to age-related macular degeneration: A paradigm for dissecting complex disease traits. *Hum Mol Genet* **16:** R174–R182.

Tang PH, Kono M, Koutalos Y, Ablonczy Z, Crouch RK. 2013. New insights into retinoid metabolism and cycling within the retina. *Prog Retin Eye Res* **32:** 48–63.

Tucker BA, Park I-H, Qi SD, Klassen HJ, Jiang C, Yao J, Redenti S, Daley GQ, Young MJ. 2011a. Transplantation of adult mouse iPS cell-derived photoreceptor precursors restores retinal structure and function in degenerative mice. *PLoS ONE* **6:** e18992.

Tucker BA, Scheetz TE, Mullins RF, DeLuca AP, Hoffmann JM, Johnston RM, Jacobson SG, Sheffield VC, Stone EM. 2011b. Exome sequencing and analysis of induced pluripotent stem cells identify the cilia-related gene male germ cell-associated kinase (MAK) as a cause of retinitis pigmentosa. *Proc Natl Acad Sci* **108:** E569–E576.

Tucker BA, Anfinson KR, Mullins RF, Stone EM, Young MJ. 2013a. Use of a synthetic xeno-free culture substrate for induced pluripotent stem cell induction and retinal differentiation. *Stem Cells Transl Med* **2:** 16–24.

Tucker BA, Mullins RF, Streb LM, Anfinson K, Eyestone ME, Kaalberg E, Riker MJ, Drack AV, Braun TA, Stone EM. 2013b. Patient-specific iPSC-derived photoreceptor precursor cells as a means to investigate retinitis pigmentosa. *eLife* **2:** e00824.

Wang S, Girman S, Lu B, Bischoff N, Holmes T, Shearer R, Wright LS, Svendsen CN, Gamm DM, Lund RD. 2008. Long-term vision rescue by human neural progenitors in a rat model of photoreceptor degeneration. *Invest Ophthalmol Vis Sci* **49:** 3201–3206.

Yamanaka S, Takahashi K. 2006. Induction of pluripotent stem cells from mouse fibroblast cultures. *Tanpakushitsu Kakusan Koso* **51:** 2346–2351.

Yang J, Li Y, Chan L, Tsai Y-T, Wu W-H, Nguyen HV, Hsu C-W, Li X, Brown LM, Egli D, et al. 2014. Validation of genome-wide association study (GWAS)-identified disease risk alleles with patient-specific stem cell lines. *Hum Mol Genet* **23:** 3445–3455.

Yao J, Tucker BA, Zhang X, Checa-Casalengua P, Herrero-Vanrell R, Young MJ. 2011. Robust cell integration from co-transplantation of biodegradable MMP2-PLGA microspheres with retinal progenitor cells. *Biomaterials* **32:** 1041–1050.

Yonehara K, Farrow K, Ghanem A, Hillier D, Balint K, Teixeira M, Jüttner J, Noda M, Neve RL, Conzelmann K-K, et al. 2013. The first stage of cardinal direction selectivity is localized to the dendrites of retinal ganglion cells. *Neuron* **79:** 1078–1085.

Zareparsi S, Branham KEH, Li M, Shah S, Klein RJ, Ott J, Hoh J, Abecasis GR, Swaroop A. 2005. Strong association of the Y402H variant in complement factor H at 1q32 with susceptibility to age-related macular degeneration. *Am J Hum Genet* **77:** 149–153.

Zhang Y, Klassen HJ, Tucker BA, Perez M-TR, Young MJ. 2007. CNS progenitor cells promote a permissive environment for neurite outgrowth via a matrix metalloproteinase-2-dependent mechanism. *J Neurosci* **27:** 4499–4506.

Zhang H, Morrison MA, Dewan A, Adams S, Andreoli M, Huynh N, Regan M, Brown A, Miller JW, Kim IK, et al. 2008. The NEI/NCBI dbGAP database: Genotypes and haplotypes that may specifically predispose to risk of neovascular age-related macular degeneration. *BMC Med Genet* **9:** 51.

Zrenner E, Bartz-Schmidt KU, Benav H, Besch D, Bruckmann A, Gabel V-P, Gekeler F, Greppmaier U, Harscher A, Kibbel S, et al. 2011. Subretinal electronic chips allow blind patients to read letters and combine them to words. *Proc Biol Sci* **278:** 1489–1497.

A Review of Secondary Photoreceptor Degenerations in Systemic Disease

Naveen Mysore[1,2], Jamie Koenekoop[2], Shen Li[2], Huanan Ren[2], Vafa Keser[2], Irma Lopez-Solache[2], and Robert K. Koenekoop[1,2,3,4]

[1]Department of Paediatric Surgery, Human Genetics and Ophthalmology, McGill University, Montreal, Quebec H3A 1A1, Canada

[2]McGill Ocular Genetics Laboratory, Montreal, Quebec H3H 1P3, Canada

[3]Faculty of Medicine, Human Genetics, McGill University, Montreal, Quebec H3A 1B1, Canada

[4]Montreal Children's Hospital Research Institute, Montreal, Quebec H3H 1P3, Canada

Correspondence: robert.koenekoop@mcgill.ca

Photoreceptor neuronal degenerations are common and incurable causes of human blindness with one in 2000 affected. Approximately, half of all patients are associated with known mutations in more than 200 disease genes. Most retinal degenerations are restricted to the retina (primary retinal degeneration) but photoreceptor degeneration can also be found in a wide variety of systemic and syndromic diseases. These are called secondary retinal degenerations. We review several well-known systemic diseases with retinal degenerations (RD). We discuss RD with hearing loss, RD with brain disease, and RD with musculoskeletal disease. We then postulate which retinal degenerations may also have previously undetected systemic features. Emerging new and exciting evidence is showing that ubiquitously expressed genes associated with multitissue syndromic disorders may also harbor mutations that cause isolated primary retinal degeneration. Examples are *RPGR, CEP290, CLN3, MFSD5,* and *HK1* mutations that cause a wide variety of primary retinal degenerations with intact systems.

RETINAL DEGENERATION AND SYSTEMIC DISEASE

Photoreceptor degeneration leads to blindness in millions of people and is thought to have a worldwide prevalence of one in 2000. Photoreceptor death and pigmentary retinal degeneration is the final common outcome in many retinal disorders (such as retinitis pigmentosa, RP) and many choroidal disorders (such as choroideremia), but it is also a common and serious manifestation of numerous metabolic, neuro-degenerative and other systemic diseases.

The evaluation of patients with pigmentary retinal degeneration is especially challenging for various reasons. First, the retinal degenerations can be found in babies and infants, and dominate the phenotype early in the disease process, whereas life threatening systemic disease follows

Cite this article as *Cold Spring Harb Perspect Med* doi: 10.1101/cshperspect.a025825

later. Second, the retinal appearance, although highly variable even within families, does not predict the genetic lesion, nor the systemic disease as the fundus picture may represent a primary eye disease, a harbinger of impending neurological disease, a remote effect of cancer, or the beginning of a full blown systemic disease. Third, the genetic heterogeneity underlying primary and secondary photoreceptor degenerations is astounding and unexpected. There are currently 260 gene or loci associated with retinal degenerations. Fourth, as a result of intense genetic, genomic, proteomic, and therapeutic research, this exciting field is rapidly changing and new concepts about the relationship between genotype and phenotype are emerging. Examples of these new concepts will be discussed in this article and include retinal diseases that were thought to be confined to the retina, but after careful phenotyping, turned out to be systemic diseases. That is, *RPGR* mutations cause X-linked RP, but were later found to associate with and cause hearing loss and sinus disease. A second new concept is the emergence of the new knowledge that ubiquitously expressed genes, associated with multisystem systemic disease, can be mutated and associated with primary retinal degeneration without the systemic features. *CEP290* mutations are an important cause of Joubert syndrome, a systemic neurological disorder. Hypomorphic alleles in *CEP290* have been identified as the most common cause of Leber congenital amaurosis (LCA), a primary photoreceptor degeneration (den Hollander et al. 2006).

The retinal dystrophies with a systemic component (sometimes called secondary retinal dystrophies or secondary pigmentary retinopathies) are extensive. We will review three categories of retinal degenerations (RD) with systemic diseases: (1) hearing loss with RD; (2) musculoskeletal disease with RD; and (3) central nervous system (CNS) disease with RD. We will then discuss several eye diseases that turn out to be systemic diseases, followed by a discussion of four ubiquitously expressed genes associated with multisystem disease that were recently found to harbor hypomorphic alleles that cause primary photoreceptor degeneration without the systemic disease.

SYSTEMIC DISEASE WITH SECONDARY RETINAL DEGENERATION

Hearing loss with pigmentary retinopathy are seen with the systemic diseases Usher syndrome (USH), Alström disease, and Refsum disease. Hearing loss is caused by loss or dysfunction of auditory hair cells, whereas vision impairment is caused by death and dysfunction of photoreceptor cells. Both cells are related, are modified ciliated cells from ciliated progenitor cells and their shared vulnerability in many important diseases is not a surprise or coincidence.

USH is the most common form of inherited deaf (hearing loss)-blindness with a worldwide prevalence of nearly one in 6000. Three clinical subtypes (USH1, USH2, and USH3) are defined according to the severity of the hearing impairment, the presence of vestibular dysfunction (ataxia), and the age of onset of the RD, in which type I is profound, type II is partial, and type III is acquired and progressive. All are inherited in an autosomal recessive manner. All three types are genetically heterogeneous conditions and currently 12 USH genes and three loci have been described (see https://sph.uth.edu/retnet/). Genetic complexity is also exhibited in the fact that USH mutations can cause diverse diseases, and genotype–phenotype correlations are not straightforward. For example, USH2A mutations can cause Usher syndrome type 2 (USH2), nonsyndromic RP without hearing loss, and nonsyndromic deafness without blindness, sometimes in the same family (Chen et al. 2014).

The Usher gene products localize to the connecting cilium and periciliary regions of photoreceptors and hair cells, and the Usher proteins form a proteomic network. Photoreceptors, auditory hair cells, and vestibular hair cells develop from ciliated progenitors and are therefore all affected by mutations in Usher proteins. Sperm motility may also be affected, leading to infertility. A generalized abnormality of all Usher disease patients is a ciliary abnormality specifically caused by the cytoskeletal structures of cilia. In mature hair cells of the ear, the disease is likely caused by defects in the Usher proteins that anchor the taller stereocilia's actin cytoskeleton core to the shorter adjacent stereocilia and to the mechanotransduction channels. All the USH1 and USH2 proteins are organized into a protein network by harmonin, whirlin, and SANS (Sorusch et al. 2014). This new proteomic information has contributed greatly to our currently improved understanding of USH protein function in the eye and the ear, and partly explains why defects in proteins of different families cause very similar phenotypes, unlike RP in which the causal genes have a wide variety of different functions (Sorusch et al. 2014). The Usher protein interactome at the periciliary region of the photoreceptor outer segment suggests that Usher proteins regulate protein trafficking between the inner and outer segments of photoreceptors as well as cytoskeletal functions and roles in molecular transport processes and ciliary cargo delivery in photoreceptor cells. USH is thus related to other ciliopathies, including nonsyndromic inner ear defects and isolated retinal dystrophies but also to kidney diseases and syndromes like the Bardet–Biedl syndrome. USH is therefore a "ciliopathy," molecularly related to other ciliopathies, which may open an avenue for common therapy strategies for all ciliopathies.

Currently, there is no treatment for Usher patients, other than augmentation of hearing with hearing aids. Oral antioxidants may slow down retinal disease progression. There is no definitive treatment for the sensory-neuronal degeneration of the eye. In very exciting new developments, gene-based therapies to halt, slow down, or cure the retinal degeneration of USH1 patients are being studied (Nagel-Wolfrum et al. 2014). Three different avenues are currently being tested: (1) USH retinal gene augmentation using recombinant adeno-associated virus; (2) genome editing by homologous recombination mediated by zinc-finger nucleases (ZFN) (Overlack et al. 2012); and (3) read-through therapy using novel designer amino glycosides (Nagel-Wolfrum et al. 2014), as in-frame nonsense mutations account for ~20% of all USH cases. These exciting therapies are slowly entering human clinical trials, and may be applicable to a wide range of ciliopathies, beyond USH. These developments can be followed on the clinical trials web site (see https://clinicaltrials.gov/ct2/search).

Alström disease is an autosomal recessive systemic single gene disorder, caused by mutations in *ALMS1* (2p13). Alström syndrome is a severe, early onset, progressive but variable multisystemic disease, with cone–rod retinal degeneration leading to juvenile blindness, sensorineural hearing loss, obesity, insulin resistance with hyperinsulinemia, and type 2 diabetes mellitus. Very high incidences of additional disease phenotypes that may severely affect prognosis and survival include endocrine abnormalities, dilated cardiomyopathy, pulmonary fibrosis and restrictive lung disease, and progressive hepatic and renal failure. Other clinical features in some patients are hypertension, hypothyroidism, hyperlipidemia, hypogonadism, urological abnormalities, adult short stature, and bone–skeletal disturbances. Most patients show normal intelligence, although some reports indicate delayed psychomotor and intellectual development (Marshall et al. 2007). The visual loss can be so severe and congenital, that it is possible to diagnose a child with severe visual loss at birth, nystagmus and normal systemic features as LCA, and subsequently see the later development of the multisystem disorder and thus Alström syndrome.

The clinical diagnosis of Alström syndrome in an infant or very young child requires the presence of a characteristic infancy onset retinal dystrophy with photodysphoria and either obesity or cardiomyopathy. In childhood, early adolescence, and adulthood, additional phenotypes evolve. Insulin resistant diabetes can occur from puberty and may be preceded by acanthosis nigricans. Triglycerides are often elevated. Many patients develop cardiomyopathy in infancy or adolescence. Recurrent lower respiratory tract infections are common in early childhood and nonalcoholic fatty liver disease develops during puberty. Chronic renal failure is seen in up to 25% of patients during the second decade. Multiple organ fibrosis is found at postmortem (Marshall et al. 2011). Recently, the protein product of the Alström gene, *ALMS1*, has also been localized to cilia and been implicated in endosome trafficking and recycling. Impaired endosome recycling has an impact on cell division, and internalization of protein and lipid products based on external cues (Collin et al. 2012). There have been 98 different disease-causing mutations described thus far including nonsense (49%), indels (43%), frameshifts, and splice site alterations (3%). Both mutations are found in 63% of patients; in 33% only one mutation is found, and in 4% no mutations are found (Marshall et al. 2011).

Finally, classic or adult onset Refsum disease (OMIM 266500) was first described by Norwegian neurologist Sigvald Refsum. It represents an autosomal recessive inborn error of lipid metabolism, classically characterized by a pentad of clinical abnormalities: pigmentary retinal degeneration; hearing loss; peripheral neuropathy; cerebellar ataxia; and elevated protein levels in the cerebrospinal fluid (CSF) without an increase in the number of cells. However, not all patients show all these features. All patients have accumulation of an unusual branched-chain fatty acid and phytanic acid in blood and tissues due a deficiency in phytanoyl-CoA hydroxylase, which is caused by mutations in *PHYH*. Other variable features include cardiac dysfunction, ichthyosis, and multiple epiphyseal dysplasia. Hence, the above clinical features are the result of a buildup of phytanic acid in neurons. As cilia (Usher and Alström) and phytanoyl-CoA hydroxylase (Refsum) are ubiquitous structures and enzymes respectively, it makes sense that these entities are systemic diseases with secondary photoreceptor degenerations. Increased levels of phytanic acid can also be found in the blood and tissues of peroxisomal biogenesis disorders, among which is the infantile Refsum disease (OMIM 601539), a distinct disorder with a different phenotype and a different genotype. However, a phenotype clinically indistinguishable from that of classic Refsum disease (OMIM 614879) but with a different biochemical profile, can be caused by mutation in the gene encoding peroxin-7 (*PEX7*) on chromosome 6q.

Eldjarn and colleagues showed that with a diet free of chlorophyll and other foods, which might contain phytol or phytanic acid, the levels of phytanic acid could be reduced in the blood and the clinical improvements can be documented (Eldjarn et al. 1966). Also, plasmapheresis performed once or twice a month can effectively remove phytanic acid from the body and prevents progression of the clinical features (Gibberd et al. 1979).

The musculoskeletal diseases with pigmentary retinopathy are usually associated with mitochondrial defects and therefore exhibit mitochondrial inheritance (maternal). The disease entities include Kearns–Sayre syndrome and mitochondrial encephalopathy with lactic acidosis and stroke-like episodes (MELAS). Kearns–Sayre syndrome includes chronic progressive external ophthalmoplegia, pigmentary retinopathy, cardiac arrhythmia, cerebellar ataxia, and dementia. MELAS is associated with elevated lactic acid, sensorineural hearing loss, Wernicke's aphasia, encephalopathy, and seizures. The mtDNA deletions that cause Kearns–Sayre syndrome result in the loss of genes important for mitochondrial protein formation and oxidative phosphorylation. The most common deletion removes 4997 nucleotides, which includes 12 mitochondrial genes. Deletions of mtDNA result in impairment of oxidative phosphorylation and a decrease in cellular energy production.

While Kearns–Sayre has typical tapetoretinal degeneration, MELAS shows a diffuse granular and choriocapillaris loss. There is significant outer retinal thinning (de Laat et al. 2013) and in vivo retinal imaging by optical coherence tomography (OCT) show occasional ovoid retinal structures with hyperreflective borders. Mutations in a particular transfer RNA gene, *MT-TL1*, cause >80% of all cases of MELAS. These mutations impair the ability of mitochondria to make proteins, use oxygen, and produce energy. Because mitochondria are found in all the cells of the human body, these defects are expected to cause multisystem disease including the photoreceptors.

The CNS conditions associated with pigmentary retinopathies are Abetalipoproteine-

 Cite this article as *Cold Spring Harb Perspect Med* doi: 10.1101/cshperspect.a025825

mia, Bardet–Biedle syndrome (BBS), Joubert syndrome, Laurence–Moon syndrome (LMS) and neuronal ceroid lipofuscinosis (NCL).

Abetalipoproteinemia (or Bassen–Kornzweig syndrome, BKS) is a monogenic, rare disease with a prevalence of one in a million caused by malabsorption of vitamins A and E in the small intestines. BKS is characterized by fat malabsorbtion, acanthocytosis, and hypocholesterolemia in infancy, with later development of a severe deficiency of fat soluble vitamins and subsequent development of atypical retinal degeneration, coagulopathy, posterior column neuropathy, and myopathy. BKS is an autosomal recessive systemic condition owing to homozygous or compound heterozygous mutations in *MTTP* gene, which encodes the microsomal triglyceride transfer protein, essential for creating beta-lipoproteins. MTTP plays a critical role in the liver and the formation of hepatic very low-density lipoproteins. Lipoproteins are essential for absorption of fats, cholesterol, and fat-soluble vitamins (A and E) from the diet. In BKS, the *MTTP* mutations result in decreased production of beta-lipoproteins in the body, and therefore poor uptake of essential vitamins A and E. Ultra-long-term intake of high dose oral vitamins, including A, E, and K has been documented to slow the progression of the neurological and the retinal degenerative diseases.

Bardet–Biedle syndrome (BBS) is an autosomal recessive and genetically heterogenous systemic syndrome associated with mental or behavioral abnormalities, truncal obesity, polydactyly, hypogonadism, severe renal dysfunction (nephrogenic diabetes insipidus), and retinal degeneration. Although there are multiple genes (currently 18 genes have been described that settle ~70%–75% of the BBS patients) associated with BBS, fundamentally the phenotype is a result of ciliary dysfunction. There are currently two known BBS protein complexes, the BBSome consisting of seven known BBS proteins, and the BBS chaperone complex consisting of three known BBS proteins. The formation of the BBSome requires the function of the BBS chaperone complex. BBS genes exhibit ciliary function, in intracellular and intraflagellar trafficking (IFT). The common primary function of BBS proteins is likely the mediation and regulation of microtubule-based intracellular and ciliary protein transport. Currently, in BBS patients, the cell types known to be impacted by the global ciliary dysfunction include renal and retinal tissues as well as the neural tube, developing limbs, pancreas, liver, spleen, bone, and several parts of the CNS (Zaghloul and Katsanis 2009). Obesity may be related to dysregulated hormonal cues for feeding (ciliary dysfunction in the hypothalamus) as well as increased adipogenesis. Cilia are required in the downstream signaling pathway for Sonic Hedgehog in limb development. In renal development, cilia are required for the cell polarity and orientation of the nephron. Ciliopathies may lead to dysfunctional neuronal migration resulting in mental retardation, however this is not very well understood. The associated retinopathy is caused by photoreceptor death secondary to connecting cilium between the inner segments of the photoreceptors, or a possible defect in vesicular transport. The Lawrence–Moon syndrome is similar phenotypically to Bardet–Biedle syndrome but individuals do not have obesity and polydactyly.

Neuronal ceroid lipofuscinosis (NCL) is a group of conditions that result in accumulation of toxic lipofuscin in neuronal tissues (including the brain, retina, and peripheral nerves). NCL is inherited in an autosomal recessive manner. Infantile NCL or Santavuori disease, caused by mutations in *CLN1* begins between 6 mo and 2 yr, and is associated with muscular hypotonia, ataxia, retinal degeneration, and progressive and rapid mental deterioration. *CLN1* encodes palmitoyl protein thioesterase 1, which participates in various cellular processes, including apoptosis, endocytosis, vesicular trafficking, synaptic function, and lipid metabolism. Palmitoyl protein thioesterase 1 (PPT1) may also be involved in cell death signaling as reduced expression of PPT1 increases the susceptibility to induced apoptosis (Jalanko and Braulke 2009). Late infantile NCL or Jansky–Bielchowsky disease, caused by mutations in *CLN2* presents between the ages 2–4 yr, and has similar findings as the infantile form. *CLN2* encodes tripeptidyl peptidase 1

(TPP1), a lysosomal hydrolase that removes tripeptides from the amino terminus of small polypeptides. The deficiency in TTP1 leads to buildup of lysosomal storage products. Juvenile NCL, caused by mutations in *CLN3* is slowly progressive, and is associated with seizures, but children have normal development. *CLN3* encodes a hydrophobic integral membrane protein. The proposed functions of CLN3 include lysosomal acidification, lysosomal arginine import, membrane fusion, vesicular transport, cytoskeletal linked function, autophagy, apoptosis, and proteolipid modification (Jalanko and Braulke 2009). A deficiency of CLN3 can thus lead to a buildup of lysosomal storage products. In all three conditions of NCL, optic atrophy and pigmentary retinopathy is seen. Interestingly, electron microscopy of skin cells reveals curvilinear bodies in the cytoplasm. In vivo retinal imaging by OCT of the retina shows small hyperreflective bodies at the level of the RPE.

Primary Retinal Degenerations That Are Actually Secondary Retinal Degenerations with Systemic Disease

Bietti's crystalline retinal dystrophy (BCD) is an autosomal recessive retinal degeneration having clinical overlap with choroideremia CHM. BCD represents a severe progressive retinal degeneration with retinal crystals caused by mutations in *CYP4V2*. BCD is a rare disease described by Bietti in 1937, characterized by multiple small crystalline intraretinal deposits (crystals), with retinal pigment epithelium (RPE) atrophy, pigment clumping, and choroidal sclerosis. The crystals are visible on clinical funduscopy, but eventually, as the disease worsens and progresses, the crystals become impossible to see and disappear. Initially thought to be restricted to the retina, BCD crystalline inclusions were surprisingly also found throughout the body, including in the cornea, peripheral blood lymphocytes, and skin fibroblasts, with elevations of fatty acid levels in the serum (Lee et al. 2001). With increased risk factors for cardiovascular disease, BCD has recently been redesignated as a systemic lipid metabolic disease with photoreceptor degeneration. Patients with BCD were found to have a significantly higher concentrations of octadecanoic acid (18:0) but lower concentration of octadecadienoic acid (18:1n-9), while the total monounsaturated fatty acid concentration was significantly lower in BCD as well as lower activity of the **Δ**-9-desaturase enzyme (Lai et al. 2010). Similar to CHM, BCD patients exhibit severe progressive chorio-retinal atrophy and degeneration. However, unlike CHM patients, BCD patients exhibit retinal crystals on fundus exam, systemic crystals, and elevated fatty acid levels.

Having reviewed secondary retinopathies and recently added BCD to the list of secondary pigment degenerations with systemic disease, we can consider the following important question. Are there other primary retinopathies that have a systemic component? In particular, we can consider gyrate atrophy and central areolar choroidal dystrophy. Gyrate atrophy is an autosomal recessive condition, caused by mutations in *OAT*, which encodes ornithine aminotransferase, a ubiquitously expressed gene. Patients with gyrate atrophy have abnormal OAT activity, resulting in elevated levels of ornithine. The retinal findings include punched out round peripheral lesions, forming a scalloped border between normal and abnormal retina. Interestingly, OCT findings reveal possible subretinal crystals (ovoid bodies with hyperreflective borders) (Sergouniotis et al. 2012). Thus, there may be systemic features in gyrate atrophy as *OAT* is expressed in many tissues. Central areolar choriodal dystrophy (CACD) has an autosomal dominant inheritance pattern with mutations in the peripherin-2 (*PRPH2*) gene. Peripherin-2 is thought to play a structural role, stabilizing photoreceptor discs (Smailhodzic et al. 2011). In the early stages of the condition, spectral domain OCT shows disorganization of the photoreceptor layer with thinning of the outer retinal layers. In advanced cases, ovoid structures with similar hyperreflective borders have also been seen (Smailhodzic et al. 2011). Currently there are no observed systemic features in CACD, but the presence of these ovoid bodies, similar to those seen in BCD, may suggest the possibility of finding systemic abnormalities.

 Cite this article as *Cold Spring Harb Perspect Med* doi: 10.1101/cshperspect.a025825

Ubiquitously Expressed Genes Associated with Complex Multitissue Systemic Disease Can Be Mutated in Primary Retinal Degeneration

RPGR Mutations Cause X-linked RP, but Can Also Cause Hearing Loss and Sinus Disease

The first and most commonly mutated gene in X-linked retinitis pigmentosa is *RPGR*, retinitis pigmentosa GTPase regulator protein gene. RPGR predominantly localizes to the transition zone of primary cilia and associates with selected ciliary and microtubule associated protein assemblies. The RPGR interactome facilitates a growing and increasing number of multiple ciliary protein complexes. RPGR is mutated in ~70% of X-linked RP patients and in 10%–20% of simplex RP males, two severe eye diseases confined to the retina. Recently Zito et al., Iannaccone et al. and Koenekoop have documented retinal degeneration patients and families, with significant hearing loss, and pseudo Usher disease, who also developed recurrent sinus disease (Iannaccone et al. 2003; Zito et al. 2003; Koenekoop 2004). In addition, Iannaccone et al. detected RPGR expression in bronchial and sinus epithelial cells. A new concept emerged that some ubiquitously expressed genes can cause isolated retinal degeneration or secondary retinal degeneration plus systemic disease. Severity, location of the mutations, the different isoforms and modifying environment, and background genetic factors may all play a role in this process.

CEP290 Mutations May Be Hypomorphic and Cause Isolated Primary Retinal Degeneration

Mutations in the gene encoding the 290 kDa centrosomal protein (CEP290) cause a surprising, wide ranging, and expanding array of debilitating human and animal diseases ranging from lethal Meckel Gruber disease (meningo-occipital encephalocele, cystic kidney dysplasia, hepatobiliary ductal plate malformation, and postaxial polydactyly), Joubert syndrome (psychomotor delay, hypotonia, ataxia, and "molar tooth sign", indicating hypoplasia of the cerebellar vermis, nephronophthisis and retinal dystrophy), Senior–Loken syndrome (nephronophtisis and retinal degeneration), and Bardet–Biedle syndrome (obesity, psychomotor delay, retinal degeneration, polydactyly, hypogonadism, and renal abnormalities). *CEP290* mutations were also discovered to be the most important and frequent cause of isolated blindness in Leber congenital amaurosis (den Hollander et al. 2006). *CEP290* positive LCA patients have no systemic disease. The type, severity, and location of the mutations in CEP290 do not explain the diversity of associated phenotypes (den Hollander et al. 2006).

How can mutations in a gene be associated with severe multisystem disease, whereas other mutations in the same gene cause isolated retinal degeneration? How the many identified mutations in *CEP290* contribute to these diverse pathologies ranging from lethal multitissue disease to isolated retinal blindness remains unknown, and the protein's normal biological role has not been well characterized. One possibility is the existence of hypomorphic alleles. In the original LCA family with the first CEP290 mutations, it was found that notably in affected patients' lymphoblastoid cell lines harboring the common c.2991 + 1655A → G mutation, a small amount of wild-type CEP290 protein product was found. This suggests that this is a hypomorphic allele, harming the retina but not the other tissues in which CEP290 is expressed (den Hollander et al. 2006).

Another explanation may be that different domains and their inactivation by mutations cause different disease entities. Drivas et al. (2013) discovered four new functional domains of the CEP290 protein. They found that CEP290 directly binds to the cell membranes, through an amino-terminal domain that includes a highly conserved motif, and to microtubules, through a domain located within its myosin-tail homology domain. They also identified that CEP290 activity was regulated by two novel auto inhibitory domains within both the amino and carboxyl termini, both of which were found to play critical roles in regulating ciliogenesis (Drivas et al. 2013). Disruption of the microtubule-binding domain in a mouse model (rd16) of LCA was sufficient to induce significant deficits in cilium formation, which led to isolated retinal degeneration. Drivas et al. (2013) showed that CEP290 is a crucial integral structural and regulatory component of the cilium. Further, their data illustrate, for the first time, that disruption of particular CEP290 functional domains lead to particular disease phenotypes. Also, truncation mutants of CEP290 lacking the inhibitory domains but maintaining the other functional regions of the protein may exhibit normal, or even enhanced, CEP290 function allowing for truncated therapeutic packages delivered by viral vectors such as AAV (Drivas et al. 2013).

In another development, Burnight et al. (2014) report the development of lentiviral vectors carrying full-length *CEP290* for the purpose of correcting the CEP290 disease-specific phenotype in human cells. A lentiviral vector containing CMV-driven human full-length *CEP290* and transduced in iPSC-derived, photoreceptor precursor cells. As CEP290 is important in ciliogenesis, the ability of fibroblast cultures from CEP290-associated LCA patients was tested. They show, for the first time, that lentiviral delivery of CEP290 rescued the ciliogenesis defect.

CLN3 Mutations Can Cause Isolated Primary Retinal Degenerations

CLN3 mutations are known to cause Batten disease, a devastating multitissue disease with neurodegeneration and intracellular accumulation of autofluorescent lipopigment storage material causing progressive dementia, seizures, and progressive visual failure. The *CLN3* gene product may function as a chaperone involved in the folding/unfolding or assembly/disassembly of other proteins, specifically subunit c of the ATP synthase complex. It is expressed ubiquitously, especially strong in the brain and neurons. Wang et al. (2014) found *CLN3* mutations in five isolated retinal degeneration patients, with normal brain and neurological systems. The patients were followed until late adulthood. Wang et al. (2014) suggest that these alleles are hypomorphic, causing retinal disease without affecting the other tissues.

MFSD8 Mutations Can Cause Primary Macular Dystrophy

MFSD8 mutations are well known causes of late infantile neuronal lipoid fuscinosis (NCL). Roosing et al. (2014) found MFSD8 mutations in isolated retinal degeneration patient without systemic disease. They identified variants in *MFSD8* as a novel cause of nonsyndromic autosomal recessive macular disease. Affected individuals showed no neurological features typical for the very late-infantile form of NCL. They propose a ("gene dosage") genotype–phenotype model in which a combination of a severe and a mild variant cause nonsyndromic macular disease, while two severe mutations cause very late infantile neuronal ceroid lipofuscinosis (Roosing et al. 2014).

HK1 Mutations Cause Dominant Retinitis Pigmentosa

HK1 encodes hexokinase 1, a well-known ubiquitous enzyme in the glycolytic pathway of all cells, which catalyzes phosphorylation of glucose to glucose-6-phosphate. HK1 mutations have been found in nonspherocytic hemolytic anemia. Sullivan et al. (2014) recently found dominant HK1 mutations in autosomal dominant retinitis pigmentosa in five families. They hypothesize that the effect of this mutation is limited to the retina, as no systemic abnormalities in glycolysis were detected and that HK1 has a novel function in retina (Sullivan et al. 2014).

In summary, in the study of primary and secondary retinal degenerations and their relationship, several new trends are emerging. Primary photoreceptor degenerations without systemic features are caused by a large number of genes that are crucial to retinal development, functioning, or maintenance. Many genes solely expressed in the eye or retina will not have systemic features, but genes that are expressed elsewhere may in fact cause systemic disease in previously thought to be isolated retinal disease. Bietti crystalline dystrophy represents an example of a primary retinal degeneration that is now known to be a systemic disease with secondary

 Cite this article as *Cold Spring Harb Perspect Med* doi: 10.1101/cshperspect.a025825

retinal degeneration. Other primary retinal degenerations may follow suit, as choroideremia and gyrate atrophy may also be secondary retinal degenerations. In a second new emerging theme, the opposite may also be true. Ubiquitously expressed genes associated with well-known multitissue syndromic disorders (NCL, BBS, JBT, SL, and others) may harbor mutations that cause isolated primary retinal degeneration. *RPGR, CEP290, CLN3, MFSD8*, and *HK1* are examples of recently identified ubiquitous genes that can cause primary isolated X-linked RP, LCA, arRP, arCRD, or adRP, respectively.

ACKNOWLEDGMENTS

We thank the patients for their participation. The authors acknowledge funding and support from Foundation Fighting Blindness (FFB) Canada, Canadian Institutes of Health Research (CIHR), National Institutes of Health (NIH), National Eye Institute (NEI), Fonds de la Recherche en Santé du Québec (FRSQ), Foundation for Retinal Research (FRR), and Reseau de Recherche en Santé de la Vision (to R.K.K.).

REFERENCES

Bietti G. 1937. Ueber familiaeres Vorkommen von 'Retinitis punctata albescens' (verbunden mit 'Dystrophia marginalis cristallinea corneae'), Glitzern des Glaskoerpers und anderen degenerativen Augenveraenderungen. *Klin. Monatsbl. Augenheilkd.* **99:** 737–757.

Burnight ER, Wiley LA, Drack AV, Braun TA, Anfinson KR, Kaalberg EE, Halder JA, Affatigato LM, Mullins RF, Stone EM, et al. 2014. CEP290 gene transfer rescues Leber congenital amaurosis cellular phenotype. *Gene Ther* **21:** 662–672.

Chen X, Sheng X, Liu X, Li H, Liu Y, Rong W, Ha S, Liu W, Kang X, Zhao K, et al. 2014. Targeted next-generation sequencing reveals novel *USH2A* mutations associated with diverse disease phenotypes: Implications for clinical and molecular diagnosis. *PLoS ONE* **9:** e105439.

Collin GB, Marshall JD, King BL, Milan G, Maffei P, Jagger DJ, Naggert JK. 2012. The Alström syndrome protein, ALMS1, interacts with α-actinin and components of the endosome recycling pathway. *PLoS ONE* **7:** e37925.

de Laat P, Smeitink JA, Janssen MC, Keunen JE, Boon CJ. 2013. Mitochondrial retinal dystrophy associated with the m.3243A>G mutation. *Ophthalmology* **120:** 2684–2696.

den Hollander AI, Koenekoop RK, Yzer S, Lopez I, Arends ML, Voesenek KE, Zonneveld MN, Strom TM, Meitinger T, Brunner HG, et al. 2006. Mutations in the *CEP290* (*NPHP6*) gene are a frequent cause of Leber congenital amaurosis. *Am J Hum Genet* **79:** 556–561.

Drivas TG, Holzbaur EL, Bennett J. 2013. Disruption of CEP290 microtubule/membrane-binding domains causes retinal degeneration. *J Clin Invest* **123:** 4525–4539.

Eldjarn L, Try K, Stokke O, Munthe-Kaas AW, Refsum S, Steinberg D, Avigan J, Mize C. 1966. Dietary effects on serum-phytanic-acid levels and on clinical manifestations in heredopathia atactica polyneuritiformis. *Lancet* **1:** 691–693.

Gibberd FB, Billimoria JD, Page NG, Retsas S. 1979. Heredopathia atactica polyneuritiformis (Refsum's disease) treated by diet and plasma-exchange. *Lancet* **1:** 575–578.

Iannaccone A, Breuer DK, Wang XF, Kuo SF, Normando EM, Filippova E, Baldi A, Hiriyanna S, MacDonald CB, Baldi F, et al. 2003. Clinical and immunohistochemical evidence for an X linked retinitis pigmentosa syndrome with recurrent infections and hearing loss in association with an *RPGR* mutation. *J Med Genet* **40:** e118.

Jalanko A, Braulke T. 2009. Neuronal ceroid lipofuscinoses. *Biochim Biophys Acta* **1793:** 697–709.

Koenekoop RK. 2004. An overview of Leber congenital amaurosis: A model to understand human retinal development. *Surv Ophthalmol* **49:** 379–398.

Lai TY, Chu KO, Chan KP, Ng TK, Yam GH, Lam DS, Pang CP. 2010. Alterations in serum fatty acid concentrations and desaturase activities in Bietti crystalline dystrophy unaffected by *CYP4V2* genotypes. *Invest Ophthalmol Vis Sci* **51:** 1092–1097.

Lee J, Jiao X, Hejtmancik JF, Kaiser-Kupfer M, Gahl WA, Markello TC, Guo J, Chader GJ. 2001. The metabolism of fatty acids in human Bietti crystalline dystrophy. *Invest Ophthalmol Vis Sci* **42:** 1707–1714.

Marshall JD, Beck S, Maffei P, Naggert JK. 2007. Alström syndrome. *Eur J Hum Genet* **15:** 1193–1202.

Marshall JD, Maffei P, Beck S, Barrett TG, Paisey RB. 2011. Clinical utility gene card for: Alström syndrome. *Eur J Hum Genet* **19:** 1108.

Nagel-Wolfrum K, Baasov T, Wolfrum U. 2014. Therapy strategies for Usher syndrome type 1C in the retina. *Adv Exp Med Biol* **801:** 741–747.

Overlack N, Goldmann T, Wolfrum U, Nagel-Wolfrum K. 2012. Gene repair of an Usher syndrome causing mutation by zinc-finger nuclease mediated homologous recombination. *Invest Ophthalmol Vis Sci* **53:** 4140–4146.

Roosing S, van den Born LI, Sangermano R, Banfi S, Koenekoop RK, Zonneveld-Vrieling MN, Klaver CC, van Lith-Verhoeven JJ, Cremers FP, den Hollander AI, et al. 2014. Mutations in MFSD8, encoding a lysosomal membrane protein, are associated with nonsyndromic autosomal recessive macular dystrophy. *Ophthalmology.* doi: 10.1016/j.ophtha.2014.07.040.

Sergouniotis PI, Davidson AE, Lenassi E, Devery SR, Moore AT, Webster AR. 2012. Retinal structure, function, and molecular pathologic features in gyrate atrophy. *Ophthalmology* **119:** 596–605.

Smailhodzic D, Fleckenstein M, Theelen T, Boon CJ, van Huet RA, van de Ven JP, Den Hollander AI, Schmitz-

Valckenberg S, Hoyng CB, Weber BH, et al. 2011. Central areolar choroidal dystrophy (CACD) and age-related macular degeneration (AMD): Differentiating characteristics in multimodal imaging. *Invest Ophthalmol Vis Sci* **52:** 8908–8918.

Sorusch N, Wunderlich K, Bauss K, Nagel-Wolfrum K, Wolfrum U. 2014. Usher syndrome protein network functions in the retina and their relation to other retinal ciliopathies. *Adv Exp Med Biol* **801:** 527–533.

Sullivan LS, Koboldt DC, Bowne SJ, Lang S, Blanton SH, Cadena EL, Avery CE, Lewis RA, Webb-Jones K, Wheaton DK, et al. 2014. A dominant mutation in hexokinase 1 (HK1) causes retinitis pigmentosa. *Invest Ophthalmol Vis Sci* doi:10.1167/iovs.14-15419.

Wang F, Wang H, Tuan HF, Nguyen DH, Sun V, Keser V, Bowne SJ, Sullivan LS, Luo H, Zhao L, et al. 2014. Next generation sequencing-based molecular diagnosis of retinitis pigmentosa: Identification of a novel genotype-phenotype correlation and clinical refinements. *Hum Genet* **133:** 331–345.

Zaghloul NA, Katsanis N. 2009. Mechanistic insights into Bardet-Biedl syndrome, a model ciliopathy. *J Clin Invest* **119:** 428–437.

Zito I, Downes SM, Patel RJ, Cheetham ME, Ebenezer ND, Jenkins SA, Bhattacharya SS, Webster AR, Holder GE, Bird AC, et al. 2003. *RPGR* mutation associated with retinitis pigmentosa, impaired hearing, and sinorespiratory infections. *J Med Genet* **40:** 609–615.

Clinical Characteristics and Current Treatment of Age-Related Macular Degeneration

Yoshihiro Yonekawa and Ivana K. Kim

Retina Service, Department of Ophthalmology, Massachusetts Eye and Ear Infirmary, Harvard Medical School, Boston, Massachusetts 02114

Correspondence: Ivana_Kim@meei.harvard.edu

Age-related macular degeneration (AMD) is a multifactorial degeneration of photoreceptors and retinal pigment epithelium. The societal impact is significant, with more than 2 million individuals in the United States alone affected by advanced stages of AMD. Recent progress in our understanding of this complex disease and parallel developments in therapeutics and imaging have translated into new management paradigms in recent years. However, there are many unanswered questions, and diagnostic and prognostic precision and treatment outcomes can still be improved. In this article, we discuss the clinical features of AMD, provide correlations with modern imaging and histopathology, and present an overview of treatment strategies.

Age-related macular degeneration (AMD) is a multifactorial maculopathy characterized by late-onset progressive neurodegeneration of photoreceptors and retinal pigment epithelium (RPE) (Miller 2013). AMD is the leading cause of irreversible blindness in older individuals of industrialized nations. In the United States alone, it was estimated that more than 9 million people had AMD in 2000, of which nearly 2 million were in advanced stages (Friedman et al. 2004). These figures were projected to more than double by 2020. The World Health Organization indicates that AMD ranks third after cataract and glaucoma as a leading cause of blindness globally (WHO 2013).

AMD is typically classified into two phenotypic categories: nonneovascular (dry; nonexudative), and neovascular (wet; exudative). Nonneovascular AMD is characterized by small, yellow, round deposits called drusen at the level of the RPE. Other changes include focal RPE hyperpigmentation and atrophy. When atrophic areas become confluent, the condition is termed geographic atrophy, which is considered an advanced stage of nonexudative AMD. Neovascular AMD is also an advanced form of AMD, and occurs when abnormal blood vessels grow beneath the neurosensory retina or RPE.

Although only 10% of patients with AMD have the neovascular form, it formerly caused ~90% of AMD-related blindness (Ferris et al. 1984). The past decade has seen revolutionary advances in the treatment of neovascular AMD with anti-vascular endothelial growth factor (VEGF) agents. Numerous basic, translational, and clinical studies are underway to further im-

Cite this article as *Cold Spring Harb Perspect Med* doi: 10.1101/cshperspect.a017178

prove these outcomes and lessen treatment burden.

RISK FACTORS

Demographic Risk Factors

Age is the strongest risk factor for development and progression of all forms of AMD. The Eye Diseases Prevalence Research Group pooled data from seven regional population-based studies and applied the rates to the 2000 United States Census (Friedman et al. 2004). The prevalence of intermediate AMD (at least one druse 125 μm or larger in one or both eyes) was 5.4% in 60- to 64-year old people, 7.4% in 65–69-year old people, 10.2% in 70–74-year old people, 14.1% in 75- to 79-year old people, and 23.6% in those 80 or older. The respective rates of geographic atrophy were 0.3%, 0.5%, 0.9%, 1.8%, and 6.9%. The respective rates of neovascular AMD were 0.4%, 0.6%, 1.2%, 2.2%, and 8.2%.

Advanced AMD (neovascular AMD and geographic atrophy) has been shown to be more frequent in Caucasians. In the Baltimore Eye Study (BES), 30% of bilateral blindness was caused by AMD in Caucasians, whereas none of the African Americans became bilaterally blind from AMD (Sommer et al. 1991). The Eye Diseases Prevalence Research Group pooled data from the Baltimore Eye Study, Barbados Eye Study, and the Salisbury Eye Evaluation Project, and showed that African Americans, similar to Caucasians, have a steady increase in large drusen and advanced AMD with age (Friedman et al. 2004). However, the exponential increase later in life is not observed in African Americans. Latinos appear to have high prevalence of early AMD but not advanced AMD (Varma et al. 2004), and Asians have relatively similar rates to Caucasians (Kawasaki et al. 2010).

Environmental Risk Factors

Smoking is an important modifiable risk factor for AMD. The Age-Related Eye Disease Study (AREDS) was a randomized study that examined the effects of high-dose antioxidants and zinc as a treatment for AMD. From the 4519 subjects enrolled in the risk factor analyses, the AREDS showed that those who had ever smoked had almost double the risk for neovascular AMD compared with those who had never smoked (AREDS-Study-Group 2000). The Physicians' Health Study involved 21,157 participants and showed that current smokers of 20 or more cigarettes per day had double the risk of developing AMD compared with never-smokers (Christen et al. 1996). The Nurses' Health Study analysis of 31,843 women showed similar findings (Seddon et al. 1996).

Systemic Risk Factors

The association between AMD and cardiovascular disease has been observed, but it remains equivocal whether cardiovascular disease is an independent risk factor for AMD. Some large studies have shown that carotid atherosclerotic lesions increase the risk for AMD (Vingerling et al. 1995), although others have not (Klein et al. 2013). Cerebrovascular disease overall does not seem to be a strong risk factor (Goldberg et al. 1988; Eye-Disease-Case-Control-Study-Group 1992; Klein et al. 1993; Vinding 1995; Vingerling et al. 1995). A larger number of epidemiological studies have implicated hypertension as a risk factor (Sperduto and Hiller 1986; Goldberg et al. 1988; Hyman et al. 2000; Klein et al. 2003; van Leeuwen et al. 2003) compared to those that did not (Eye-Disease-Case-Control-Study-Group 1992; Klein et al. 1993). Studies investigating gene-environment interactions may provide a better understanding of the role of cardiovascular disease in AMD (Feehan et al. 2011).

CLINICAL FEATURES

Normal Aging

The macula undergoes a spectrum of subclinical changes in the normally aging eye. In a subset of individuals, these changes progress to more pathologically significant findings and manifest clinically as AMD (Zarbin 2004). Healthy young maculae normally have a sharp foveal light reflex on biomicroscopy, caused by the concave shape of the fovea. As the macula ages, this reflex becomes blunted, possibly owing to the decrease in photoreceptor density, shallowing of the foveal pit, and enlargement of the capillary-free zone (Laatikainen and Larinkari 1977). Several small, well-defined drusen will usually be present in the elderly (Klein et al. 1992). Irregularity of the RPE also causes a stippled background of varying degrees.

Morphologic changes are abundant in the normally aging macula. The photoreceptor drop-out during aging is mostly caused by loss of rods (Curcio et al. 1993); foveal cone density appears to remain constant until beyond the ninth decade (Feeney-Burns et al. 1990; Curcio et al. 1993). The outer segments of the rods become disorganized and may accumulate at the apices of the RPE (Feeney-Burns et al. 1990).

The RPE is vulnerable to age-related changes because it is a nonreplicating tissue. For the entire lifespan of the eye, it continually engulfs photoreceptor discs and material from surrounding photoreceptors and RPE cells; it also undergoes autophagy of its cellular contents. Undigested material remains as lipofuscin, a granular lipid-containing pigment containing a mixture of fluorescent cellular byproducts, which exponentially increases with aging (Feeney-Burns et al. 1980). As lipofuscin accumulates in the RPE, cytoplasmic space and metabolic capacity become limited, and the RPE deteriorates over time (Panda-Jonas et al. 1996).

The basal infoldings of the RPE are also reduced from striated cuticular or basal laminar deposits (BLamD) that start to accumulate between the RPE basal plasma membrane and the underlying basement membrane. BLamD are uniformly seen by the seventh decade of life (Sarks 1976) and are composed of lipoproteins and amyloid β. They are considered normal aging changes if they are focal lesions (Miller 2013). Clinically, early forms of BLamD can appear as small, well-circumscribed, "hard" drusen. They may have a translucent appearance if clustered together and viewed with retroillumination on biomicroscopy for middle-aged individuals. However, BLamD are often not directly visible on clinical funduscopy and represent more of a histopathologic finding. An eye with early BLamD typically has a normal clinical fundus appearance. BLamD are distinct from basal linear deposits (BLinD), which are specific histopathologic findings of AMD. Whereas BLamD accumulate between the RPE plasma membrane and the RPE basement membrane (in the sub-RPE space), BLinD are located deeper beneath the RPE basement membrane at the level of Bruch's membrane (Miller 2013).

Early and Intermediate AMD

The aforementioned morphologic changes of the aging fundus are clinically benign. There are several features that characterize the tipping point toward the pathologic state of AMD. In AMD with RPE degeneration, the patchy BLamD seen in normal aging develop an overlying layer of a diffuse, thick, amorphous, hyalinized material, which can become nodular elevations (Bressler et al. 1994). Clinical correlation of this late form of BLamD has not been accurately established, but its presence can be inferred by pigmentary changes (Sarks et al. 2007). Focal areas of hyperpigmentation correlate histologically with RPE hypertrophy and pigmented cells that migrate to the sub-RPE and subretinal space. These pigmented cells may also migrate into the outer nuclear layer, and represent compromised RPE cells that can no longer support photoreceptors.

BLinD form layers of membranous debris within Bruch's membrane, between the RPE basement membrane and the inner collagenous layer. BLinD are thought to be primarily composed of lipoprotein particles (Sarks et al. 1980). These layers accumulate and clinically appear as soft drusen that are characteristic of AMD (Fig. 1) (Sarks et al. 2007). Multilayered BLinD cause a separation of the RPE from Bruch's membrane, and blood, serous fluid, and choroidal neovascular membranes can make their way into this space. However, BLinD can also accumulate as focal aggregations of basal mounds between the RPE basement membrane and plasma membrane (Sarks et al. 1988). BLinD do not manifest as drusen in this type of accumulation, but may cause pigmentary changes and primary geographic atrophy without drusen on clinical examination (Sarks et al. 2007).

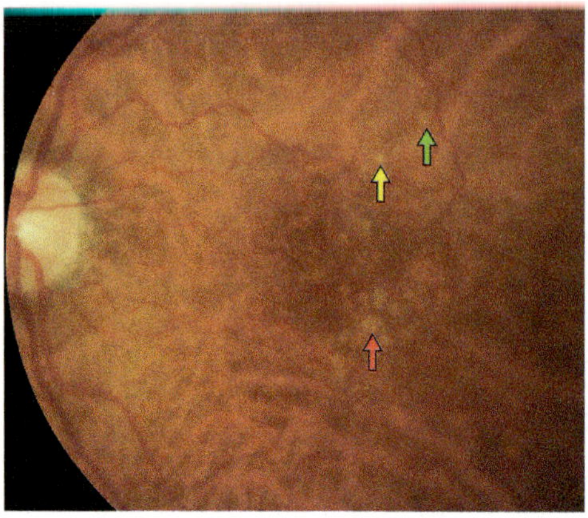

Figure 1. Color fundus photograph of drusen in nonneovascular age-related macular degeneration. There are small (<63 μm, green arrow), intermediate (63–124 μm, yellow arrow), and large (≥125 μm [average diameter of retinal venule at the optic disc margin], red arrow) drusen.

Reticular Pseudodrusen

Reticular pseudodrusen (or subretinal drusenoid deposits) represent a subphenotype of AMD that was first identified on blue-light (red-free) fundus photography (Mimoun et al. 1990). They clinically appear as yellowish, faint, interlacing networks that most commonly occur along the arcades, and do not fluoresce on fluorescein angiography. Fluorescein sodium is a yellow, synthetic salt dye. Its molecules excite when exposed to blue light (wavelengths 485–500 nm), and emit a green light (520–535 nm) as it returns to its original state. For retinal imaging, fluorescein is injected intravenously, and serial fundus photographs or videos are taken using a green filter.

Imaging with optical coherence tomography (OCT), particularly spectral domain OCT, (SD-OCT) has been shown to be effective at detecting reticular pseudodrusen. OCT is a noncontact imaging apparatus that projects infrared light onto the retina and detects backscattered light, which is converted into high-resolution cross-sectional images that can be reconstructed into three dimensional thickness maps. SD-OCT systems have scanning rates of 20,000–40,000 axial scans per sec, with axial resolution of 5 μm. Hyperreflective materials include the nerve fiber layer, plexiform layers, RPE, and blood, whereas the nuclear layers, photoreceptors, and fluid appear hyporeflective. In patients with AMD, intraretinal fluid, subretinal fluid, and pigment epithelial detachments can be visualized with exquisite detail not previously possible with biomicroscopy.

SD-OCT imaging of reticular pseudodrusen shows numerous drusenoid deposits above the RPE in the subretinal space (Fig. 2) (Schmitz-Valckenberg et al. 2010; Zweifel et al. 2010). This is contrary to previous histopathologic studies that localized the changes to the choroid. The origin of these lesions remains unclear, but may represent direct photoreceptor damage. Reticular pseudodrusen were initially associated with neovascular AMD (Arnold et al. 1995; Cohen et al. 2007), but recent studies show that they also represent a risk factor for progression to geographic atrophy (Klein et al. 2008b; Pumariega et al. 2011).

Geographic Atrophy

Geographic atrophy is a late manifestation of nonneovascular AMD and is clinically characterized by a sharply delineated area of depigmentation revealing the underlying choroidal vasculature (Fig. 3). Most cases of geographic atrophy develop in areas previously noted to have large drusen. The life cycle of long-standing drusen is commonly characterized by the initial development of hyperpigmentation, followed by hypopigmentation as the drusen regress, and finally geographic atrophy (Klein et al. 2008a). In the AREDS, sites that developed geographic atrophy were preceded by drusen in 100%, large drusen in 96%, confluent drusen in 94%, hyperpigmentation in 96%, hypopigmentation in 82%, and refractile bodies in 23% of patients. The time of progression to geographic atrophy varied from 5.9 yr for confluent drusen to 2.5 yr for hypopigmentation or refractile bodies. The spread of atrophy can progress around the fovea in a continuous ring or in several patches perifoveally. Geographic atrophy usually does not affect the center of vision (fixation) until later stages.

Geographic atrophy on fluorescein angiography appears as sharply demarcated areas of

Cite this article as *Cold Spring Harb Perspect Med* doi: 10.1101/cshperspect.a017178

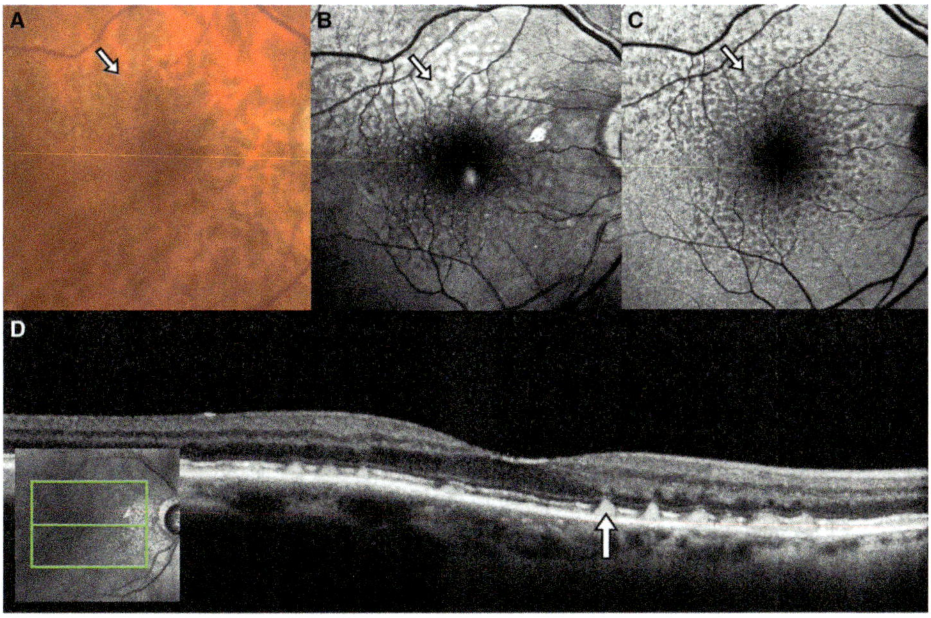

Figure 2. Multimodal imaging of reticular pseudodrusen (arrows). (*A*) Color fundus photograph showing yellowish interlacing networks that extend to the vascular arcades. (*B*) Red-free fundus photography most clearly demonstrates the pseudodrusen as bright spots and the interlacing networks that appear hyporeflective. (*C*) Fundus autofluorescence shows that the lesions are hypoautofluorescent. (*D*) Spectral-domain optical coherence tomography demonstrates that the pseudodrusen are located between the retina and retinal pigment epithelium (RPE), rather than the sub-RPE localization of typical drusen.

hyperfluorescence during the transit phase because of transmission from the underlying choroidal vasculature. On SD-OCT, areas of geography atrophy are characterized by loss of the external limiting membrane, inner/outer segment junction (or ellipsoid zone), and the RPE-Bruch's membrane complex. Because of the lack of RPE, there is often enhancement of the underlying choroidal reflectivity.

Fundus autofluorescence has been popularized as an accurate tool for monitoring the progression of geographic atrophy (Fig. 3). Autofluorescence refers to light-emitting properties of certain tissues in their natural state. The main fluorophore of RPE lipofuscin is A2E, a pyridinium bisretinoid conjugate containing two vitamin A aldehyde molecules and one ethanolamine molecule. Lipofuscin can respond to excitation by wavelengths 300–500 nm, with emission of 620–630 nm. Autofluorescence can be captured with a fundus camera equipped with the appropriate filters or more commonly now with a scanning laser ophthalmoscope. Lesions with increased lipofuscin result in hyperautofluorescence, and a decrease of lipofuscin or absence of RPE results in hypoautofluorescence. In geographic atrophy, the atrophic areas appear as sharply demarcated areas of loss of autofluorescence, corresponding to areas of RPE loss and therefore lack of lipofuscin. Studies have demonstrated that hyperautofluorescence of the junction between atrophic and nonatrophic areas is predictive of subsequent enlargement of the geographic atrophy, and that patches of hyperautofluorescence in the posterior pole precede new areas of atrophy (Holz et al. 2001; Schmitz-Valckenberg et al. 2006). This is thought to be from lipofuscin overload in dysfunctional RPE cells.

Neovascular AMD

Choroidal neovascularization (CNV) is the defining characteristic of neovascular AMD. The

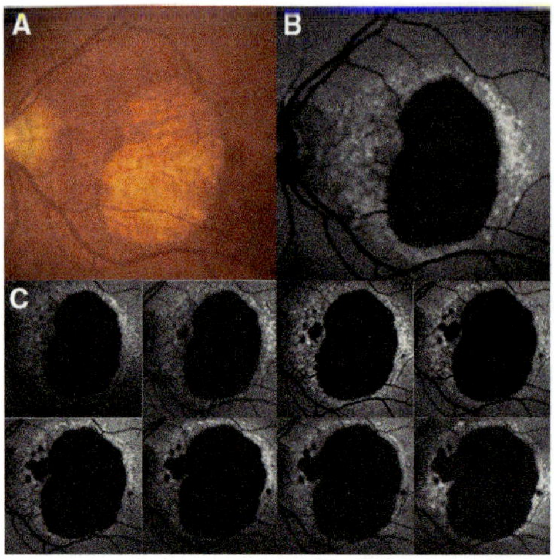

Figure 3. Geographic atrophy in advanced nonneovascular age-related macular degeneration. (*A*) Color fundus photograph of central geographic atrophy. (*B*) The corresponding fundus autofluorescence delineates the kidney-shaped area of atrophy as hypoautofluorescent (dark). However, it also shows that the surrounding clinically normal-appearing retina is hyperautofluorescent, which indicates an accumulation of lipofuscin. (*C*) Over the course of the next 6 years, the geographic atrophy gradually extends to the areas that were hyperautofluorescent in (*B*). (Reprinted, with permission, from Schmitz-Valckenberg et al. 2009.)

CNV grows through breaks in Bruch's membrane and expands beneath the RPE (type I CNV), or between the RPE and photoreceptors (type II CNV). The incompetent endothelial cells of the new vasculature cause fluid leakage and accumulation of proteins and lipids. The new friable vessels are also prone to hemorrhage. Type I CNV typically manifests clinically as a fibrovascular retinal pigment epithelial detachment (PED). The typical clinical appearance of type II CNV is a gray-green lesion beneath the retina with overlying retinal thickening. Subretinal and intraretinal fluid, lipid exudates, and subretinal hemorrhage may accompany both types of CNV.

Fluorescein angiography is the gold standard for diagnosing CNV. Angiography can provide valuable data in distinguishing CNV from other potential causes of retinal edema such as diabetic macular edema and pseudophakic cystoid macular edema. The angiographic term "classic" CNV refers to a well-demarcated area of hyperfluorescence that manifests in the early phases of the angiography. In the intermediate and late phases, there is typically intense leakage from the lesion (Fig. 4A–C). This pattern correlates with type II CNV. "Occult" (type I) CNV has two patterns: (1) fibrovascular PEDs or (2) leakage from an undetermined source, characterized by an ill-defined focus of choroidal leakage without identifiable classic CNV or fibrovascular PED (Fig. 4D–F).

PEDs are focal areas that appear as elevations of the RPE on bimicroscopy. Visual acuity is relatively preserved compared with neurosensory detachments, as long as there is no overlying neurosensory detachment. There are several different types of PED: fibrovascular, drusenoid, and serous. Fibrovascular PEDs are associated with underlying CNV, whereas drusenoid PEDs are not, and serous PEDs may be seen in both scenarios.

Fibrovascular PEDs demonstrate early mottled or granular hyperfluorescence on fluorescein angiography with mild late leakage. Fibrovascular PEDs may be associated with blood. Hemorrhage localized to the sub-RPE space of the PED will appear as dark greenish-red elevations, but the blood may also track into the subretinal space and, rarely, into the vitreous. Patients with predominantly hemorrhagic PEDs often present with poor visual acuity (Bressler et al. 2004).

Drusenoid PEDs are slowly enlarging; shallow elevations of the RPE with scalloped borders that are thought to develop from the coalescence of soft drusen. They have better short-term visual outcomes compared to the other types of PEDs (Hartnett et al. 1992), but 42% of eyes with drusenoid PEDs eventually progressed to either geographic atrophy or neovascular AMD by 5 yr in the AREDS, with associated decline in vision (Cukras et al. 2010). On fluorescein angiography, there is delayed, gradual, mild staining deep to the RPE with no leakage, and drusenoid PEDs do not become intensely fluorescent as do serous PEDs. Compared with fibrovascular PEDs, drusenoid PEDs are smaller, shallower, and have irregular borders.

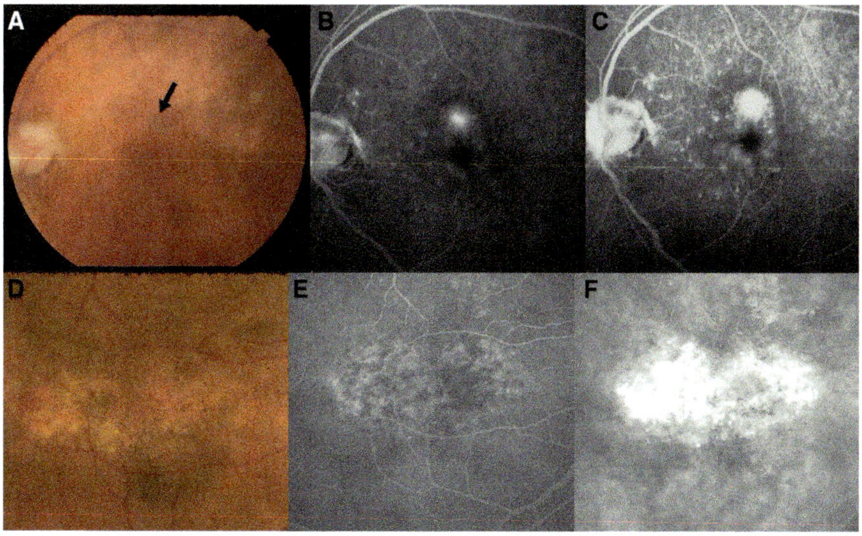

Figure 4. Classic and occult choroidal neovascularization (CNV) in neovascular age-related macular degeneration. (*A*) Color fundus photograph shows a greenish lesion deep to the retina (arrow). (*B*) Fluorescein angiography shows a focal well-demarcated hyperfluorescence of the CNV that leaks in later (*C*) frames. There are also scattered drusen that also appear bright. (*D*) Color fundus photograph shows drusen, pigmentary changes, and a diffusely mottled appearance of the retinal pigment epithelium. Fluorescein angiography demonstrates an ill-defined area of hyperfluoresence (*E*) that leaks diffusely in mid to late frames (*F*).

Serous PEDs are sharply demarcated, dome-shaped RPE elevations. Fluorescein pools in the lesions briskly, uniformly, and intensely, without leakage. These lesions may interfere with visualization of underlying CNV on fluorescein angiography. OCT and indocyanine green angiography (see section on Polypoidal Choroidal Vasculopathy) may be useful adjunctive tools in such cases. The natural history of all types of PEDs involves eventual collapse. Geographic atrophy can develop after the collapse of PEDs, especially with large drusenoid PEDs. Tears of the RPE may mimic geographic atrophy, but the former is usually characterized by fluid overlying the tear and intense hyperfluorescence on fluorescein angiography.

OCT, especially SD-OCT, provides detailed anatomical characterization of eyes with neovascular AMD. The ease and speed of acquiring the images has made it the most frequently used imaging modality to follow AMD patients. CNV appears as hyperreflective membranes deep to the RPE or in the subretinal space with associated intraretinal or subretinal fluid. Three-dimensional OCT reconstructions of CNV lesions have been shown to correlate with fluorescein findings (Malamos et al. 2009). One study showed that fluorescein angiography is superior to time-domain OCT in detecting new-onset CNV (Do et al. 2012), but it is not yet known whether this holds true with the higher-resolution SD-OCT (Khurana et al. 2010).

SD-OCT allows high-resolution imaging of the exudative fluid associated with CNV (Sayanagi et al. 2009). PEDs appear as elevation of the RPE from Bruch's membrane. Serous PEDs appear dome-shaped, with homogeneously hyporeflective material (optically empty) and good visualization of the underlying choroidal structures. Drusenoid PEDs typically have smooth surface contours with homogeneously hyperreflective material within the PED. Fibrovascular PEDs can have surfaces that are either smooth or irregular, and have heterogeneous material within the PED (Fig. 5). OCT software algorithms are under development to allow automated classification of the type of PED (Lee et al. 2012a).

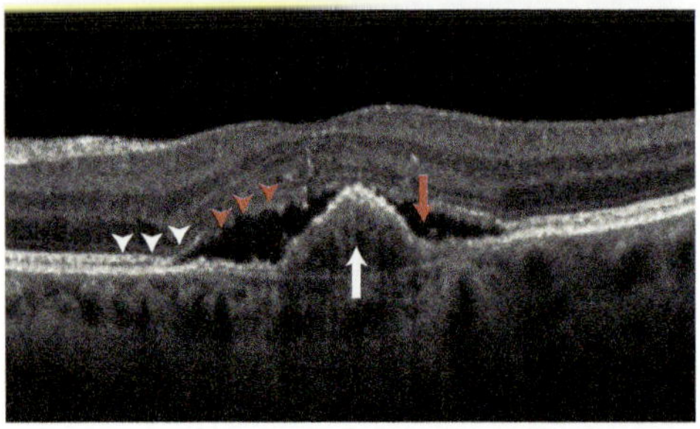

Figure 5. Spectral-domain optical coherence tomography of a central fibrovascular pigment epithelial detachment (white arrow) with overlying subretinal fluid (red arrow). The inner-segment/outer-segment junction of the photoreceptors (white arrowheads) has become disrupted in the area overlying the lesion (red arrowheads).

Subretinal fluid on SD-OCT appears as darkly hyporeflective spaces beneath the retina, and intraretinal fluid commonly presents as hyporeflective cystic spaces within the retina. Degenerative cystic changes can be seen in long-standing disease, but these findings do not signify active exudation. These cystic lesions are often sharply demarcated and static. Outer retinal tubulation is another finding in advanced AMD, consisting of round or ovoid, relatively hyporeflective spaces with hyperreflective borders (Fig. 6) (Zweifel et al. 2009). These structures are thought to represent cross sections of tubular branches of degenerating photoreceptors. It is important to recognize degenerative cysts and outer retinal tubulation, because these findings may be misinterpreted as active intraretinal fluid and may prompt unnecessary treatment.

The end-stage result of neovascular AMD is a subretinal, fibrovascular, disciform scar that causes deterioration of the overlying sensory retina. Disciform scars usually appear white to yellow and may have areas of hyperpigmentation caused by RPE hyperplasia. Depending on the extent of RPE hyperplasia within the scar, angiography may show staining or blockage. These fibrovascular scars may continue to grow, with new neovascularization along the borders of the lesions. The late-stage appearance can be very variable. Some heavily pigmented, elevated scars may mimic choroidal tumors, whereas others may develop substantial lipid deposition to mimic Coats' disease and rarely, massive exudation of fluid may cause a large serous retinal detachment.

Polypoidal Choroidal Vasculopathy

Polypoidal choroidal vasculopathy (PCV) is proposed to be a variant of type I CNV (Imamura et al. 2010). Abnormal tubular and polyp-shaped vascular channels deep to the RPE characterize PCV. It is generally seen in Asian, Hispanic, and black populations. One study from Japan showed that approximately half of patients with neovascular AMD had PCV (Maruko et al. 2007). It is now recognized that PCV also affects white populations, albeit to a lesser degree (Imamura et al. 2010). PCV occurs more often in younger patients, may not always be associated with drusen, and often contains a hemorrhagic component. Large polyps may be visible on clinical examination, but fundoscopy,

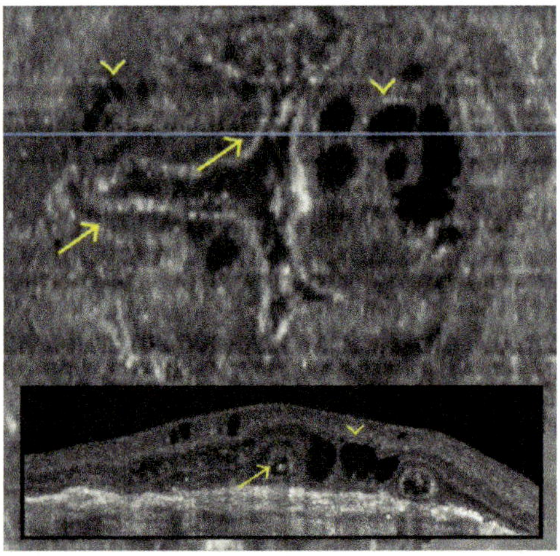

Figure 6. Outer retinal tubulation (arrows) and degenerative cystic cavities (arrowheads) located above a fibrovascular scar. The "en face" optical coherence tomography (OCT) demonstrates that the tubulations form a branching network. The corresponding B-scan OCT (inset) shows the tubulations as round and ovoid hyporeflective spaces with a ring of hyperreflectivity, and the degenerative cysts as sharply demarcated cavities. (Adapted, with permission, from Wolff et al. 2012.)

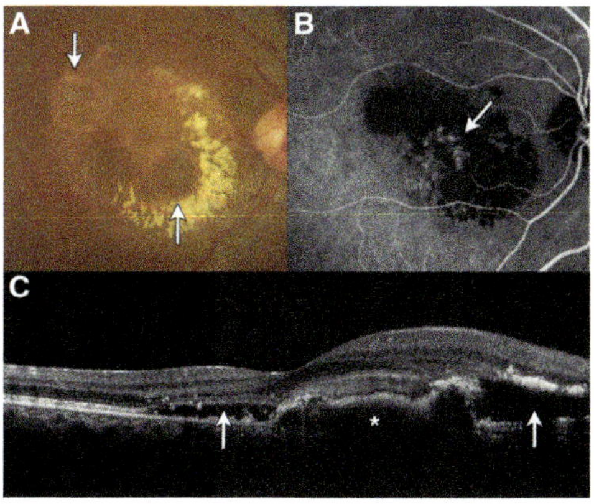

Figure 7. Polypoidal choroidal vasculopathy. (*A*) Color fundus photograph showing two pigment epithelial detachments (PED; arrows) with circinate exudation and subretinal fluid. (*B*) Indocyanine green angiography showing hyperfluorescent polypoidal lesions in the choroidal vasculature (arrow). (*C*) The corresponding spectral domain optical coherence tomography shows the subretinal fluid (arrows) and elevation of the retinal pigment epithelium (asterisk). (Adapted, with permission, from Yonekawa 2013.)

OCT, and fluorescein angiography are often not able to distinguish PCV from typical AMD. Indocyanine green (ICG) angiography is the definitive method to image the polypoidal vascular structures in the choroid (Fig. 7).

ICG angiography uses a high-molecular weight dye with infrared emission (830–840 nm). A confocal laser applies an infrared 790 nm light beam and photographs/video are taken similarly to fluorescein angiography. The ICG dye has strong protein-binding properties, and the large size of the ICG-protein complexes reduces the amount of extravasation from the choriocapillaris, which allows superior visualization of the choroidal circulation. Compared with the visible light used for fluorescein, the infrared spectrum allows deeper penetration through the retina and RPE, as well as through media opacities such as cataract and hemorrhage.

Retinal Angiomatous Proliferation

Retinal angiomatous proliferation is another variant of neovascular AMD that is characterized by intraretinal neovascularization. Other names for this entity include "retinal angiomatous lesion," "deep retinal vascular anomalous complex," "retinal anastomosis to the lesion," "retinal vascular anomalous complex," "retinal choroidal anastomosis," and "type III neovascularization" (Yannuzzi et al. 2001; Freund et al. 2008). As the multiple names suggest, there is much debate over its pathogenesis and natural history. Yannuzzi and colleagues introduced the most commonly used term "retinal angiomatous proliferation (RAP)" in 2001 to describe a neovascular process that originated within the neurosensory retina (Yannuzzi et al. 2001). The intraretinal neovascularization was then thought to extend posteriorly into the subretinal space, create a PED, and merge with underlying type I CNV. Gass and colleagues proposed an alternative theory in 2003, describing a process in which the initial pathologic stimulus is an occult type I CNV with associated superficial retinal hemorrhages between the outer retinal capillaries and the CNV (Gass et al. 2003). This was thought to be followed by choroidal-retinal anastomoses, resulting in a "piggy-back" type II CNV overlying the type I CNV.

Clinically, RAP lesions are commonly characterized by intraretinal hemorrhage overlying a retinal vessel that acutely dives in toward the RPE (Fig. 8). Lesions are often located in the paramacular area. Angiomatous tissue with surrounding capillary telangiectasia and dilated perfusing arterioles or draining venules can be seen in early stages. Subretinal fluid and/or hemorrhage are seen if type II neovascularization has occurred. ICG plays an important role in distinguishing RAP from PCV and occult CNV. ICG angiography allows visualization of the anastomotic connections between the retinal and choroidal circulation characteristic of RAP. However, anastomotic connections may also be seen in end-stage neovascular AMD or disciform scarring. The visual prognosis of RAP lesions was conventionally thought to be poor, but subgroup analysis of the Verteporfin in Photodynamic Therapy (VIP) trial showed that the natural history is in fact quite variable, as in typical neovascular AMD, and the lesions responded well to photodynamic therapy (Scott and Bressler 2010).

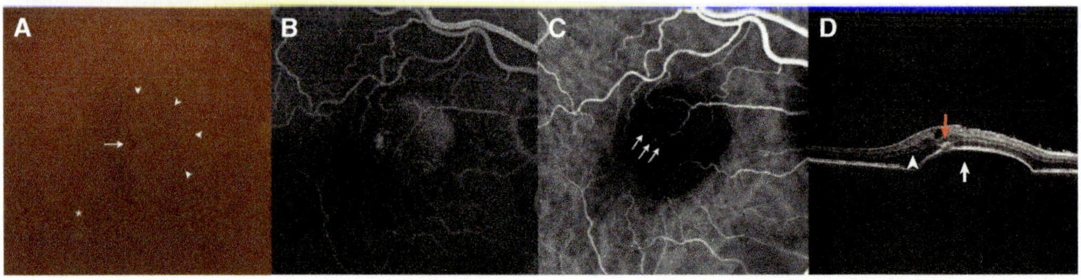

Figure 8. Retinal angiomatous proliferation (RAP). (*A*) Color fundus photograph showing focal intraretinal hemorrhage (arrow) and an underlying pigment epithelial detachment (PED) (arrowheads). There are also drusen (asterisk). (*B*) Fluorescein angiography shows a focal hyperfluorescence and the underlying PED. (*C*) Indocyanine green angiography reveals an anastomotic lesion connecting retinal vasculature (arrows). (*D*) Spectral-domain optical coherence tomography also shows that there is intraretinal fluid (arrowhead) in addition to the PED (white arrow). A hyperreflective focus on the surface of the PED corresponds to the RAP lesion (red arrow).

TREATMENT OF NONNEOVASCULAR AMD

AREDS was a randomized, double-masked clinical trial, which examined the effect of antioxidant and zinc supplementation on progression of AMD. (AREDS Study Group 2000; AREDS Study Group 2001). It enrolled 3640 participants who were stratified into four categories of severity. Category 1: essentially no AMD, with total drusen area less than 5 small drusen (<63 μm); Category 2: mild AMD with multiple small drusen or single/scattered intermediate drusen (63–124 μm), and/or pigmentary changes; Category 3: at least one large druse (≥125 μm) and/or extensive intermediate drusen and/or geographic atrophy not involving the central macula; Category 4: advanced AMD in the fellow nonstudy eye. Participants were randomized to one of four treatment arms: oral daily supplementation with (1) antioxidants (vitamin C 500 mg, vitamin E 400 IU, β-carotene 15 mg), (2) zinc (zinc oxide 80 mg and copper 2 mg), (3) the combination of antioxidants and zinc, or (4) placebo.

Control patients in Category 2 had a 1.3% probability of progressing to advanced AMD in 5 yr. Category 3 had 18% likelihood, and Category 4 had 43%. The largest risk reduction was seen in Category 3 and 4 participants who were randomized to take both antioxidants and zinc (odds radio 0.66, or 34% odds reduction; $p = 0.001$). This group also had the largest reduction in loss of 15 letters or more with an odds ratio of 0.73 ($p = 0.008$), corresponding to a 27% risk reduction. Based on these findings, it was recommended that patients in Category 3 and 4 would benefit from antioxidant and zinc supplementation. Current and former heavy smokers were urged to take a regimen free of β-carotene, which has been shown by epidemiologic studies to increase the risk of lung cancer in smokers.

The AREDS investigators initiated AREDS 2 in 2006 (AREDS2 Study Group 2013). The goal was to determine whether adding omega-3 fatty acids (docosahexanoic acid [DHA] and its precursor eicosapentanoic acid [EPA]) and/or lutein and zeaxanthin to the original AREDS formulation would further reduce the risk of advanced AMD. 4203 participants with either bilateral large drusen or large drusen in one eye and advanced AMD in the fellow eye were randomized into four arms: (1) original AREDS, (2) AREDS + lutein 10 mg + zeaxanthin 2 mg, (3) AREDS + DHA 350 mg + EPA 650 mg, and (4) AREDS + DHA/EPA + lutein/zeaxanthin. In a secondary randomization, participants were randomized to the original AREDS formulation with or without β-carotene, and standard or lower doses of zinc.

The results (AREDS2 Study Group 2013) showed that there was no further benefit in adding DHA/EPA or lutein/zeaxanthin to the original AREDS formulation. However, it was found that participants who took the original AREDS formulation without β-carotene but with lutein and zeaxanthin and had slightly lower rates of progression to advanced AMD, compared to those taking the original formulation with β-carotene (hazard ratio 0.82; $p = 0.02$). Therefore it was suggested that lutein/zeaxanthin could be substituted for β-carotene.

Treatments in Development

The complement pathway has been implicated in the pathogenesis of AMD and many clinical trials are under way to investigate whether complement inhibitors can slow the progression of nonneovascular AMD. Studies of a systemically administered anti-C5 antibody, eculizumab, failed to show efficacy in reducing drusen volume or progression of geographic atrophy. (Garcia Filho et al. 2014; Yehoshua et al. 2014). A Phase II sham-controlled, randomized study that enrolled 129 patients with bilateral geographic atrophy, and showed that monthly intravitreal injections of lampalizumab (antifactor D, Roche/Genentech) resulted in a 20% reduction in the rate of growth geographic atrophy at 18 mo (Regillo 2013). Of note, patients positive for a specific complement factor I polymorphism (57% of the study participants) benefited from a 44% growth reduction. Many other trials of complement inhibitors are also in progress (Miller 2013).

Other potential therapeutic strategies in development include targeting inflammasomes, visual cycle modulation, and neuroprotection. Inflammasomes are multiprotein complexes that activate inflammatory cascades, and have been identified as potential targets for both nonneovascular (Tarallo et al. 2012) and neovascular (Doyle et al. 2012) AMD. Interrupting the photoreceptor light cycle to decrease the accumulation of A2E, a toxic component of lipofuscin, is another avenue under investigation. Early trials indicate that visual cycle modulators may have a role in slowing the progression of geographic atrophy (Kubota et al. 2012; Mata et al. 2013). Research in neuroprotection aims to identify agents that will interfere with cell death pathways and inhibit the loss of neural retina that is the ultimate cause of vision loss in AMD as well as many other disorders. (Trichonas et al. 2010; Wong et al. 2010; Zhang et al. 2011a; Miller 2013; Tsai 2013). Subretinal transplantation of stem cells is also being investigated as a means of regenerating RPE cells and eventually, perhaps photoreceptors as well (Schwartz et al. 2012).

TREATMENT OF NEOVASCULAR AMD

Photocoagulation

The Macular Photocoagulation Study (MPS) demonstrated the efficacy of argon photocoagulation for extrafoveal CNV (MPS Study Group 1982; MPS Study Group 1986). However, this treatment modality has been largely abandoned because of frequent recurrences and limited applicability.

Macular Surgery

Submacular surgery to directly remove neovascular membranes evolved in the 1990s as an alternative to observation or photocoagulation. The Submacular Surgery Trials showed that there was no benefit in visual outcomes in patients with subfoveal CNV treated with submacular surgery (Hawkins et al. 2004). However, treated lesions that were predominantly hemorrhagic lost less vision compared with observation (Bressler et al. 2004), although this did not translate into improved quality of life (Childs et al. 2004).

Macular translocation is a surgical procedure in which CNV is typically removed and the macula is displaced so that the fovea overlies normal RPE (Machemer and Steinhorst 1993; Ninomiya et al. 1996; de Juan et al. 1998; Lai et al. 2002; Mruthyunjaya et al. 2004). Limited macular translocation involves partially detaching the retina via injection of subretinal fluid and shifting the inferior retina downward with the help of a gas bubble to create a retinal fold. Another translocation technique involves 360° peripheral retinectomy to fully detach and rotate the entire retina. Since the emergence of pharmacological therapies, surgical techniques are rarely used in management of neovascular AMD.

The current primary indication for surgical intervention in neovascular AMD is management of large submacular hemorrhages. Displacement of such hemorrhage is often attempted with vitrectomy and subretinal injection of tissue plasminogen activator and intravitreal gas (Hassan et al. 1999; Hattenbach et al. 2001; Haupert et al. 2001; Olivier et al. 2004; Singh et al. 2006). Successful pneumatic displacement with intravitreal gas injection, injections without vitrectomy and with or without tissue plasminogen activator, have also been reported (Ohji et al. 1998; Daneshvar et al. 1999; Ron et al. 2007; Mizutani et al. 2011).

Photodynamic Therapy

Photodynamic therapy (PDT) using verteporfin (Visudyne; Valeant Ophthalmics, Bridgewater, NJ) was approved by the United States Food and Drug Administration (FDA) for the treatment of neovascular AMD in 2000. PDT uses intravenously administered photosensitizing molecules that can be activated by photons in specific wavelengths, which allows photochemical damage by the generation of free radicals. An advantage over photocoagulation is the relative sparing of normal tissue, because only tissues that accumulate the photosensitizers are directly affected.

The Treatment of AMD with Photodynamic Therapy (TAP) trial was the phase III study that established the efficacy of PDT for neovascular AMD (TAP-Study-Group 1999). It randomized 609 participants with subfoveal neovascular AMD with a predominantly classic component, to verteporfin PDT or placebo. More eyes treated with PDT lost less than 15 letters of visual acuity at 12 mo (61% vs. 46%; $p < 0.001$). Eyes with predominantly classic lesions benefited the most. The benefits were sustained at two (Bressler 2001) and three years (Blumenkranz et al. 2002).

The VIP study examined verteporfin PDT for the treatment of subfoveal occult-only lesions and classic lesions with good visual acuities (VIP Study Group 2001). Eyes treated with PDT experienced less vision loss of 15 or more letters (54% vs 67%; $p = 0.023$) at two years compared with placebo. The VIO trial also randomized patients with occult lesions to PDT or placebo, but showed only a trend favoring PDT that was not statistically significant (Kaiser 2009).

Anti-VEGF Therapy

Pegaptanib

Pegaptanib sodium (Macugen; Valeant Ophthalmics, Bridgewater, NJ) is a pegylated RNA aptamer that selectively binds $VEGF_{165}$, which is thought to be one of the primary pathologic VEGF isoforms. Pegaptanib became the first anti-VEGF agent approved by the FDA for treatment of neovascular AMD based on the VISION studies (Gragoudas et al. 2004) which demonstrated that pegaptanib 0.3 mg given intravitreally every 6 wk resulted in 70% of patients losing fewer than 15 letters of visual acuity, compared to 55% of controls ($p < 0.001$). However, use of pegaptanib has been largely replaced by the pan-VEGF-A inhibitors.

Ranibizumab

Ranibizumab (Lucentis; Genentech, South San Francisco, CA) is a humanized monoclonal Fab fragment that neutralizes all active isoforms of VEGF-A. Its efficacy was demonstrated in the ANCHOR (Brown et al. 2009) and MARINA (Rosenfeld et al. 2006) trials, and it was FDA approved for the treatment of neovascular AMD in 2006.

The ANCHOR study randomized 430 participants with predominantly classic CNV to monthly 0.3 mg ranibizumab, 0.5 mg ranibizumab, or verteporfin PDT (Brown et al. 2009). The primary outcome of loss of fewer than 15 letters at 12 mo was met (94.3%, 96.4%, and 64.3%, respectively; $p < 0.001$) and sustained at 24 mo. Visual acuity improved by 15 letters or more in 35.7%, 40.3%, and 5.6%, respectively ($p < 0.001$), at 12 mo, and similarly at 24 mo. At 12 mo, the mean letters gained or lost were +8.5, +11.3, and −9.5, respectively ($p < 0.001$), and this difference was comparable at 24 mo.

The MARINA trial randomized 716 participants with minimally classic or occult CNV with evidence of recent progression to 0.3 mg ranibizumab, 0.5 mg ranibizumab, or sham injections (Rosenfeld et al. 2006). At 12 mo, <15 letters were lost in 94.5%, 94.6%, and 62.2% of patients, respectively ($p < 0.001$). Visual acuity improved by 15 or more letters in 24.8%, 33.8%, and 5.0% of patients, respectively ($p < 0.001$). Mean letters gained or lost were +6.5, +7.2, and −10.4, respectively ($p < 0.001$). The benefits were sustained at 24 mo.

Bevacizumab

Bevacizumab (Avastin; Genentech, South San Francisco, CA), a monoclonal anti-VEGF-A antibody, is the parent molecule of ranibizumab. It is FDA approved for the treatment of several systemic malignancies, but is used off-label as a cost-effective anti-VEGF agent for various ophthalmic conditions. The Comparison of AMD Treatment Trials (CATT) study was a federally funded, multicenter, noninferiority trial that randomized 1208 participants with neovascular AMD to receive ranibizumab or bevacizumab on either a monthly schedule or "as needed." (Martin et al. 2011, 2012). Monthly bevacizumab and monthly ranibizumab had similar efficacies, with a mean of 8.0 and 8.5 letters gained, respectively. The as-needed schedules were also comparable, with 5.9 and 6.8 letters gained, respectively. The difference between monthly and as-needed regimens did not reach statistical significance.

Aflibercept

Aflibercept (Eylea; Regeneron, Tarrytown, NY) is a recombinant fusion protein of the ligand-binding elements of VEGF receptors 1 and 2, which are fused to the Fc portion of human IgG1. It blocks all VEGF-A isoforms, VEGF-B and placental growth factor (Browning et al. 2012; Stewart 2012). The benefit of aflibercept over previous agents is its demonstrated efficacy when given on a less frequent bimonthly injection schedule (Papadopoulos et al. 2012). Aflibercept was FDA approved in 2011 after the results of the VIEW 1 and VIEW 2 studies, which were two parallel phase III trials that randomized 2419 patients to 0.5 mg monthly aflibercept, 2.0 mg monthly aflibercept, 2.0 mg aflibercept every 2 mo after three initial monthly doses, or monthly 0.5 mg ranibizumab (Heier et al. 2012). All aflibercept groups were comparable to monthly ranibizumab for the primary endpoint (proportion of patients losing <15 letters at 1 yr). The letters gained and anatomic measures as seen on OCT were also comparable.

Combination Therapy

The role of PDT in treating typical neovascular AMD has become limited to refractory cases given the superior results obtained with anti-VEGF therapy. Studies investigating combination PDT and anti-VEGF therapy for AMD did not show benefit with respect to visual acuity or significant reduction in number of injections (Kaiser et al. 2012; Larsen et al. 2012).

PDT, however, still plays an important role in the treatment of PCV (Kurashige et al. 2008; Kang et al. 2013; Yamashita et al. 2013). Anti-VEGF agents can decrease the exudation associated with PCV to improve visual acuity, but often do not close the polypoidal vascular abnormalities (Gomi et al. 2008; Koizumi et al. 2011); the local photochemical damage of PDT can directly close these channels (Koh et al. 2012). Combining PDT with anti-VEGF agents appears to be an effective approach (Kim and Yu 2011; Koh et al. 2012; Lee et al. 2012b; Tomita et al. 2012). The EVEREST study randomized 61 patients with PCV to verteporfin PDT, ranibizumab 0.5 mg, or the combination, and showed that PDT with ranibizumab or PDT alone was superior to ranibizumab monotherapy in achieving polyp regression at 6 mo ($p < 0.01$) (Koh et al. 2012).

Despite the success of current pharmacotherapies for neovascular AMD, better visual results and more durable therapies remain goals to be achieved. Strategies under investigation include inhibition of platelet-derived growth factor (Boyer 2013), and other mechanisms of VEGF blockade including anti-VEGF gene therapy. (Lukason et al. 2011; Zhang et al. 2011b; Campochiaro et al. 2013).

CONCLUDING REMARKS

Many recent advances in ophthalmology have been in the arena of AMD. From genetic studies to new imaging technology, breakthroughs in treatment, and gains in the fundamental understanding of its pathophysiology, the strides made in AMD research have prevented blindness in millions of individuals. However, better and further-reaching treatments are needed. Directions for ongoing and future research that will help achieve such treatments include more precise phenotyping of AMD utilizing modern imaging capabilities combined with genotyping, a deeper understanding of AMD pathophysiology, improved disease models, further insight into pharmacogenomic interactions, and new drug delivery technology.

REFERENCES

AREDS Study Group. 2000. Risk factors associated with age-related macular degeneration. A case-control study in the age-related eye disease study: Age-Related Eye Disease Study Report Number 3. *Ophthalmology* **107:** 2224–2232.

AREDS Study Group. 2001. A randomized, placebo-controlled, clinical trial of high-dose supplementation with vitamins C and E, β carotene, and zinc for age-related macular degeneration and vision loss: AREDS report no. 8. *Arch Ophthalmol* **119:** 1417–1436.

AREDS2 Study Group. 2013. Lutein + zeaxanthin and omega-3 fatty acids for age-related macular degeneration: the Age-Related Eye Disease Study 2 (AREDS2) randomized clinical trial. *JAMA* **309:** 2005–2015.

Arnold JJ, Sarks SH, Killingsworth MC, Sarks JP. 1995. Reticular pseudodrusen. A risk factor in age-related maculopathy. *Retina* **15:** 183–191.

Blumenkranz MS, Bressler NM, Bressler SB, Donati G, Fish GE, Haynes LA, Lewis H, Miller JW, Mones JM, Potter MJ, et al. 2002. Verteporfin therapy for subfoveal choroidal neovascularization in age-related macular degeneration: Three-year results of an open-label extension of 2 randomized clinical trials—TAP Report no. 5. *Arch Ophthalmol* **120:** 1307–1314.

Boyer D. 2013. A phase 2b study of Fovista™, a platelet derived growth factor (PDGF) inhibitor in combination with a vascular endothelial growth factor (VEGF) inhibitor for neovascular age-related macular degeneration (AMD). *Association for Research in Vision and Ophthalmology Annual Meeting*, Abstract 2175. Seattle, May 5–9.

Bressler NM, TAP Study Group. 2001. Photodynamic therapy of subfoveal choroidal neovascularization in age-related macular degeneration with verteporfin: Two-year results of 2 randomized clinical trials-tap report 2. *Arch Ophthalmol* **119:** 198–207.

Bressler NM, Silva JC, Bressler SB, Fine SL, Green WR. 1994. Clinicopathologic correlation of drusen and retinal pigment epithelial abnormalities in age-related macular degeneration. *Retina* **14:** 130–142.

Bressler NM, Bressler SB, Childs AL, Haller JA, Hawkins BS, Lewis H, MacCumber MW, Marsh MJ, Redford M, Sternberg P Jr, et al. 2004. Surgery for hemorrhagic choroidal neovascular lesions of age-related macular degeneration: Ophthalmic findings: SST report no. 13. *Ophthalmology* **111:** 1993–2006.

Brown DM, Michels M, Kaiser PK, Heier JS, Sy JP, Ianchulev T. 2009. Ranibizumab versus verteporfin photodynamic therapy for neovascular age-related macular degeneration: Two-year results of the ANCHOR study. *Ophthalmology* **116:** 57–65, e55.

Browning DJ, Kaiser PK, Rosenfeld PJ, Stewart MW. 2012. Aflibercept for age-related macular degeneration: A game-changer or quiet addition? *Am J Ophthalmol* **154:** 222–226.

Campochiaro PA, Channa R, Berger BB, Heier JS, Brown DM, Fiedler U, Hepp J, Stumpp MT. 2013. Treatment of diabetic macular edema with a designed ankyrin repeat protein that binds vascular endothelial growth factor: A phase I/II study. *Am J Ophthalmol* **155:** 697–704, 704 e691–e692.

Childs AL, Bressler NM, Bass EB, Hawkins BS, Mangione CM, Marsh MJ, Miskala PH. 2004. Surgery for hemorrhagic choroidal neovascular lesions of age-related macular degeneration: Quality-of-life findings: SST report no. 14. *Ophthalmology* **111:** 2007–2014.

Christen WG, Glynn RJ, Manson JE, Ajani UA, Buring JE. 1996. A prospective study of cigarette smoking and risk of age-related macular degeneration in men. *JAMA* **276:** 1147–1151.

Cohen SY, Dubois L, Tadayoni R, Delahaye-Mazza C, Debibie C, Quentel G. 2007. Prevalence of reticular pseudodrusen in age-related macular degeneration with newly diagnosed choroidal neovascularisation. *Br J Ophthalmol* **91:** 354–359.

Cukras C, Agron E, Klein ML, Ferris FL 3rd, Chew EY, Gensler G, Wong WT. 2010. Natural history of drusenoid pigment epithelial detachment in age-related macular degeneration: Age-Related Eye Disease Study Report No. 28. *Ophthalmology* **117:** 489–499.

Curcio CA, Millican CL, Allen KA, Kalina RE. 1993. Aging of the human photoreceptor mosaic: Evidence for selective vulnerability of rods in central retina. *Invest Ophthalmol Vis Sci* **34:** 3278–3296.

Daneshvar H, Kertes PJ, Leonard BC, Peyman GA. 1999. Management of submacular hemorrhage with intravitreal sulfur hexafluoride: A pilot study. *Can J Ophthalmol* **34:** 385–388.

de Juan E Jr, Loewenstein A, Bressler NM, Alexander J. 1998. Translocation of the retina for management of subfoveal choroidal neovascularization II: A preliminary report in humans. *Am J Ophthalmol* **125:** 635–646.

Do DV, Gower EW, Cassard SD, Boyer D, Bressler NM, Bressler SB, Heier JS, Jefferys JL, Singerman LJ, Solomon SD. 2012. Detection of new-onset choroidal neovascularization using optical coherence tomography: The AMD DOC Study. *Ophthalmology* **119:** 771–778.

Doyle SL, Campbell M, Ozaki E, Salomon RG, Mori A, Kenna PF, Farrar GJ, Kiang AS, Humphries MM, Lavelle EC, et al. 2012. NLRP3 has a protective role in age-related macular degeneration through the induction of IL-18 by drusen components. *Nat Med* **18:** 791–798.

Eye-Disease-Case-Control-Study-Group. 1992. Risk factors for neovascular age-related macular degeneration. *Arch Ophthalmol* **110:** 1701–1708.

Feehan M, Hartman J, Durante R, Morrison MA, Miller JW, Kim IK, DeAngelis MM. 2011. Identifying subtypes of patients with neovascular age-related macular degeneration by genotypic and cardiovascular risk characteristics. *BMC Med Genet* **12:** 83.

Feeney-Burns L, Berman ER, Rothman H. 1980. Lipofuscin of human retinal pigment epithelium. *Am J Ophthalmol* **90:** 783–791.

Feeney-Burns L, Burns RP, Gao CL. 1990. Age-related macular changes in humans over 90 years old. *Am J Ophthalmol* **109:** 265–278.

Ferris FL III, Fine SL, Hyman L. 1984. Age-related macular degeneration and blindness due to neovascular maculopathy. *Arch Ophthalmol* **102:** 1640–1642.

Freund KB, Ho IV, Barbazetto IA, Koizumi H, Laud K, Ferrara D, Matsumoto Y, Sorenson JA, Yannuzzi L. 2008. Type 3 neovascularization: The expanded spectrum of retinal angiomatous proliferation. *Retina* **28:** 201–211.

Friedman DS, O'Colmain BJ, Munoz B, Tomany SC, McCarty C, de Jong PT, Nemesure B, Mitchell P, Kempen J. 2004. Prevalence of age-related macular degeneration in the United States. *Arch Ophthalmol* **122:** 564–572.

Garcia Filho CA, Yehoshua Z, Gregori G, Nunes RP, Penha FM, Moshfeghi AA, Zhang K, Feuer W, Rosenfeld PJ. 2014. Change in drusen volume as a novel clinical trial endpoint for the study of complement inhibition in age-related macular degeneration. *Ophthalmic Surg Lasers Imaging Retina* **45:** 18–31.

Gass JD, Agarwal A, Lavina AM, Tawansy KA. 2003. Focal inner retinal hemorrhages in patients with drusen: An early sign of occult choroidal neovascularization and chorioretinal anastomosis. *Retina* **23:** 741–751.

Goldberg J, Flowerdew G, Smith E, Brody JA, Tso MO. 1988. Factors associated with age-related macular degeneration. An analysis of data from the first National Health and Nutrition Examination Survey. *Am J Epidemiol* **128:** 700–710.

Gomi F, Sawa M, Sakaguchi H, Tsujikawa M, Oshima Y, Kamei M, Tano Y. 2008. Efficacy of intravitreal bevacizumab for polypoidal choroidal vasculopathy. *Br J Ophthalmol* **92:** 70–73.

Gragoudas ES, Adamis AP, Cunningham ET Jr, Feinsod M, Guyer DR. 2004. Pegaptanib for neovascular age-related macular degeneration. *N Engl J Med* **351:** 2805–2816.

Hartnett ME, Weiter JJ, Garsd A, Jalkh AE. 1992. Classification of retinal pigment epithelial detachments associated with drusen. *Graefes Arch Clin Exp Ophthalmol* **230:** 11–19.

Hassan AS, Johnson MW, Schneiderman TE, Regillo CD, Tornambe PE, Poliner LS, Blodi BA, Elner SG. 1999. Management of submacular hemorrhage with intravitreous tissue plasminogen activator injection and pneumatic displacement. *Ophthalmology* **106:** 1900–1907.

Hattenbach LO, Klais C, Koch FH, Gumbel HO. 2001. Intravitreous injection of tissue plasminogen activator and gas in the treatment of submacular hemorrhage under various conditions. *Ophthalmology* **108:** 1485–1492.

Haupert CL, McCuen BW II, Jaffe GJ, Steuer ER, Cox TA, Toth CA, Fekrat S, Postel EA. 2001. Pars plana vitrectomy, subretinal injection of tissue plasminogen activator, and fluid-gas exchange for displacement of thick submacular hemorrhage in age-related macular degeneration. *Am J Ophthalmol* **131:** 208–215.

Hawkins BS, Bressler NM, Miskala PH, Bressler SB, Holekamp NM, Marsh MJ, Redford M, Schwartz SD, Sternberg P Jr, Thomas MA, et al. 2004. Surgery for subfoveal choroidal neovascularization in age-related macular degeneration: Ophthalmic findings: SST report no. 11. *Ophthalmology* **111:** 1967–1980.

Heier JS, Brown DM, Chong V, Korobelnik J-F, Kaiser PK, Nguyen QD, Kirchhof B, Ho A, Ogura Y, Yancopoulos GD, et al. 2012. Intravitreal aflibercept (VEGF Trap-Eye) in wet age-related macular degeneration. *Ophthalmology* **119:** 2537–2548.

Holz FG, Bellman C, Staudt S, Schutt F, Volcker HE. 2001. Fundus autofluorescence and development of geographic atrophy in age-related macular degeneration. *Invest Ophthalmol Vis Sci* **42:** 1051–1056.

Hyman L, Schachat AP, He Q, Leske MC. 2000. Hypertension, cardiovascular disease, and age-related macular degeneration. Age-Related Macular Degeneration Risk Factors Study Group. *Arch Ophthalmol* **118:** 351–358.

Imamura Y, Engelbert M, Iida T, Freund KB, Yannuzzi LA. 2010. Polypoidal choroidal vasculopathy: A review. *Surv Ophthalmol* **55:** 501–515.

Kaiser PK. 2009. Verteporfin PDT for subfoveal occult CNV in AMD: Two-year results of a randomized trial. *Curr Med Res Opin* **25:** 1853–1860.

Kaiser PK, Boyer DS, Cruess AF, Slakter JS, Pilz S, Weisberger A. 2012. Verteporfin plus ranibizumab for choroidal neovascularization in age-related macular degeneration: Twelve-month results of the DENALI study. *Ophthalmology* **119:** 1001–1010.

Kang HM, Kim YM, Koh HJ. 2013. Five-year follow-up results of photodynamic therapy for polypoidal choroidal vasculopathy. *Am J Ophthalmol* **155:** 438–447, e431.

Kawasaki R, Yasuda M, Song SJ, Chen SJ, Jonas JB, Wang JJ, Mitchell P, Wong TY. 2010. The prevalence of age-related macular degeneration in Asians: A systematic review and meta-analysis. *Ophthalmology* **117:** 921–927.

Khurana RN, Dupas B, Bressler NM. 2010. Agreement of time-domain and spectral-domain optical coherence tomography with fluorescein leakage from choroidal neovascularization. *Ophthalmology* **117:** 1376–1380.

Kim SJ, Yu HG. 2011. Efficacy of combined photodynamic therapy and intravitreal bevacizumab injection versus photodynamic therapy alone in polypoidal choroidal vasculopathy. *Retina* **31:** 1827–1834.

Klein R, Klein BE, Linton KL. 1992. Prevalence of age-related maculopathy. The Beaver Dam Eye Study. *Ophthalmology* **99:** 933–943.

Klein R, Klein BE, Franke T. 1993. The relationship of cardiovascular disease and its risk factors to age-related maculopathy. The Beaver Dam Eye Study. *Ophthalmology* **100:** 406–414.

Klein R, Klein BE, Tomany SC, Cruickshanks KJ. 2003. The association of cardiovascular disease with the long-term incidence of age-related maculopathy: The Beaver Dam Eye Study. *Ophthalmology* **110:** 1273–1280.

Klein ML, Ferris FL III, Armstrong J, Hwang TS, Chew EY, Bressler SB, Chandra SR. 2008a. Retinal precursors and the development of geographic atrophy in age-related macular degeneration. *Ophthalmology* **115:** 1026–1031.

Klein R, Meuer SM, Knudtson MD, Iyengar SK, Klein BE. 2008b. The epidemiology of retinal reticular drusen. *Am J Ophthalmol* **145:** 317–326.

Klein R, Cruickshanks KJ, Myers CE, Sivakumaran TA, Iyengar SK, Meuer SM, Schubert CR, Gangnon RE, Klein BE. 2013. The relationship of atherosclerosis to the 10-year cumulative incidence of age-related macular degeneration: The Beaver Dam studies. *Ophthalmology* **120:** 1012–1019.

Koh A, Lee WK, Chen LJ, Chen SJ, Hashad Y, Kim H, Lai TY, Pilz S, Ruamviboonsuk P, Tokaji E, et al. 2012. EVEREST study: Efficacy and safety of verteporfin photodynamic therapy in combination with ranibizumab or alone versus ranibizumab monotherapy in patients with symptomatic macular polypoidal choroidal vasculopathy. *Retina* **32:** 1453–1464.

Koizumi H, Yamagishi T, Yamazaki T, Kinoshita S. 2011. Predictive factors of resolved retinal fluid after intravitreal ranibizumab for polypoidal choroidal vasculopathy. *Br J Ophthalmol* **95:** 1555–1559.

Kubota R, Boman NL, David R, Mallikaarjun S, Patil S, Birch D. 2012. Safety and effect on rod function of ACU-4429, a novel small-molecule visual cycle modulator. *Retina* **32:** 183–188.

Kurashige Y, Otani A, Sasahara M, Yodoi Y, Tamura H, Tsujikawa A, Yoshimura N. 2008. Two-year results of photodynamic therapy for polypoidal choroidal vasculopathy. *Am J Ophthalmol* **146:** 513–519.

Laatikainen L, Larinkari J. 1977. Capillary-free area of the fovea with advancing age. *Invest Ophthalmol Vis Sci* **16:** 1154–1157.

Lai JC, Lapolice DJ, Stinnett SS, Meyer CH, Arieu LM, Keller MA, Toth CA. 2002. Visual outcomes following macular translocation with 360-degree peripheral retinectomy. *Arch Ophthalmol* **120:** 1317–1324.

Larsen M, Schmidt-Erfurth U, Lanzetta P, Wolf S, Simader C, Tokaji E, Pilz S, Weisberger A. 2012. Verteporfin plus ranibizumab for choroidal neovascularization in age-related macular degeneration: Twelve-month MONT BLANC study results. *Ophthalmology* **119:** 992–1000.

Lee SY, Stetson PF, Ruiz-Garcia H, Heussen FM, Sadda SR. 2012a. Automated characterization of pigment epithelial detachment by optical coherence tomography. *Invest Ophthalmol Vis Sci* **53:** 164–170.

Lee YA, Yang CH, Yang CM, Ho TC, Lin CP, Huang JS, Chen MS. 2012b. Photodynamic therapy with or without intravitreal bevacizumab for polypoidal choroidal vasculopathy: Two years of follow-up. *Am J Ophthalmol* **154:** 872–880, e872.

Lukason M, DuFresne E, Rubin H, Pechan P, Li Q, Kim I, Kiss S, Flaxel C, Collins M, Miller J, et al. 2011. Inhibition of choroidal neovascularization in a nonhuman primate model by intravitreal administration of an AAV2 vector expressing a novel anti-VEGF molecule. *Mol Ther* **19:** 260–265.

Machemer R, Steinhorst UH. 1993. Retinal separation, retinotomy, and macular relocation: II. A surgical approach for age-related macular degeneration? *Graefes Arch Clin Exp Ophthalmol* **231:** 635–641.

Malamos P, Sacu S, Georgopoulos M, Kiss C, Pruente C, Schmidt-Erfurth U. 2009. Correlation of high-definition optical coherence tomography and fluorescein angiography imaging in neovascular macular degeneration. *Invest Ophthalmol Vis Sci* **50:** 4926–4933.

Martin DF, Maguire MG, Ying GS, Grunwald JE, Fine SL, Jaffe GJ. 2011. Ranibizumab and bevacizumab for neovascular age-related macular degeneration. *N Engl J Med* **364:** 1897–1908.

Martin DF, Maguire MG, Fine SL, Ying GS, Jaffe GJ, Grunwald JE, Toth C, Redford M, Ferris FL III. 2012. Ranibizumab and bevacizumab for treatment of neovascular age-related macular degeneration: Two-year results. *Ophthalmology* **119:** 1388–1398.

Maruko I, Iida T, Saito M, Nagayama D, Saito K. 2007. Clinical characteristics of exudative age-related macular degeneration in Japanese patients. *Am J Ophthalmol* **144:** 15–22.

Mata NL, Lichter JB, Vogel R, Han Y, Bui TV, Singerman LJ. 2013. Investigation of oral fenretinide for treatment of geographic atrophy in age-related macular degeneration. *Retina* **33:** 498–507.

Miller JW. 2013. Age-related macular degeneration revisited—Piecing the puzzle: The LXIX Edward Jackson memorial lecture. *Am J Ophthalmol* **155:** 1–35, e13.

Mimoun G, Soubrane G, Coscas G. 1990. Macular drusen. *J Fr Ophtalmol* **13:** 511–530.

Mizutani T, Yasukawa T, Ito Y, Takase A, Hirano Y, Yoshida M, Ogura Y. 2011. Pneumatic displacement of submacular hemorrhage with or without tissue plasminogen activator. *Graefes Arch Clin Exp Ophthalmol* **249:** 1153–1157.

MPS Study Group. 1982. Argon laser photocoagulation for senile macular degeneration. Results of a randomized clinical trial. *Arch Ophthalmol* **100:** 912–918.

MPS Study Group. 1986. Argon laser photocoagulation for neovascular maculopathy. Three-year results from randomized clinical trials. *Arch Ophthalmol* **104:** 694–701.

Mruthyunjaya P, Stinnett SS, Toth CA. 2004. Change in visual function after macular translocation with 360° retinectomy for neovascular age-related macular degeneration. *Ophthalmology* **111:** 1715–1724.

Ninomiya Y, Lewis JM, Hasegawa T, Tano Y. 1996. Retinotomy and foveal translocation for surgical management of subfoveal choroidal neovascular membranes. *Am J Ophthalmol* **122:** 613–621.

Ohji M, Saito Y, Hayashi A, Lewis JM, Tano Y. 1998. Pneumatic displacement of subretinal hemorrhage without tissue plasminogen activator. *Arch Ophthalmol* **116:** 1326–1332.

Olivier S, Chow DR, Packo KH, MacCumber MW, Awh CC. 2004. Subretinal recombinant tissue plasminogen activator injection and pneumatic displacement of thick submacular hemorrhage in age-related macular degeneration. *Ophthalmology* **111:** 1201–1208.

Panda-Jonas S, Jonas JB, Jakobczyk-Zmija M. 1996. Retinal pigment epithelial cell count, distribution, and correlations in normal human eyes. *Am J Ophthalmol* **121:** 181–189.

Papadopoulos N, Martin J, Ruan Q, Rafique A, Rosconi MP, Shi E, Pyles EA, Yancopoulos GD, Stahl N, Wiegand SJ. 2012. Binding and neutralization of vascular endothelial growth factor (VEGF) and related ligands by VEGF Trap, ranibizumab and bevacizumab. *Angiogenesis* **15:** 171–185.

Pumariega NM, Smith RT, Sohrab MA, Letien V, Souied EH. 2011. A prospective study of reticular macular disease. *Ophthalmology* **118:** 1619–1625.

Regillo CD. 2013. Lampalizumab (anti-factor D) in patients with geography atrophy: The MAHALO phase 2 results. *Annual Meeting of the American Academy of Ophthalmology*, New Orleans, November 16–19.

Ron Y, Ehrlich R, Axer-Siegel R, Rosenblatt I, Weinberger D. 2007. Pneumatic displacement of submacular hemorrhage due to age-related macular degeneration. *Ophthalmologica* **221:** 57–61.

Rosenfeld PJ, Brown DM, Heier JS, Boyer DS, Kaiser PK, Chung CY, Kim RY. 2006. Ranibizumab for neovascular age-related macular degeneration. *N Engl J Med* **355:** 1419–1431.

Sarks SH. 1976. Ageing and degeneration in the macular region: a clinico-pathological study. *Br J Ophthalmol* **60:** 324–341.

Sarks SH, Van Driel D, Maxwell L, Killingsworth M. 1980. Softening of drusen and subretinal neovascularization. *Trans Ophthalmol Soc U K* **100:** 414–422.

Sarks JP, Sarks SH, Killingsworth MC. 1988. Evolution of geographic atrophy of the retinal pigment epithelium. *Eye (Lond)* **2** (Pt 5): 552–577.

Sarks S, Cherepanoff S, Killingsworth M, Sarks J. 2007. Relationship of Basal laminar deposit and membranous debris to the clinical presentation of early age-related macular degeneration. *Invest Ophthalmol Vis Sci* **48:** 968–977.

Sayanagi K, Sharma S, Yamamoto T, Kaiser PK. 2009. Comparison of spectral-domain versus time-domain optical coherence tomography in management of age-related macular degeneration with ranibizumab. *Ophthalmology* **116:** 947–955.

Schmitz-Valckenberg S, Bindewald-Wittich A, Dolar-Szczasny J, Dreyhaupt J, Wolf S, Scholl HP, Holz FG. 2006. Correlation between the area of increased autofluorescence surrounding geographic atrophy and disease progression in patients with AMD. *Invest Ophthalmol Vis Sci* **47:** 2648–2654.

Schmitz-Valckenberg S, Fleckenstein M, Scholl HP, Holz FG. 2009. Fundus autofluorescence and progression of age-related macular degeneration. *Surv Ophthalmol* **54:** 96–117.

Schmitz-Valckenberg S, Steinberg JS, Fleckenstein M, Visvalingam S, Brinkmann CK, Holz FG. 2010. Combined confocal scanning laser ophthalmoscopy and spectral-domain optical coherence tomography imaging of reticular drusen associated with age-related macular degeneration. *Ophthalmology* **117:** 1169–1176.

Schwartz SD, Hubschman JP, Heilwell G, Franco-Cardenas V, Pan CK, Ostrick RM, Mickunas E, Gay R, Klimanskaya I, Lanza R. 2012. Embryonic stem cell trials for macular degeneration: a preliminary report. *Lancet* **379:** 713–720.

Scott AW, Bressler SB. 2010. Retinal angiomatous proliferation or retinal anastomosis to the lesion. *Eye (Lond)* **24:** 491–496.

Seddon JM, Willett WC, Speizer FE, Hankinson SE. 1996. A prospective study of cigarette smoking and age-related macular degeneration in women. *JAMA* **276:** 1141–1146.

Singh RP, Patel C, Sears JE. 2006. Management of subretinal macular haemorrhage by direct administration of tissue plasminogen activator. *Br J Ophthalmol* **90:** 429–431.

Sommer A, Tielsch JM, Katz J, Quigley HA, Gottsch JD, Javitt JC, Martone JF, Royall RM, Witt KA, Ezrine S. 1991. Racial differences in the cause-specific prevalence of blindness in East Baltimore. *N Engl J Med* **325:** 1412–1417.

Sperduto RD, Hiller R. 1986. Systemic hypertension and age-related maculopathy in the Framingham Study. *Arch Ophthalmol* **104:** 216–219.

Stewart MW. 2012. Aflibercept (VEGF Trap-eye): The newest anti-VEGF drug. *Br J Ophthalmol* **96:** 1157–1158.

TAP Study Group. 1999. Photodynamic therapy of subfoveal choroidal neovascularization in age-related macular degeneration with verteporfin: One-year results of 2 randomized clinical trials—TAP report. *Arch Ophthalmol* **117:** 1329–1345.

Tarallo V, Hirano Y, Gelfand BD, Dridi S, Kerur N, Kim Y, Cho WG, Kaneko H, Fowler BJ, Bogdanovich S, et al. 2012. DICER1 loss and *Alu* RNA induce age-related macular degeneration via the NLRP3 inflammasome and MyD88. *Cell* **149:** 847–859.

Tomita K, Tsujikawa A, Yamashiro K, Ooto S, Tamura H, Otani A, Nakayama Y, Yoshimura N. 2012. Treatment of polypoidal choroidal vasculopathy with photodynamic therapy combined with intravitreal injections of ranibizumab. *Am J Ophthalmol* **153:** 68–80, e61.

Trichonas G, Murakami Y, Thanos A, Morizane Y, Kayama M, Debouck CM, Hisatomi T, Miller JW, Vavvas DG. 2010. Receptor interacting protein kinases mediate retinal detachment-induced photoreceptor necrosis and compensate for inhibition of apoptosis. *Proc Natl Acad Sci* **107:** 21695–21700.

Tsai JC. 2013. Canadian Journal of Ophthalmology Lecture: Translational research advances in glaucoma neuroprotection. *Can J Ophthalmol* **48:** 141–145.

van Leeuwen R, Ikram MK, Vingerling JR, Witteman JC, Hofman A, de Jong PT. 2003. Blood pressure, atherosclerosis, and the incidence of age-related maculopathy: The Rotterdam Study. *Invest Ophthalmol Vis Sci* **44:** 3771–3777.

Varma R, Fraser-Bell S, Tan S, Klein R, Azen SP. 2004. Prevalence of age-related macular degeneration in Latinos: the Los Angeles Latino eye study. *Ophthalmology* **111:** 1288–1297.

Vinding T. 1995. Age-related macular degeneration. An epidemiological study of 1000 elderly individuals. With reference to prevalence, funduscopic findings, visual impairment and risk factors. *Acta Ophthalmol Scand Suppl*: 1–32.

Vingerling JR, Dielemans I, Bots ML, Hofman A, Grobbee DE, de Jong PT. 1995. Age-related macular degeneration is associated with atherosclerosis. The Rotterdam Study. *Am J Epidemiol* **142:** 404–409.

VIP Study Group. 2001. Verteporfin therapy of subfoveal choroidal neovascularization in age-related macular degeneration: Two-year results of a randomized clinical trial including lesions with occult with no classic choroidal neovascularization—Verteporfin in photodynamic therapy report 2. *Am J Ophthalmol* **131:** 541–560.

WHO. 2013. Prevention of blindness and visual impairment; priority eye diseases (http://www.who.int/blindness/causes/priority/en/index7.html).

Wolff B, Matet A, Vasseur V, Sahel JA, Mauget-Faysse M. 2012. En face OCT imaging for the diagnosis of outer retinal tubulations in age-related macular degeneration. *J Ophthalmol* **2012:** 542417.

Wong WT, Kam W, Cunningham D, Harrington M, Hammel K, Meyerle CB, Cukras C, Chew EY, Sadda SR, Ferris FL. 2010. Treatment of geographic atrophy by the topical administration of OT-551: Results of a phase II clinical trial. *Invest Ophthalmol Vis Sci* **51:** 6131–6139.

Yamashita A, Shiraga F, Shiragami C, Shirakata Y, Fujiwara A. 2013. Two-year results of reduced-fluence photodynamic therapy for polypoidal choroidal vasculopathy. *Am J Ophthalmol* **155:** 96–102, e101.

Yannuzzi LA, Negrao S, Iida T, Carvalho C, Rodriguez-Coleman H, Slakter J, Freund KB, Sorenson J, Orlock D, Borodoker N. 2001. Retinal angiomatous proliferation in age-related macular degeneration. *Retina* **21:** 416–434.

Yehoshua Z, de Amorim Garcia Filho CA, Nunes RP, Gregori G, Penha FM, Moshfeghi AA, Zhang K, Sadda S, Feuer W, Rosenfeld PJ. 2014. Systemic complement inhibition with eculizumab for geographic atrophy in age-related macular degeneration: The COMPLETE study. *Ophthalmology* **121:** 693–701.

Yonekawa Y. 2013. Aflibercept for the treatment of refractory polypoidal choroidal vasculopathy. *Can J Ophthalmol* **48:** e59–e60.

Zarbin MA. 2004. Current concepts in the pathogenesis of age-related macular degeneration. *Arch Ophthalmol* **122:** 598–614.

Zhang K, Hopkins JJ, Heier JS, Birch DG, Halperin LS, Albini TA, Brown DM, Jaffe GJ, Tao W, Williams GA. 2011a. Ciliary neurotrophic factor delivered by encapsulated cell intraocular implants for treatment of geographic atrophy in age-related macular degeneration. *Proc Natl Acad Sci* **108:** 6241–6245.

Zhang M, Zhang J, Yan M, Luo D, Zhu W, Kaiser PK, Yu DC. 2011b. A phase 1 study of KH902, a vascular endothelial growth factor receptor decoy, for exudative age-related macular degeneration. *Ophthalmology* **118:** 672–678.

Zweifel SA, Engelbert M, Laud K, Margolis R, Spaide RF, Freund KB. 2009. Outer retinal tubulation: A novel optical coherence tomography finding. *Arch Ophthalmol* **127:** 1596–1602.

Zweifel SA, Imamura Y, Spaide TC, Fujiwara T, Spaide RF. 2010. Prevalence and significance of subretinal drusenoid deposits (reticular pseudodrusen) in age-related macular degeneration. *Ophthalmology* **117:** 1775–1781.

Genome-Wide Association Studies: Getting to Pathogenesis, the Role of Inflammation/Complement in Age-Related Macular Degeneration

Jessica N. Cooke Bailey[1], Margaret A. Pericak-Vance[2], and Jonathan L. Haines[1]

[1]Department of Epidemiology and Biostatistics, Case Western Reserve University Medical Center, Cleveland, Ohio 44106

[2]Hussman Institute of Human Genomics, Miller School of Medicine, University of Miami, Miami, Florida 33136

Correspondence: jonathan.haines@case.edu

Age-related macular degeneration (AMD) is a chronic, degenerative, and significant cause of visual impairment and blindness in the elderly. Genetic and epidemiological studies have confirmed that AMD has a strong genetic component, which has encouraged the application of increasingly sophisticated genetic techniques to uncover the important underlying genetic variants. Although various genes and pathways have been implicated in the risk for AMD, complement activation has been emphasized repeatedly throughout the literature as having a major role both physiologically and genetically in susceptibility to and pathogenesis of this disease. This article explores the research efforts that brought about the discovery and characterization of the role of inflammatory and immune processes (specifically complement) in AMD. The focus herein is on the genetic evidence for the role of complement in AMD as supported specifically by genome-wide association (GWA) studies, which interrogate hundreds of thousands of variants across the genome in a hypothesis-free approach, and other genetic interrogation methods.

The complement system is a key mediator of three central physiologic activities including host defense against infection, waste disposal, and the overlap between innate and adaptive immunity (Walport 2001a). The more than 40 proteins and regulators that comprise this system are found in the systemic circulation (Khandhadia et al. 2012). There are three complement pathways, each with a unique activator. The classical pathway is triggered by an antibody–antigen complex, the alternative pathway is activated by host cell or pathogen surface binding, and the lectin pathway is triggered by surface polysaccharides of microbes (Khandhadia et al. 2012). For an extensive review of the complement system, the reader is referred to other published reviews (Morgan 1995; Hageman et al. 2001; Walport 2001a,b; Anderson et al. 2002). Disorders of the complement system have been implicated in numerous diseases including atypical hemolytic uremia, systemic lupus erythematosus-like syndrome, multiple

Cite this article as *Cold Spring Harb Perspect Med* doi: 10.1101/cshperspect.a017186

autoimmune diseases, and age-related macular degeneration (AMD) (Degn et al. 2011). We focus herein on the role of genetic mediators in the complement system implicated in AMD.

Although the current understanding of AMD etiology is far from complete, research has established that it is a heterogeneous disease with early and late stages and multiple subtypes. Early AMD is defined by the presence of drusen, visible on ophthalmoscopy as focal yellow deposits of acellular, polymorphous debris, along with focal hyperpigmentation of the retinal pigment epithelium (RPE) and pathologic alterations to the RPE and Bruch's membrane (reviewed in Miller 2013; Ratnapriya and Chew 2013). Progression from early to late AMD varies between patients (Klein and Klein 2007; Tikellis et al. 2007), although the underlying reasons for this variation have not yet been elucidated. Advanced AMD is characterized by choroidal neovascularization, geographic atrophy, or both. Neovascular or "wet" AMD is distinguishable by formation and leakage of new blood vessels under or within the retina. Nonneovascular "dry" AMD is characterized by progressive RPE and outer retinal atrophy. Both forms can lead to irreversible vision loss, and current clinical management lacks the promise of full visual restoration. Current treatment for neovascular AMD consists of intraocular injections of antiangiogenic agents that target vascular endothelial growth factor (VEGF), a secreted endothelial mitogen that is the key regulator of angiogenesis and vascular permeability and has been implicated as an important factor in development and progression of neovascular AMD (reviewed in Ratnapriya and Chew 2013). There is currently limited therapy for nonneovascular AMD.

AMD susceptibility and pathogenesis are influenced by multiple factors, as highlighted in Fig. 1, including genetic polymorphisms, environmental factors, and interactions between them (reviewed in DeAngelis et al. 2011). The undisputable contribution of genetic variation to AMD is supported by several lines of evidence including increased risk for AMD among relatives of patients (Klaver et al. 1998; Clemons

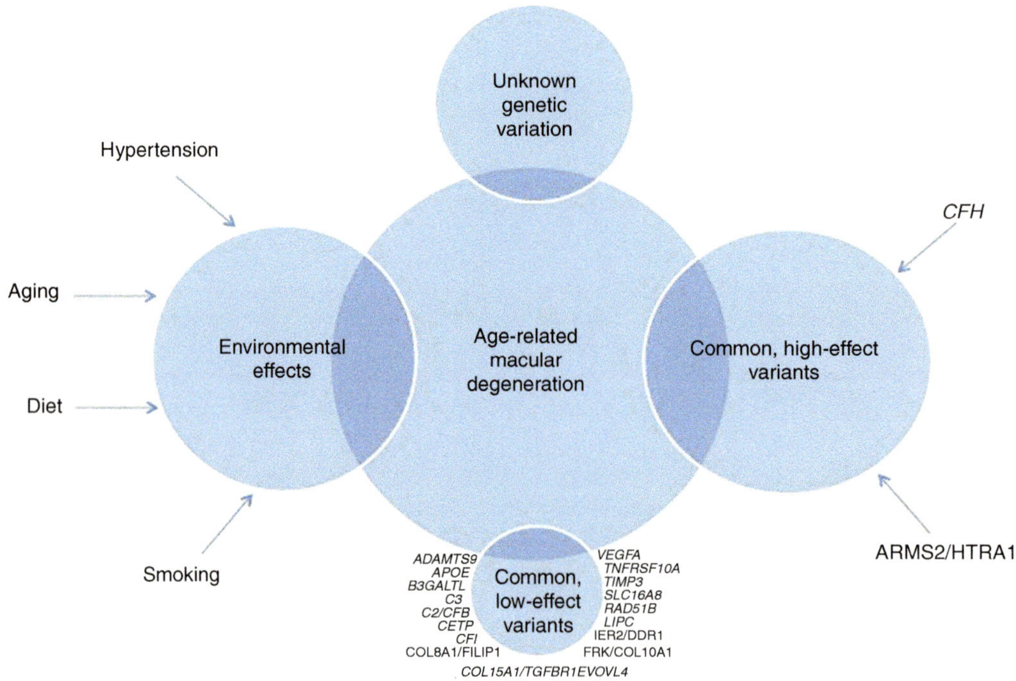

Figure 1. Representation of the genetic and environmental influences on AMD susceptibility.

et al. 2005; Swaroop et al. 2007) and twin studies reporting higher rates in monozygotic versus dizygotic twin pairs (Klein et al. 1994; Meyers 1994; Meyers et al. 1995; Klaver et al. 1998; Hammond et al. 2002). Extensive genetic studies of AMD, including genome-wide linkage screens, candidate gene studies, and genome-wide association (GWA) studies, have identified multiple variants that alter AMD risk (e.g., Weeks et al. 2000, 2001, 2004; Majewski et al. 2003; Schick et al. 2003; Seddon et al. 2003; Iyengar et al. 2004; Fisher et al. 2005). Major risk-modifying loci include variants in the *CFH* gene on chromosome 1 (e.g., Edwards et al. 2005; Hageman et al. 2005; Haines et al. 2005; Klein et al. 2005; Souied et al. 2005; Zareparsi et al. 2005; Baird et al. 2006; Conley et al. 2006; Hughes et al. 2006) and the *ARMS2-HTRA1* locus on chromosome 10 (e.g., Jakobsdottir et al. 2005; Rivera et al. 2005; Maller et al. 2006; Schmidt et al. 2006; Yang et al. 2006; Shuler Jr. et al. 2007; Fritsche et al. 2008). Additional AMD-associated variants are located in several other complement genes including *C3* (Maller et al. 2007; Yates et al. 2007; Spencer et al. 2008b), *CFI* (Fagerness et al. 2009), and two genes located in the major histocompatibility complex class III region (*C2* and *CFB*) (Gold et al. 2006; Spencer et al. 2007).

The two major genetic contributors to AMD are variants in the *CFH* and *ARMS2/HTRA1* genes. We will expand further on the *CFH* and other complement genes associated with AMD in the remainder of the article; however, it is important to note that signals in additional genes have been identified. Briefly, a high-effect locus on chromosome 10q26 was first implicated by linkage analysis in 2004 (Weeks et al. 2004; Fisher et al. 2005) and later confirmed to be associated with AMD (e.g., Jakobsdottir et al. 2005; Rivera et al. 2005; Schmidt et al. 2006; Schwartz et al. 2012). This locus contains three genes, *PLEKHA1* (pleckstrin homology domain-containing family A member 1), *ARMS2* (age-related maculopathy susceptibility 2; formerly *LOC387715*), and *HTRA1* (HtrA serine peptidase 1), which encompass variants that are strongly associated with AMD (odds ratios exceeding 10 [e.g., Dewan et al. 2006]). Because of the strong linkage disequilibrium across this region, discerning the true associated variant(s) continues to prove difficult (for a recent and comprehensive review, refer to Wang 2014). Additionally, the function of ARMS2 remains largely unknown and functional studies have been inconsistent regarding the role of this protein in AMD (reviewed in Wang 2014). Although the function of HTRA1 is better understood and it can be argued that it makes a better functional candidate, results from functional analyses of the implicated variants have been largely inconsistent as well (reviewed in Wang 2014).

More recently discovered variants associated with AMD reside within and/or near genes *ADAMTS9, B3GALTL, CETP, COL8A1-FILIP1L, IER3-DDR1, LIPC, RAD51B, SLC16A8, TGFBR1*, and *TIMP3* (for more information, refer to Chen et al. 2010; Neale et al. 2010; Fritsche et al. 2013). We focus the remainder of the article specifically on genetic contributors to AMD that are related to the complement system.

It has been well established that inflammatory and immunologic mediators play key roles in the pathogenesis of AMD (e.g., Penfold et al. 1985; Hageman et al. 2001; Anderson et al. 2002, 2010; Patel and Chan 2008; Ding et al. 2009). In 1985, Penfold and colleagues detected inflammatory and immunologic hallmarks in lesions of AMD (Penfold et al. 1985). Since then, the role of immunological events and inflammatory mediators in AMD has been well studied both from functional and genetic aspects. Hallmarks of advanced AMD, including drusen and retinal lesions, promote inflammatory and immune responses including recruitment of macrophages, accumulation of microglia cells, activation of complement, release of cytokines and chemokines, and oxidative stress (Tuo et al. 2012).

Following the functional implication for the complement system in AMD, genetic studies of this relationship exploded. However, the success of these studies was limited. Targeted candidate gene studies seeking to reveal genetic differences accounting for the high prevalence of AMD by analyzing variants in suspected disease genes were unsuccessful (Tuo et al. 2004). Multiple family-based whole-genome linkage scans localized chromosomal regions with evidence of linkage to AMD (Klein et al. 1998; Weeks et al. 2000, 2001, 2004; Majewski et al. 2003; Seddon et al. 2003; Abecasis et al. 2004; Iyengar et al. 2004), including specifically the chromosome 1q25-q32 region first identified by Klein and colleagues (Klein et al. 1998). In this study, a linkage peak on chromosome 1q25-q31 was identified in a large family with high prevalence of AMD. This region was later repeatedly confirmed by additional linkage studies (Majewski et al. 2003; Seddon et al. 2003; Abecasis et al. 2004; Iyengar et al. 2004; Weeks et al. 2004), which also implicated this region of chromosome 1 (also known as *ARMD1*) as having a role in AMD. With few exceptions (such as chromosome 1), these multitudes of genetic linkage studies did not confirm each other's results, and the overall genetic picture remained unclear. Fortunately, when these studies were combined into a large scale meta-analysis, some consistently supported regions were identified, including chromosomes 1, 4, 10, and 16 (Fisher et al. 2005).

Following these linkage study reports, multiple research groups began to explore additional methods for more focused detection of disease-associated variants. The convergence of four different approaches led to the discovery and confirmation of the first AMD-associated gene on chromosome 1, *CFH*, which encodes the complement factor H protein (Fig. 2). In one of the first GWA studies ever performed and reported, implementing a hypothesis-free approach of interrogating large numbers of single nucleotide polymorphisms (SNPs) for association with AMD, Klein et al. (2005) screened 96 AMD cases and 50 non-AMD controls to evaluate variants associated with disease. The data set was derived from part of the age-related eye disease study (AREDS 1999) and the individuals were of self-reported non-Hispanic white ethnicity. This analysis interrogated >116,000 SNPs across the genome. Of the 116,204 successfully genotyped SNPs, intronic SNP rs380390, located within *CFH* on chromosome 1q31, was strongly associated with AMD ($P < 10^{-7}$). Linkage disequilibrium analysis of SNPs in the large 41 kb haplotype block revealed a risk haplotype that increases the risk for AMD by a factor of 7.4. To further localize the signal detected, *CFH* exons and the intronic region containing rs380390 were resequenced to isolate potential functional polymorphisms in the region. The most strongly associated nonsynonymous SNP implicated in this analysis was rs1061170; this polymorphism causes the substitution of a histidine for a tyrosine at amino acid 402 (Y402H) in exon 9 of *CFH*.

Simultaneously and independently, a second study implemented a completely different study design that used a purely locational genomic approach. It also implicated the Y402H variant in AMD (Haines et al. 2005). Focusing on the 24 Mb region implicated in several linkage

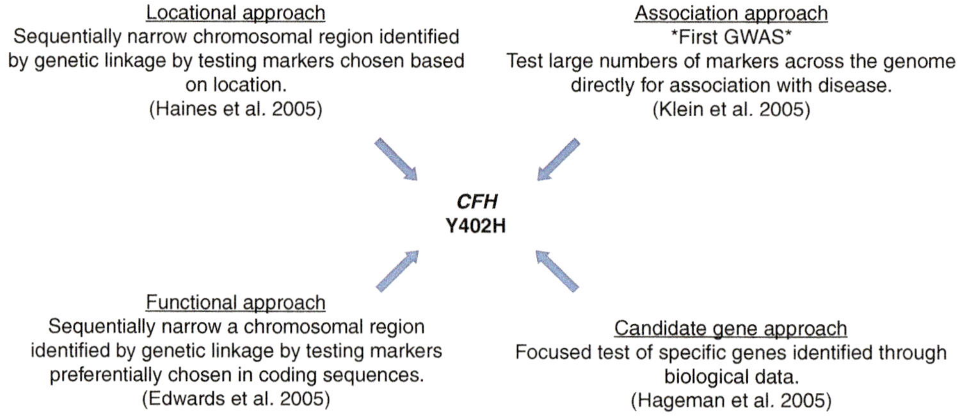

Figure 2. Four genetic approaches converge to facilitate the discovery of the *CFH* Y402H AMD susceptibility variant.

studies of AMD (Abecasis et al. 2004; Iyengar et al. 2004; Weeks et al. 2004) and extending slightly beyond this region, this study genotyped 61 SNPs in two independent data sets comprised of family-based and case-control samples. A five-SNP haplotype spanning a 261 kb region and encompassing the regulators of complement activation (RCA) gene cluster was associated in both the family and case-control data sets. They next screened the coding region of *CFH* for risk variants by sequencing 48 individuals homozygous for the associated haplotype. In this analysis, which included 24 AMD cases and 24 non-AMD controls, 11 variants were detected, including rs1061170 (Y402H), which was by far the most significantly associated with AMD. When the sequencing data was expanded and Y402H genotyped in the full family and an independent case-control data set, it was significantly associated with AMD ($P = 6 \times 10^{-5}$). Interestingly, the odds ratio for AMD in carriers of one C allele was 2.45 (95% confidence interval [CI]: 1.41–4.25), whereas in homozygous C carriers, the odds ratio was 3.33 (CI: 1.79–6.20). When restricted to only individuals with neovascular AMD, odds ratios increased to 3.45 (95% CI: 1.72–6.92) and 5.57 (95% CI: 2.52–12.27), respectively, for heterozygous and homozygous risk allele carriers. The population attributable risk (PAR) for carrying one or more risk alleles was 43% (95% CI: 23%–68%), indicating that quite a large portion of AMD could be attributed specifically to this variant.

Also simultaneously and using yet another independent and complimentary approach, Edwards and colleagues (Edwards et al. 2005) also identified the Y402H variant. This group applied a focused fine-mapping method centered on the chromosome 1 *ARMD1* region, which had been previously implicated in a linkage study of AMD (Edwards et al. 2005) but, unlike the Haines et al. (2005) study, this group focused preferentially on markers in coding sequences. The region was interrogated with a total of 86 SNPs spanning the RCA locus in a discovery sample of 224 cases and 133 controls. Of the associated variants, all 29 were located within the RCA; the most significant polymorphism was rs1061170 (Y402H) in *CFH*. Confirmatory support for this SNP's involvement in AMD was evident in replication analysis in which 14 SNPs were genotyped in 176 cases and 68 controls, and rs1061170 was again associated. The attributable fraction for rs1061170 in this study was 50%, indicating that individuals carrying the C allele accounted for approximately half of AMD cases.

Hageman and colleagues (2005) again confirmed the Y402H variant, applying yet a fourth genetic analysis method. They applied their prior knowledge of the involvement of *CFH* (also called HF1) in membranoproliferative glomerulonephritis (MPGN) type II (MPGNII). These patients develop ocular drusen similar to those found in AMD patients, and the genetic lesion for MPGNII also resides within the 1q31-32 region. Thus they evaluated *CFH* (HF1) sequence variants for association with AMD in addition to examining gene transcription and protein distribution in the macular RPE/choroid complex from controls and AMD patients (Hageman et al. 2005). Evaluating two samples of unrelated individuals including 404 and 550 cases and 131 and 275 controls, respectively, for variation in *CFH* associated with AMD, their results implicated two common missense variants that showed highly significant associations (I62 V, $P = 3.2 \times 10^{-7}$; and Y402H, $P = 1.6 \times 10^{-13}$). Thus, these results again supported the involvement of Y402H in AMD but also indicated that multiple CFH variants mediate risk for AMD. Functional evaluation of macula from controls and AMD patients indicated that CFH accumulates within drusen and is synthesized by the RPE, thus further supporting the physiologic role of CFH in AMD.

These four complimentary studies provided confirmation and signal localization for the chromosome 1 regions highlighted in linkage studies of AMD (Abecasis et al. 2004; Iyengar et al. 2004; Weeks et al. 2004). In addition to the pivotal knowledge gained from the four approaches, these studies also supported the novel genetic analysis approach known as the GWA study by confirming not only the same region, but the same SNP, as being associated with AMD. The convergence of these four different and independently performed studies provided the field of genetics and disease gene discovery with the necessary confidence in the newly defined GWA method to encourage its application to numerous other diseases. More than 2000 GWA studies have now been published (Welter et al. 2014).

The discovery of the *CFH* variant, which so powerfully influences AMD risk, spurred various analyses of this and additional complement genes in attempts to elucidate variants mediating AMD risk beyond the initially implicated Y402H in *CFH*. Multiple additional studies explored the *CFH* region, with varied success. Seeking to confirm the *CFH* signal, Maller and colleagues evaluated a sample of 2172 unrelated European-descended individuals including 1238 AMD cases and reported a second signal in a *CFH* intron (rs1410996, $P = 2.65 \times 10^{-61}$) that remained associated ($P < 10^{-9}$) after conditioning on Y402H (Maller et al. 2006). Although they performed dense mapping of this region, no other SNPs remained associated after conditioning on Y402H and rs1410996.

To characterize the genetic architecture of *CFH* and five *CFH*-related genes (*CFHR1-5*), Hughes et al. genotyped a region spanning these genes in 173 severe neovascular AMD cases and 170 elderly AMD-free controls; this analysis confirmed two strongly associated haplotypes that appeared to be conferring protection from AMD (Hughes et al. 2006). Haplotype 5, which was detected in ~20% of control and only 7.8% of case chromosomes in their discovery sample, was independent of the risk variant Y402H (Hughes et al. 2006). Genotyping Y402H and haplotype 5 SNPs in an additional sample of 192 AMD cases and 192 elderly controls confirmed the haplotype 5 frequency in each group (Hughes et al. 2006). In an effort to determine the source of the haplotype 5 protective effect, exon sequencing was performed on *CFH* and *CFHR1*; this analysis detected a deletion of *CFHR1* and *CFHR3* (Hughes et al. 2006). The encoded proteins were absent from the serum of individuals homozygous for the protective haplotype 5 (Hughes et al. 2006). Further analyses confirmed this protective effect and the independence of this effect from the Y402H variant (e.g., Spencer et al. 2008a; Fritsche et al. 2010; Sawitzke et al. 2011), although results for the level of significance the deletion contributes to protection from AMD varied (e.g., Spencer et al. 2008b). Further exploring *CFH*, Spencer and colleagues evaluated previously reported (Hageman et al. 2005) *CFH* haplotypes and the interaction of smoking status with these in a sample of 584 AMD cases and 248 controls and an additional analysis of 201 families (Spencer et al. 2007). They identified and confirmed two *CFH* haplotypes associated ($P = 0.001$, $P = 0.077$, respectively) with protection from AMD and also detected nominal evidence ($P = 0.04$) for an interaction between smoking and a protective haplotype, thus providing evidence for the involvement of interaction between a complement component and smoking in AMD risk.

Beyond *CFH*, various studies sought to evaluate the role of additional compliment mediators in AMD. Because CFH is an activator of the alternative complement pathway, Gold et al. (2006) hypothesized that other activators of this pathway might also be associated with AMD. Initially scanning 18 exons of the factor B-encoding gene *BF*, which is paralogous to complement component 2 (*C2*), in 180 AMD cases and controls, this group detected two sequence variants that were more frequent in controls—the L9H and R32Q mutations. The L9H variant in *BF* is in near complete linkage disequilibrium (i.e., is always inherited together with the E318D *C2* variant). Additionally, the R32Q variant is in nearly complete linkage disequilibrium with intronic *C2* SNP rs547154; these variants are highly protective against AMD, which was supported by replication analysis performed by this group. Combined analysis of BF/C2 variation in combination with the *CFH* Y402H variant indicated that 74% of cases and 56% of controls were predictable when these data were available. These variants were confirmed shortly thereafter by Maller and colleagues (2006), who further investigated the evolutionary history of the alleles and determined that the rare, protective variants arose on two distinct haplotypes and likely independently influence AMD risk for AMD.

Exploring complement cascade components beyond *CFH* and *C2/CFB* for involvement in AMD, Yates et al. (2007) genotyped 13 SNPs in *C3* and *C5*, key complement cascade proteins, in three European case-control groups. Evaluating two data sets of English ancestry with a total of 603 cases and 350 controls, no variants in *C5* were associated with AMD; however, strong evidence of association was detected at rs2230199, which encodes amino acid substitution R120G ($P = 5.9 \times 10^{-5}$) in C3. The variant replicated in a Scottish cohort of 244 cases and 351 controls ($P = 5.0 \times 10^{-5}$); odds ratios for risk allele heterozygotes and homozygotes, were 1.7 (95% CI 1.3–2.1) and 2.6 (95% CI 1.6–4.1), respectively, with an estimated population attributable risk of 22%, thus implicating *C3* and further supporting the role of the complement pathway in AMD pathogenesis. This variant again replicated in an independent sample of 2172 primarily European descent individuals including 1238 cases (Maller et al. 2007). Resequencing of *C3* identified a nonsynonymous SNP in moderate linkage disequilibrium ($r^2 = \sim 0.53$ in this data set) with R80G (rs1047286, L314P) (Maller et al. 2007); conditional analysis confirmed that the R102G polymorphism is likely the causal variant in *C3* (Spencer et al. 2008b).

Also seeking to evaluate complement components potentially involved in AMD beyond the previously implicated ones, Fagerness and colleagues performed targeted genotyping of 1500 SNPs in genes falling under suggestive linkage peaks identified in Fisher et al. (2005) as well as complement genes not in those regions (Fagerness et al. 2009). This analysis was performed in a study population of 2053 unrelated Caucasians $\geq$60 years of age including 1228 dry and wet AMD cases. The most significantly associated variant, which was surrounded by suggestively associated SNPs, was rs10033900 ($P = 9.11 \times 10^{-8}$), which is 2.8 kb upstream of the 3′ UTR of the complement factor I (*CFI*) gene. Dense follow-up genotyping in the region surrounding rs10033900 followed by conditional association analysis did not reveal any variants with greater significance than the original associated SNP. Haplotype analysis in the region implicated rs13117504 and rs10033900 together ($P = 1.18 \times 10^{-8}$) were more strongly associated with AMD than the single SNP, although neither SNP is thought to be functional.

Another group seeking to clarify the role of additional complement genes in AMD, Stanton and colleagues explored the role of complement factor D (*CFD*) in AMD by genotyping two SNPs in six separate case-control samples of European descent (Stanton et al. 2011). Their analysis of a total of 4765 individuals including 2833 AMD cases detected that rs3826945 was associated with AMD, although it replicated almost solely in females.

Additional approaches to clarify the role of complement in AMD have not all been met with success. Further exploring the AMD association with additional complement pathway genes beyond those thus far described has been a major focus for groups seeking to genetically explain AMD risk and pathogenesis. Implementing a candidate gene approach and exploring 20 SNPs in four complement genes—*CFP*, *CD46*, *CD55*, and *CD59* in 446 AMD cases and 262 controls, Cipriani and colleagues (2012) did not detect association.

Additional GWA studies on individual data sets beyond the first reported in AMD have been met with limited success beyond replication of known signals. Ryu and colleagues (2010) performed a GWA study in 593 non-Hispanic white subjects from the age-related eye disease study (AREDS) in which 109,270 SNPs were interrogated and analyzed for association with AMD. Replication was performed in an independent data set of 444 AMD cases and 300 non-AMD controls. Loci in previously implicated complement genes *CFH*, *CFB*, and *C3* replicated association in this analysis, although no novel variants were detected. A recently reported GWA study examined 400 AMD cases with an interesting set of controls—400 individuals with primary open angle glaucoma (POAG) with no history, clinical signs, or symptoms of AMD (Scheetz et al. 2013). Samples were genotyped at 500,000 loci on the Affymetrix 500 k and Mapping 5.0 arrays; this method, although presenting its own challenges in terms of disease phase of given association, is a time- and cost-effective approach. Although previously detected loci in *CFH* and *ARMS2-HTRA1-PLEKHA1* were associated in this analysis along with several other previously implicated loci, no novel associations were detected.

META-ANALYSIS OF GWA STUDIES

Although the GWA approach has been informative for numerous studies since those first reported in the mid-2000s (Welter et al. 2014), a substantial proportion of genetic etiology of GWAS studied diseases has yet to be explained; this is true for AMD, in which identified risk variants are estimated to account for 15%–65% of the genetic portion of AMD (Manolio et al. 2009). Approaches to enhance the detection of genetic variation associated with disease have grown beyond the traditional GWA approach and include imputing variants using known genetic information for a reference sample, performing conditional analyses, and implementing pathway analyses.

Increasing sample size of studies is crucial, as large sample sizes of cases and controls accelerate the identification of genetic variation associated with the disease of interest. Beyond increasing the number of samples tested, increasing the number of variants tested has also become a more attainable goal by performing imputation on GWA data. Imputation is a technique that greatly increases the number of tested variants beyond those interrogated in a GWA study by inferring genotypes of untyped SNPs. Combining known genotypes at GWA-interrogated SNPs with DNA sequences from a reference panel, genotypes at numerous SNPs can then be inferred with varying degrees of confidence and accuracy. Imputation not only increases the power of GWA studies by increasing the number of SNPs that can be tested, it can also lead to more efficient identification of causal variants and/or SNPs in high-linkage disequilibrium with a causal variant (Marchini and Howie 2010; Li et al. 2009). Imputation has been implemented in several studies of AMD to enhance the ability to detect associated variants (Fritsche et al. 2013; Helgason et al. 2013; Seddon et al. 2013).

Studies that bring together the described techniques substantially increase the value of GWA data. In the most recent publication from the AMD Gene Consortium (Fritsche et al. 2013), seven novel variants were detected by using GWA data beyond traditionally implemented methods. Using GWA data from 7650 advanced AMD cases and 51,844 controls and imputing to the HapMap II human variation reference dataset (Frazer et al. 2007), the Consortium evaluated nearly 2.5 million total SNPs. Of these, 32 were further evaluated in an additional 9531 cases and 8230 controls. Joint analysis detected 19 total loci attaining genome-wide significance at $P < 5 \times 10^{-8}$. Significant loci included 12 previously identified variants in *ARMS2-HTRA1, CFH, C2-CFB, C3, TIMP3, APOE, CETP, VEGFA, TNFRSF10A, LIPC, CFI,* and *COL10A1*, with odds ratios ranging from 1.13 (*COL10A1*) to 2.71 (*ARMS2-HTRA1*). An additional seven variants in *COL8A1-FILIP1L, IER3-DDR1, SLC16A8, TGFBR1, RAD51B, ADAMTS9,* and *B3GALTL* met genome-wide significance for the first time, with odds ratios ranging from 1.11 (*RAD51B*) to 1.28 (*COL8A10-FILIP1L*) (Fritsche et al. 2013).

This study also went beyond traditional GWA methods by exploring stratification by AMD subtype, gender, and ancestry. Of particular interest, *CFH* risk alleles associated preferentially with geographic atrophy risk when compared with choroidal neovascularization, and had stronger evidence of association in Europeans compared with Asians. Interaction analyses, which explored whether pairs of risk alleles occurring together conferred higher risk than alleles occurring alone, highlighted one interaction between SNPs near *CFH* and *C2-CFB* in which carriers of risk alleles at both loci were at slightly higher risk for AMD than what would normally be expected. These results further confirmed the importance of the complement system in AMD and provided the best overall estimates of the effect sizes for each of the implicated variants to date.

Pathway enrichment analyses are used to identify biological relationships between biologically associated genetic signals and pathways of interest in a particular disease. These are implemented by evaluating GWA results for SNPs to assess overrepresentation in particular biological pathways and serve to evaluate signals that could be biologically meaningful but are overlooked amidst numerous potentially false-positive results (Yaspan et al. 2011). Thus, pathway analyses provide insight to the functional aspects of a disease by evaluating GWA results in a broader manner than single-SNP analyses, and can identify potentially meaningful relationships for SNPs other than those attaining a specific p-value cutoff. Such results may highlight additional small and/or interactive effects that are important to evaluate in addition to and in the context of the overall GWA results. The most recent publication of the AMD Gene Consortium reported implementing INRICH (Interval-based Enrichment Analysis Tool for Genome Wide Association Studies) pathway analysis (Lee et al. 2012) to evaluate overall results (Fritsche et al. 2013). While confirming previously implicated AMD pathways, this analysis also highlighted additional pathways of interest; among the seven new loci, there was enrichment for genes encoding proteins in the complement and atherosclerotic pathways in addition to genes encoding collagen and extracellular region proteins, complement and coagulation cascades, lipoprotein metabolism, and regulation of apoptosis (Fritsche et al. 2013).

BEYOND GWA STUDIES

Whole exome and whole genome sequencing are additional approaches that investigate far beyond the genome-wide arrays, and their utility is just starting to be realized in AMD. These confer the ability to evaluate rare and low-frequency variants, which have been implicated as a potential source of missing heritability in many diseases with a genetic component (Manolio et al. 2009). AMD, having nearly one-third of the genetic component of the disease unexplained, has been investigated in several rare variant studies (e.g., Raychaudhuri et al. 2011; Gu et al. 2013; Helgason et al. 2013; Seddon et al. 2013; van de Ven et al. 2013; Zhan et al. 2013). In two recent publications, the role of rare variation was explored on a large scale. Helgason et al. whole-genome sequenced 2230 Icelandic samples and used these data to impute 34.2 million SNPs and short insertions/deletions using Illumina array data from 95,085 Icelanders. Variants were then tested for association with AMD in 1143 Icelanders with AMD and 51,435 controls; no new loci were detected that attained genome-wide significance thresholds. Applying conditional analyses to previously implicated loci, they searched for independent signals and detected a rare variant in *C3*, rs147859257, which codes for a Lys155Gln substitution, present at <1% frequency in their sample, that appears to be independent of previously reported Arg102-Gly and Pro314Leu (Helgason et al. 2013) variants. This type of analysis is important for deciphering residual signals at previously reported loci—as evidenced by the lack of significant signals after conditioning on both the Pro314Leu and newly discovered Lys155Gln variants.

Another recent study discovered rare variants in three genes, *CFI, C3,* and *C9* that are associated with AMD by applying targeted next-generation sequencing to coding regions of candidate genes in AMD-associated loci and pathways (Seddon et al. 2013). This analysis evaluated 681 genes in 1676 AMD cases prioritized for extreme phenotype (severe disease, familial disease, and early age of onset), 745 controls and 36 siblings discordant for AMD (Seddon et al. 2013). Evaluating coding variants present at <1% frequency and applying burden testing identified *CFI* as having an increased burden of rare variation in cases compared with controls, independent of the known rs4698775 risk variant. They additionally tested 1824 rare (frequency <1% variants present at least five times) individually for association with AMD; 11 variants were followed up in an independent sample of 2227 cases and 2888 controls.

ADDITIONAL FUNCTIONAL STUDIES

The ability to relate functional data to genetic data can greatly increase the interpretation of the genetic data. The AMD Gene Consortium found that *CFH* mRNA was differentially expressed in postmortem retina of young and elderly individuals (Fritsche et al. 2013). In addition, *C3* expression was higher in adult compared with fetal RPE, and all complement genes that were expressed at detectable levels in the retina or RPE were expressed at higher levels in tissue from older individuals. Thus, functional data linked with genetic data is incredibly informative and clearly still implicates the complement system in AMD pathogenesis.

Current efforts in genetic studies of AMD require implementation of all described methods, in addition to developing new analyses and experiments for further parsing out the role of complement and other biological systems in AMD susceptibility and pathogenesis. Analysis of data from exome chips, designed to jointly interrogate data relevant to association studies of common variants and sequencing studies of rare variants, will improve various aspects of genetic analysis of AMD. These data will provide greater coverage of known disease susceptibility loci via fine mapping, improve discovery of novel disease loci, and provide means for rare coding and copy number variant analysis. With new technology undoubtedly comes the challenge of implementing new analysis methods. For instance, most variants interrogated on exome arrays are quite rare; therefore, single variant analysis may not yield results that are truly representative of the impact of a specific region on disease risk. To address this challenge, data will be evaluated by aggregating sets of low-frequency variants associated with disease (e.g., applying burden testing). One particular method for burden testing designed to detect association signals distributed over multiple variants is the sequence kernel association test (SKAT) method, which allows for the incorporation of flexible weight functions, thereby allowing, for example, one to increase the weight of variants with lower minor allele frequencies and decrease the weight of variants inferred with lower confidence (in the case of imputed data) (Wu et al. 2011). Such analysis techniques will be crucial to moving forward future analyses that will clarify the molecular mechanisms linking known loci to disease.

The goal of the above described and additional ongoing studies is to improve the current comprehension of new and existing disease loci, as well as to improve the prediction of individual phenotypes to increase the knowledge of AMD biology in hopes of ultimately facilitating the development of better strategies for disease treatment and prevention.

GENETIC RISK SCORES

As the focus of biomedical research transitions toward personalized medicine, genetic studies now have the task of not only detecting variants that mediate disease risk but also assessing whether those variants interact with known environmental and clinical factors (and whether there is clinical utility for this knowledge in the current or future medical setting). The most comprehensive case-control analysis in AMD in a recent report from the AMD Gene Consortium indicates that risk scores based on the now 19 known common SNPs mediating risk for AMD are able to distinguish fairly well between case and control individuals (Fritsche et al. 2013), although it is not clear that the most recently identified variants contribute a great deal of information regarding disease risk beyond what prior known SNPs indicate. Other studies have evaluated the utility of categorized risk intervals based on genetic variation solely and in addition to known environmental contributors with generally positive results (e.g., Ho et al. 2011; Spencer et al. 2011; Grassmann et al. 2012). Beyond simple genetic risk score analysis, the interaction of genetic risk with environmental factors is also valuable not only clinically but to further elucidate mechanisms of disease susceptibility and pathogenesis. For example, Spencer and colleagues developed an algorithm using genetic profile and smoking history that was able to categorize individuals into high- and low-risk profiles for AMD (Spencer et al. 2011). In addition, Buitendijk et al. (2013) show that, although the difference is perhaps not clinically significant, the best statistical model for predicting AMD is attained when genetic as well as environmental factors are included. This type of model does not add a

 Cite this article as *Cold Spring Harb Perspect Med* doi: 10.1101/cshperspect.a017186

great deal of information beyond what is indicated from a clinically integrated evaluation that includes only age, sex, AMD baseline grade, smoking, and BMI, although the difference is statistically significant (Buitendijk et al. 2013). As phenotyping improves, additional genetic variants involved in AMD will likely be detected, and their role in disease more clearly defined (Ratnapriya and Chew 2013). Additionally, the role of environmental factors and their interactions with genetic variation must continue to be elucidated; thus, before the full utility of genetic risk scores can be applied in AMD, the genetic architecture must continue to be unraveled (Ratnapriya and Chew 2013), within and beyond the contribution of complement and other known genetic mediators of disease.

CONCLUDING REMARKS

That there is a role for complement in AMD is overwhelmingly supported by genetic and physiologic evidence. As biomedical research continues to elucidate the mechanisms by which complement contributes to the pathology of this disease, increasingly sophisticated techniques will be applied to analyzing and interpreting genetic data. Ongoing and planned studies interrogate the entire exome, even the entire genome, in hopes of gaining additional knowledge pertinent to the pathophysiology of AMD. Additionally, better characterizing the contributions of known risk loci will be important to continue to clarify the molecular mechanisms linking these to disease. The ultimate overall goal of these efforts is to increase the understanding of AMD biology so that better strategies for disease treatment and prevention can be developed and implemented.

ACKNOWLEDGMENTS

This work was supported by the National Institutes of Health grants EY012118 (J.L.H., M.A.P.V.), EY023164 (J.L.H., M.A.P.V.), T32 EY007157 (J.N.C.B.), and T32 EY21453-2 (J.N.C.B.).

REFERENCES

Abecasis GR, Yashar BM, Zhao Y, Ghiasvand NM, Zareparsi S, Branham KE, Reddick AC, Trager EH, Yoshida S, Bahling J, et al. 2004. Age-related macular degeneration: A high-resolution genome scan for susceptibility loci in a population enriched for late-stage disease. *Am J Hum Genet* **74:** 482–494.

Age-Related Eye Disease Study Research Group. 1999. The age-related eye disease study (AREDS): Design implications. AREDS report no. 11. *Control Clin Trials* **20:** 573–600.

Anderson DH, Mullins RD, Hageman GS, Johnson LV. 2002. A role for local inflammation in the formation of drusen in the aging eye. *Am J Ophthalmol* **134:** 411–431.

Anderson DH, Radeke MJ, Gallo NB, Chapin EA, Johnson PT, Curletti CR, Hancox LS, Hu J, Ebright JN, Malek G, et al. 2010. The pivotal role of the complement system in aging and age-related macular degeneration: Hypothesis re-visited. *Prog Retin Eye Res* **29:** 95–112.

Baird PN, Islam FM, Richardson AJ, Cain M, Hunt N, Guymer R. 2006. Analysis of the Y402H variant of the complement factor H gene in age-related macular degeneration. *Invest Ophthalmol Vis Sci* **47:** 4194–4198.

Buitendijk GH, Rochtchina E, Myers C, van Duijn CM, Lee KE, Klein BE, Meuer SM, de Jong PT, Holliday EG, Tan AG, et al. 2013. Prediction of age-related macular degeneration in the general population: The three continent AMD consortium. *Ophthalmology* **120:** 2644–2655.

Chen W, Stambolian D, Edwards AO, Branham KE, Othman M, Jakobsdottir J, Tosakulwong N, Pericak-Vance MA, Campochiaro PA, Klein ML, et al. 2010. Genetic variants near *TIMP3* and high-density lipoprotein-associated loci influence susceptibility to age-related macular degeneration. *Proc Natl Acad Sci* **107:** 7401–7406.

Cipriani V, Matharu BK, Khan JC, Shahid H, Stanton CM, Hayward C, Wright AF, Bunce C, Clayton DG, Moore AT, et al. 2012. Genetic variation in complement regulators and susceptibility to age-related macular degeneration. *Immunobiology* **217:** 158–161.

Clemons TE, Milton RC, Klein R, Seddon JM, Ferris FL III. 2005. Risk factors for the incidence of advanced age-related macular degeneration in the age-related eye disease study (AREDS) AREDS report no. 19. *Ophthalmology* **112:** 533–539.

Conley YP, Jakobsdottir J, Mah T, Weeks DE, Klein R, Kuller L, Ferrell RE, Gorin MB. 2006. *CFH*, *ELOVL4*, *PLEKHA1* and *LOC387715* genes and susceptibility to age-related maculopathy: AREDS and CHS cohorts and meta-analyses. *Hum Mol Genet* **15:** 3206–3218.

DeAngelis MM, Silveira AC, Carr EA, Kim IK. 2011. Genetics of age-related macular degeneration: Current concepts, future directions. *Semin Ophthalmol* **26:** 77–93.

Degn SE, Jensenius JC, Thiel S. 2011. Disease-causing mutations in genes of the complement system. *Am J Hum Genet* **88:** 689–705.

Dewan A, Liu M, Hartman S, Zhang SS, Liu DT, Zhao C, Tam PO, Chan WM, Lam DS, Snyder M, et al. 2006. *HTRA1* promoter polymorphism in wet age-related macular degeneration. *Science* **314:** 989–992.

Ding X, Patel M, Chan CC. 2009. Molecular pathology of age-related macular degeneration. *Prog Retin Eye Res* **28:** 1–18.

Edwards AO, Ritter R III, Abel KJ, Manning A, Panhuysen C, Farrer LA. 2005. Complement factor H polymorphism and age-related macular degeneration. *Science* **308:** 421–424.

Fagerness JA, Maller JB, Neale BM, Reynolds RC, Daly MJ, Seddon JM. 2009. Variation near complement factor I is associated with risk of advanced AMD. *Eur J Hum Genet* **17:** 100–104.

Fisher SA, Abecasis GR, Yashar BM, Zareparsi S, Swaroop A, Iyengar SK, Klein BE, Klein R, Lee KE, Majewski J, et al. 2005. Meta-analysis of genome scans of age-related macular degeneration. *Hum Mol Genet* **14:** 2257–2264.

Frazer KA, Ballinger DG, Cox DR, Hinds DA, Stuve LL, Gibbs RA, Belmont JW, Boudreau A, Hardenbol P, Leal SM, et al. 2007. A second generation human haplotype map of over 3.1 million SNPs. *Nature* **449:** 851–861.

Fritsche LG, Loenhardt T, Janssen A, Fisher SA, Rivera A, Keilhauer CN, Weber BH. 2008. Age-related macular degeneration is associated with an unstable *ARMS2* (*LOC387715*) mRNA. *Nat Genet* **40:** 892–896.

Fritsche LG, Lauer N, Hartmann A, Stippa S, Keilhauer CN, Oppermann M, Pandey MK, Kohl J, Zipfel PF, Weber BH, et al. 2010. An imbalance of human complement regulatory proteins CFHR1, CFHR3 and factor H influences risk for age-related macular degeneration (AMD). *Hum Mol Genet* **19:** 4694–4704.

Fritsche LG, Chen W, Schu M, Yaspan BL, Yu Y, Thorleifsson G, Zack DJ, Arakawa S, Cipriani V, Ripke S, et al. 2013. Seven new loci associated with age-related macular degeneration. *Nat Genet* **45:** 433–432.

Gold B, Merriam JE, Zernant J, Hancox LS, Taiber AJ, Gehrs K, Cramer K, Neel J, Bergeron J, Barile GR, et al. 2006. Variation in factor B (*BF*) and complement component 2 (*C2*) genes is associated with age-related macular degeneration. *Nat Genet* **38:** 458–462.

Grassmann F, Fritsche LG, Keilhauer CN, Heid IM, Weber BH. 2012. Modelling the genetic risk in age-related macular degeneration. *PLoS ONE* **7:** e37979.

Gu BJ, Baird PN, Vessey KA, Skarratt KK, Fletcher EL, Fuller SJ, Richardson AJ, Guymer RH, Wiley JS. 2013. A rare functional haplotype of the *P2RX4* and *P2RX7* genes leads to loss of innate phagocytosis and confers increased risk of age-related macular degeneration. *FASEB J* **27:** 1479–1487.

Hageman GS, Luthert PJ, Victor Chong NH, Johnson LV, Anderson DH, Mullins RF. 2001. An integrated hypothesis that considers drusen as biomarkers of immune-mediated processes at the RPE-Bruch's membrane interface in aging and age-related macular degeneration. *Prog Retin Eye Res* **20:** 705–732.

Hageman GS, Anderson DH, Johnson LV, Hancox LS, Taiber AJ, Hardisty LI, Hageman JL, Stockman HA, Borchardt JD, Gehrs KM, et al. 2005. A common haplotype in the complement regulatory gene factor H (*HF1/CFH*) predisposes individuals to age-related macular degeneration. *Proc Natl Acad Sci* **102:** 7227–7232.

Haines JL, Hauser MA, Schmidt S, Scott WK, Olson LM, Gallins P, Spencer KL, Kwan SY, Noureddine M, Gilbert JR, et al. 2005. Complement factor H variant increases the risk of age-related macular degeneration. *Science* **308:** 419–421.

Hammond CJ, Webster AR, Snieder H, Bird AC, Gilbert CE, Spector TD. 2002. Genetic influence on early age-related maculopathy: A twin study. *Ophthalmology* **109:** 730–736.

Helgason H, Sulem P, Duvvari MR, Luo H, Thorleifsson G, Stefansson H, Jonsdottir I, Masson G, Gudbjartsson DF, Walters GB, et al. 2013. A rare nonsynonymous sequence variant in *C3* is associated with high risk of age-related macular degeneration. *Nat Genet* **45:** 1371–1374.

Ho L, van LR, Witteman JC, van Duijn CM, Uitterlinden AG, Hofman A, de Jong PT, Vingerling JR, Klaver CC. 2011. Reducing the genetic risk of age-related macular degeneration with dietary antioxidants, zinc, and ω-3 fatty acids: The Rotterdam study. *Arch Ophthalmol* **129:** 758–766.

Hughes AE, Orr N, Esfandiary H, Diaz-Torres M, Goodship T, Chakravarthy U. 2006. A common *CFH* haplotype, with deletion of *CFHR1* and *CFHR3*, is associated with lower risk of age-related macular degeneration. *Nat Genet* **38:** 1173–1177.

Iyengar SK, Song D, Klein BE, Klein R, Schick JH, Humphrey J, Millard C, Liptak R, Russo K, Jun G, et al. 2004. Dissection of genomewide-scan data in extended families reveals a major locus and oligogenic susceptibility for age-related macular degeneration. *Am J Hum Genet* **74:** 20–39.

Jakobsdottir J, Conley YP, Weeks DE, Mah TS, Ferrell RE, Gorin MB. 2005. Susceptibility genes for age-related maculopathy on chromosome 10q26. *Am J Hum Genet* **77:** 389–407.

Khandhadia S, Cipriani V, Yates JR, Lotery AJ. 2012. Age-related macular degeneration and the complement system. *Immunobiology* **217:** 127–146.

Klaver CC, Wolfs RC, Assink JJ, van Duijn CM, Hofman A, de Jong PT. 1998. Genetic risk of age-related maculopathy. Population-based familial aggregation study. *Arch Ophthalmol* **116:** 1646–1651.

Klein BE, Klein R. 2007. Lifestyle exposures and eye diseases in adults. *Am J Ophthalmol* **144:** 961–969.

Klein ML, Mauldin WM, Stoumbos VD. 1994. Heredity and age-related macular degeneration. Observations in monozygotic twins. *Arch Ophthalmol* **112:** 932–937.

Klein ML, Schultz DW, Edwards A, Matise TC, Rust K, Berselli CB, Trzupek K, Weleber RG, Ott J, Wirtz MK, et al. 1998. Age-related macular degeneration. Clinical features in a large family and linkage to chromosome 1q. *Arch Ophthalmol* **116:** 1082–1088.

Klein RJ, Zeiss C, Chew EY, Tsai JY, Sackler RS, Haynes C, Henning AK, SanGiovanni JP, Mane SM, Mayne ST, et al. 2005. Complement factor H polymorphism in age-related macular degeneration. *Science* **308:** 385–389.

Lee PH, O'Dushlaine C, Thomas B, Purcell SM. 2012. INRICH: Interval-based enrichment analysis for genome-wide association studies. *Bioinformatics* **28:** 1797–1799.

Li Y, Willer C, Sanna S, Abecassis G. 2009. Genotype imputation. *Ann Rev Hum Genet* **10:** 387–406.

Majewski J, Schultz DW, Weleber RG, Schain MB, Edwards AO, Matise TC, Acott TS, Ott J, Klein ML. 2003. Age-related macular degeneration—A genome scan in extended families. *Am J Hum Genet* **73:** 540–550.

Maller J, George S, Purcell S, Fagerness J, Altshuler D, Daly MJ, Seddon JM. 2006. Common variation in three genes, including a noncoding variant in *CFH*, strongly influences risk of age-related macular degeneration. *Nat Genet* **38:** 1055–1059.

Maller JB, Fagerness JA, Reynolds RC, Neale BM, Daly MJ, Seddon JM. 2007. Variation in complement factor 3 is associated with risk of age-related macular degeneration. *Nat Genet* **39:** 1200–1201.

Manolio TA, Collins FS, Cox NJ, Goldstein DB, Hindorff LA, Hunter DJ, McCarthy MI, Ramos EM, Cardon LR, Chakravarti A, et al. 2009. Finding the missing heritability of complex diseases. *Nature* **461:** 747–753.

Marchini J, Howie B. 2010. Genotype imputation for genome-wide association studies. *Nat Rev Genet* **11:** 499–511.

Meyers SM. 1994. A twin study on age-related macular degeneration. *Trans Am Ophthalmol Soc* **92:** 775–843.

Meyers SM, Greene T, Gutman FA. 1995. A twin study of age-related macular degeneration. *Am J Ophthalmol* **120:** 757–766.

Miller JW. 2013. Age-related macular degeneration revisited—Piecing the puzzle: The LXIX Edward Jackson memorial lecture. *Am J Ophthalmol* **155:** 1–35.

Morgan BP. 1995. Physiology and pathophysiology of complement: Progress and trends. *Crit Rev Clin Lab Sci* **32:** 265–298.

Neale BM, Fagerness J, Reynolds R, Sobrin L, Parker M, Raychaudhuri S, Tan PL, Oh EC, Merriam JE, Souied E, et al. 2010. Genome-wide association study of advanced age-related macular degeneration identifies a role of the hepatic lipase gene (*LIPC*). *Proc Natl Acad Sci* **107:** 7395–7400.

Patel M, Chan CC. 2008. Immunopathological aspects of age-related macular degeneration. *Semin Immunopathol* **30:** 97–110.

Penfold PL, Killingsworth MC, Sarks SH. 1985. Senile macular degeneration: The involvement of immunocompetent cells. *Graefes Arch Clin Exp Ophthalmol* **223:** 69–76.

Ratnapriya R, Chew EY. 2013. Age-related macular degeneration—Clinical review and genetics update. *Clin Genet* **84:** 160–166.

Raychaudhuri S, Iartchouk O, Chin K, Tan PL, Tai AK, Ripke S, Gowrisankar S, Vemuri S, Montgomery K, Yu Y, et al. 2011. A rare penetrant mutation in *CFH* confers high risk of age-related macular degeneration. *Nat Genet* **43:** 1232–1236.

Rivera A, Fisher SA, Fritsche LG, Keilhauer CN, Lichtner P, Meitinger T, Weber BH. 2005. Hypothetical *LOC387715* is a second major susceptibility gene for age-related macular degeneration, contributing independently of complement factor H to disease risk. *Hum Mol Genet* **14:** 3227–3236.

Ryu E, Fridley BL, Tosakulwong N, Bailey KR, Edwards AO. 2010. Genome-wide association analyses of genetic, phenotypic, and environmental risks in the age-related eye disease study. *Mol Vis* **16:** 2811–2821.

Sawitzke J, Im KM, Kostiha B, Dean M, Gold B. 2011. Association assessment of copy number polymorphism and risk of age-related macular degeneration. *Ophthalmology* **118:** 2442–2446.

Scheetz TE, Fingert JH, Wang K, Kuehn MH, Knudtson KL, Alward WL, Boldt HC, Russell SR, Folk JC, Casavant TL, et al. 2013. A genome-wide association study for primary open angle glaucoma and macular degeneration reveals novel loci. *PLoS ONE* **8:** e58657.

Schick JH, Iyengar SK, Klein BE, Klein R, Reading K, Liptak R, Millard C, Lee KE, Tomany SC, Moore EL, et al. 2003. A whole-genome screen of a quantitative trait of age-related maculopathy in sibships from the Beaver Dam Eye Study. *Am J Hum Genet* **72:** 1412–1424.

Schmidt S, Hauser MA, Scott WK, Postel EA, Agarwal A, Gallins P, Wong F, Chen YS, Spencer K, Schnetz-Boutaud N, et al. 2006. Cigarette smoking strongly modifies the association of *LOC387715* and age-related macular degeneration. *Am J Hum Genet* **78:** 852–864.

Schwartz SG, Agarwal A, Kovach JL, Gallins PJ, Cade W, Postel EA, Wang G, Ayala-Haedo J, Spencer KM, Haines JL, et al. 2012. The *ARMS2* A69S variant and bilateral advanced age-related macular degeneration. *Retina* **32:** 1486–1491.

Seddon JM, Santangelo SL, Book K, Chong S, Cote J. 2003. A genomewide scan for age-related macular degeneration provides evidence for linkage to several chromosomal regions. *Am J Hum Genet* **73:** 780–790.

Seddon JM, Yu Y, Miller EC, Reynolds R, Tan PL, Gowrisankar S, Goldstein JI, Triebwasser M, Anderson HE, Zerbib J, et al. 2013. Rare variants in *CFI*, *C3* and *C9* are associated with high risk of advanced age-related macular degeneration. *Nat Genet* **45:** 1366–1370.

Shuler RK Jr, Hauser MA, Caldwell J, Gallins P, Schmidt S, Scott WK, Agarwal A, Haines JL, Pericak-Vance MA, Postel EA. 2007. Neovascular age-related macular degeneration and its association with *LOC387715* and complement factor H polymorphism. *Arch Ophthalmol* **125:** 63–67.

Souied EH, Leveziel N, Richard F, Dragon-Durey MA, Coscas G, Soubrane G, Benlian P, Fremeaux-Bacchi V. 2005. Y402H complement factor H polymorphism associated with exudative age-related macular degeneration in the French population. *Mol Vis* **11:** 1135–1140.

Spencer KL, Hauser MA, Olson LM, Schmidt S, Scott WK, Gallins P, Agarwal A, Postel EA, Pericak-Vance MA, Haines JL. 2007. Protective effect of complement factor B and complement component 2 variants in age-related macular degeneration. *Hum Mol Genet* **16:** 1986–1992.

Spencer KL, Hauser MA, Olson LM, Schmidt S, Scott WK, Gallins P, Agarwal A, Postel EA, Pericak-Vance MA, Haines JL. 2008a. Deletion of *CFHR3* and *CFHR1* genes in age-related macular degeneration. *Hum Mol Genet* **17:** 971–977.

Spencer KL, Olson LM, Anderson BM, Schnetz-Boutaud N, Scott WK, Gallins P, Agarwal A, Postel EA, Pericak-Vance MA, Haines JL. 2008b. *C3* R102G polymorphism increases risk of age-related macular degeneration. *Hum Mol Genet* **17:** 1821–1824.

Spencer KL, Olson LM, Schnetz-Boutaud N, Gallins P, Agarwal A, Iannaccone A, Kritchevsky SB, Garcia M, Nalls MA, Newman AB, et al. 2011. Using genetic variation and environmental risk factor data to identify individuals at high risk for age-related macular degeneration. *PLoS ONE* **6:** e17784.

Stanton CM, Yates JR, den Hollander AI, Seddon JM, Swaroop A, Stambolian D, Fauser S, Hoyng C, Yu Y, Atsuhiro K, et al. 2011. Complement factor D in age-related macular degeneration. *Invest Ophthalmol Vis Sci* **52:** 8828–8834.

Swaroop A, Branham KE, Chen W, Abecasis G. 2007. Genetic susceptibility to age-related macular degeneration: A paradigm for dissecting complex disease traits. *Hum Mol Genet* **16:** R174–R182.

Tikellis G, Robman LD, Dimitrov P, Nicolas C, McCarty CA, Guymer RH. 2007. Characteristics of progression of early age-related macular degeneration: The cardiovascular health and age-related maculopathy study. *Eye (Lond)* **21:** 169–176.

Tuo J, Bojanowski CM, Chan CC. 2004. Genetic factors of age-related macular degeneration. *Prog Retin Eye Res* **23:** 229–249.

Tuo J, Grob S, Zhang K, Chan CC. 2012. Genetics of immunological and inflammatory components in age-related macular degeneration. *Ocul Immunol Inflamm* **20:** 27–36.

van de Ven JP, Nilsson SC, Tan PL, Buitendijk GH, Ristau T, Mohlin TC, Nabuurs SB, Schoenmaker-Koller FE, Smailhodzic D, Campochiaro PA, et al. 2013. A functional variant in the *CFI* gene confers a high risk of age-related macular degeneration. *Nat Genet* **45:** 813–817.

Walport MJ. 2001a. Complement. First of two parts. *N Engl J Med* **344:** 1058–1066.

Walport MJ. 2001b. Complement. Second of two parts. *N Engl J Med* **344:** 1140–1144.

Wang G. 2014. Chromosome 10q26 locus and age-related macular degeneration: A progress update. *Exp Eye Res* **119:** 1–7.

Weeks DE, Conley YP, Mah TS, Paul TO, Morse L, Ngo-Chang J, Dailey JP, Ferrell RE, Gorin MB. 2000. A full genome scan for age-related maculopathy. *Hum Mol Genet* **9:** 1329–1349.

Weeks DE, Conley YP, Tsai HL, Mah TS, Rosenfeld PJ, Paul TO, Eller AW, Morse LS, Dailey JP, Ferrell RE, et al. 2001. Age-related maculopathy: An expanded genome-wide scan with evidence of susceptibility loci within the 1q31 and 17q25 regions. *Am J Ophthalmol* **132:** 682–692.

Weeks DE, Conley YP, Tsai HJ, Mah TS, Schmidt S, Postel EA, Agarwal A, Haines JL, Pericak-Vance MA, Rosenfeld PJ, et al. 2004. Age-related maculopathy: A genomewide scan with continued evidence of susceptibility loci within the 1q31, 10q26, and 17q25 regions 16. *Am J Hum Genet* **75:** 174–189.

Welter D, Macarthur J, Morales J, Burdett T, Hall P, Junkins H, Klemm A, Flicek P, Manolio T, Hindorff L, et al. 2014. The NHGRI GWAS Catalog, a curated resource of SNP-trait associations. *Nucleic Acids Res* **42:** D1001–D1006.

Wu MC, Lee S, Cai T, Li Y, Boehnke M, Lin X. 2011. Rare-variant association testing for sequencing data with the sequence kernel association test. *Am J Hum Genet* **89:** 82–93.

Yang Z, Camp NJ, Sun H, Tong Z, Gibbs D, Cameron DJ, Chen H, Zhao Y, Pearson E, Li X, et al. 2006. A variant of the *HTRA1* gene increases susceptibility to age-related macular degeneration. *Science* **314:** 992–993.

Yaspan BL, Bush WS, Torstenson ES, Ma D, Pericak-Vance MA, Ritchie MD, Sutcliffe JS, Haines JL. 2011. Genetic analysis of biological pathway data through genomic randomization. *Hum Genet* **129:** 563–571.

Yates JR, Sepp T, Matharu BK, Khan JC, Thurlby DA, Shahid H, Clayton DG, Hayward C, Morgan J, Wright AF, et al. 2007. Complement *C3* variant and the risk of age-related macular degeneration. *N Engl J Med* **357:** 553–561.

Zareparsi S, Branham KE, Li M, Shah S, Klein RJ, Ott J, Hoh J, Abecasis GR, Swaroop A. 2005. Strong association of the Y402H variant in complement factor H at 1q32 with susceptibility to age-related macular degeneration. *Am J Hum Genet* **77:** 149–153.

Zhan X, Larson DE, Wang C, Koboldt DC, Sergeev YV, Fulton RS, Fulton LL, Fronick CC, Branham KE, Bragg-Gresham J, et al. 2013. Identification of a rare coding variant in complement 3 associated with age-related macular degeneration 5. *Nat Genet* **45:** 1375–1379.

The Proteomics of Drusen

John W. Crabb

Cole Eye Institute, Cleveland Clinic, Cleveland, Ohio 44195

Correspondence: crabbj@ccf.org

The formation of extracellular deposits known as drusen below the macular region of the retina correlates with increased risk of severe visual loss from age-related macular degeneration (AMD). Inflammation and complement dysregulation contribute to AMD progression; however, disease mechanisms remain incompletely defined. Multiple genetic and environmental factors influence AMD pathology, and although immune system processes play a central role, multiple molecular mechanisms appear to be involved. Drusen proteomics, including the analyses of constituent proteins, oxidative protein modifications, and pattern recognition receptors, provide a foundation for deciphering mechanisms of drusen biogenesis and AMD pathology.

Drusen are extracellular deposits of debris that accumulate with age on Bruch's membrane below the retinal pigment epithelium (RPE) and are considered clinical hallmarks of age-related macular degeneration (AMD). AMD, the leading cause of blindness in the elderly worldwide, is a complex disease involving inflammation and, in part, dysregulation of the complement system (Jager et al. 2008; Ding et al. 2009; Anderson et al. 2010). To date, 19 genetic loci (Fritsche et al. 2013) and multiple environmental factors, including diet and smoking, have been associated with AMD risk (Jager et al. 2008; Ding et al. 2009). Clinicians refer to drusen as either "soft" or "hard" in describing their relative shape and size, with hard drusen being nodular and generally smaller than soft drusen, which have a more diffuse appearance (Hageman et al. 2001). The presence of numerous and/or confluent soft drusen in the macula is considered a major risk factor for development of advanced AMD with severe visual loss (Fig. 1). Only 10%–20% of cases of early/mid-stage AMD (also known as "dry" AMD) progress to advanced AMD, with neovascular or "wet" AMD (characterized by choroidal neovascularization) being the more prevalent form of advanced AMD (Ferris et al. 1984; Zarbin 2004). Geographic atrophy, also known as advanced dry AMD, is characterized by focal atrophy of the RPE and loss of macular photoreceptors, whereas choroidal neovascularization involves abnormal blood vessel growth from the choriocapillaris through the RPE, resulting in possible hemorrhage, exudation, scarring, and/or retinal detachment. It is possible for the two forms of advanced AMD to occur at the same time in separate eyes of an individual. Antivascular endothelial growth factor (VEGF) treatments can slow the progression of choroidal neovascularization (Jager et al. 2008), but universally effective therapies for geographic at-

Cite this article as *Cold Spring Harb Perspect Med* doi: 10.1101/cshperspect.a017194

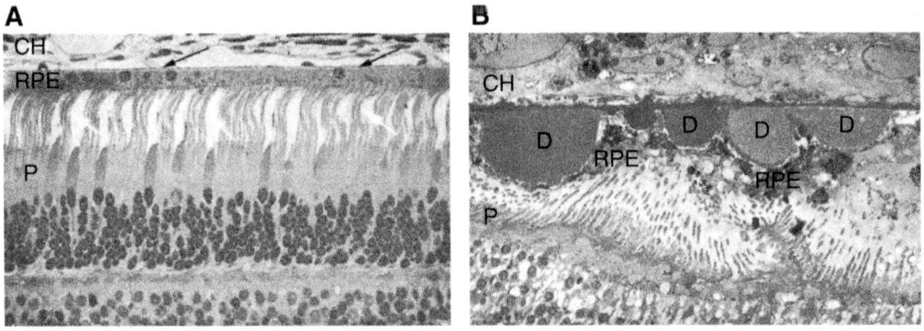

Figure 1. Comparison of ocular tissues containing drusen from normal eyes and eyes from AMD patients. In the normal retina (*A*), the photoreceptor cells (P) are highly organized, and their light-sensitive outer segments (white arrows) are in close contact with the RPE. Bruch's membrane (dark arrows), a thin layer of extracellular matrix between the RPE and choriocapillaris (CH), is barely visible at this magnification. In the AMD retina (*B*), photoreceptors are highly disorganized because of the presence of drusen (D), which also distorts the RPE and Bruch's membrane. (From Bok 2002; reproduced, with permission from National Academy of Sciences USA © 2002.)

rophy or for the prevention of wet or dry AMD have yet to be developed.

Drusen are widely accepted as contributors to the progression of AMD but the molecular mechanics of drusen formation are not yet well defined. Many components of drusen have been identified however the details of drusen biogenesis continue to be sought for molecular insights into AMD prevention and therapy. Histochemical and immunohistochemical studies have shown that drusen contain a variety of lipids, polysaccharides, glycosaminoglycans and proteins (Abdelsalam et al. 1999; Hageman et al. 1999, 2001; Kamei and Hollyfield 1999; Mullins et al. 2000; Malek et al. 2003; Anderson et al. 2004; Curcio et al. 2005a,b; Luibl et al. 2006; Wang et al. 2010; Jiang et al. 2012). Proteomic studies, both qualitative and quantitative, have expanded the repertoire of proteins and protein modifications associated with drusen (Crabb et al. 2002a; Umeda et al. 2005; Yuan et al. 2010; Garland et al. 2013). This review focuses on the proteomic components of drusen, and their potential impacts on drusen biogenesis and AMD pathology.

QUALITATIVE PROTEOMIC STUDIES

By the year 2000, about 20 protein components of human drusen had been identified by immunohistochemistry, including several immune system proteins, leading to the hypothesis that drusen formation involves inflammatory and immune responses to RPE damage (Hageman et al. 1999; Johnson et al. 2000; Mullins et al. 2000). In 2002, unbiased proteomic analysis by liquid chromatography tandem mass spectrometry (LC MS/MS) identified 129 proteins from isolated human drusen (Crabb et al. 2002a). Drusen are often found in the retinal periphery of normal aged eyes, and this early qualitative proteomic analysis included drusen isolated from 18 normal donors and 5 AMD donors. Based on the frequency of detection, common proteins found in both AMD drusen and normal donor drusen included tissue inhibitor of metalloproteinase 3 (TIMP3), clusterin, vitronectin, serum albumin, and crystallins, with crystallins detected more frequently in AMD donor drusen than in normal donor drusen. Significant proteomic heterogeneity was also apparent, with about a third of the proteins detected in AMD drusen not observed in normal donor drusen. To date, this study remains the only reported LC MS/MS proteomic comparison of human drusen purified from AMD eyes and normal eyes, in part because of the difficulty in obtaining AMD specimens and to the laborious drusen isolation procedure (Crabb et al. 2002a). Another mass spectrometric study has identified 60 proteins from drusen isolated from cynomolgus monkeys (*Macaca fascicula-*

ris) exhibiting macular degeneration (Umeda et al. 2005). About 50% of the monkey proteins were identical to or homologous with human drusen components. The currently identified proteins from isolated primate drusen constitute a subset of the drusen proteome, as many other proteins could be present as shown by the quantitative proteomic studies discussed below.

Immunocytochemical evidence has corroborated the drusen localization of several of the proteins identified by LC MS/MS, including annexins I and VI, proteins S100 A7, S100 A8, and S100 A9 (Crabb et al. 2002a), clusterin (Sakaguchi et al. 2002), TIMP3 (Kamei and Hollyfield 1999), vitronectin (Hageman et al. 1999), amyloid A, amyloid P, α1-antitrypsin, α1-antichymotrypsin, apolipoprotein A1, apolipoprotein E (APOE), multiple complement components (C3, C5, and C9), fibrinogen, immunoglobulin κ, immunoglobulin λ, and ubiquitin (Mullins et al. 2000). Annexin II, identified by LC MS/MS, was localized to the basal plasma membrane of the RPE adhering to drusen (Crabb et al. 2002a). Among the primate drusen proteins identified by LC MS/MS, it is possible that others may also belong to the RPE or Bruch's membrane. Nevertheless, this proteome supports the idea that drusen proteins come from several sources including the RPE, choroidal vasculature (Hageman et al. 2001; Penfold et al. 2001), and the systemic circulation.

QUANTITATIVE PROTEOMIC STUDIES

Two quantitative proteomic studies provide additional insights into mechanisms of drusen formation and macular degeneration. These studies include an analysis of the macular region of the Bruch's membrane/choroid complex from human AMD donors and normal donors (Yuan et al. 2010), and a proteomic analysis of Bruch's membrane/choroid from a mouse model of Doyne honeycomb retinal dystrophy/malattia Leventinese (Garland et al. 2013). Bruch's membrane is an important extracellular, semipermeable support for the RPE, influences the diffusion of nutrients and waste products between the RPE and the choroidal bloodstream, and restricts cell migration (Goldberg 1976). It is composed of the basement membranes of the RPE and choriocapillaris, inner and outer collagenous layers, and a central elastin zone (Booij et al. 2010). AMD pathology typically involves thickening and decreased permeability of Bruch's membrane (Goldberg 1976), thought to be caused in part by accumulation of collagen, lipids, advanced glycation endproducts (AGEs), RPE waste products and cross-links that covalently trap debris (Booij et al. 2010).

AMD-Associated Protein Alterations in Human Macular Bruch's Membrane/Choroid

LC MS/MS isobaric tags for relative and absolute quantitation (iTRAQ) technology has been used to quantify proteins in the macular region of the Bruch's membrane/choroid complex from human postmortem eyes (10 with early/mid dry AMD, six with advanced dry AMD, eight with wet AMD, and 25 normal eyes) (Yuan et al. 2010). A total of 901 proteins was quantified, the majority of which differed little in amount between AMD and controls and thus provide a partial proteome of normal human macular tissues of average age 81. Ninety-nine proteins were identified with significantly altered amounts in AMD macular tissues relative to normal controls, including 56 elevated and 43 reduced proteins. Consistent with proposed mechanisms of Bruch's membrane thickening (Booij et al. 2010), the relative amounts of 13 different collagens and protein-glutamine γ-glutamyltransferase 2, a cross-linking enzyme, were elevated in AMD tissues (Yuan et al. 2010). About 60% of the elevated proteins were immune response and host defense proteins, including many complement proteins and complement-associated proteins (e.g., C3, C4A, C5, C6, C7, C8γ, C9, complement factor B, complement factor H (CFH), and clusterin). Also among the elevated proteins were several damage-associated molecular pattern proteins (DAMPs) such as α-defensins 1-3, protein S100-A8, protein S100-A9, α-crystallin A, α-crystallin B, histones and galectin-3. DAMPs are endogenous proteins released by damaged cells and capable of activating pattern recognition receptors (Lotze et al. 2007). Not surprisingly, several proteins identified in isolated drusen were elevated in the macular AMD tissues (Table 1).

Inflammatory response proteins were found to be elevated in multiple categories of AMD progression, supporting the idea that inflammatory processes are involved in both initiating events of AMD and progression to advanced AMD. Four retinoid processing proteins (retinal pigment epithelium-specific 65 kDa protein, cellular retinoic acid-binding protein 1, cellular retinaldehyde binding protein, and interphotoreceptor retinoid binding protein) were found uniquely elevated in early/mid stage AMD, suggesting that retinoid metabolism contributes to AMD initiation, likely through mechanisms involving RPE lipofuscin (Eldred and Lasky 1993; Sakai et al. 1996; Sparrow and Boulton 2005; Kim et al. 2007; Sparrow 2007; Ng et al. 2008; Wu et al. 2010). AGE receptor 3 (also known as galectin-3) was the most significantly elevated protein in advanced dry AMD, implicating a role for AGEs in geographic atrophy. The remaining ~40% of the elevated proteins were associated with other regulatory functions and specialized metabolic or housekeeping processes. Elevated regulatory proteins included the protease inhibitors TIMP3 and α-1-microglobulin as well as pigment epithelium-derived factor, a neurotrophic antiangiogenic protein, all of which were also detected in purified drusen (Crabb et al. 2002a). Other elevated regulatory proteins in macular Bruch's/choroid included phosphatidylethanol-amine binding protein 1, a serine protease inhibitor; Rho GDP-dissociation inhibitor 1, a cell adhesion regulator; reticulon-4, a cell migration regulator; and voltage-dependent anion-selective channel protein 3, a diffusion regulator of small molecules. Consistent with proposed roles for mitochondrial dysfunction in aging (Knott et al. 2008) and AMD pathology (Nordgaard et al. 2008), mitochondrial cytochrome c oxidase subunit 5B, 2-oxoglutarate/malate carrier protein, and mitochondrial aldehyde dehydrogenase were elevated in the macular AMD Bruch's membrane/choroid complex in AMD.

Significantly reduced proteins accounted for a small fraction (<2%) of the proteins quantified in the macular region of the Bruch's/choroid complex in AMD. Over half of these proteins can be associated with cell adhesion and protein interactions (asporin, nidogen-2, Protein FAM 10A4, CD9), or vascularization and angiogenesis (tryptase α1, plasmalemma vesicle associated protein, caveolin-1, β2-glycoprotein 1). Proteins decreased only in early/mid stage AMD implicate hematologic malfunctions, reduced extracellular matrix integrity, and weakened cellular interactions. Proteins uniquely decreased in advanced dry AMD included β-crystallin B2, carbonic anhydrase 4, ubiquitin, and haptoglobin. Neuroblast differentiation-associated protein, a membrane remodeling and repair protein also known as desmoyokin, was decreased in advanced dry AMD but elevated in neovascular AMD. Proteins uniquely reduced in neovascular AMD included two histones, CD 9, three glycolytic enzymes, mitochondrial trifunctional enzyme β, creatine kinase B and ferritin light chain. Interphotorecepetor retinoid binding protein was reduced in both advanced dry and wet AMD. While reduced protein abundance in advanced AMD could reflect disease consequences (e.g., cell death), the majority of elevated proteins were different in geographic atrophy compared with neovascular AMD, implicating multiple mechanisms of AMD progression.

Proteins in the Bruch's Membrane/Choroid in *Efemp1*$^{R345W/R345W}$ Mice

Doyne honeycomb retinal dystrophy/malattia Leventinese is an inherited macular dystrophy caused by a point mutation (R345W) in the gene that encodes epidermal growth-factor-containing fibulin-like extracellular matrix protein 1 (EFEMP1), yielding a human phenotype similar to dry AMD with extensive drusen (Stone et al. 1999, 2004; Marmorstein 2002; Michaelides et al. 2006; Fu et al. 2007). Gene-targeted *Efemp1*$^{R345W/R345W}$mice provide an animal model that with age exhibit a macular degeneration-like phenotype and extensive formation of extracellular basal laminar deposits under the RPE (Fu et al. 2007; Marmorstein et al. 2007). Such basal deposits have long been con-

Table 1 Drusen proteins found in elevated amounts in macular Bruch's membrane/choroid of AMD eyes

			All AMD			Early/mid stage AMD			Advanced dry AMD			Advanced wet AMD		
SwissProt accession	Protein	Subcellular source	Mean protein ratio	Donors total = 24	*P* value	Mean protein ratio	Donors total = 10 value	*P* value	Mean protein ratio	Donors total = 6	*P* value	Mean protein ratio	Donors total = 8	*P* value
P05109	Protein S100-A8	Cytoplasmic	1.7	12	<0.01	1.6	5	<0.01				1.7	4	0.02
P07360	Complement C8γ	Secreted	1.7	7	0.04									
P13671	Complement C6	Secreted	1.6	4	0.03									
P10643	Complement C7	Secreted	1.6	8	<0.01	2.0	3	0.03						
P02763	α1-acid glycoprotein 1	Secreted	1.5	9	<0.01	1.5	4	<0.01				1.6	3	0.03
P06702	Protein S100-A9	Cytoplasmic	1.4	12	<0.01				1.7	3	0.02	1.9	4	0.01
P35625	TIMP3	Secreted	1.4	24	<0.01	1.4	10	<0.01	1.3	6	0.02	1.4	8	<0.01
P02489	α-Crystallin A	Cytoplasmic	1.3	13	<0.01	1.6	6	0.05						
P02760	AM BP protein	Secreted	1.3	3	0.04									
P01031	Complement C5	Secreted	1.3	10	<0.01	1.5	5	<0.01						
P06899	Histone H2B type 1-J	Nuclear	1.2	9	<0.01	1.2	3	0.02	1.2	3	0.04			
P04004	Vitronectin	Secreted	1.2	24	<0.01							1.3	8	<0.01
P36955	Pigment epithelium-derived factor	Secreted	1.2	8	0.01									
P02748	Complement C9	Secreted	1.2	24	0.01	1.2	10	0.03				1.5	8	0.01
P10909	Clusterin	Secreted	1.1	24	<0.01				1.2	6	0.04			
P02511	α-Crystailin B	Cytoplasmic	1.1	24	<0.01	1.3	10	<0.01						
P01011	α1-antichymotrypsin	Secreted	1.1	24	0.07	1.2	10	0.05				1.2	8	0.05
P01024	Complement C3	Secreted	1.1	22	0.02							1.2	7	0.01

Proteins were identified in isolated human drusen (Crabb et al. 2002a) and quantified in separate analysis of human macular Bruch's membrane/choroid from 24 AMD donors and 25 normal control donors (Yuan et al. 2010).

Mean protein ratios (AMD/control), donor frequency and *p* values (*t*-test) are shown. Proteins were considered significantly elevated if quantified in ≥3 donor specimens per group with protein ratios > 1 standard deviation above the group mean protein ratio and with *P* values ≤ 0.05.

sidered potential precursors of drusen (Sarks 1976; Green and Enger 1993; Spraul and Grossniklaus 1997; Curcio and Millican 1999; Sarks et al. 2007).

Quantitative proteomic analysis of basal deposits in the *Efemp1*$^{R345W/R345W}$ mouse model has revealed important clues to mechanisms of basal deposit formation (Garland et al. 2013). Bruch's membrane/choroid specimens from three ages of mutant and control mice (8, 14, and 24 mo) were analyzed to detect protein changes from early through extensive basal deposit formation. Bruch's membrane specimens without RPE or choroid were analyzed at 24 mo to more closely measure the basal deposit proteome. About 780 proteins per animal were identified, yielding a total of 1062 proteins quantified using LC MS/MS spectral counting methods. Major changes in protein abundance in the mutant mice were found associated with immune system processes. Notably, 11 complement components were detected in the samples from *Efemp1*$^{R345W/R345W}$ mice, with significant increases relative to controls in the abundance of complement components C3 and C4 in both 24-mo Bruch's membrane samples and in Bruch's/choroid specimens by 14 mo. The functional role of the complement system in basal deposit formation was further tested by generating homozygous *Efemp1*$^{R345W/R345W}$:*C3*$^{-/-}$ double mutant mice that expressed the R345W point mutation but lacked C3 expression. Histological analyses showed that basal deposits were markedly reduced in the double mutant mice, demonstrating that an active complement system plays an important role in basal deposit formation in this mouse model. The molecular details of this process, however, remain to be determined.

Quantitative proteomic changes in *Efemp1*$^{R345W/R345W}$mutant mice highlighted three other major biological processes that potentially contribute to basal deposit formation, namely cell–cell and cell–matrix adhesion, signal transduction, and intracellular transport (Garland et al. 2013). Four proteins exhibiting large increases in the Bruch's membrane of mutant mice and of possible pathological significance were EFEMP1, thrombospondin 1, milk-fat globule-EGF factor 8, and collagen VI, each of which can be associated with multiple processes and/or extracellular matrix structure function. No new or unusual proteins were identified, suggesting that normal extracellular matrix components in altered amounts or structure contribute to basal deposit formation. Similarities in the proteomic results from Bruch's membrane/choroid from *Efemp1*$^{R345W/R345W}$ mice (Garland et al. 2013) and human AMD donors (Yuan et al. 2010) were significant. About 50% of the proteins identified in the human study were also detected in the mouse samples, with remarkable quantitative agreement between select proteins, including C3, C4, vitronectin, galectin-3, and Ig μ chain C region, which were increased in both advanced AMD patients and the mutant mice.

OXIDATIVE PROTEIN MODIFICATIONS IN DRUSEN

Oxidative stress has long been considered a major contributor to AMD pathology (Seddon et al. 1996; Beatty et al. 2000; AREDS 2001; Hageman et al. 2001). Because of high oxygen tension and light exposure, the RPE/Bruch's/choroid interface is an extreme environment that facilitates the production of reactive oxygen species and nitrogen species that can stimulate inflammatory and immune responses (Verhasselt et al. 1998; Matsue et al. 2003; Hazen 2008; Hagenow et al. 2009). Moreover, in this extreme environment, photoreceptor outer segment tips phagocytized daily by the RPE are highly susceptible to oxidation, resulting in the production of reactive cleavage fragments from lipids, sugars, and retinoids, and subsequent oxidative modifications. A host of elevated protein modifications derived from lipoxidation and glycoxidation have been associated with AMD ocular tissues (Crabb 2012), and several have been demonstrated in drusen.

Oxidative protein modifications have the potential to mask proteolytic cleavage sites, inactivate enzymes (Crabb et al. 2002b), and contribute to the accumulation of cross-linked intracellular debris that copurifies with RPE lipofuscin granules (Chio et al. 1969; Schutt et al.

2003; Ng et al. 2008) and with extracellular debris in drusen (Crabb et al. 2002a). For example, several drusen proteins have been shown to migrate in multiple mass ranges in SDS gel electrophoresis, from the top to the bottom of the gel (Crabb et al. 2002a). The higher-mass components containing TIMP3, vitronectin, and C9 suggest the presence of covalent cross-links caused by reactive oxidation fragments from lipids and/or carbohydrates (Friguet et al. 1994; Elgawish et al. 1996).

Carboxymethyllysine was the first oxidative protein modification reported in drusen (Fig. 2). Greater immunoreactivity for carboxymethyllysine was detected in basal laminar and basal linear deposits, soft macular drusen, and choroidal neovascular membranes from AMD eyes compared to control eyes (Ishibashi et al. 1998). Carboxymethyllysine is a lysine glycoxidation modification formed through the nonenzymatic Maillard reaction, which combines sugar carbonyls with primary amino groups to form Amadori products. Amadori products undergo subsequent nonenzymatic reactions, including oxidative decomposition, to form a heterogeneous group of modifications known as AGEs (Baynes 2001). The presence of AGEs in aging ocular tissues is well-established (Ishibashi et al. 1998; Farboud et al. 1999; Hammes et al. 1999; Handa et al. 1999; Crabb et al. 2002a; Howes et al. 2004; Glenn et al. 2007, 2009). Pentosidine, another AGE in drusen, forms fluorescent lysine–arginine cross-links (Handa et al. 1999; Glenn et al. 2007). Advanced glycation occurs slowly over time, and long-lived proteins (e.g., collagens) in extracellular matrices such as Bruch's membrane are particularly susceptible to modification. AGE modifications promote protein denaturation, decreased solubility, decreased flexibility, and increased resistance to proteolytic degradation. Several studies have demonstrated that carboxymethyllysine induces VEGF expression in vitro in a variety of cell types, (Hirata et al. 1997; Lu et al. 1998; Treins et al. 2001; Hoffmann et al. 2002; Urata et al. 2002) and stimulates neovascularization in vivo

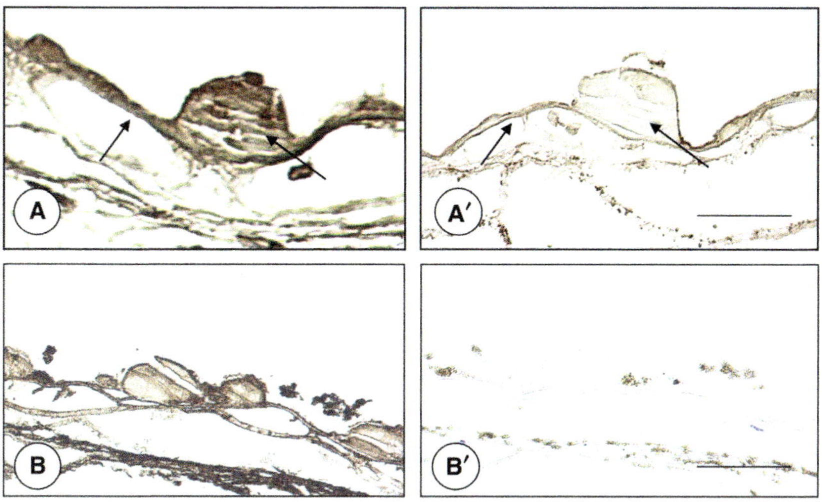

Figure 2. Oxidative protein modifications in human drusen and Bruch's membrane. (*A*) Immunohistochemical analysis of Bruch's membrane/choroid tissue with anticarboxyethylpyrrole monoclonal antibody. (*A′*) Control section, probed with preimmune IgG. (Arrows indicate Bruch's membrane and drusen; scale bar, 50 μm). (*B*) Immunohistochemical analysis with anticarboxymethyllysine monoclonal antibody. (*B′*) Control consecutive section treated with normal mouse IgG. This figure demonstrates the lipoxidation product carboxyethylpyrrole and the glycoxidation product carboxymethyllysine associated with drusen and Bruch's membrane. (Scale bar, 50 μm). (From Crabb et al. 2002a; reproduced, with permission from National Academy of Sciences USA © 2002.)

(Okamoto et al. 2002). Plasma levels of both carboxymethyllysine and pentosidine are elevated in AMD (Ni et al. 2009).

Several receptors modulate the biological effects of AGEs (Goh and Cooper 2008), including receptor of AGEs (RAGE), a pattern-recognition receptor that binds a variety of ligands, including DAMPs. RAGE ligands vary in their proinflammatory potential, but carboxymethyllysine is a strong inducer of RAGE signaling (Herold et al. 2007). Drusen proteins S100A8 and S100A9 (Crabb et al. 2002a; Yuan et al. 2010) are DAMPs thought to be activators of RAGE (Sparvero et al. 2009). Treatment of cultured RPE cells with AGEs, including carboxymethyllysine, has been shown to upregulate RAGE, resulting in apoptotic RPE cell death (Howes et al. 2004).

Multiple lipoxidation products are present in drusen, Bruch's membrane, and the cellular debris that copurifies with RPE lipofuscin granules (Crabb et al. 2002a; Gu et al. 2003a; Schutt et al. 2003; Shen et al. 2007; Ng et al. 2008; Weismann et al. 2011; Shaw et al. 2012). Lipoxidation in drusen is not surprising given the high amounts of cholesterol esters and phospholipids in drusen (Wang et al. 2010). Reactive lipid fragments can form Schiff base linkages with primary amino groups, resulting in the formation of a variety of adducts (Esterbauer et al. 1991; Gu et al. 2003b). Carboxyethylpyrrole was the first lipoxidation product identified in drusen (Fig. 2) and has been shown to be significantly more abundant in AMD ocular tissues and blood than in normal tissues (Crabb et al. 2002a; Gu et al. 2009). Carboxyethylpyrrole adducts are generated by the covalent reaction of primary amino groups (e.g., protein ε-lysyl NH_2) with 4-hydroxy-7-oxohept-5-enoic acid, a reactive fragment derived uniquely from oxidative cleavage of docosahexaenoate (DHA)-containing lipids (Gu et al. 2003b). DHA is abundant in the retina (Fliesler and Anderson 1983) and concentrated in the photoreceptor outer segments and the RPE (Wang and Anderson 1992; Alvarez et al. 1994). Mass spectrometric analysis of carboxyethylpyrrole-immunoreactive 2D gel spots has identified albumin and α1-antitrypsin as likely carboxyethylpyrrole-modified proteins in the Bruch's membrane/choroid/RPE complex in AMD; both of these proteins have been found in drusen (Crabb et al. 2002a).

Carboxyethylpyrrole adducts stimulate angiogenesis *in vivo* through toll-like receptor 2 (TLR2), another pattern recognition receptor. In contrast to neovascularization induced by carboxymethyllysine, carboxyethylpyrrole stimulates angiogenesis independent of VEGF (Ebrahem et al. 2006; West et al. 2010). Similar to complement and RAGE, TLR2 binds multiple ligands and initiates inflammatory and immune responses (Zahringer et al. 2008). At low concentrations, carboxyethylpyrrole adducts are hypothesized to contribute to wound healing, but at high concentrations may catalyze amplified TLR2 signaling and excessive neovascularization (West et al. 2010). Carboxyethylpyrrole protein adducts have also been shown to promote platelet activation and aggregation in vitro and thrombosis in vivo through toll-like receptor 9 (TLR9) (Panigrahi et al. 2013). Mice immunized with carboxyethylpyrrole-adducted mouse albumin develop focal changes in the RPE resembling those in advanced dry AMD, exhibit monocyte and macrophage migration into the interphotoreceptor matrix and also exhibit elevated complement deposition in Bruch's membrane (Hollyfield et al. 2008). Carboxyethylpyrrole adducts appear to be initiators of immune responses capable of contributing to either dry or wet AMD-like phenotypes.

Other lipoxidation products in drusen appear to be ligands for CFH, including malondialdehyde (Weismann et al. 2011) and 1-palmitoyl-2-(5′-oxo-valeroyl)-*sn*-glycero-3-phosphocholine (POVPC) (Shaw et al. 2012). CFH exhibiting the AMD risk 402H polymorphism was found to bind malondialdehyde or POVPC with less affinity than the CFH 402Y nonrisk variant (Weismann et al. 2011; Shaw et al. 2012). These independent studies also reported that inflammatory responses stimulated by malondialdehyde and POVPC in vitro and in vivo were stronger with the AMD risk variant of CFH than with the nonrisk CFH isoform, suggesting that the nonrisk isoform may help dampen inflammatory responses induced by oxidative modifications. These observations add support to the hypothesized central role of oxidative modifications in the pathology of AMD and justify further mechanistic studies.

DRUSEN FORMATION

Immune-mediated events have long been thought to play a role in drusen formation due to the presence of proteins in drusen upregulated during inflammatory responses (Johnson et al. 2000; Hageman et al. 2001). Growing evidence supports this hypothesis. Consistent with early drusen studies, several genes involved in inflammation, and/or the immune system have now been associated with AMD risk. These include CFH (Edwards et al. 2005; Hageman et al. 2005; Haines et al. 2005; Klein et al. 2005), complement factor B (Gold et al. 2006), complement C3 (Yates et al. 2007), APOE (Zareparsi et al. 2004; Baird et al. 2006), toll-like receptor 4 (Zareparsi et al. 2005), LOC387715/ARMS2 (Rivera et al. 2005; Kanda et al. 2007), HTRA1 (Dewan et al. 2006; Yang et al. 2006), and ABCA4 (Allikmets 2000). In a human RPE cell culture model mimicking early AMD, drusen biogenesis was reported to involve select serum protein interactions with APOE-rich sub-RPE deposits, which subsequently activate the complement cascade and the deposition of complement complexes (Johnson et al. 2011). Amyloid β (Aβ) may also play a role in drusen formation (Johnson 2002; Dentchev et al. 2003; Anderson et al. 2004; Luibl et al. 2006; Isas et al. 2010). Notably, drusen-like deposits develop below the RPE following Aβ treatment of mice lacking the Aβ-degrading enzyme neprilysin (Yoshida et al. 2005). In the human *APOE4-knockin* mouse model of AMD, Aβ is found in sub-RPE deposits and neovascular lesions (Malek et al. 2005; Ding et al. 2008), and anti-Aβ therapy blocks histopathologic changes (Ding et al. 2011). In human drusen, Aβ has been colocalized with activated complement (Johnson 2002; Dentchev et al. 2003; Anderson et al. 2004). Aβ has also been reported to activate complement (Rogers et al. 1992; Jiang et al. 1994) and other pattern recognition receptors, including RAGE (Chen et al. 2007; Schmidt et al. 2009) and toll-like receptors (Fassbender et al. 2004; Liu et al. 2005). As recently reported and described above, an active complement system has an important function in basal deposit formation in *Efemp1*$^{R345W/R345W}$ mutant mice (Garland et al. 2013). While specific molecular mechanisms remain to be defined, immune system processes appear to play a major role in drusen formation.

CONCLUDING REMARKS

Drusen, when concentrated on Bruch's membrane in the macular region, are major risk factors for AMD progression to advanced disease. Early immunohistochemical studies suggested that inflammatory and immune response processes after RPE injury contribute to drusen formation, a hypothesis that has gained significant support. Qualitative proteomic analysis of isolated drusen using mass spectrometry has made important contributions toward understanding drusen formation, including the identification of multiple immune responses and cellular defense proteins, and support for multiple sources of drusen components, including the RPE, choroidal vasculature, and the systemic circulation. Quantitative proteomic analysis of the human Bruch's membrane/choroid complex has identified 99 proteins significantly altered in abundance in the macular region of AMD tissues, many of which are involved in immune system and cellular defense processes, and also were previously identified in isolated human drusen. Quantitative proteomics and genomics have also demonstrated a critical role for the complement system in basal deposit formation in a mouse model of Doyne honeycomb retinal dystrophy/malattia Leventinese, with remarkable quantitative agreement between select proteins from human and mouse Bruch's membrane/choroid complex. Double mutant mice expressing the disease-causing variant of EFEMP1 protein but not expressing C3 exhibited markedly reduced basal deposit formation, demonstrating that in this mouse model, the immune system plays a major role in basal deposit formation.

Immune system processes involving pattern recognition receptors other than the complement system may also contribute to AMD pathology. Several studies have shown that drusen and ocular tissues from AMD donors contain a variety of oxidative protein modifications, including lipoxidation products (e.g., carboxyethylpyrrole, malondialdehyde, and POVPC), glycoxidation products (e.g., carboxymethyllysine and pentosidine), and protein cross-links. Whereas CFH has been reported to bind malondialdehyde and POVPC, oxidative modifications such as carboxymethyllysine and carboxyethylpyrrole trigger immune responses through other pattern recognition receptors such as RAGE, TLR2, and TLR9. Drusen and the macular Bruch's membrane/choroid complex from AMD donors contain elevated levels of several DAMPS (e.g., protein S100s, crystallins, and histones) that may also trigger pattern recognition receptors. Other proteins such as Aβ and the cross-linking enzyme protein-glutamine γ-glutamyltransferase 2 also may have important roles in drusen formation. Multiple molecular mechanisms appear to be involved and more work is required to fully understand drusen biogenesis.

ACKNOWLEDGMENTS

Supported in part by NIH grants EY021840, EY022134, EY14239, EY15638, Ohio Biomedical Research Technology Transfer grant 05-29, a Research Center grant from The Foundation Fighting Blindness, an unrestricted grant from Research to Prevent Blindness (RPB), an RPB Senior Investigator Award, a Steinbach Award, and The Cleveland Clinic Foundation.

REFERENCES

Abdelsalam A, Del Priore L, Zarbin MA. 1999. Drusen in age-related macular degeneration: Pathogenesis, natural course, and laser photocoagulation-induced regression. *Surv Ophthalmol* **44:** 1–29.

Age Related Eye Disease Study Group. 2001. A randomized, placebo-controlled, clinical trial of high-dose supplementation with vitamins C and E, β carotene, and zinc for age-related macular degeneration and vision loss: AREDS report no. 8. *Arch Ophthalmol* **119:** 1417–1436.

Allikmets R. 2000. Further evidence for an association of *ABCR* alleles with age-related macular degeneration. The International ABCR Screening Consortium. *Am J Hum Genet* **67:** 487–491.

Alvarez R, Aguirre G, Acland G, Anderson R. 1994. Docosapentaenoic acid is converted to docosahexaenoic acid in the retinas of normal and *prcd*-affected miniature poodle dogs. *Invest Ophthalmol Vis Sci* **35:** 402–408.

Anderson DH, Talaga KC, Rivest AJ, Barron E, Hageman GS, Johnson LV. 2004. Characterization of β amyloid assemblies in drusen: The deposits associated with aging and age-related macular degeneration. *Exp Eye Res* **78:** 243–256.

Anderson DH, Radeke MJ, Gallo NB, Chapin EA, Johnson PT, Curletti CR, Hancox LS, Hu J, Ebright JN, Malek G, et al. 2010. The pivotal role of the complement system in aging and age-related macular degeneration: Hypothesis re-visited. *Prog Retin Eye Res* **29:** 95–112.

Baird PN, Richardson AJ, Robman LD, Dimitrov PN, Tikellis G, McCarty CA, Guymer RH. 2006. Apolipoprotein (APOE) gene is associated with progression of age-related macular degeneration (AMD). *Hum Mutat* **27:** 337–342.

Baynes JW. 2001. The role of AGEs in aging: Causation or correlation. *Exp Gerontol* **36:** 1527–1537.

Beatty S, Koh H, Phil M, Henson D, Boulton M. 2000. The role of oxidative stress in the pathogenesis of age-related macular degeneration. *Surv Ophthalmol* **45:** 115–134.

Bok D. 2002. New insights and new approaches toward the study of age-related macular degeneration. *Proc Natl Acad Sci* **99:** 14619–14621.

Booij JC, Baas DC, Beisekeeva J, Gorgels TG, Bergen AA. 2010. The dynamic nature of Bruch's membrane. *Prog Retin Eye Res* **29:** 1–18.

Chen X, Walker DG, Schmidt AM, Arancio O, Lue LF, Yan SD. 2007. RAGE: A potential target for Aβ-mediated cellular perturbation in Alzheimer's disease. *Curr Mol Med* **7:** 735–742.

Chio KS, Reiss U, Fletcher B, Tappel AL. 1969. Peroxidation of subcellular organelles: Formation of lipofuscinlike fluorescent pigments. *Science* **166:** 1535–1536.

Crabb JW. 2012. Oxidative modifications as triggers of AMD pathology. In *Studies on Retinal and Choroidal Disorders* (ed. Stratton R, Hauswirth W, Gardiner T), pp. 65–84. Humana Press.

Crabb JW, Miyagi M, Gu X, Shadrach K, West KA, Sakaguchi H, Kamei M, Hasan A, Yan L, Rayborn ME, et al. 2002a. Drusen proteome analysis: An approach to the etiology of age-related macular degeneration. *Proc Natl Acad Sci* **99:** 14682–14687.

Crabb JW, O'Neil J, Miyagi M, West K, Hoff HF. 2002b. Hydroxynonenal inactivates cathepsin B by forming Michael adducts with active site residues. *Protein Sci* **11:** 831–840.

Curcio CA, Millican CL. 1999. Basal linear deposit and large drusen are specific for early age-related maculopathy. *Arch Ophthalmol* **117:** 329–339.

Curcio CA, Presley JB, Malek G, Medeiros NE, Avery DV, Kruth HS. 2005a. Esterified and unesterified cholesterol in drusen and basal deposits of eyes with age-related maculopathy. *Exp Eye Res* **81:** 731–741.

Curcio CA, Presley JB, Millican CL, Medeiros NE. 2005b. Basal deposits and drusen in eyes with age-related maculopathy: Evidence for solid lipid particles. *Exp Eye Res* **80:** 761–775.

Dentchev T, Milam AH, Lee VM, Trojanowski JQ, Dunaief JL. 2003. Amyloid-β is found in drusen from some age-related macular degeneration retinas, but not in drusen from normal retinas. *Mol Vis* **9:** 184–190.

Dewan A, Liu M, Hartman S, Zhang S, Liu D, Zhao C, Tam P, Chan W, Lam D, Snyder M, et al. 2006. *HTRA1*promoter polymorphism in wet age-related macular degeneration. *Science* **314:** 989–992.

Ding X, Patel M, Chan CC. 2009. Molecular pathology of age-related macular degeneration. *Prog Retin Eye Res* **28:** 1–18.

Ding JD, Johnson LV, Herrmann R, Farsiu S, Smith SG, Groelle M, Mace BE, Sullivan P, Jamison JA, Kelly U, et al. 2011. Anti-amyloid therapy protects against retinal pigmented epithelium damage and vision loss in a model of age-related macular degeneration. *Proc Natl Acad Sci* **108:** E279–E287.

Ding JD, Lin J, Mace BE, Herrmann R, Sullivan P, Bowes Rickman C. 2008. Targeting age-related macular degeneration with Alzheimer's disease based immunotherapies: Anti-amyloid-β antibody attenuates pathologies in an age-related macular degeneration mouse model. *Vision Res* **48:** 339–345.

Ebrahem Q, Renganathan K, Sears J, Vasanji A, Gu X, Lu L, Salomon RG, Crabb JW, Anand-Apte B. 2006. Carboxyethylpyrrole oxidative protein modifications stimulate neovascularization: Implications for age-related macular degeneration. *Proc Natl Acad Sci* **103:** 13480–13484.

Edwards A, Ritter R, Abel K, Manning A, Panhuysen C, Farrer L. 2005. Complement factor H polymorphism and age-related macular degeneration. *Science* **308:** 421–424.

Eldred GE, Lasky MR. 1993. Retinal age pigments generated by self-assembling lysosomotropic detergents. *Nature* **361:** 724–726.

Elgawish A, Glomb M, Friedlander M, Monnier VM. 1996. Involvement of hydrogen peroxide in collagen cross-linking by high glucose in vitro and in vivo. *J Biol Chem* **271:** 12964–12971.

Esterbauer H, Schaur RJ, Zollner H. 1991. Chemistry and biochemistry of 4-hydroxynonenal, malonaldehyde and related aldehydes. *Free Radic Biol Med* **11:** 81–128.

Farboud B, Aotaki-Keen A, Miyata T, Hjelmeland LM, Handa JT. 1999. Development of a polyclonal antibody with broad epitope specificity for advanced glycation endproducts and localization of these epitopes in Bruch's membrane of the aging eye. *Mol Vis* **5:** 11.

Fassbender K, Walter S, Kuhl S, Landmann R, Ishii K, Bertsch T, Stalder AK, Muehlhauser F, Liu Y, Ulmer AJ, et al. 2004. The LPS receptor (CD14) links innate immunity with Alzheimer's disease. *FASEB J* **18:** 203–205.

Ferris FL III, Fine SL, Hyman L. 1984. Age-related macular degeneration and blindness due to neovascular maculopathy. *Arch Ophthalmol* **102:** 1640–1642.

Fliesler SJ, Anderson RE. 1983. Chemistry and metabolism of lipids in the vertebrate retina. *Prog Lipid Res* **22:** 79–131.

Friguet B, Stadtman ER, Szweda LI. 1994. Modification of glucose-6-phosphate dehydrogenase by 4-hydroxy-2-nonenal. Formation of cross-linked protein that inhibits the multicatalytic protease. *J Biol Chem* **269:** 21639–21643.

Fritsche LG, Chen W, Schu M, Yaspan BL, Yu Y, Thorleifsson G, Zack DJ, Arakawa S, Cipriani V, Ripke S, et al. 2013. Seven new loci associated with age-related macular degeneration. *Nat Genet* **45:** 433–439.

Fu L, Garland D, Yang Z, Shukla D, Rajendran A, Pearson E, Stone EM, Zhang K, Pierce EA. 2007. The R345W mutation in *EFEMP1* is pathogenic and causes AMD-like deposits in mice. *Hum Mol Genet* **16:** 2411–2422.

Garland DL, Fernandez-Godino R, Kaur I, Speicher KD, Harnly JM, Lambris JD, Speicher DW, Pierce EA. 2013. Mouse genetics and proteomic analyses demonstrate a critical role for complement in a model of DHRD/ML, an inherited macular degeneration. *Hum Mol Genet* **23:** 52–68.

Glenn JV, Beattie JR, Barrett L, Frizzell N, Thorpe SR, Boulton ME, McGarvey JJ, Stitt AW. 2007. Confocal Raman microscopy can quantify advanced glycation end product (AGE) modifications in Bruch's membrane leading to accurate, nondestructive prediction of ocular aging. *FASEB J* **21:** 3542–3552.

Glenn JV, Mahaffy H, Wu K, Smith G, Nagai R, Simpson DA, Boulton ME, Stitt AW. 2009. Advanced glycation end product (AGE) accumulation on Bruch's membrane: Links to age-related RPE dysfunction. *Invest Ophthalmol Vis Sci* **50:** 441–451.

Goh SY, Cooper ME. 2008. Clinical review: The role of advanced glycation end products in progression and complications of diabetes. *J Clin Endocrinol Metab* **93:** 1143–1152.

Gold B, Merriam JE, Zernant J, Hancox LS, Taiber AJ, Gehrs K, Cramer K, Neel J, Bergeron J, Barile GR, et al. 2006. Variation in factor B (*BF*) and complement component 2 (*C2*) genes is associated with age-related macular degeneration. *Nat Genet* **38:** 458–462.

Goldberg MF. 1976. Bruch's membrane and vascular gowth. *Invest Ophthalmol Vis Sci* **15:** 443–446.

Green WR, Enger C. 1993. Age-related macular degeneration histopathologic studies. The 1992 Lorenz E. Zimmerman Lecture. *Ophthalmology* **100:** 1519–1535.

Gu X, Meer SG, Miyagi M, Rayborn ME, Hollyfield JG, Crabb JW, Salomon RG. 2003a. Carboxyethylpyrrole protein adducts and autoantibodies, biomarkers for age-related macular degeneration. *J Biol Chem* **278:** 42027–42035.

Gu X, Sun M, Gugiu B, Hazen S, Crabb JW, Salomon RG. 2003b. Oxidatively truncated docosahexaenoate phospholipids: Total synthesis, generation, and peptide adduction chemistry. *J Org Chem* **68:** 3749–3761.

Gu J, Paeur GJ, Yue X, Narendra U, Sturgill GM, Bena J, Gu X, Peachey NS, Salomon RG, Hagstrom SA, et al. 2009. Assessing susceptibility to age-related macular degeneration with proteomic and genomic biomarkers. *Molecular & Cellular Proteomics* **8:** 1338–1349.

Hageman G, Mullins R, Russell S, Johnson L, Anderson D. 1999. Vitronectin is a constituent of ocular drusen and the vitronectin gene is expressed in human retinal pigmented epithelial cells. *FASEB J* **13:** 477–484.

Hageman GS, Anderson DH, Johnson LV, Hancox LS, Taiber AJ, Hardisty LI, Hageman JL, Stockman HA, Borchardt

JD, Gehrs KM, et al. 2005. A common haplotype in the complement regulatory gene factor H (*HF1/CFH*) predisposes individuals to age-related macular degeneration. *Proc Natl Acad Sci* **102:** 7227–7232.

Hageman GS, Luthert PJ, Victor Chong NH, Johnson LV, Anderson DH, Mullins RF. 2001. An integrated hypothesis that considers drusen as biomarkers of immune-mediated processes at the RPE-Bruch's membrane interface in aging and age-related macular degeneration. *Prog Retin Eye Res* **20:** 705–732.

Hagenow K, Gelderman KA, Hultqvist M, Merky P, Backlund J, Frey O, Kamradt T, Holmdahl R. 2009. Ncf1-associated reduced oxidative burst promotes IL-33R$^+$ T cell-mediated adjuvant-free arthritis in mice. *J Immunol* **183:** 874–881.

Haines J, Hauser M, Schmidt S, Scott W, Olson L, Gallins P, Spencer K, Kwan S, Noureddine M, Gilbert J, et al. 2005. Complement factor H variant increases the risk of age-related macular degeneration. *Science* **308:** 419–421.

Hammes HP, Hoerauf H, Alt A, Schleicher E, Clausen JT, Bretzel RG, Laqua H. 1999. N(ε)(Carboxymethyl)lysin and the AGE receptor RAGE colocalize in age-related macular degeneration. *Invest Ophthalmol Vis Sci* **40:** 1855–1859.

Handa JT, Verzijl N, Matsunaga H, Aotaki-Keen A, Lutty GA, te Koppele JM, Miyata T, Hjelmeland LM. 1999. Increase in the advanced glycation end product pentosidine in Bruch's membrane with age. *Invest Ophthalmol Vis Sci* **40:** 775–779.

Hazen SL. 2008. Oxidized phospholipids as endogenous pattern recognition ligands in innate immunity. *J Biol Chem* **283:** 15527–15531.

Herold K, Moser B, Chen Y, Zeng S, Yan SF, Ramasamy R, Emond J, Clynes R, Schmidt AM. 2007. Receptor for advanced glycation end products (RAGE) in a dash to the rescue: Inflammatory signals gone awry in the primal response to stress. *J Leukoc Biol* **82:** 204–212.

Hirata C, Nakano K, Nakamura N, Kitagawa Y, Shigeta H, Hasegawa G, Ogata M, Ikeda T, Sawa H, Nakamura K, et al. 1997. Advanced glycation end products induce expression of vascular endothelial growth factor by retinal Müller cells. *Biochem Biophys Res Commun* **236:** 712–715.

Hoffmann S, Friedrichs U, Eichler W, Rosenthal A, Wiedemann P. 2002. Advanced glycation end products induce choroidal endothelial cell proliferation, matrix metalloproteinase-2 and VEGF upregulation in vitro. *Graefes Arch Clin Exp Ophthalmol* **240:** 996–1002.

Hollyfield JG, Bonilha VL, Rayborn ME, Yang X, Shadrach KG, Lu L, Ufret RL, Salomon RG, Perez VL. 2008. Oxidative damage-induced inflammation initiates age-related macular degeneration. *Nat Med* **14:** 194–198.

Howes KA, Liu Y, Dunaief JL, Milam A, Frederick JM, Marks A, Baehr W. 2004. Receptor for advanced glycation end products and age-related macular degeneration. *Invest Ophthalmol Vis Sci* **45:** 3713–3720.

Isas JM, Luibl V, Johnson LV, Kayed R, Wetzel R, Glabe CG, Langen R, Chen J. 2010. Soluble and mature amyloid fibrils in drusen deposits. *Invest Ophthalmol Vis Sci* **51:** 1304–1310.

Ishibashi T, Murata T, Hangai M, Nagai R, Horiuchi S, Lopez PF, Hinton DR, Ryan SJ. 1998. Advanced glycation end products in age-related macular degeneration. *Arch Ophthalmol* **116:** 1629–1632.

Jager R, Mieler W, Miller J. 2008. Age-related macular degeneration. *N Engl J Med* **358:** 2606–2617.

Jiang H, Burdick D, Glabe CG, Cotman CW, Tenner AJ. 1994. β-Amyloid activates complement by binding to a specific region of the collagen-like domain of the C1q A chain. *J Immunol* **152:** 5050–5059.

Jiang K, To E, Cui JZ, Cao SJG, Matsubara JA. 2012. Drusen and pro-inflammatory mediators in the post-mortem human eye. *J Clinic Experiment Ophthalmol* **3:** 208–216.

Johnson LV. 2002. The Alzheimer's Aβ-peptide is deposited at sites of complement activation in pathologic deposits associated with aging and age-related macular degeneration. *Proc Natl Acad Sci* **99:** 11830–11835.

Johnson LV, Ozaki S, Staples MK, Erickson PA, Anderson DH. 2000. A potential role for immune complex pathogenesis in drusen formation. *Exp Eye Res* **70:** 441–449.

Johnson LV, Forest DL, Banna CD, Radeke CM, Maloney MA, Hu J, Spencer CN, Walker AM, Tsie MS, Bok D, et al. 2011. Cell culture model that mimics drusen formation and triggers complement activation associated with age-related macular degeneration. *Proc Natl Acad Sci* **108:** 18277–18282.

Kamei M, Hollyfield JG. 1999. TIMP-3 in Bruch's membrane: Changes during aging and in age-related macular degeneration. *Invest Ophthalmol Vis Sci* **40:** 2367–2375.

Kanda A, Chen W, Othman M, Branham KE, Brooks M, Khanna R, He S, Lyons R, Abecasis GR, Swaroop A. 2007. A variant of mitochondrial protein LOC387715/ARMS2, not HTRA1, is strongly associated with age-related macular degeneration. *Proc Natl Acad Sci* **104:** 16227–16232.

Kim SR, Jang YP, Jockusch S, Fishkin NE, Turro NJ, Sparrow JR. 2007. The all-trans-retinal dimer series of lipofuscin pigments in retinal pigment epithelial cells in a recessive Stargardt disease model. *Proc Natl Acad Sci* **104:** 19273–19278.

Klein R, Zeiss C, Chew E, Tsai J, Sackler R, Haynes C, Henning A, SanGiovanni J, Mane S, Mayne S, et al. 2005. Complement factor H polymorphism in age-related macular degeneration. *Science* **308:** 385–389.

Knott AB, Perkins G, Schwarzenbacher R, Bossy-Wetzel E. 2008. Mitochondrial fragmentation in neurodegeneration. *Nat Rev Neurosci* **9:** 505–518.

Liu Y, Walter S, Stagi M, Cherny D, Letiembre M, Schulz-Schaeffer W, Heine H, Penke B, Neumann H, Fassbender K. 2005. LPS receptor (CD14): A receptor for phagocytosis of Alzheimer's amyloid peptide. *Brain* **128:** 1778–1789.

Lotze MT, Zeh HJ, Rubartelli A, Sparvero LJ, Amoscato AA, Washburn NR, Devera ME, Liang X, Tor M, Billiar T. 2007. The grateful dead: Damage-associated molecular pattern molecules and reduction/oxidation regulate immunity. *Immunol Rev* **220:** 60–81.

Lu M, Kuroki M, Amano S, Tolentino M, Keough K, Kim I, Bucala R, Adamis AP. 1998. Advanced glycation end products increase retinal vascular endothelial growth factor expression. *J Clin Invest* **101:** 1219–1224.

Luibl V, Isas JM, Kayed R, Glabe CG, Langen R, Chen J. 2006. Drusen deposits associated with aging and age-related macular degeneration contain nonfibrillar amyloid oligomers. *J Clin Invest* **116:** 378–385.

Malek G, Li CM, Guidry C, Medeiros NE, Curcio CA. 2003. Apolipoprotein B in cholesterol-containing drusen and basal deposits of human eyes with age-related maculopathy. *Am J Pathol* **162:** 413–425.

Malek G, Johnson LV, Mace BE, Saloupis P, Schmechel DE, Rickman DW, Toth CA, Sullivan PM, Bowes Rickman C. 2005. Apolipoprotein E allele-dependent pathogenesis: A model for age-related retinal degeneration. *Proc Natl Acad Sci* **102:** 11900–11905.

Marmorstein LY. 2002. Aberrant accumulation of EFEMP1 underlies drusen formation in Malattia Leventinese and age-related macular degeneration. *Proc Natl Acad Sci* **99:** 13067–13072.

Marmorstein LY, McLaughlin PJ, Peachey NS, Sasaki T, Marmorstein AD. 2007. Formation and progression of sub-retinal pigment epithelium deposits in *Efemp1* mutation knock-in mice: A model for the early pathogenic course of macular degeneration. *Hum Mol Genet* **16:** 2423–2432.

Matsue H, Edelbaum D, Shalhevet D, Mizumoto N, Yang C, Mummert ME, Oeda J, Masayasu H, Takashima A. 2003. Generation and function of reactive oxygen species in dendritic cells during antigen presentation. *J Immunol* **171:** 3010–3018.

Michaelides M, Jenkins SA, Brantley MA Jr, Andrews RM, Waseem N, Luong V, Gregory-Evans K, Bhattacharya SS, Fitzke FW, Webster AR. 2006. Maculopathy due to the R345W substitution in fibulin-3: Distinct clinical features, disease variability, and extent of retinal dysfunction. *Invest Ophthalmol Vis Sci* **47:** 3085–3097.

Mullins R, Russell S, Anderson D, Hageman G. 2000. Drusen associated with aging and age-related macular degeneration contain proteins common to extracellular deposits associated with atherosclerosis, elastosis, amyloidosis, and dense deposit disease. *FASEB J* **14:** 835–846.

Ng KP, Gugiu B, Renganathan K, Davies MW, Gu X, Crabb JS, Kim SR, Rozanowska MB, Bonilha VL, Rayborn ME, et al. 2008. Retinal pigment epithelium lipofuscin proteomics. *Mol Cell Proteomics* **7:** 1397–1405.

Ni J, Yuan X, Gu J, Yue X, Gu X, Nagaraj RH, Crabb JW, Group. TCGaPAS. 2009. Plasma protein pentosidine and carboxymethyllysine, biomarkers for age-related macular degeneration. *Mol Cell Proteomics* **8:** 1921–1933.

Nordgaard CL, Karunadharma PP, Feng X, Olsen TW, Ferrington DA. 2008. Mitochondrial proteomics of the retinal pigment epithelium at progressive stages of age-related macular degeneration. *Invest Ophthalmol Vis Sci* **49:** 2848–2855.

Okamoto T, Tanaka S, Stan AC, Koike T, Kase M, Makita Z, Sawa H, Nagashima K. 2002. Advanced glycation end products induce angiogenesis in vivo. *Microvasc Res* **63:** 186–195.

Panigrahi S, Ma Y, Hong L, Gao D, West XZ, Salomon RG, Byzova TV, Podrez EA. 2013. Engagement of platelet toll-like receptor 9 by novel endogenous ligands promotes platelet hyperreactivity and thrombosis. *Circ Res* **112:** 103–112.

Penfold PL, Madigan MC, Gillies MC, Provis JM. 2001. Immunological and aetiological aspects of macular degeneration. *Prog Retin Eye Res* **20:** 385–414.

Rivera A, Fisher SA, Fritsche LG, Keilhauer CN, Lichtner P, Meitinger T, Weber BH. 2005. Hypothetical *LOC387715* is a second major susceptibility gene for age-related macular degeneration, contributing independently of complement factor H to disease risk. *Hum Mol Genet* **14:** 3227–3236.

Rogers J, Cooper NR, Webster S, Schultz J, McGeer PL, Styren SD, Civin WH, Brachova L, Bradt B, Ward P, et al. 1992. Complement activation by β-amyloid in Alzheimer disease. *Proc Natl Acad Sci* **89:** 10016–10020.

Sakaguchi H, Miyagi M, Shadrach KG, Rayborn ME, Crabb JW, Hollyfield JG. 2002. Clusterin is present in drusen in age-related macular degeneration. *Exp Eye Res* **74:** 547–549.

Sakai N, Decatur J, Nakanishi K, Eldred GE. 1996. Ocular age pigment "A2-E": An unprecedented pyridinium bis-retinoid. *J Am Chem Soc* **118:** 1559–1560.

Sarks S. 1976. Aging and degeneration in the macular region: A clinico-pathological study. *Br J Ophthalmol* **60:** 324–328.

Sarks S, Cherepanoff S, Killingsworth M, Sarks J. 2007. Relationship of basal laminar deposit and membranous debris to the clinical presentation of early age-related macular degeneration. *Invest Ophthalmol Vis Sci* **48:** 968–977.

Schmidt AM, Sahagan B, Nelson RB, Selmer J, Rothlein R, Bell JM. 2009. The role of RAGE in amyloid-β peptide-mediated pathology in Alzheimer's disease. *Curr Opin Investig Drugs* **10:** 672–680.

Schutt F, Bergmann M, Holz FG, Kopitz J. 2003. Proteins modified by malondialdehyde, 4-hydroxynonenal, or advanced glycation end products in lipofuscin of human retinal pigment epithelium. *Invest Ophthalmol Vis Sci* **44:** 3663–3668.

Seddon JM, Willett WC, Speizer FE, Hankinson SE. 1996. A prospective study of cigarette smoking and age-related macular degeneration in women. *JAMA* **276:** 1141–1146.

Shaw PX, Zhang L, Zhang M, Du H, Zhao L, Lee C, Grob S, Lim SL, Hughes G, Lee J, et al. 2012. Complement factor H genotypes impact risk of age-related macular degeneration by interaction with oxidized phospholipids. *Proc Natl Acad Sci* **109:** 13757–13762.

Shen JK, Dong A, Hackett SF, Bell WR, Green WR, Campochiaro PA. 2007. Oxidative damage in age-related macular degeneration. *Histol Histopathol* **22:** 1301–1308.

Sparrow JR. 2007. RPE lipofuscin: formation, properties, and relevance to retinal degeneration. In *Retinal Degenerations: Biology, Diagnostics and Therapeutics* (ed. Tombran-Tink J, Barnstable CJ), pp. 213–236. Human Press, Totowa, NJ.

Sparrow JR, Boulton M. 2005. RPE lipofuscin and its role in retinal pathobiology. *Exp Eye Res* **80:** 595–606.

Sparvero LJ, Asafu-Adjei D, Kang R, Tang D, Amin N, Im J, Rutledge R, Lin B, Amoscato AA, Zeh HJ, et al. 2009. RAGE (Receptor for Advanced Glycation Endproducts), RAGE ligands, and their role in cancer and inflammation. *J Transl Med* **7:** 17.

Spraul C, Grossniklaus H. 1997. Characteristics of drusen and Bruch's membrane in postmortem eyes with age-related macular degeneration. *Ophthalmology* **115:** 267–273.

Stone EM, Lotery AJ, Munier FL, Heon E, Piguet B, Guymer RH, Vandenburgh K, Cousin P, Nishimura D, Swiderski RE, et al. 1999. A single *EFEMP1* mutation associated with both Malattia Leventinese and Doyne honeycomb retinal dystrophy. *Nat Genet* **22:** 199–202.

Stone EM, Braun TA, Russell SR, Kuehn MH, Lotery AJ, Moore PA, Eastman CG, Casavant TL, Sheffield VC. 2004. Missense variations in the fibulin 5 gene and age-related macular degeneration. *N Engl J Med* **351:** 346–353.

Treins C, Giorgetti-Peraldi S, Murdaca J, Van Obberghen E. 2001. Regulation of vascular endothelial growth factor expression by advanced glycation end products. *J Biol Chem* **276:** 43836–43841.

Umeda S, Suzuki M, Okamoto H, Ono F, Mizota A, Terao K, Yoshikawa Y, Tanaka Y, Iwata T. 2005. Molecular composition of drusen and possible involvement of anti-retinal autoimmunity in two different forms of macular degeneration in cynomolgus monkey (*Macaca fascicularis*). *FASEB J* **19:** 1683–1685.

Urata Y, Yamaguchi M, Higashiyama Y, Ihara Y, Goto S, Kuwano M, Horiuchi S, Sumikawa K, Kondo T. 2002. Reactive oxygen species accelerate production of vascular endothelial growth factor by advanced glycation end products in RAW264.7 mouse macrophages. *Free Radic Biol Med* **32:** 688–701.

Verhasselt V, Goldman M, Willems F. 1998. Oxidative stress up-regulates IL-8 and TNF-α synthesis by human dendritic cells. *Eur J Immunol* **28:** 3886–3890.

Wang N, Anderson RE. 1992. Enrichment of polyunsaturated fatty acids from rat retinal pigment epithelium to rod outer segments. *Curr Eye Res* **11:** 783–791.

Wang L, Clark M, Crossman D, Kojima K, Messinger J, Mobley J, Curcio C. 2010. Abundant lipid and protein components of drusen. *PLoS ONE* **5:** e10329.

Weismann D, Hartvigsen K, Lauer N, Bennett KL, Scholl HP, Charbel Issa P, Cano M, Brandstatter H, Tsimikas S, Skerka C, et al. 2011. Complement factor H binds malondialdehyde epitopes and protects from oxidative stress. *Nature* **478:** 76–81.

West XZ, Malinin NL, Merkulova AA, Tischenko M, Kerr BA, Borden EC, Podrez EA, Salomon RG, Byzova TV. 2010. Oxidative stress induces angiogenesis by activating TLR2 with novel endogenous ligands. *Nature* **467:** 972–976.

Wu Y, Yanase E, Feng X, Siegel MM, Sparrow JR. 2010. Structural characterization of bisretinoid A2E photocleavage products and implications for age-related macular degeneration. *Proc Natl Acad Sci* **107:** 7275–7280.

Yang Z, Camp NJ, Sun H, Tong Z, Gibbs D, Cameron DJ, Chen H, Zhao Y, Pearson E, Li X, et al. 2006. A variant of the *HTRA1* gene increases susceptibility to age-related macular degeneration. *Science* **314:** 992–993.

Yates J, Sepp T, Matharu B, Khan J, Thurlby D, Shahid H, Clayton D, Hayward C, Morgan J, Wright A, et al. 2007. Complement C3 variant and the risk of age-related macular degeneration. *N Engl J Med* **357:** 553–561.

Yoshida T, Ohno-Matsui K, Ichinose S, Sato T, Iwata N, Saido TC, Hisatomi T, Mochizuki M, Morita I. 2005. The potential role of amyloid β in the pathogenesis of age-related macular degeneration. *J Clin Invest* **115:** 2793–2800.

Yuan X, Gu X, Crabb JS, Yue X, Shadrach K, Hollyfield JG, Crabb JW. 2010. Quantitative proteomics: Comparison of the macular Bruch membrane/choroid complex from age-related macular degeneration and normal eyes. *Mol Cell Proteomics* **9:** 1031–1046.

Zahringer U, Lindner B, Inamura S, Heine H, Alexander C. 2008. TLR2—promiscuous or specific? A critical re-evaluation of a receptor expressing apparent broad specificity. *Immunobiology* **213:** 205–224.

Zarbin MA. 2004. Current concepts in the pathogenesis of age-related macular degeneration. *Arch Ophthalmol* **122:** 598–614.

Zareparsi S, Reddick AC, Branham KE, Moore KB, Jessup L, Thoms S, Smith-Wheelock M, Yashar BM, Swaroop A. 2004. Association of apolipoprotein E alleles with susceptibility to age-related macular degeneration in a large cohort from a single center. *Invest Ophthalmol Vis Sci* **45:** 1306–1310.

Zareparsi S, Buraczynska M, Branham KE, Shah S, Eng D, Li M, Pawar H, Yashar BM, Moroi SE, Lichter PR, et al. 2005. Toll-like receptor 4 variant D299G is associated with susceptibility to age-related macular degeneration. *Hum Mol Genet* **14:** 1449–1455.

Highly Penetrant Alleles in Age-Related Macular Degeneration

Anneke I. den Hollander and Eiko K. de Jong

Department of Ophthalmology and Department of Human Genetics, Radboud University Medical Centre, Nijmegen, The Netherlands

Correspondence: Anneke.denHollander@radboudumc.nl

Age-related macular degeneration (AMD) is a complex disease caused by a combination of genetic and environmental factors. Genome-wide association studies have identified several common genetic variants associated with AMD, which together account for 15%–65% of the heritability of AMD. Multiple hypotheses to clarify the unexplained portion of genetic variance have been proposed, such as gene–gene interactions, gene–environment interactions, structural variations, epigenetics, and rare variants. Several studies support a role for rare variants with large effect sizes in the pathogenesis of AMD. In this work, we review the methods that can be used to detect rare variants in common diseases, as well as the recent progress that has been made in the identification of rare variants in AMD. In addition, the relevance of these rare variants for diagnosis, prognosis, and treatment of AMD is highlighted.

Age-related macular degeneration (AMD) is a complex, multifactorial disease caused by a combination of genetic and environmental factors. The most commonly associated environmental risk factor is smoking (Thornton et al. 2005). Evidence for a strong genetic component in AMD comes from familial and twin-based studies (Seddon et al. 1997, 2005). The proportion of variability in the risk of AMD that is attributed to genetic makeup, or heritability, is ~45%–70% (Seddon et al. 2005).

Genome-wide association studies and candidate gene approaches have identified several common genetic variants (with a minor allele frequency [MAF] >5%) that are associated with AMD (Fig. 1). A significant breakthrough in the AMD field came with the identification of a strong association between AMD and a coding variant (rs1061170; p.Tyr402His) and several noncoding variants in the complement factor H (*CFH*) gene, which encodes a primary regulator of the alternative complement pathway (Edwards et al. 2005; Hageman et al. 2005; Haines et al. 2005). A strong association has also been identified between AMD and a haplotype on chromosome 10q26, which contains the *ARMS2* and *HTRA1* genes (Jakobsdottir et al. 2005; Rivera et al. 2005; Dewan et al. 2006). In addition, several genetic variants with smaller effect sizes have been identified in other complement factor genes (*CFB*/*C2*, *C3*, and *CFI*) (Gold et al. 2006; Yates et al. 2007; Fagerness et al. 2009) as well as in genes encoding members of the high-density lipoprotein cholesterol pathway

Cite this article as *Cold Spring Harb Perspect Med* doi: 10.1101/cshperspect.a017202

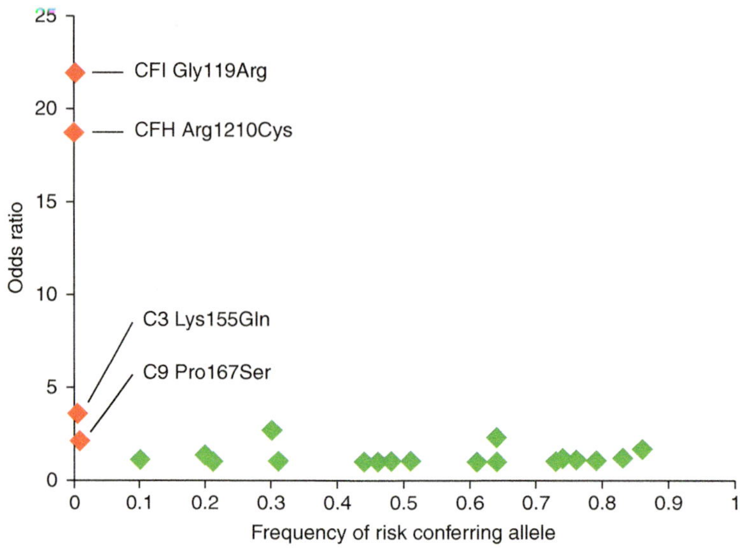

Figure 1. Effect sizes (odds ratios) of common and rare variants associated with AMD. Common variants with relatively small effect sizes at loci recently described in (Fritsche et al. 2013) are indicated in green. Rare variants with low population allele frequencies and large effect sizes are indicated in red: *CFI* Gly119Arg (MAF 0.001, OR 22) (van de Ven et al. 2013); *CFH* Arg1210Cys (MAF 0.0002, OR 18.8) calculated from (Raychaudhuri et al. 2011); *C3* Lys155Gln (MAF 0.004, OR 3.7) (Helgason et al. 2013); *C9* Pro167Ser (MAF 0.008, OR 2.2) (Seddon et al. 2013). MAF calculated from NHLBI exome sequencing project, alleles from European ancestry.

(*APOE*, *LIPC*, *CETP*), components of the extracellular collagen matrix (*TIMP3*, *COL8A1*, *COL10A1*), and proteins promoting angiogenesis (*VEGFA*, *TGFBR1*) (Yu et al. 2011; Fritsche et al. 2013). The most comprehensive genome-wide association study performed thus far involved 18 international research groups, and included >17,000 advanced AMD cases and >60,000 controls of European and Asian ancestry (Fritsche et al. 2013).

Although common variants in the *CFH* gene and at the *ARMS2/HTRA1* locus exert a relatively large effect, increasing disease risk by two- to threefold, most common variants individually confer relatively small increments in risk (Fig. 1) (Fritsche et al. 2013). Together, the common variants identified thus far account for 15%–65% of the heritability of AMD (Manolio et al. 2009). Although genome-wide association studies with even larger samples sizes might elucidate additional common variants with smaller effect sizes, it is clear that a significant proportion of the missing heritability remains unexplained. Multiple hypotheses to clarify the unexplained portion of genetic variance have been proposed, such as gene–gene interactions, gene–environment interactions, structural variations, epigenetics, and rare variants (Liu and Leal 2012; Liu et al. 2012). Current efforts in complex disease genetics are shifting to investigate the "common disease, rare variant" hypothesis to determine whether rare variants (with a MAF ≤1%) and low-frequency variants (with a MAF 1%–5%) explain the remaining fraction of the missing heritability (Pritchard 2001; Bodmer and Bonilla 2008). Such rare and low-frequency variants would need to have large effect sizes to be detected, because those with small effect sizes will be very difficult or impossible to detect by genetic means (Manolio et al. 2009).

Several studies support a role for rare variants with large effect sizes in the pathogenesis of AMD. First of all, the risk of AMD is greatly increased (by 16-fold) by having an affected first-degree relative (Shahid et al. 2012). Second, relatives of AMD patients do not only have an increased risk, but also have an earlier onset of the disease (Klaver et al. 1998b). Finally, a recent study reported that the aggregation of AMD in densely affected families is not sufficiently explained by the genotypic load of the common genetic risk variants for AMD. Simulation studies suggested that rare, highly penetrant variants are likely to explain the heritability in these families (Sobrin et al. 2010). In this article, we review the methods that can be used to detect rare variants in common disease, as well as the recent progress that has been made in the identification of rare variants in AMD. In addition, the relevance of these rare variants for diagnosis, prognosis, and treatment of AMD is highlighted.

METHODS TO IDENTIFY RARE VARIANTS IN COMMON DISEASE

Linkage Analysis in Families

For some common diseases, such as Alzheimer disease, rare familial forms exist that are caused by rare, highly penetrant alleles. The genes involved in such inherited (or Mendelian) diseases have traditionally been mapped using linkage analysis in families with several affected family members. Linkage analysis attempts to identify a region (or locus) in the genome associated with the disease by identifying alleles that are present only in affected members of the family (Mayeux 2005). A genome-wide segregation analysis is performed with polymorphic markers spread throughout the genome. In the past, sets of variable number of tandem repeats (VNTR) or microsatellite markers have been used, whereas more recently, microarrays containing 6000–10,000 single nucleotide polymorphisms (SNPs) have efficiently been used for genome-wide mapping.

A way to determine whether the identified locus is potentially relevant to the disease is to calculate the logarithm of odds (LOD) score, which compares the probability of the observation assuming a degree of linkage to the probability of obtaining the same observation without any linkage. For significant locus assignment by genome-wide genotyping, a minimum LOD score of 3.3 must be obtained, and a LOD score of 1.86 is suggestive for linkage (Lander and Kruglyak 1995). A locus of interest can be mapped in more detail to narrow down the region, and subsequently the genes in the identified chromosomal interval can be analyzed for the causative mutation.

A benefit of linkage analysis in families is that the technique is suitable for identifying causal mutations in large families that show clear and penetrant Mendelian inheritance patterns. A potential drawback, especially in the case of age-related complex disorders, is that the disease is not always fully penetrant in some individuals. Furthermore, there may be a considerable contribution of other genetic and environmental factors to the development of the disease in other individuals. Thus, incomplete cosegregation of an allele within a family does not exclude the possibility that the allele can be causal in some individuals (Cirulli and Goldstein 2010).

Candidate Gene Analysis

Another approach that can be used to identify rare variants in common diseases is by sequencing one or more candidate genes in a case-control setting. A critical step in the study design is the selection of appropriate candidate genes for the disease of interest. Potential candidate genes are those that have been identified in familial forms of the disease, genes at or near common variants that have been identified to be associated with the disease by genome-wide association studies, or genes known to be involved in the biology of the disease based on biochemical and physiological studies (Bodmer and Bonilla 2008; Cirulli and Goldstein 2010).

In the past decades, DNA sequence analysis was based on the chain termination method described by Sanger (Sanger et al. 1977). Sanger sequencing can be used to sequence one or a limited number of genes in a limited number of samples, and is therefore not the most suitable approach to identify rare variants in common diseases. In the past five years, new sequence technologies (next-generation sequencing) have been developed, allowing the analysis of larger amounts of sequence data with higher speed and at much lower costs compared with

Sanger sequencing. Various target enrichment strategies exist that can enrich a specific target (targeted next-generation sequencing of one or more genes), the exons of all human genes (exome sequencing), or even the entire genome (whole-genome sequencing).

A challenge in the design of candidate gene studies is the extremely large sample sizes that are required to implicate single genes in a complex disease. This can be overcome by target enrichment using molecular inversion probes, which allows candidate resequencing in very large cohorts at ultra-low costs per sample (O'Roak et al. 2012).

Exome Chip Analysis

Genome-wide association studies with SNP microarrays can successfully identify associations with common variants with a MAF of >5% in the general population, whereas exome sequencing can identify very rare and even unique coding variants. Because exome sequencing of very large numbers of samples is currently very expensive, an intermediate experiment can be designed for a fraction of the cost using exome chips containing >100,000 rare and low-frequency variants. These arrays contain coding variants that have been identified several times in existing sequence data sets. This line of thought implicitly underlies the 1000 Genomes Project, which is extending the catalogue of known human variants down to a frequency of near 1%. Exome chips will allow a new wave of genome-wide association studies that can identify rare and low-frequency variants contributing to common traits (Cirulli and Goldstein 2010; Huyghe et al. 2013). In an ongoing worldwide effort to identify rare and low-frequency variants in AMD, >50,000 samples are currently being genotyped with exome chips containing 103,947 rare and low-frequency variants by the International AMD Genomics Consortium.

Exome and Whole-Genome Sequencing

The most comprehensive study to identify rare variants in complex diseases involves exome sequencing or, preferably, whole-genome sequencing of very large sample sizes. Because these technologies are currently very expensive to apply to large numbers of samples, two designs can be used to enrich the study population for rare variants, which would require smaller sample sizes. The first design involves family-based sequencing, in which selected families with multiple affected individuals are analyzed. The second approach involves selecting individuals that are at the extreme ends of a trait distribution (Cirulli and Goldstein 2010).

When designing an exome or whole-genome sequencing study aimed to identify rare variants, important considerations are sufficient coverage (at least 40-fold), and preferably analyzing all samples (both cases and controls) together as a set. This ensures a high-quality data set, which is of utmost importance for downstream analyses. Exome and whole-genome sequencing generate a tremendous amount of data, which can make association analyses complex. To discern relevant from irrelevant effects, bioinformatics software can be used to predict the effect of amino acid changes, allowing researchers to distinguish whether a variant is or is not likely to be deleterious. Because deleterious variants are often rare, it is difficult to detect association using single-variant analyses. Statistical tests (e.g., burden tests) are available that collapse variants across a gene or pathway, resulting in a gene-based or pathway-based test. The burden test compares frequencies of damaging variants in a gene or pathway between cases and controls. Variants can be weighted using external information, such as pathogenicity prediction scores. Other statistical tests (such as the C-alpha test, the sequence kernel association test, and the estimated regression coefficient test) can also take the direction of the effect (i.e., deleterious or protective) into account (Kiezun et al. 2012; Goldstein et al. 2013).

RARE VARIANTS IN AMD

Complement Component C3

C3 is a central component of the complement cascade. Cleavage of C3 into C3a and C3b is the central step in complement activation. In a feed-forward mechanism, C3b activation amplifies further cleavage of C3 and leads to cleavage of C5 via the generation of C3 and C5 convertase complexes, respectively. Subsequently, components C6 through C9 are recruited to form a large molecular pore (the membrane attack complex) on target membranes, resulting in cell lysis (Walport 2001a,b). Because these activation fragments are nondiscriminatory, the complement system is tightly regulated by several inhibitory proteins, including CFH and complement factor I (CFI), which protect the host cells from complement attack.

A common variant (Arg102Gly; rs2230199) in the *C3* gene has been significantly associated with AMD (Yates et al. 2007). To search for rare and low-frequency variants in the previously identified AMD loci, whole-genome sequencing of 2230 Icelanders was performed and identified sequence variants were predicted (imputed) for a larger cohort of Icelanders genotyped with SNP microarrays. A rare missense variant (Lys155Gln; rs14785925) was identified that is highly associated with AMD ($p = 8.8 \times 10^{-16}$, odds ratio = 3.65 [95% CI 2.66–5.00]) (Fig. 1). The association of the rare Lys155Gln variant with AMD is independent of the common Arg102Gly variant (Helgason et al. 2013). The Lys155Gln variant was also identified by next generation sequencing of AMD genes and related pathways in two independent studies ($p = 5.2 \times 10^{-9}$, odds ratio = 3.8 [95% CI 2.3–6.1], and $p = 2.8 \times 10^{-5}$, odds ratio = 2.68]) (Seddon et al. 2013; Zhan et al. 2013).

The Lys155Gln variant localizes to the C3b fragment of the C3 protein. The presence of the Lys155Gln variant in the C3b protein causes reduced binding to the complement inhibitor molecule CFH. C3b becomes resistant to decay, which in turn leads to a gain of function of the C3 convertase activity (Miller 2012). A lower ability to degrade C3b, resulting in sustained complement attack in the macula, is the proposed disease mechanism for this rare variant.

Complement Component C9

Sequence analysis of 681 genes within all reported AMD loci and related pathways in 2493 cases and controls identified a rare missense variant in the *C9* gene (Pro167Ser) to be associated with AMD ($p = 6.5 \times 10^{-7}$, odds ratio 2.2 [95% CI 1.6–3.0]) (Seddon et al. 2013). Variants in the *C9* gene have not previously been associated with AMD, and this therefore for the first time links a component of the membrane attack complex with the pathogenesis of AMD. The functional effect of the Pro167Ser variant on the activity of the membrane attack complex remains to be determined.

CFH

CFH is the primary inhibitor of the alternative complement pathway. Genetic studies identified strong associations between AMD and a coding variant (Tyr402His; rs1061170) and several noncoding variants in the *CFH* gene (Edwards et al. 2005; Hageman et al. 2005; Haines et al. 2005). In addition to these common genetic variants, rare variants with an even larger effect have been identified in the *CFH* gene (Fig. 2A).

Heterozygous nonsense and frameshift mutations have been identified in the *CFH* gene among family members with cuticular drusen, a clinical subtype of AMD (Boon et al. 2008; van de Ven et al. 2012a). These mutations are predicted to lead to reduced levels of functional CFH protein. A recessive disease model was initially suggested in which patients were thought to develop cuticular drusen in the presence of a severe *CFH* mutation on one allele and the *CFH* Tyr402His risk variant on the other allele (Boon et al. 2008). A second study found that single heterozygous loss-of-function mutations in the *CFH* gene are sufficient for developing cuticular drusen, even in the absence of the Tyr402His risk allele (van de Ven et al. 2012a).

Another study identified a rare, highly penetrant missense variant (Arg1210Cys, rs121 913059) in 40 out of 2423 AMD patients, compared with only one out of 1122 control individuals ($p = 8.0 \times 10^{-5}$) (Fig. 1) (Raychaudhuri et al. 2011). The Arg1210Cys variant conferred risk independently of the common Tyr402His variant. The AMD patients who carried the Arg1210Cys variant had a significantly younger age of disease onset than did AMD patients

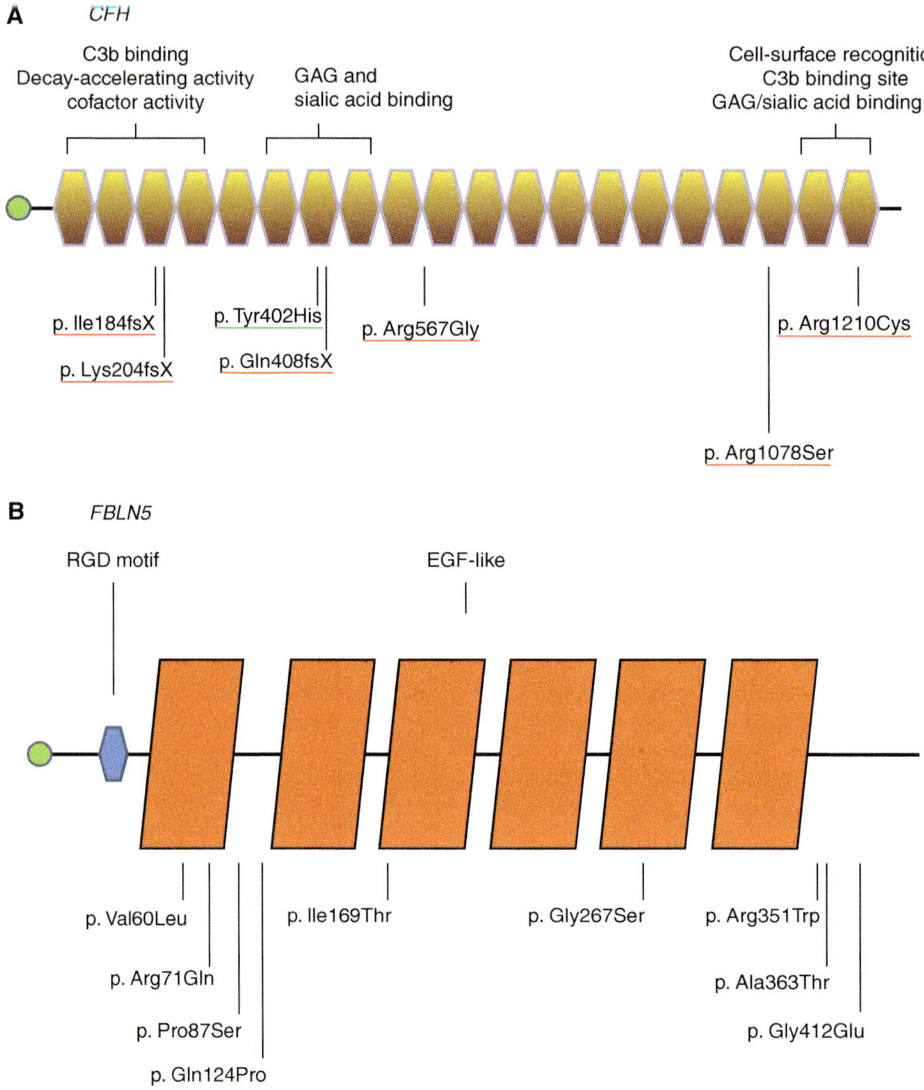

Figure 2. Overview of rare variants identified in complement factor H (*CFH*) and fibulin-5 (*FBLN5*) in AMD. (*A*) Location of rare variants in *CFH*. After an initial signal peptide, CFH consists of 20 adjacently positioned complement control protein (CCP, or sushi) domains that have differential affinity for C3 and/or cell surface structures. Underlined in green is the common variant Tyr402His. Underlined in red are rare variants in *CFH* that have been identified in AMD. GAG, glycosaminoglycans. (*B*) Location of rare variants in *FBLN5*. After an initial signal peptide, FBLN5 has one cell adhesion or integrin-binding motif (RGD, Arginyl-glycyl-aspartic acid), followed by six epidermal growth factor (EGF)-like domains.

without this mutation. The CFH Arg1210Cys amino acid substitution causes reduced binding to C3d, C3b, heparin, and endothelial cells (Manuelian et al. 2003; Ferreira et al. 2009). In addition, the Arg1210Cys mutant protein forms a covalent interaction with human serum albumin, which is likely caused by the introduction of an additional cysteine residue at this position (Sanchez-Corral et al. 2002).

These highly penetrant variants lead to impaired function and/or decreased levels of CFH, subsequently leading to a decreased ability to

 Cite this article as *Cold Spring Harb Perspect Med* doi: 10.1101/cshperspect.a017202

inhibit the complement system. Because CFH is expressed by the retinal pigment epithelium and the choroid (Anderson et al. 2010), the protection of these cells against complement activation is compromised in individuals carrying these rare variants. Several factors have been proposed to trigger complement activation in the macula, such as photooxidative stress caused by high sunlight exposure (Anderson et al. 2010). Individuals with insufficient complement-modulating activity can experience sustained complement attack, resulting in injury of the retinal pigment epithelium and subsequent formation of drusen (Anderson et al. 2010).

CFI

Similar to CFH, CFI is also required to maintain complement homeostasis and to restrict complement activation. Recently, rare variants in the *CFI* gene were found to confer a high risk of the development of AMD (van de Ven et al. 2013). Sequence analysis of a cohort of AMD patients identified two missense variants, Gly119Arg (rs141853578) and Gly188Ala. The Gly188Ala variant was found in four affected family members of one family. The Gly119Arg variant was identified in 20 out of 3567 unrelated AMD cases compared with only one out of 3937 controls, consistent with Gly119Arg conferring a high risk for developing AMD ($p = 3.79 \times 10^{-6}$, odds ratio = 22.20 [95% CI = 2.98–164.49]) (Fig. 1). Fundus fluorescein angiography revealed that carriers of the Gly119Arg and Gly188Ala variants had the cuticular drusen subtype of AMD (Boon et al. 2013). In addition, an increased burden of rare missense variants in *CFI* was observed in cases compared with controls. Rare missense variants were detected in 7.8% of AMD compared with 2.3% of controls ($p = 2 \times 10^{-8}$, odds ratio = 3.6) (Seddon et al. 2013).

The Gly119Arg and Gly188Ala variants severely impair the expression and secretion of the mutant CFI protein (van de Ven et al. 2013). As a result, patients carrying the CFI Gly119Arg or Gly188Ala variant have significantly lower plasma CFI levels than both controls and AMD patients who do not carry this CFI variant. Consequently, these mutation carriers have a significantly lower ability to degrade C3b, leading to sustained complement activation (van de Ven et al. 2013). In individuals with impaired CFI levels, a similar disease mechanism is proposed as for individuals carrying highly penetrant variants in the *CFH* gene, in which insufficient complement-modulating activity results in sustained complement attack and injury of the macula.

ATP-Binding Cassette A4 (ABCA4)

The *ABCA4* gene encodes an ATP-binding cassette transporter that is expressed in retinal photoreceptor cells. ABCA4 actively flips *N*-retinylidene-phosphatidylethanolamine from the lumen to the cytoplasmic leaflet of disc membranes, thereby facilitating the removal of potentially toxic retinoid compounds from photoreceptors (Quazi et al. 2012). Mutations in the *ABCA4* gene are found in Stargardt disease, an autosomal recessive retinal disorder characterized by a juvenile-onset macular dystrophy, delayed dark adaptation, and subretinal deposition of lipofuscin-like material (Allikmets 1997). Because of the phenotypic similarities between Stargardt disease and AMD, the *ABCA4* gene was considered a candidate gene for AMD.

Several rare *ABCA4* variants were detected in AMD patients (Allikmets et al. 1997), but the finding was criticized by several researchers (Dryja et al. 1998; Klaver et al. 1998a). Two rare variants (Gly1961Glu and Asp2177Asn), which lead to altered ATPase activity of the ABCA4 protein (Sun et al. 2000), were found to be significantly associated with AMD (Allikmets 2000). The association of *ABCA4* alleles with AMD was not confirmed by others (De La Paz et al. 1999; Rivera et al. 2000; Guymer et al. 2001; Webster et al. 2001), but this does not rule out that *ABCA4* may play a role in some cases of AMD (De La Paz et al. 1999).

In recent studies, a subgroup of AMD patients with a fine granular pattern with peripheral punctate spots, also referred to as late-onset Stargardt disease, was found to be significantly associated with rare *ABCA4* variants (Burke et al. 2012; Fritsche et al. 2012; Westeneng-van

Haaften et al. 2012). The differential diagnosis between this group of patients and AMD may be challenging, and it is plausible that such patients have been randomly included in some AMD cohorts, possibly explaining the previously described associations (Fritsche et al. 2012).

Fibulin-5 (FBLN5)

The *FBLN5* gene encodes a member of the fibulin family of extracellular matrix proteins. The fibulin proteins are involved in the formation and stabilization of supramolecular extracellular matrix complexes and are widely expressed in the basement membrane of epithelia and blood vessels. The fibulin genes were considered attractive candidate genes for AMD because a mutation in the fibulin-3 gene (also known as *EFEMP1*) causes Doyne honeycomb retinal dystrophy/malattia Leventinese, a Mendelian macular disease with an age of onset in early to mid-adulthood that shares phenotypic similarities with AMD (Stone et al. 1999).

Sequence analysis of all fibulin genes in a cohort of 402 AMD patients identified heterozygous amino acid variants in the *FBLN5* gene in seven patients, whereas none were observed among 429 control subjects ($p < 0.01$) (Fig. 2B) (Stone et al. 2004). Interestingly, all seven of these patients had cuticular drusen, a clinical subtype of AMD (Stone et al. 2004). In a follow-up study, an analysis of the *FBLN5* gene in 805 AMD cases and 279 controls identified two heterozygous amino acid variants in three patients (Fig. 2B). Two of these patients also had cuticular drusen (Lotery et al. 2006).

In the eye, fibulin-5 is located in Bruch's membrane (Mullins et al. 2007), a pentalaminar elastin- and collagen-rich extracellular matrix located between the retinal pigment epithelium and the choroid. Fibulin-5 is believed to serve a key role in elastogenesis by interacting with fibrillin, tropoelastin, and LOX-like protein, thereby bringing these proteins in close proximity (Schneider et al. 2010). Fibulin-5 also contains an amino-terminal Arg-Gly-Asp (RGD) motif that binds to cell-surface integrins and may facilitate the anchoring of elastic fibers to the cell surface (Schneider et al. 2010).

Four variants (Gly412Glu, Gly267Ser, Ile169Thr, Gln124Pro) in fibulin-5 that have been associated with AMD dramatically reduce the protein's secretion, and a similar effect was observed for mutations that have been linked to cutis laxa, a rare connective tissue disorder that is characterized by loose, sagging, inelastic skin that can present together with developmental emphysema and major defects in the systemic and pulmonary arteries (Lotery et al. 2006; Schneider et al. 2010). The Gly412Glu variant causes aggregation of the protein (Jones et al. 2010), and the Gly267Ser variant causes extensive misfolding (Schneider et al. 2010), which may explain the reduced secretion of these mutant proteins. Two other variants (Val60Leu and Arg71Gln) affecting residues close to the integrin-binding motif have insignificant effects on fibulin-5 aggregation (Jones et al. 2010); these variants might disrupt integrin binding or they may interfere with other intermolecular interactions.

The pathogenic effects of AMD-associated variants may stem from the long-term cumulative effects of subtle changes in Bruch's membrane over the individual's lifetime (Jones et al. 2010). A restricted availability of functional fibulin-5 during elastogenesis may lead to changes in the biophysical and biochemical properties of Bruch's membrane (Mullins et al. 2007; Schneider et al. 2010). Elastin is a principal component of Bruch's membrane, and reduced levels of functional fibulin-5 protein in the extracellular matrix may impair the normal assembly of elastin within Bruch's membrane (Stone et al. 2004). Interestingly, overexpression of HTRA1, which has been associated with AMD pathogenesis (Yang et al. 2010), has been shown to alter elastogenesis in Bruch's membrane through cleaving fibulin-5 (Yang et al. 2010; Vierkotten et al. 2011). Alternatively, interference with another function of fibulin-5 (for example, integrin-mediated cell attachment) may contribute to the pathogenic mechanism underlying fibulin-5 variants (Stone et al. 2004). Impeding normal elastic lamina formation in Bruch's membrane and/or attachment of the RPE to Bruch's membrane could make this structure susceptible to deposit formation (Mullins et al. 2007).

 Cite this article as *Cold Spring Harb Perspect Med* doi: 10.1101/cshperspect.a017202

Hemicentin-1 (HMCN1)

The *HMCN1* gene encodes an extracellular matrix protein with similarities to fibulins, and is therefore also referred to as fibulin-6. Linkage analysis in a large family with AMD identified a locus on chromosome 1q25-q31 encompassing 50 genes with a LOD score of 3.0 (Klein et al. 1998). Sequence analysis of 20 genes in the interval identified 29 exonic variants, with only one rare variant (Gln5345Arg) in the *HMCN1* gene that exclusively segregates with the disease in the family. The glutamine at position 5345 in hemicentin-1 is highly conserved among mammalian species, suggesting that it may have an important functional role (Schultz et al. 2003). It has been suggested that mutations in fibulins may alter the assembly or stability of elastin fibers and could disturb normal adhesion of the retinal pigment epithelium to Bruch's membrane (Schultz et al. 2005), which would fit with the disease pathogenesis of AMD.

However, the rare Gln5345Arg variant in the *HMCN1* gene was not found to be significantly associated with AMD in several case-control studies, even if the results of all studies are combined (Hayashi et al. 2004; McKay et al. 2004; Schultz et al. 2005). In this light, it should be noted that in the large AMD family, besides the Gln5345Arg variant in the *HMCN1* gene, 10 exonic variants were also identified in the *CFH* gene, which resides in the same linkage interval (Schultz et al. 2003). Considering the well-recognized role of *CFH* in the pathogenesis of AMD, it is plausible that one or more of the *CFH* variants, rather than the *HMCN1* Gln5354Arg variant, underlie the disease in this large AMD family. Even if these *CFH* variants do not completely segregate in the family, this does not exclude them as the cause of AMD in at least some of the affected individuals.

RELEVANCE OF RARE VARIANTS IN AMD

Predictive Testing

The first predictive tests for AMD based on a small number of common variants have been offered directly to consumers via the internet (23andMe, deCODEme, Navigenics, Sequenom, ArcticDx, Genetic Testing Laboratories, EasyDNA) (Kalf et al. 2014). However, the reliability and predictive value of these tests have been debated. The predictive ability of genetic risk models can be quantified by the area under the receiver operating characteristic curve (AUC). An AUC of 0.5 means that the test has no predictive value (like flipping a coin), whereas a model with an AUC of 1 provides a perfect prediction. The predictive tests offered by 23andMe (based on 3 common variants), deCODEme and Navigenics (both based on 6 common variants) had an AUC value around 0.80 (Kalf et al. 2014). Therefore, the predictive value of these tests was intermediate, performing better than flipping a coin but far from a perfect prediction. The predicted risks reported to individual consumers differed substantially among the three companies. For 20% of individuals, opposing risks for AMD were predicted by at least two companies (Kalf et al. 2014). Therefore, the results of the predictive tests that have been offered to consumers should be interpreted with great caution.

Because these predictive tests were based on a small number of common variants, they were not reliable in individuals carrying rare variants conferring high risk of AMD. It is essential to understand the role of rare variants in the genetic architecture of AMD before reliable genetic tests can be developed. To provide timely and effective treatments, reliable predictive tests are necessary to determine who is at high risk of developing AMD. These tests should not only be based on a small number of common variants, but also need to address rare, highly penetrant variants (van de Ven et al. 2013), for example, by including sequence analysis of all coding exons of the *C3*, *C9*, *CFH*, *CFI*, *ABCA4*, and *FBLN5* genes. This is particularly true for AMD cases in densely affected families, which are likely to be caused by rare, highly penetrant variants (Sobrin et al. 2010), and for whom this question is most urgent.

Genetic testing for AMD is currently not recommended by professional organizations, such as The American Academy of Ophthalmology Task Force on Genetic Testing (Stone et al. 2012), because the assessment of a small number of common genetic variants cannot reliably predict the development of the disease. Genetic testing for complex diseases will become relevant to routine clinical practice as soon as clinical trials can show that patients with specific genotypes benefit from specific types of therapy or surveillance. Until such benefits can be shown, routine genetic testing of patients with AMD or their family members is not recommended (Stone et al. 2012). Recently, companies offering direct-to-consumer tests have been directed by the U.S. Food and Drug Administration to stop marketing and selling direct-to-consumer genetic testing owing to concerns about public health consequences of inaccurate results (Park 2013; Annas and Elias 2014).

Recognition of Clinical Subtypes of AMD

Interestingly, several patients carrying rare variants in the *CFH*, *CFI*, and *FBLN5* genes have been reported to have cuticular drusen (Stone et al. 2004; Lotery et al. 2006; Boon et al. 2008, 2013; van de Ven et al. 2012a). This clinical subtype of AMD presents at an earlier age than typical AMD, has a strong familial component, and it has been proposed that genetic factors may play a more important role in its development than in the general AMD population (Grassi et al. 2007; van de Ven et al. 2012b; Boon et al. 2013). Cuticular drusen can be visualized by fluorescein angiography, even in individuals as young as 18 yr old, before any visual complaints have occurred. Patients with variants in the *ABCA4* gene can be distinguished by a fine granular pattern with peripheral punctate spots on fundus autofluorescence, also described as late-onset Stargardt disease (Fritsche et al. 2012; Westeneng-van Haaften et al. 2012). This implies that predictive tests may be improved by integrating results of clinical and genetic analyses, and that these tests can facilitate the recognition of clinical subtypes of AMD.

Development of Personalized Treatments for AMD

There is a need for treatment options that can stop the progression of AMD to advanced stages, rather than attempting to control end-stage complications. Elucidating rare, causal variants, for example in genes encoding components of the complement cascade, will enable a more-targeted therapeutic strategy in individual patients. The strong involvement of the complement system in AMD has prompted researchers to target complement activation in AMD. Complement-based therapeutics may have the potential to allow clinicians to intervene earlier in the disease process than current treatment options. Several compounds that target the complement pathway are currently being investigated, some of which are already in clinical trials. However, a phase 2 clinical trial with eculizumab, a systemic inhibitor of complement component C5, appeared not to effectively restrict geographic atrophy in AMD patients (Yehoshua et al. 2014). It has been speculated that complement inhibitors are more likely to be effective in individuals carrying rare variants conferring a large effect on complement activation as opposed to AMD patients in general (van de Ven et al. 2013).

CONCLUDING REMARKS

Genome-wide association studies have identified a number of common genetic variations to be associated with AMD, which together are estimated to account for 15%–65% of the genetic variance of AMD (Manolio et al. 2009; Fritsche et al. 2013). Recent studies suggest that at least a fraction of the "missing heritability" of AMD may be explained by rare variants with large effect sizes (Fig. 1) (Raychaudhuri et al. 2011; Seddon et al. 2013; van de Ven et al. 2013; Zhan et al. 2013). This shapes a new genetic architecture for AMD, encompassing both common genetic variants with relatively small effect sizes and rare genetic variants with large effect sizes. Further identification of such rare variants is important to improve predictive testing, to unravel the pathogenic mechanisms in different subgroups

 Cite this article as *Cold Spring Harb Perspect Med* doi: 10.1101/cshperspect.a017202

of AMD patients, and to develop personalized medicine for individual AMD patients tailored to his or her genetic background.

ACKNOWLEDGMENTS

This work was supported by research grants from the Macula Vision Research Foundation and the Netherlands Organisation for Scientific Research (016.096.309).

REFERENCES

Allikmets R. 1997. A photoreceptor cell-specific ATP-binding transporter gene (*ABCR*) is mutated in recessive Stargardt macular dystrophy. *Nat Genet* **17:** 122.

Allikmets R, The International ABCR Screening Consortium. 2000. Further evidence for an association of *ABCR* alleles with age-related macular degeneration. *Am J Hum Genet* **67:** 487–491.

Allikmets R, Shroyer NF, Singh N, Seddon JM, Lewis RA, Bernstein PS, Peiffer A, Zabriskie NA, Li Y, Hutchinson A, et al. 1997. Mutation of the Stargardt disease gene (*ABCR*) in age-related macular degeneration. *Science* **277:** 1805–1807.

Anderson DH, Radeke MJ, Gallo NB, Chapin EA, Johnson PT, Curletti CR, Hancox LS, Hu J, Ebright JN, Malek G, et al. 2010. The pivotal role of the complement system in aging and age-related macular degeneration: Hypothesis re-visited. *Prog Retin Eye Res* **29:** 95–112.

Annas GJ, Elias S. 2014. 23andMe and the FDA. *N Engl J Med* **370:** 985–988.

Bodmer W, Bonilla C. 2008. Common and rare variants in multifactorial susceptibility to common diseases. *Nat Genet* **40:** 695–701.

Boon CJ, Klevering BJ, Hoyng CB, Zonneveld-Vrieling MN, Nabuurs SB, Blokland E, Cremers FP, den Hollander AI. 2008. Basal laminar drusen caused by compound heterozygous variants in the *CFH* gene. *Am J Hum Genet* **82:** 516–523.

Boon CJ, van de Ven JP, Hoyng CB, den Hollander AI, Klevering BJ. 2013. Cuticular drusen: Stars in the sky. *Prog Retin Eye Res* **37:** 90–113.

Burke TR, Fishman GA, Zernant J, Schubert C, Tsang SH, Smith RT, Ayyagari R, Koenekoop RK, Umfress A, Ciccarelli ML, et al. 2012. Retinal phenotypes in patients homozygous for the G1961E mutation in the *ABCA4* gene. *Invest Ophthalmol Vis Sci* **53:** 4458–4467.

Cirulli ET, Goldstein DB. 2010. Uncovering the roles of rare variants in common disease through whole-genome sequencing. *Nat Rev Genet* **11:** 415–425.

De La Paz MA, Guy VK, Abou-Donia S, Heinis R, Bracken B, Vance JM, Gilbert JR, Gass JD, Haines JL, Pericak-Vance MA. 1999. Analysis of the Stargardt disease gene (*ABCR*) in age-related macular degeneration. *Ophthalmology* **106:** 1531–1536.

Dewan A, Liu M, Hartman S, Zhang SS, Liu DT, Zhao C, Tam PO, Chan WM, Lam DS, Snyder M, et al. 2006. *HTRA1* promoter polymorphism in wet age-related macular degeneration. *Science* **314:** 989–992.

Dryja TP, Berson EL, Rosenfeld PJ, Abitbol M. 1998. *ABCR* gene and age-related macular degeneration. *Science* **279.**

Edwards AO, Ritter R III, Abel KJ, Manning A, Panhuysen C, Farrer LA. 2005. Complement factor H polymorphism and age-related macular degeneration. *Science* **308:** 421–424.

Fagerness JA, Maller JB, Neale BM, Reynolds RC, Daly MJ, Seddon JM. 2009. Variation near complement factor I is associated with risk of advanced AMD. *Eur J Hum Genet* **17:** 100–104.

Ferreira VP, Herbert AP, Cortes C, McKee KA, Blaum BS, Esswein ST, Uhrin D, Barlow PN, Pangburn MK, Kavanagh D. 2009. The binding of factor H to a complex of physiological polyanions and C3b on cells is impaired in atypical hemolytic uremic syndrome. *J Immunol* **182:** 7009–7018.

Fritsche LG, Fleckenstein M, Fiebig BS, Schmitz-Valckenberg S, Bindewald-Wittich A, Keilhauer CN, Renner AB, Mackensen F, Mossner A, Pauleikhoff D, et al. 2012. A subgroup of age-related macular degeneration is associated with mono-allelic sequence variants in the *ABCA4* gene. *Invest Ophthalmol Vis Sci* **53:** 2112–2118.

Fritsche LG, Chen W, Schu M, Yaspan BL, Yu Y, Thorleifsson G, Zack DJ, Arakawa S, Cipriani V, Ripke S, et al. 2013. Seven new loci associated with age-related macular degeneration. *Nat Genet* **45:** 433–439.

Gold B, Merriam JE, Zernant J, Hancox LS, Taiber AJ, Gehrs K, Cramer K, Neel J, Bergeron J, Barile GR, et al. 2006. Variation in factor B (*BF*) and complement component 2 (*C2*) genes is associated with age-related macular degeneration. *Nat Genet* **38:** 458–462.

Goldstein DB, Allen A, Keebler J, Margulies EH, Petrou S, Petrovski S, Sunyaev S. 2013. Sequencing studies in human genetics: Design and interpretation. *Nat Rev Genet* **14:** 460–470.

Grassi MA, Folk JC, Scheetz TE, Taylor CM, Sheffield VC, Stone EM. 2007. Complement factor H polymorphism p.Tyr402His and cuticular drusen. *Arch Ophthalmol* **125:** 93–97.

Guymer RH, Heon E, Lotery AJ, Munier FL, Schorderet DF, Baird PN, McNeil RJ, Haines H, Sheffield VC, Stone EM. 2001. Variation of codons 1961 and 2177 of the Stargardt disease gene is not associated with age-related macular degeneration. *Arch Ophthalmol* **119:** 745–751.

Hageman GS, Anderson DH, Johnson LV, Hancox LS, Taiber AJ, Hardisty LI, Hageman JL, Stockman HA, Borchardt JD, Gehrs KM, et al. 2005. A common haplotype in the complement regulatory gene factor H (*HF1/CFH*) predisposes individuals to age-related macular degeneration. *Proc Natl Acad Sci* **102:** 7227–7232.

Haines JL, Hauser MA, Schmidt S, Scott WK, Olson LM, Gallins P, Spencer KL, Kwan SY, Noureddine M, Gilbert JR, et al. 2005. Complement factor H variant increases the risk of age-related macular degeneration. *Science* **308:** 419–421.

Hayashi M, Merriam JE, Klaver CC, Zernant J, Bergen AA, Smith RT, Chang S, Merriam JC, Allikmets R. 2004. Evaluation of the *ARMD1* locus on 1q25–31 in patients with age-related maculopathy: Genetic variation in laminin genes and in exon 104 of *HEMICENTIN-1*. *Ophthal Genet* **25:** 111–119.

Helgason H, Sulem P, Duvvari MR, Luo H, Thorleifsson G, Stefansson H, Jonsdottir I, Masson G, Gudbjartsson DF, Walters GB, et al. 2013. A rare nonsynonymous sequence variant in *C3* is associated with high risk of age-related macular degeneration. *Nat Genet* **45:** 1371–1374.

Huyghe JR, Jackson AU, Fogarty MP, Buchkovich ML, Stancakova A, Stringham HM, Sim X, Yang L, Fuchsberger C, Cederberg H, et al. 2013. Exome array analysis identifies new loci and low-frequency variants influencing insulin processing and secretion. *Nat Genet* **45:** 197–201.

Jakobsdottir J, Conley YP, Weeks DE, Mah TS, Ferrell RE, Gorin MB. 2005. Susceptibility genes for age-related maculopathy on chromosome 10q26. *Am J Hum Genet* **77:** 389–407.

Jones RP, Ridley C, Jowitt TA, Wang MC, Howard M, Bobola N, Wang T, Bishop PN, Kielty CM, Baldock C, et al. 2010. Structural effects of fibulin 5 missense mutations associated with age-related macular degeneration and cutis laxa. *Invest Ophthalmol Vis Sci* **51:** 2356–2362.

Kalf RR, Mihaescu R, Kundu S, de Knijff P, Green RC, Janssens AC. 2014. Variations in predicted risks in personal genome testing for common complex diseases. *Genet Med* **16:** 85–91.

Kiezun A, Garimella K, Do R, Stitziel NO, Neale BM, McLaren PJ, Gupta N, Sklar P, Sullivan PF, Moran JL, et al. 2012. Exome sequencing and the genetic basis of complex traits. *Nat Genet* **44:** 623–630.

Klaver CC, Bergen AA, van Duijn CM. 1998a. *ABCR* gene and age-related macular degeneration. *Science* **279**.

Klaver CC, Wolfs RC, Assink JJ, van Duijn CM, Hofman A, de Jong PT. 1998b. Genetic risk of age-related maculopathy. Population-based familial aggregation study. *Arch Ophthalmol* **116:** 1646–1651.

Klein ML, Schultz DW, Edwards A, Matise TC, Rust K, Berselli CB, Trzupek K, Weleber RG, Ott J, Wirtz MK, et al. 1998. Age-related macular degeneration. Clinical features in a large family and linkage to chromosome 1q. *Arch Ophthalmol* **116:** 1082–1088.

Lander E, Kruglyak L. 1995. Genetic dissection of complex traits: Guidelines for interpreting and reporting linkage results. *Nat Genet* **11:** 241–247.

Liu DJ, Leal SM. 2012. Estimating genetic effects and quantifying missing heritability explained by identified rare-variant associations. *Am J Hum Genet* **91:** 585–596.

Liu MM, Chan CC, Tuo J. 2012. Genetic mechanisms and age-related macular degeneration: Common variants, rare variants, copy number variations, epigenetics, and mitochondrial genetics. *Hum Genom* **6:** 13.

Lotery AJ, Baas D, Ridley C, Jones RP, Klaver CC, Stone E, Nakamura T, Luff A, Griffiths H, Wang T, et al. 2006. Reduced secretion of fibulin 5 in age-related macular degeneration and cutis laxa. *Hum Mutat* **27:** 568–574.

Manolio TA, Collins FS, Cox NJ, Goldstein DB, Hindorff LA, Hunter DJ, McCarthy MI, Ramos EM, Cardon LR, Chakravarti A, et al. 2009. Finding the missing heritability of complex diseases. *Nature* **461:** 747–753.

Manuelian T, Hellwage J, Meri S, Caprioli J, Noris M, Heinen S, Jozsi M, Neumann HP, Remuzzi G, Zipfel PF. 2003. Mutations in factor H reduce binding affinity to C3b and heparin and surface attachment to endothelial cells in hemolytic uremic syndrome. *J Clin Invest* **111:** 1181–1190.

Mayeux R. 2005. Mapping the new frontier: Complex genetic disorders. *J Clin Invest* **115:** 1404–1407.

McKay GJ, Clarke S, Hughes A, McConnell V, Schultz DW, Klein ML, Silvestri G, Simpson DA. 2004. A novel diagnostic test detects a low frequency of the hemicentin Gln5345Arg variant among Northern Irish age related macular degeneration patients. *Mol Vis* **10:** 682–687.

Miller E. 2012. Characterization of complement C3 dysregulation predisposing to two human disease states. PhD thesis, Washington University, St Louis.

Mullins RF, Olvera MA, Clark AF, Stone EM. 2007. Fibulin-5 distribution in human eyes: Relevance to age-related macular degeneration. *Exp Eye Res* **84:** 378–380.

O'Roak BJ, Vives L, Fu W, Egertson JD, Stanaway IB, Phelps IG, Carvill G, Kumar A, Lee C, Ankenman K, et al. 2012. Multiplex targeted sequencing identifies recurrently mutated genes in autism spectrum disorders. *Science* **338:** 1619–1622.

Park A. 2013. FDA halts 23andMe genetic tests. *Time* **182:** 18.

Pritchard JK. 2001. Are rare variants responsible for susceptibility to complex diseases? *Am J Hum Genet* **69:** 124–137.

Quazi F, Lenevich S, Molday RS. 2012. ABCA4 is an *N*-retinylidene-phosphatidylethanolamine and phosphatidylethanolamine importer. *Nat Commun* **3:** 925.

Raychaudhuri S, Iartchouk O, Chin K, Tan PL, Tai AK, Ripke S, Gowrisankar S, Vemuri S, Montgomery K, Yu Y, et al. 2011. A rare penetrant mutation in *CFH* confers high risk of age-related macular degeneration. *Nat Genet* **43:** 1232–1236.

Rivera A, White K, Stohr H, Steiner K, Hemmrich N, Grimm T, Jurklies B, Lorenz B, Scholl HP, Apfelstedt-Sylla E, et al. 2000. A comprehensive survey of sequence variation in the *ABCA4* (*ABCR*) gene in Stargardt disease and age-related macular degeneration. *Am J Hum Genet* **67:** 800–813.

Rivera A, Fisher SA, Fritsche LG, Keilhauer CN, Lichtner P, Meitinger T, Weber BH. 2005. Hypothetical *LOC387715* is a second major susceptibility gene for age-related macular degeneration, contributing independently of complement factor H to disease risk. *Hum Mol Genet* **14:** 3227–3236.

Sanchez-Corral P, Perez-Caballero D, Huarte O, Simckes AM, Goicoechea E, Lopez-Trascasa M, de Cordoba SR. 2002. Structural and functional characterization of factor H mutations associated with atypical hemolytic uremic syndrome. *Am J Hum Genet* **71:** 1285–1295.

Sanger F, Nicklen S, Coulson AR. 1977. DNA sequencing with chain-terminating inhibitors. *Proc Natl Acad Sci* **74:** 5463–5467.

Schneider R, Jensen SA, Whiteman P, McCullagh JS, Redfield C, Handford PA. 2010. Biophysical characterisation of fibulin-5 proteins associated with disease. *J Mol Biol* **401:** 605–617.

Schultz DW, Klein ML, Humpert AJ, Luzier CW, Persun V, Schain M, Mahan A, Runckel C, Cassera M, Vittal V, et al. 2003. Analysis of the *ARMD1* locus: Evidence that a mutation in *HEMICENTIN-1* is associated with age-related macular degeneration in a large family. *Hum Mol Genet* **12:** 3315–3323.

Schultz DW, Weleber RG, Lawrence G, Barral S, Majewski J, Acott TS, Klein ML. 2005. *HEMICENTIN-1* (FIBULIN-6) and the 1q31 AMD locus in the context of complex disease: Review and perspective. *Ophthal Genet* **26:** 101–105.

Seddon JM, Ajani UA, Mitchell BD. 1997. Familial aggregation of age-related maculopathy. *Am J Ophthalmol* **123:** 199–206.

Seddon JM, Cote J, Page WF, Aggen SH, Neale MC. 2005. The US twin study of age-related macular degeneration: Relative roles of genetic and environmental influences. *Arch Ophthalmol* **123:** 321–327.

Seddon JM, Yu Y, Miller EC, Reynolds R, Tan PL, Gowrisankar S, Goldstein JI, Triebwasser M, Anderson HE, Zerbib J, et al. 2013. Rare variants in *CFI*, *C3* and *C9* are associated with high risk of advanced age-related macular degeneration. *Nat Genet* **45:** 1366–1370.

Shahid H, Khan JC, Cipriani V, Sepp T, Matharu BK, Bunce C, Harding SP, Clayton DG, Moore AT, Yates JR, et al. 2012. Age-related macular degeneration: The importance of family history as a risk factor. *Br J Ophthalmol* **96:** 427–431.

Sobrin L, Maller JB, Neale BM, Reynolds RC, Fagerness JA, Daly MJ, Seddon JM. 2010. Genetic profile for five common variants associated with age-related macular degeneration in densely affected families: A novel analytic approach. *Eur J Hum Genet* **18:** 496–501.

Stone EM, Lotery AJ, Munier FL, Heon E, Piguet B, Guymer RH, Vandenburgh K, Cousin P, Nishimura D, Swiderski RE, et al. 1999. A single *EFEMP1* mutation associated with both Malattia Leventinese and Doyne honeycomb retinal dystrophy. *Nat Genet* **22:** 199–202.

Stone EM, Braun TA, Russell SR, Kuehn MH, Lotery AJ, Moore PA, Eastman CG, Casavant TL, Sheffield VC. 2004. Missense variations in the fibulin 5 gene and age-related macular degeneration. *N Engl J Med* **351:** 346–353.

Stone EM, Aldave AJ, Drack AV, Maccumber MW, Sheffield VC, Traboulsi E, Weleber RG. 2012. Recommendations for genetic testing of inherited eye diseases: Report of the American Academy of Ophthalmology task force on genetic testing. *Ophthalmology* **119:** 2408–2410.

Sun H, Smallwood PM, Nathans J. 2000. Biochemical defects in ABCR protein variants associated with human retinopathies. *Nat Genet* **26:** 242–246.

Thornton J, Edwards R, Mitchell P, Harrison RA, Buchan I, Kelly SP. 2005. Smoking and age-related macular degeneration: A review of association. *Eye* **19:** 935–944.

van de Ven JP, Boon CJ, Fauser S, Hoefsloot LH, Smailhodzic D, Schoenmaker-Koller F, Klevering J, Klaver CC, den Hollander AI, Hoyng CB. 2012a. Clinical evaluation of 3 families with basal laminar drusen caused by novel mutations in the complement factor H gene. *Arch Ophthalmol* **130:** 1038–1047.

van de Ven JP, Smailhodzic D, Boon CJ, Fauser S, Groenewoud JM, Chong NV, Hoyng CB, Klevering BJ, den Hollander AI. 2012b. Association analysis of genetic and environmental risk factors in the cuticular drusen subtype of age-related macular degeneration. *Mol Vis* **18:** 2271–2278.

van de Ven JP, Nilsson SC, Tan PL, Buitendijk GH, Ristau T, Mohlin FC, Nabuurs SB, Schoenmaker-Koller FE, Smailhodzic D, Campochiaro PA, et al. 2013. A functional variant in the *CFI* gene confers a high risk of age-related macular degeneration. *Nat Genet* **45:** 813–817.

Vierkotten S, Muether PS, Fauser S. 2011. Overexpression of HTRA1 leads to ultrastructural changes in the elastic layer of Bruch's membrane via cleavage of extracellular matrix components. *PLoS ONE* **6:** e22959.

Walport MJ. 2001a. Complement. First of two parts. *N Engl J Med* **344:** 1058–1066.

Walport MJ. 2001b. Complement. Second of two parts. *N Engl J Med* **344:** 1140–1144.

Webster AR, Heon E, Lotery AJ, Vandenburgh K, Casavant TL, Oh KT, Beck G, Fishman GA, Lam BL, Levin A, et al. 2001. An analysis of allelic variation in the *ABCA4* gene. *Invest Ophthalmol Vis Sci* **42:** 1179–1189.

Westeneng-van Haaften SC, Boon CJ, Cremers FP, Hoefsloot LH, den Hollander AI, Hoyng CB. 2012. Clinical and genetic characteristics of late-onset Stargardt's disease. *Ophthalmology* **119:** 1199–1210.

Yang Z, Tong Z, Chen Y, Zeng J, Lu F, Sun X, Zhao C, Wang K, Davey L, Chen H, et al. 2010. Genetic and functional dissection of *HTRA1* and *LOC387715* in age-related macular degeneration. *PLoS Genet* **6:** e1000836.

Yates JR, Sepp T, Matharu BK, Khan JC, Thurlby DA, Shahid H, Clayton DG, Hayward C, Morgan J, Wright AF, et al. 2007. Complement *C3* variant and the risk of age-related macular degeneration. *N Engl J Med* **357:** 553–561.

Yehoshua Z, de Amorim Garcia Filho CA, Nunes RP, Gregori G, Penha FM, Moshfeghi AA, Zhang K, Sadda S, Feuer W, Rosenfeld PJ. 2014. Systemic complement inhibition with eculizumab for geographic atrophy in age-related macular degeneration: The COMPLETE study. *Ophthalmology* **121:** 693–701.

Yu Y, Bhangale TR, Fagerness J, Ripke S, Thorleifsson G, Tan PL, Souied EH, Richardson AJ, Merriam JE, Buitendijk GH, et al. 2011. Common variants near *FRK/COL10A1* and *VEGFA* are associated with advanced age-related macular degeneration. *Hum Mol Genet* **20:** 3699–3709.

Zhan X, Larson DE, Wang C, Koboldt DC, Sergeev YV, Fulton RS, Fulton LL, Fronick CC, Branham KE, Bragg-Gresham J, et al. 2013. Identification of a rare coding variant in complement 3 associated with age-related macular degeneration. *Nat Genet* **45:** 1375–1379.

Differential Gene Expression in Age-Related Macular Degeneration

Denise J. Morgan and Margaret M. DeAngelis

Department of Ophthalmology and Visual Sciences, John A. Moran Eye Center, University of Utah School of Medicine, Salt Lake City, Utah 84132

Correspondence: margaret.deangelis@utah.edu

Gene expression is the first step in ascribing function between an associated gene and disease. Understanding how variation in a gene influences expression, particularly in tissues affected by the disease, may help elucidate what influences the phenotypic outcome of that disease. Previous studies of the genetics of age-related macular degeneration (AMD) have identified several risk factors, but have not yet bridged the gap between gene association and identifying a specific mechanism or function that is involved in the pathogenesis of AMD. Advances in genomic technologies, such as RNA sequencing (RNA-seq), single cell RNA-seq, bilsulfite sequencing, and/or whole genome methylation, will be powerful tools for identifying genes/pathways that are differentially expressed in those with AMD versus those without AMD. These technologies should advance the field of AMD research so that appropriate preventive and therapeutic targets can be developed.

Age-related macular degeneration (AMD) is a multifactorial, complex disorder that affects the retinal pigment epithelium (RPE) with the accompanying loss of the overlying photoreceptors in the neural retina. The hallmark of AMD is the deposition of drusen, subretinal yellowish deposits accompanied by hypo- or hyperpigmentary changes of the RPE. The number, size, and area of drusen, along with the presence or absence of these pigmentary changes of the RPE, determine the severity of AMD in the early or intermediate stages (Ferris et al. 2005). These changes, which typically occur after the age of 40 yr, can occur in both the macula and extra macula but mostly concentrate in the macula (Curcio et al. 1996; Klein et al. 1997). The reasons why are not entirely clear. As AMD is a progressive degenerative disease, having the intermediate stage puts one at risk for the advanced forms of the disease. Clinically, two forms of advanced AMD are recognized: geographic atrophy; and neovascular AMD. Geographic atrophy represents an area of loss of the RPE and choroid resulting in the gradual loss of photoreceptors. Neovascular or "wet" AMD is characterized by the growth of abnormal new blood vessels from the choroid into sub-RPE and subretinal regions and that can cause severe and rapid vision loss owing to hemorrhage and exudation. It is neovascular AMD that is responsible for the majority of debilitating vision loss because of AMD. Because the

Cite this article as *Cold Spring Harb Perspect Med* doi: 10.1101/cshperspect.a017210

macula is primarily affected, central vision loss results, with reduced quality of life manifesting as impaired ability to read, drive, and recognize faces. It is estimated that nearly 10 million U.S. citizens have some type of AMD in at least one eye, with the expectation that the contralateral eye will also be affected within 5 yr. Unfortunately, degeneration of the macula and/or the retina has generally begun by the time the patient is diagnosed with some form of AMD in the clinical setting. Additionally, most current treatments (which are directed against the advanced stage of AMD) are limited in their applicability and cannot reverse vision loss over the long term. Understanding which genes mechanistically underlie the pathophysiology of AMD could help us to identify biomarkers and/or predictors of disease onset, and to prevent progression to the intermediate and more advanced stages of AMD.

The genetic and epidemiological factors that contribute to overall AMD risk have been well studied, and it is likely that an individual's susceptibility to the disease is influenced by a combination of many different genetic and environmental factors (for reviews, see DeAngelis et al. 2011; Gorin 2012; Miller 2013; Fritsche et al. 2014). The architecture of AMD genetics has been expanded by the discovery of 19 loci associated with AMD with genome-wide significance (Fritsche et al. 2013) and the ongoing exome chip experiment efforts by the International AMD Genomics Consortium (IAMDGC) to identify rare AMD coding variants along with common variation. Consistently, ARMS2/HTRA1 on chromosome 10q26 and CFH on chromosome 1q32 remain the most strongly associated loci with genetic risk of AMD (Fritsche et al. 2013). Whereas the role of complement factor H (CFH) in the complement pathway is well known, the roles of ARMS2/HTRA1 are not as clear. Based on efforts by the IAMDGC, the seven novel loci (COL8A1/FILIP1L, IER3/DDR1, SLC16A8, TGFBR1, RAD51B, ADAMTS9/MIR548A2, and B3GALTL), which reached genome-wide significance, strengthened our knowledge base from a genetic perspective. Common variation in these genes confirmed pathways and risk factors already associated with AMD pathogenesis, including collagen biogenesis (Zarbin et al. 2014), lipid metabolism (Pikuleva and Curcio 2014), cardiovascular risk factors (Chakravarthy et al. 2010), and apoptotic regulation (Payne et al. 2013). However, there remains a gap in our knowledge about the biological significance of these novel genes, as well as previously identified genes and their functions in AMD pathophysiology. From these genome-wide association (GWA) studies or candidate gene association studies, one can surmise what the function of a gene may be based on what tissues in which it is expressed, or if the gene has been associated with diseases with overlapping pathophysiology (e.g., cardiovascular disease or Alzheimer disease) (McKay et al. 2011; Cougnard-Grégoire et al. 2014; Klein et al. 2014; Logue et al. 2014). Given the limited resources of fresh human donor eye tissue for benchtop studies of gene expression, another approach is to use public databases (see Table 1) to determine tissue expression of a given gene. However, there is little information about how expression patterns differ between those with disease and those without, and whether or not

Table 1. Gene expression resources

Database	Website	Eye tissue data sets
Gene expression omnibus (GEO)	http://www.ncbi.nlm.nih.gov/geo/	GEO:GSE29801 (Newman et al. 2012), GEO:GSE40524 (Farkas et al. 2013)
Serial analysis of gene expression (SAGE)	http://cgap.nci.nih.gov/SAGE	
BioGPS	http://biogps.org/	
RNA-seq atlas	http://medicalgenomics.org/rna_seq_atlas/data	
EMBL-EBI Expression atlas	http://www.ebi.ac.uk/gxa/home	

 Cite this article as *Cold Spring Harb Perspect Med* doi: 10.1101/cshperspect.a017210

that pattern of expression differs between the various disease phenotypes. Studies of gene expression with regards to AMD phenotype are becoming increasingly important in assessing the relevance and possible functions of AMD risk loci and moving beyond genetic association to uncovering the specific pathways involved in the development and progression of the disease.

CONSIDERATIONS FOR AMD GENE EXPRESSION STUDY SAMPLES

Because AMD is a disease that affects the RPE/choroid and the photoreceptors of the neural retina, these tissues should be the primary focus of gene expression studies in AMD. Ideally, tissues should be from both the macula and extramacula regions of donor eyes with and without AMD (see Fig. 1). Moreover, because we do not know if this is a localized or systemic disease, venous blood samples collected from the donor of the eye tissue can also be useful in gene expression studies. Things to consider when conducting gene expression studies include the postmortem time, death-to-preservation time, how the tissue is dissected, which tissues to study (RPE/choroid and retina), postmortem ophthalmic imaging, and rigorous phenotyping. Furthermore, both ophthalmic records and medical records should be obtained whenever possible. As we have learned during our own experience from the creation of a fresh donor eye repository in the DeAngelis laboratory, many donor eyes have pathological signs of

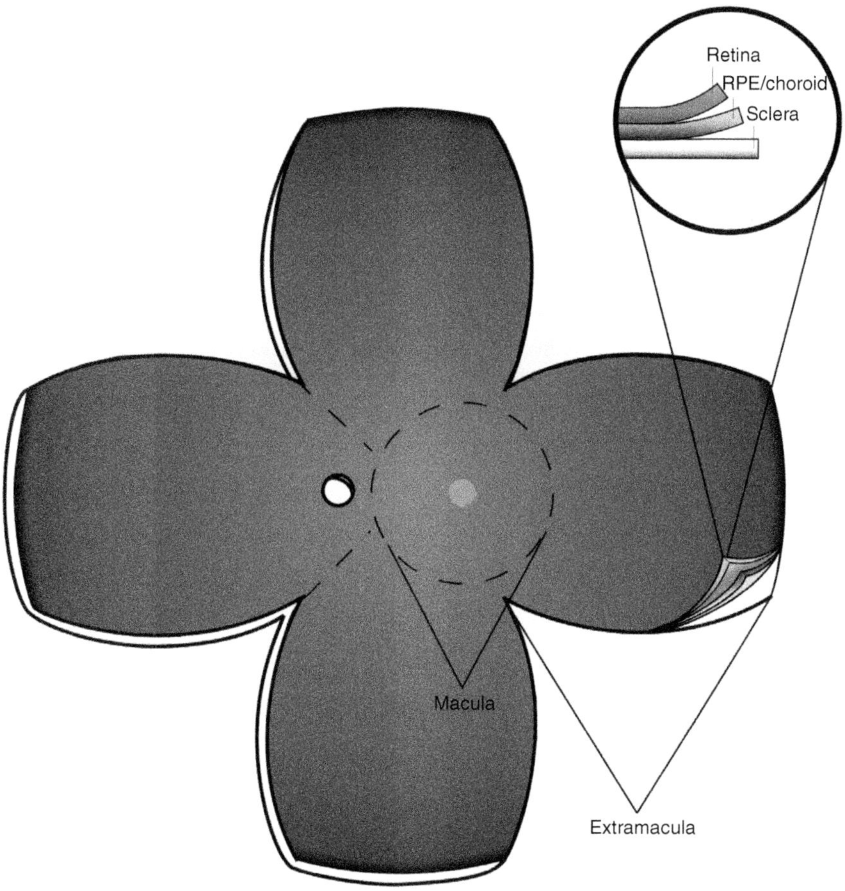

Figure 1. Geographical regions and tissue types isolated from human donor eye tissue for gene expression studies.

AMD during postmortem imaging in one or both eyes that was not documented in available records. Additionally, many donors have discordant phenotypes between eyes.

FACTORS AFFECTING GENE EXPRESSION IN AMD

There are many factors that can affect the expression of a particular gene. Genetic variation, regulatory RNAs, and epigenetic modifications can all influence gene expression and have all been implicated in AMD pathophysiology.

Genetic Variation

The mechanisms by which AMD-associated genetic variations influence AMD risk are poorly understood. Because many of the AMD gene association studies published to date are GWA studies (Fritsche et al. 2013), and most of the variants that are investigated are tagging single-nucleotide polymorphisms (SNPs) or noncoding SNPs in large intergenic regions, it can be difficult to ascribe function to any particular associated variant. Coding variants located in the exons of genes usually have a predictable effect on the genes in which they are located. These variations can cause truncated or missense transcripts that can affect protein function or stability. To date, both common coding variations and rare coding variations have been reported in AMD-associated risk genes in the complement pathway (Edwards et al. 2005; Haines et al. 2005; Klein et al. 2005; Yates et al. 2007; Helgason et al. 2013; Zhan et al. 2013; Seddon et al. 2014; Yu et al. 2014). However, for AMD-associated variants that are coding, such as the ARMS2 A69S variant (Jakobsdottir et al. 2005; Rivera et al. 2005), it is not entirely clear how the variant affects the mRNA transcript or protein. Variations that modify gene expression are likely more important in the development of complex diseases such as AMD (Cookson et al. 2009; Silveira et al. 2010; DeAngelis et al. 2011).

When mRNA abundance is studied as a quantitative trait, it is possible to identify genetic variants that regulate gene expression. These expression quantitative trait loci (eQTLs) can influence gene expression at the level of transcription or translation (Majewski and Pastinen 2011), and act in *cis* (locally) or *trans* (distantly). SNPs located in promoter regions may affect gene expression at the level of transcription. In contrast, SNPs located in splice sites, miRNAs, or in miRNA-binding sites may have a posttranscriptional effect. A study by Lalonde and colleagues used RNA sequencing (RNA-seq) data from breast cancer cell lines, and concluded that the majority of eQTLs modify gene expression at the level of transcription, with ~25% controlling their targets co- or posttranscriptionally (Lalonde et al. 2011).

To maximize their expression data, Li et al. (2014) integrated genetic variation data with expression data generated via RNA-seq. Specifically, they generated genotypes using a SNP chip on peripheral blood from each human eye donor to examine whether or not the previously identified SNPs also associated with ophthalmic diseases (including AMD), and showed allele-specific expression (ASE) in their RNA-seq data. Simply stated, the purpose of ASE analysis is to show which variants can regulate a gene in *cis*, using individuals who are heterozygous at a given SNP (Stevenson et al. 2013; Zhang et al. 2014). They identified three previously known common coding variants in the complement pathway that have also been associated with AMD risk (Fritshe et al. 2013). This shows that these disease-associated variants influence gene expression in tissues in which AMD is expected to manifest.

A few studies have looked at the effect of an AMD-associated SNP that lies in the promoter of HTRA1 (rs11200638) on gene expression. An early study on HTRA1 mRNA levels in blood lymphocytes found increased expression in individuals homozygous for the risk allele at rs11200638 (Yang et al. 2006). An additional study of cultured human RPE cells showed a twofold increase in HTRA1 expression for cells homozygous for the risk allele (An et al. 2010). However, the trend toward increased HTRA1 expression in relationship to the rs11200638 genotype was not seen in a study of human retina tissue. In fact, this study reported no observed differences in HTRA1 expression in human neural retina tissue with regards to age, AMD status, or genetic risk alleles (Kanda et al. 2010).

Alternative Splicing

Alternative splicing has been shown to be an important mechanism of gene expression regulation (Lalonde et al. 2011). A SNP located in a spice site can interfere with splice site recognition, preventing proper splicing and targeting a transcript for degradation (or otherwise blocking the translation of a particular transcript or splice variant). Although alternative splicing has been shown to occur in donor aging eye tissue of RPE/choroid/sclera (Li et al. 2014) and donor AMD retina (Karunakaran et al. 2013), it is still an understudied area in AMD pathophysiology.

Noncoding RNAs (ncRNAs)

Noncoding RNAs (ncRNAs) are involved in posttranscriptional gene modulation and are estimated to regulate translation of possibly 60% of protein-coding genes (for review, see Esteller 2011). ncRNAs also may provide a target for therapeutics in treating neurodegenerative, cardiovascular, and autoimmune diseases.

There are two primary classes of ncRNAs that can influence gene expression: microRNAs (miRNAs); and long intergenic noncoding RNAs (lincRNAs). miRNAs are generally 19 to 24 nucleotides in length and are important for posttranscriptional regulation of mRNA transcripts. It is estimated that they target up to a third of all human mRNAs, and are known to mediate their effect on mRNAs through translational repression or mRNA degradation (Gamazon et al. 2012). miRNAs are largely derived from introns of protein coding or noncoding genes. Mutations in the 2–8 bp "seed" region of the mRNA binding site, located in the 3′ UTR of the target gene, can prevent miRNA binding to target mRNA, likely resulting in increased target expression (Smith et al. 2012). Multiple studies have suggested a role for miRNA in AMD pathogenesis and as potential therapeutic targets (Lin et al. 2011; Haque et al. 2012; Hou et al. 2013; Zhou et al. 2014). lincRNAs, as their name implies, are >200 nucleotides in length and have no coding capabilities. lincRNAs can interact with DNA, other RNAs, and/or proteins; furthermore, they may control transcriptional silencing via epigenetic regulation and chromatin remodeling. For example, in body fluids such as serum from patients with neuropsychiatric disorders, ncRNAs show altered expression when compared with controls, and therefore may be used as biomarkers to predict disease development (Mamdani et al. 2013). Similarly, for onset and progression of diseases such as AMD, miRNAs are proposed to be useful biomarkers (Hrdlickova et al. 2014) as they may be specific to body fluids.

Epigenetics

The definition of epigenetics refers to heritable changes in gene expression without changes to DNA sequence. Epigenetic regulation can involve processes such as DNA methylation, histone modification, and chromatin remodeling (Bock 2012; Heard and Martienssen 2014). There is increasing evidence that in complex diseases such as AMD, DNA methylation may contribute to gene expression variation (Petronis 2010). ncRNAs are abundant in the human genome and may be susceptible to environmental changes, and, through DNA methylation, ncRNAs can be involved in gene regulation by either silencing or up-regulating expression. Specifically, lincRNAs are believed to direct methylation to a specific gene (Peschansky and Wahlestedt 2014). Similar to gene expression patterns in tissues, methylation patterns can vary by tissue type, so patterns observed in peripheral blood from a patient with AMD may not translate to eye tissue. Moreover, methylation patterns that influence gene expression may differ between tissue subtypes within the posterior eye (e.g., RPE/choroid versus neural retina). Because the largest GWA study to date has yet to show a difference in genetic architecture between subtypes of AMD (Fritsche et al. 2013), it is possible that the differences in methylation could explain why the same genes are associated with different AMD phenotypes.

Methylation levels generally decrease with aging (Bollati et al. 2009; Brunet and Berger 2014). This is not surprising, given that the effects of environmental factors, (such as nutrition, diet, medications, toxins, etc.) accumulate as we age. An example of this was demonstrated by showing that epigenetic factors control lipid variation. Specifically, methylation levels in carnitine palmitolytransferase 1A were associated with fasting very low-density lipoprotein C and triglyceride levels in 991 middle aged adults. Further, this association was found to be independent of genetic variation (Irvin et al. 2014). In another study the quality and amount of dietary fat in one's diet could influence methylation of metabolic pathways. For example, by examining ratios of monounsaturated fatty acids, polyunsaturated fatty acids, and saturated fatty acids Voisin et al. (2014) showed that methylation of genes in several metabolic pathways including leptin was associated with overall fat intake but not cholesterol intake in preadolescents.

As oxidative stress is believed to be one of the mechanisms underlying AMD pathophysiology, Hunter et al. (2012) examined the glutathione S-transferase genes, GSTM1 and GSTM5, which function in detoxification and antioxidation. They used gene expression and methylation microarray data to show that GSTM1 and GSTM5 are differentially expressed in donor eyes with and without AMD and that this corresponds to changes in promoter methylation. Specifically, the mRNA levels of GSTM1 and GSTM5 were significantly reduced in donor eyes with AMD compared with age-matched controls in both the RPE/choroid and neural retina, which corresponded to hypermethylation of the GSTM1 promoter (Hunter et al. 2012). In another example of expression and methylation in peripheral blood from patients with AMD, Wei et al. (2012) found that hypomethylation in the promoter region of the interleukin 17 receptor C gene, IL17RC, correlated with up-regulation of IL17RC expression of mRNA in peripheral blood from a twin cohort with AMD. The up-regulation in IL7RC expression was also observed in retina and RPE/choroid from donor eyes with AMD. However, DNA methylation patterns from eye tissues were not examined, so, although expression pattern between peripheral blood and eye tissue could be correlated, methylation pattern status was not determined (Wei et al. 2012). Another study by Oliver and colleagues could not replicate these findings in peripheral blood from two cohorts comprised of unrelated case controls with and without AMD and concluded that decreased methylation in the IL7 RC promoter was not useful as a biomarker for AMD (Oliver et al. 2013). Ideally, future studies will need to incorporate RPE/choroid, neural retina and blood from the same donor into studies of both expression and methylation to elucidate mechanisms underlying normal aging compared with AMD. In this manner, appropriate therapeutic targets should begin to emerge.

GENE EXPRESSION MICROARRAY AND RNA-seq STUDIES

Microarray technology has been used in multiple studies to characterize the expression profiles of normal human eye tissues (Yoshida et al. 2002; Bowes Rickman et al. 2006; Radeke et al. 2007; Booij et al. 2010; Strunnikova et al. 2010; Zhang et al. 2012) and to identify genes that are differentially expressed both systemically, and in eye tissues of those with AMD (see Table 2) (Chowers et al. 2006; Radeke et al. 2007; Anderson et al. 2010; Silveira et al. 2010; Hunter et al. 2012; Newman et al. 2012). Notably, Silveira et al. (2010) used microarray analysis of lymphoblastoid cell line RNA from an extremely discordant sibling cohort to identify genes that are differentially expressed in neovascular AMD. They combined linkage and gene expression data to identify RAR-related orphan receptor A (RORA) as an AMD-associated gene that is expressed in lower levels in individuals with neovascular AMD compared with their unaffected siblings (Silveira et al. 2010). Also of note is a study by Newman and colleagues, who performed transcriptome analysis of AMD versus normal eye tissue. This study identified multiple genes differentially expressed in AMD tissues. Specifically, they showed overexpression of cell-mediated immune response genes in RPE/choroid from AMD eyes, overexpression

Table 2. Studies of gene expression in AMD

Study	Methodology	Sample source	Death to preservation	Molecules/pathways identified
Chowers et al. 2006	Microarray	Retina tissue	Not provided	Increased transferrin expression in AMD vs. normal retina
Silveira et al. 2010	Microarray	Lymphoblastoid cell lines	Not applicable	Decreased RORA expression in AMD patients
Kurji et al. 2010	Microarray	Cultured RPE cells	Not applicable	Differential expression of immune response, inflammation, and cytokine and interferon signaling pathway genes in RPE cells stimulated with Aβ 1–40, a component of drusen
Newman et al. 2012	Microarray	Retina and RPE tissue	Iowa tissue: 4 h, Oregon: <8.7 h	Overexpression of cell-mediated immune response genes in RPE/choroid from AMD eyes, overexpression of apoptosis genes in GA and overexpression of genes involved in angiogenesis in neovascular AMD
Hunter et al. 2012	Microarray	Retina and RPE tissue	Average 5.2 h (range 2.5–9.0 h)	Reduced GSTM1 and GSTM5 expression in AMD vs. normal
An et al. 2010	Targeted rt-pcr	Cultured RPE cells	Not applicable	Increased HTRA1 expression in RPE cells from individuals homozygous for the risk allele at HTRA1 promoter SNP rs11200638
Yang et al. 2006	Targeted rt-pcr	Blood lymphocytes	Not applicable	Increased HTRA1 expression in lymphocytes from individuals homozygous for the risk allele at HTRA1 promoter SNP rs11200638
Kanda et al. 2010	Targeted rt-pcr	Retina tissue	<6 h	No differential expression of ARMS2 and HTRA1 in human retina with regards to age, AMD status, or risk alleles at chromosome 10
Tou et al. 2004	Targeted rt-pcr	Paraffin-embedded retina and RPE tissue	Not applicable	Decreased CX3CR1 expression in AMD eyes
Anderson et al. 2010	Targeted rt-pcr	Retina, RPE, various other tissue types	0.5–6 h	No differential expression of complement genes in regards to AMD status was detected.

of apoptosis genes in eyes with geographic atrophy (GA), and overexpression of genes involved in angiogenesis in neovascular AMD (Newman et al. 2012).

More recently RNA-seq has allowed examination of the transcriptome of the tissues that the disease affects in an unbiased manner. However, unlike prior studies of traditional human gene expression, RNA-seq gives a more accurate assessment by measuring gene expression abundance. Moreover, RNA-seq can also assess the isoform structure of each gene, alternative splicing events, novel and rare transcripts, and the role of ncRNAs between disease phenotypes and tissue types relevant to gene function. Compared with traditional gene expression microarrays, RNA-seq also has a lower frequency of false-positive findings and a higher reproducibility as measured by validation because of less technical variation (Twine et al. 2011; Yendrek et al. 2012; Potok et al. 2013).

To date, only two studies have used RNA-seq to study eye tissue (Farkas et al. 2013; Li et al. 2014). Specifically, Farkas et al. (2013) examined retinal tissue from three donors in their 40s with normal phenotype as defined by no known ocular history. They identified 116 putative novel genes and ~22,000 alternative splice sites. Li et al. (2014) studied eight eyes over the age of 60 yr defined as normal by phenotyping the fellow eye by retinal imaging, optical coherence tomography (OCT), and histological examination. Using RNA-seq they were able to show differential expression between the transcriptome of the neural retina and RPE/choroid/sclera.

At a minimum, the results generated from these studies have catalogued the transcribed mRNAs and novel genes of the neural retina and RPE/choroid/sclera specific to the normal eye as well as the normal aging eye. It will be important to see how this translates to the transcriptomic differences in the pathological eye with AMD and its subtypes as we and other laboratories are currently pursuing. The retina, RPE, and choroid are heterogeneous tissue composed of multiple cell types, including photoreceptors, Müller, microglial, and astrocytes (for reviews on the retina and RPE cellular composition, see Cepko 2012; Masland 2012). Single-cell RNA-seq (Shalek et al. 2014; Trombetta et al. 2014) will be needed to fully elucidate the biological variation in the complex cell types of these tissues. Conducting single-cell RNA-seq experiments on robustly defined AMD phenotypes and normal eyes will hopefully define the contributions of the cell types.

SUMMARY

In summary, gene expression studies in human eye tissue are an initial step in determining function for a putatively associated AMD risk gene. There are many challenges in obtaining and processing donor eye tissue. As discussed above, expression can be influenced by many factors, including methylation. Moreover, the most optimal study designs will include both peripheral blood and eye tissue from donors with and without AMD as well as robust phenotyping to pinpoint disease causality associated with a gene variant. These resources, combined with new genomic technologies, will help to identify therapeutic targets for the prevention and treatment particularly of the early forms of AMD.

ACKNOWLEDGMENTS

This work is supported by National Institutes of Health Grant EY-014458, the ALSAM Foundation, the Edward N. & Della L. Thome Memorial Fund, Carl Marshall Reeves & Mildred Almen Reeves Foundation, and an unrestricted grant from the Research to Prevent Blindness Foundation to the University of Utah Department of Ophthalmology and Visual Sciences.

REFERENCES

An E, Sen S, Park SK, Gordish-Dressman H, Hathout Y. 2010. Identification of novel substrates for the serine protease HTRA1 in the human RPE secretome. *Invest Ophthalmol Vis Sci* **51:** 3379–3386.

Anderson DH, Radeke MJ, Gallo NB, Chapin EA, Johnson PT, Curletti CR, Hancox LS, Hu J, Ebright JN, Malek G, et al. 2010. The pivotal role of the complement system in aging and age-related macular degeneration: Hypothesis re-visited. *Prog Retin Eye Res* **29:** 95–112.

Bock C. 2012. Analysing and interpreting DNA methylation data. *Nat Rev Genet* **13:** 705–719.

Bollati V, Schwartz J, Wright R, Litonjua A, Tarantini L, Suh H, Sparrow D, Vokonas P, Baccarelli A. 2009. Decline in genomic DNA methylation through aging in a cohort of elderly subjects. *Mech Ageing Dev* **130:** 234–239.

Booij JC, ten Brink JB, Swagemakers SMA, Verkerk AJMH, Essing AHW, van der Spek PJ, Bergen AAB. 2010. A new strategy to identify and annotate human RPE-specific gene expression. *PLoS ONE* **5:** e9341.

Bowes Rickman C, Ebright JN, Zavodni ZJ, Yu L, Wang T, Daiger SP, Wistow G, Boon K, Hauser MA. 2006. Defining the human macula transcriptome and candidate retinal disease genes using *EyeSAGE*. *Invest Ophthalmol Vis Sci* **47:** 2305–2316.

Brunet A, Berger SL. 2014. Epigenetics of aging and aging-related disease. *J Gerontol A Biol Sci Med Sci* **69:** S17–S20.

Cepko CL. 2012. Emerging gene therapies for retinal degenerations. *J Neurosci Off J Soc Neurosci* **32:** 6415–6420.

Chakravarthy U, Wong TY, Fletcher A, Piault E, Evans C, Zlateva G, Buggage R, Pleil A, Mitchell P. 2010. Clinical risk factors for age-related macular degeneration: A systematic review and meta-analysis. *BMC Ophthalmol* **10:** 31.

Chowers I, Wong R, Dentchev T, Farkas RH, Iacovelli J, Gunatilaka TL, Medeiros NE, Presley JB, Campochiaro PA, Curcio CA, et al. 2006. The iron carrier transferrin is upregulated in retinas from patients with age-related macular degeneration. *Invest Ophthalmol Vis Sci* **47:** 2135–2140.

Cookson W, Liang L, Abecasis G, Moffatt M, Lathrop M. 2009. Mapping complex disease traits with global gene expression. *Nat Rev Genet* **10:** 184–194.

Cougnard-Grégoire A, Delyfer M-N, Korobelnik J-F, Rougier M-B, Le Goff M, Dartigues J-F, Barberger-Gateau P, Delcourt C. 2014. Elevated high-density lipoprotein cholesterol and age-related macular degeneration: The Alienor study. *PLoS ONE* **9:** e90973.

Curcio CA, Medeiros NE, Millican CL. 1996. Photoreceptor loss in age-related macular degeneration. *Invest Ophthalmol Vis Sci* **37:** 1236–1249.

DeAngelis MM, Silveira AC, Carr EA, Kim IK. 2011. Genetics of age-related macular degeneration: Current concepts, future directions. *Semin Ophthalmol* **26:** 77–93.

Edwards AO, Ritter R, Abel KJ, Manning A, Panhuysen C, Farrer LA. 2005. Complement factor H polymorphism and age-related macular degeneration. *Science* **308:** 421–424.

Esteller M. 2011. Non-coding RNAs in human disease. *Nat Rev Genet* **12:** 861–874.

Farkas MH, Grant GR, White JA, Sousa ME, Consugar MB, Pierce EA. 2013. Transcriptome analyses of the human retina identify unprecedented transcript diversity and 3.5 Mb of novel transcribed sequence via significant alternative splicing and novel genes. *BMC Genomics* **14:** 486.

Ferris FL, Davis MD, Clemons TE, Lee L-Y, Chew EY, Lindblad AS, Milton RC, Bressler SB, Klein R, Age-Related Eye Disease Study (AREDS), et al. 2005. A simplified severity scale for age-related macular degeneration: AREDS Report No. 18. *Arch Ophthalmol* **123:** 1570–1574.

Fritsche LG, Chen W, Schu M, Yaspan BL, Yu Y, Thorleifsson G, Zack DJ, Arakawa S, Cipriani V, Ripke S, et al. 2013. Seven new loci associated with age-related macular degeneration. *Nat Genet* **45:** 433–439, 439e1–2.

Fritsche LG, Fariss RN, Stambolian D, Abecasis GR, Curcio CA, Swaroop A. 2014. Age-related macular degeneration: Genetics and biology coming together. *Annu Rev Genomics Hum Genet* doi: 10.1146/annurev-genom-090413-025610.

Gamazon ER, Ziliak D, Im HK, LaCroix B, Park DS, Cox NJ, Huang RS. 2012. Genetic architecture of microRNA expression: Implications for the transcriptome and complex traits. *Am J Hum Genet* **90:** 1046–1063.

Gorin MB. 2012. Genetic insights into age-related macular degeneration: Controversies addressing risk, causality, and therapeutics. *Mol Aspects Med* **33:** 467–486.

Haines JL, Hauser MA, Schmidt S, Scott WK, Olson LM, Gallins P, Spencer KL, Kwan SY, Noureddine M, Gilbert JR, et al. 2005. Complement factor H variant increases the risk of age-related macular degeneration. *Science* **308:** 419–421.

Haque R, Chun E, Howell JC, Sengupta T, Chen D, Kim H. 2012. MicroRNA-30b-mediated regulation of catalase expression in human ARPE-19 cells. *PLoS ONE* **7:** e42542.

Heard E, Martienssen RA. 2014. Transgenerational epigenetic inheritance: Myths and mechanisms. *Cell* **157:** 95–109.

Helgason H, Sulem P, Duvvari MR, Luo H, Thorleifsson G, Stefansson H, Jonsdottir I, Masson G, Gudbjartsson DF, Walters GB, et al. 2013. A rare nonsynonymous sequence variant in *C3* is associated with high risk of age-related macular degeneration. *Nat Genet* **45:** 1371–1374.

Hou Q, Tang J, Wang Z, Wang C, Chen X, Hou L, Dong XD, Tu L. 2013. Inhibitory effect of microRNA-34a on retinal pigment epithelial cell proliferation and migration. *Invest Ophthalmol Vis Sci* **54:** 6481–6488.

Hrdlickova B, de Almeida RC, Borek Z, Withoff S. 2014. Genetic variation in the non-coding genome: Involvement of micro-RNAs and long non-coding RNAs in disease. *Biochim Biophys Acta* doi: 10.1016/j.bbadis.2014.03.011.

Hunter A, Spechler PA, Cwanger A, Song Y, Zhang Z, Ying G-S, Hunter AK, Dezoeten E, Dunaief JL. 2012. DNA methylation is associated with altered gene expression in AMD. *Invest Ophthalmol Vis Sci* **53:** 2089–2105.

Irvin MR, Zhi D, Joehanes R, Mendelson M, Aslibekyan S, Claas SA, Thibeault KS, Patel N, Day K, Waite Jones L, et al. 2014. Epigenome-wide association study of fasting blood lipids in the Genetics of Lipid Lowering Drugs and Diet Network Study. *Circulation* **130:** 565–572.

Jakobsdottir J, Conley YP, Weeks DE, Mah TS, Ferrell RE, Gorin MB. 2005. Susceptibility genes for age-related maculopathy on chromosome 10q26. *Am J Hum Genet* **77:** 389–407.

Kanda A, Stambolian D, Chen W, Curcio CA, Abecasis GR, Swaroop A. 2010. Age-related macular degeneration-associated variants at chromosome 10q26 do not significantly alter *ARMS2* and *HTRA1* transcript levels in the human retina. *Mol Vis* **16:** 1317–1323.

Karunakaran DKP, Banday AR, Wu Q, Kanadia R. 2013. Expression analysis of an evolutionarily conserved alternative splicing factor, Sfrs10, in age-related macular degeneration. *PLoS ONE* **8:** e75964.

Klein R, Klein BE, Jensen SC, Meuer SM. 1997. The five-year incidence and progression of age-related maculopathy: The Beaver Dam Eye Study. *Ophthalmology* **104:** 7–21.

Klein RJ, Zeiss C, Chew EY, Tsai J-Y, Sackler RS, Haynes C, Henning AK, SanGiovanni JP, Mane SM, Mayne ST, et al. 2005. Complement factor H polymorphism in age-related macular degeneration. *Science* **308:** 385–389.

Klein R, Myers CE, Klein BEK. 2014. Vasodilators, blood pressure-lowering medications, and age-related macular degeneration: The Beaver Dam Eye Study. *Ophthalmology* **121:** 1604–1611

Kurji KH, Cui JZ, Lin T, Harriman D, Prasad SS, Kojic L, Matsubara JA. 2010. Microarray analysis identifies changes in inflammatory gene expression in response to amyloid-beta stimulation of cultured human retinal pigment epithelial cells. *Invest Ophthalmol Vis Sci* **51:** 1151–1163.

Lalonde E, Ha KCH, Wang Z, Bemmo A, Kleinman CL, Kwan T, Pastinen T, Majewski J. 2011. RNA sequencing reveals the role of splicing polymorphisms in regulating human gene expression. *Genome Res* **21:** 545–554.

Li M, Jia C, Kazmierkiewicz KL, Bowman AS, Tian L, Liu Y, Gupta NA, Gudsieva HV, Yee SS, Kim M, et al. 2014. Comprehensive analysis of gene expression in human retina and supporting tissues. *Hum Mol Genet* **23:** 4001–4014.

Lin H, Qian J, Castillo AC, Long B, Keyes KT, Chen G, Ye Y. 2011. Effect of miR-23 on oxidant-induced injury in human retinal pigment epithelial cells. *Invest Ophthalmol Vis Sci* **52:** 6308–6314.

Logue MW, Schu M, Vardarajan BN, Farrell J, Lunetta KL, Jun G, Baldwin CT, DeAngelis MM, Farrer LA. 2014. A search for age-related macular degeneration risk variants in Alzheimer disease genes and pathways. *Neurobiol Aging* **35:** 1510.e7–e18.

Majewski J, Pastinen T. 2011. The study of eQTL variations by RNA-seq: From SNPs to phenotypes. *Trends Genet TIG* **27:** 72–79.

Mamdani F, Martin MV, Lencz T, Rollins B, Robinson DG, Moon EA, Malhotra AK, Vawter MP. 2013. Coding and noncoding gene expression biomarkers in mood disorders and schizophrenia. *Dis Markers* **35:** 11–21.

Masland RH. 2012. The neuronal organization of the retina. *Neuron* **76:** 266–280.

McKay GJ, Patterson CC, Chakravarthy U, Dasari S, Klaver CC, Vingerling JR, Ho L, de Jong PTVM, Fletcher AE, Young IS, et al. 2011. Evidence of association of *APOE* with age-related macular degeneration: A pooled analysis of 15 studies. *Hum Mutat* **32:** 1407–1416.

Miller JW. 2013. Age-related macular degeneration revisited—Piecing the puzzle: The LXIX Edward Jackson memorial lecture. *Am J Ophthalmol* **155:** 1–35.e13.

Newman AM, Gallo NB, Hancox LS, Miller NJ, Radeke CM, Maloney MA, Cooper JB, Hageman GS, Anderson DH, Johnson LV, et al. 2012. Systems-level analysis of age-related macular degeneration reveals global biomarkers and phenotype-specific functional networks. *Genome Med* **4:** 16.

Oliver VF, Franchina M, Jaffe AE, Branham KE, Othman M, Heckenlively JR, Swaroop A, Campochiaro B, Vote BJ, Craig JE, et al. 2013. Hypomethylation of the *IL17RC* promoter in peripheral blood leukocytes is not a hallmark of age-related macular degeneration. *Cell Rep* **5:** 1527–1535.

Payne AJ, Kaja S, Sabates NR, Koulen P. 2013. A case for neuroprotection in ophthalmology: Developments in translational research. *Mo Med* **110:** 429–436.

Peschansky VJ, Wahlestedt C. 2014. Non-coding RNAs as direct and indirect modulators of epigenetic regulation. *Epigenetics* **9:** 3–12.

Petronis A. 2010. Epigenetics as a unifying principle in the aetiology of complex traits and diseases. *Nature* **465:** 721–727.

Pikuleva IA, Curcio CA. 2014. Cholesterol in the retina: The best is yet to come. *Prog Retin Eye Res* **41C:** 64–89.

Potok ME, Nix DA, Parnell TJ, Cairns BR. 2013. Reprogramming the maternal zebrafish genome after fertilization to match the paternal methylation pattern. *Cell* **153:** 759–772.

Radeke MJ, Peterson KE, Johnson LV, Anderson DH. 2007. Disease susceptibility of the human macula: Differential gene transcription in the retinal pigmented epithelium/choroid. *Exp Eye Res* **85:** 366–380.

Rivera A, Fisher SA, Fritsche LG, Keilhauer CN, Lichtner P, Meitinger T, Weber BHF. 2005. Hypothetical *LOC387715* is a second major susceptibility gene for age-related macular degeneration, contributing independently of complement factor H to disease risk. *Hum Mol Genet* **14:** 3227–3236.

Seddon JM, Reynolds R, Yu Y, Rosner B. 2014. Three new genetic loci (R1210C in *CFH*, variants in *COL8A1* and *RAD51B*) are independently related to progression to advanced macular degeneration. *PLoS ONE* **9:** e87047.

Shalek AK, Satija R, Shuga J, Trombetta JJ, Gennert D, Lu D, Chen P, Gertner RS, Gaublomme JT, Yosef N, et al. 2014. Single-cell RNA-seq reveals dynamic paracrine control of cellular variation. *Nature* **509:** 363–369.

Silveira AC, Morrison MA, Ji F, Xu H, Reinecke JB, Adams SM, Arneberg TM, Janssian M, Lee J-E, Yuan Y, et al. 2010. Convergence of linkage, gene expression and association data demonstrates the influence of the RAR-related orphan receptor α (*RORA*) gene on neovascular AMD: A systems biology based approach. *Vision Res* **50:** 698–715.

Smith RP, Lam ET, Markova S, Yee SW, Ahituv N. 2012. Pharmacogene regulatory elements: From discovery to applications. *Genome Med* **4:** 45.

Stevenson KR, Coolon JD, Wittkopp PJ. 2013. Sources of bias in measures of allele-specific expression derived from RNA-sequence data aligned to a single reference genome. *BMC Genomics* **14:** 536.

Strunnikova NV, Maminishkis A, Barb JJ, Wang F, Zhi C, Sergeev Y, Chen W, Edwards AO, Stambolian D, Abecasis G, et al. 2010. Transcriptome analysis and molecular signature of human retinal pigment epithelium. *Hum Mol Genet* **19:** 2468–2486.

Trombetta JJ, Gennert D, Lu D, Satija R, Shalek AK, Regev A. 2014. Preparation of single-cell RNA-seq libraries for next generation sequencing. *Curr Protoc Mol Biol* **107:** 4.22.1–4.22.17.

Tuo J, Smith BC, Bojanowski CM, Meleth AD, Gery I, Csaky KG, Chew EY, Chan C-C. 2004. The involvement of sequence variation and expression of CX3CR1 in the pathogenesis of age-related macular degeneration. FASEB J. http://www.fasebj.org/content/early/2004/07/30/fj.04-1862fje (Accessed June 25, 2014).

Twine NA, Janitz K, Wilkins MR, Janitz M. 2011. Whole transcriptome sequencing reveals gene expression and splicing differences in brain regions affected by Alzheimer's disease. *PLoS ONE* **6:** e16266.

Voisin S, Almén MS, Moschonis G, Chrousos GP, Manios Y, Schiöth HB. 2014. Dietary fat quality impacts genome-wide DNA methylation patterns in a cross-sectional study of Greek preadolescents. *Eur J Hum Genet* doi: 10.1038/ejhg.2014.139.

Wei L, Liu B, Tuo J, Shen D, Chen P, Li Z, Liu X, Ni J, Dagur P, Sen HN, et al. 2012. Hypomethylation of the *IL17RC* promoter associates with age-related macular degeneration. *Cell Rep* **2:** 1151–1158.

Yang Z, Camp NJ, Sun H, Tong Z, Gibbs D, Cameron DJ, Chen H, Zhao Y, Pearson E, Li X, et al. 2006. A variant of the *HTRA1* gene increases susceptibility to age-related macular degeneration. *Science* **314:** 992–993.

Yates JRW, Sepp T, Matharu BK, Khan JC, Thurlby DA, Shahid H, Clayton DG, Hayward C, Morgan J, Wright AF, et al. 2007. Complement C3 variant and the risk of age-related macular degeneration. *N Engl J Med* **357:** 553–561.

Yendrek CR, Ainsworth EA, Thimmapuram J. 2012. The bench scientist's guide to statistical analysis of RNA-Seq data. *BMC Res Notes* **5:** 506.

Yoshida S, Yashar BM, Hiriyanna S, Swaroop A. 2002. Microarray analysis of gene expression in the aging human retina. *Invest Ophthalmol Vis Sci* **43:** 2554–2560.

Yu Y, Triebwasser MP, Wong EKS, Schramm EC, Thomas B, Reynolds R, Mardis ER, Atkinson JP, Daly M, Raychaudhuri S, et al. 2014. Whole-exome sequencing identifies rare, functional *CFH* variants in families with macular degeneration. *Hum Mol Genet* doi: 10.1093/hmg/ddu226.

Zarbin MA, Casaroli-Marano RP, Rosenfeld PJ. 2014. Age-related macular degeneration: Clinical findings, histopathology and imaging techniques. *Dev Ophthalmol* **53:** 1–32.

Zhan X, Larson DE, Wang C, Koboldt DC, Sergeev YV, Fulton RS, Fulton LL, Fronick CC, Branham KE, Bragg-Gresham J, et al. 2013. Identification of a rare coding variant in complement 3 associated with age-related macular degeneration. *Nat Genet* **45:** 1375–1379.

Zhang Z, Zhang Y, Xiao H, Liang X, Sun D, Peng S. 2012. A gene expression profile of the developing human retinal pigment epithelium. *Mol Vis* **18:** 2961–2975.

Zhang S, Wang F, Wang H, Zhang F, Xu B, Li X, Wang Y. 2014. Genome-wide identification of allele-specific effects on gene expression for single and multiple individuals. *Gene* **533:** 366–373.

Zhou Q, Anderson C, Zhang H, Li X, Inglis F, Jayagopal A, Wang S. 2014. Repression of choroidal neovascularization through actin cytoskeleton pathways by microRNA-24. *Mol Ther* **22:** 378–389.

Clinical Applications of Age-Related Macular Degeneration Genetics

John Paul SanGiovanni and Emily Y. Chew

National Eye Institute, Clinical Trials Branch, Division of Epidemiology and Clinical Applications, National Eye Institute, National Institutes of Health, Bethesda, Maryland 20892

Correspondence: echew@nei.nih.gov; jpsangio@post.harvard.edu

Understanding genetic causes of age-related macular degeneration (AMD) will eventually yield effective discoveries and improvements in predictive/prognostic methods. These include, but are not limited to, reliable disease prediction (screening for increased discrimination of clinical risk), differential classification of AMD subtypes with biomarkers (development of risk-linked molecular taxonomies), selection of optimal preventive and therapeutic interventions (guided by a biologically meaningful understanding of treatment response), and drug dosing. In this review, we discuss clinical applications informed by key findings in AMD genetics, and provide commentary on leveraging extant and forthcoming evidence to improve AMD risk prediction, AMD classification, and knowledge on the genetic basis of drug activity and toxicity. Advances in translating AMD genetics findings for AMD risk prediction require development of a genetics-based causality for AMD incidence and progression. Molecular subtyping of AMD phenotypes requires a set of dynamic biomarkers presenting prognostic value; although these have yet to be identified, the formation of multidisciplinary teams and their participation in large-scale consortia may yield promising results. Drugs targeting complement and vascular endothelial growth factor (VEGF) systems are under evaluation, and forthcoming work on rare variants and noncoding DNA in AMD pathogenesis will likely reveal biochemical pathways enriched with AMD-associated genetic variants. Pharmacologic targets in these pathways may inform a rational and effective therapeutic approach to preventing and treating this sight-threatening disease.

Age-related macular degeneration (AMD) is a complex sight-threatening disease of public health significance (Miller 2013). Knowledge on the nature of AMD phenotypes and related pathogenic processes (as well as on constraints in approaches to investigation) has influenced our ability to make inferences on a genetics-based causality of this disease. Such inferences are necessary in the development of feasible clinic-based approaches for effective AMD prevention, prognosis, and treatment (Gorin 2012). In this review we discuss clinical applications informed by key findings in AMD genetics, and provide commentary on leveraging extant and forthcoming evidence to improve AMD risk prediction, classification, and knowledge on the genetic basis of drug activity and toxicity. We start with a definition of AMD phenotypes and follow with an overview of what research in AMD genetics has told us about the nature and

Cite this article as *Cold Spring Harb Perspect Med* doi: 10.1101/cshperspect.a017228

pathogenesis of the disease. These sections are followed by examples of clinical applications in AMD, informed by the aggregate of genetic findings from allied fields of molecular biology, biochemistry, biophysics, cell biology, and bioinformatics. We conclude with commentary on the opportunity for translating existing and emerging results for the purpose of improving clinical care.

AMD PHENOTYPES

Features of advanced, late stages of sight-threatening AMD include pathologic neurodegenerative and/or vasoproliferative changes to the interfaces between the photoreceptors, retinal pigment epithelium (RPE), and choroid vascular network. Neurodegenerative AMD (geographic atrophy) is characterized by one or more notable regions ($\geq$175 μm) of RPE depigmentation or loss, with concomitant degeneration in the choriocapillaris. Atrophic AMD subtypes are represented by abnormal focal, banded, patchy, or diffuse patterns on fundus autofluorescence measurements (Bindewald et al. 2005). Neovascular AMD involves abnormal development of nascent vessels projecting from the choriocapillaris to the subretinal (Type 1) and/or sub-RPE space (Type 2). Polypoidal choroidal vasculopathy is a subtype of neovascular AMD with clusters of spheroid, choroid-derived vessels typically settling in the sub-RPE space. Retinal angiomatous proliferation is also a discrete neovascular AMD subtype; in this condition, intraretinal neovascular lesions connect with vessels from the choroidal circulations. The Beckman Initiative for Macular Research has published a phenotypic classification of AMD based on consensus of 30 opinion leaders in the field (Ferris et al. 2013). A current goal of AMD genetics is to identify biomarkers that can be used to distinguish these heterogeneous clinical subtypes (Gorin 2012).

STATE OF SCIENCE IN AMD GENETICS

Observations on familial associations in AMD were published by Gass nearly four decades ago (reviewed in Miller 2013), and broadly projected the concept of a hereditary component to the disease. Relative risk of developing AMD among first-degree relatives is 6–12 times higher than in the general population (Klaver et al. 1998), and findings from family-based studies on sibling recurrence risk and disease coincidence in twins suggest that the proportion of variability in AMD risk attributed to heritability ranges from 45% to 70% (Seddon et al. 2005). Details on the large body of results from familial aggregation, segregation, linkage, and twin study approaches are presented by Haddad et al. (2006) and Lim et al. (2012). The key message is that hereditary forms of AMD have shown linkage peaks on at least 17 chromosomes (Gorin 2012); in at least 15 instances, these loci contain common AMD-associated DNA sequence variants present in sporadic (nonfamilial) cases of the disease (Gorin 2012; Fritsche et al. 2013).

Disease–gene relationships in sporadic cases of AMD have been investigated most commonly using the genome-wide association (GWA) study approach paired with linkage disequilibrium mapping. This approach involves broad DNA scans on hundreds of thousands of common sequence variants in thousands of people for the purpose of mapping disease-related loci, and is predicated on the idea that differences between healthy and complex disease states may be partially manifested by multiple common DNA sequence variants—a concept known as the "common disease-common variants hypothesis" (Lander 1996; Manolio et al. 2009). In 2005, the value of the GWA design for efficiently and reliably identifying disease-associated loci (from common sequence variants) was shown in the first set of reports implicating the complement factor H (*CFH*) Y402H variant (chromosome 1q31 locus) in advanced AMD (Klein et al. 2005). These findings, and those describing common variants within another prominent AMD-associated linkage peak on chromosome 10q26, have been replicated in numerous cohorts of subjects with American, Asian, or European ancestry (Haddad et al. 2006; Gorin 2012; Fritsche et al. 2013). In 2013, researchers from a multinational consortium reported results on 19 common susceptibility loci for AMD from analyses on nearly 80,000 people; in aggregate, these loci explain 10%–30% of phenotypic variation in the disease (Fritsche et al. 2013).

The 19 AMD susceptibility loci were identified with the GWA study approach and have shown characteristics (presented below) of other large-scale efforts noted by Manolio et al. (2009) four years following publication of the initial AMD-Y402H findings. From this study and follow-up commentaries on the topic (Manolio and Green 2011; Manolio 2013), a key message emerges: The many robust relationships elucidated by the GWA approach have offered meaningful guidance on the underlying biology of complex diseases. Furthermore, by amplifying GWA-derived signals with a careful curation process (leading to a more complete annotation of noncoding DNA overlapping regulatory elements, rare/low frequency variants, and structural variants), one may develop meaningful clinical applications. To adequately inform a translation to the clinic, these efforts require extended work (beyond annotation) aimed to identify disease-associated rare, structural, and regulatory variants. Strengths and limitations to inference based on the method are (1) the GWA approach has been successful in identifying novel susceptibility loci for guiding efficient searches on plausible etiologic processes and strengthening insights on phenotypes (Cichon et al. 2009); (2) the magnitude of effects in GWA-based disease-gene associations have been modest (in the range of a 10%–50% change in disease likelihood for the presence of each risk allele) due to aspects of disease biology and chip design constraints—chips carry probes mainly for common single-nucleotide polymorphisms (SNPs), rather than rare SNPs or structural variants, which include copy number variants, inversions, deletions and insertions; (3) individual GWA studies are generally underpowered to detect modest effect sizes typically observed for common variants, which may lead to underestimates of the number of disease–gene relationships, whereas combining data from multiple studies has produced informative and independently replicated findings (Fritsche et al. 2013); (4) positional information yielded by GWA studies has almost never directly identified a causal variant (Gorin 2012); (5) the range of associated "functional" SNPs (those that lead to changes in processing or expression of the gene transcript or structural and subsequent functional integrity of the protein) coinherited with an AMD-associated SNP may extend 100 kb, and these are candidate regions for fine mapping or resequencing, copy number variants, and promoter regions; and (6) a region may house multiple independent risk variants.

Disease-associated rare variants typically show larger effect sizes and higher predictive value than those of common variants; accordingly, a number of well-funded groups are now directing their efforts to searching for rare variants (McCarthy et al. 2008; Gorin 2012; Manolio et al. 2013). The Seddon group presented the first major finding on a rare and highly penetrant AMD-associated variant in the *CFH* locus (Raychaudhuri et al. 2011). The complement component 3 (*C3*) gene was recently shown to contain a rare AMD-associated variant yielding a greater effect size than those attributed to common AMD-associated variants in the gene; these discoveries were made efficiently after results from GWA studies identified regions for deep sequencing to be used in a cohort large enough to attain stable estimates of effect (Seddon et al. 2013). Gorin offers detailed commentary on the importance of investigating rare variants in complex disease, acknowledging the possibility that genes encoding key etiologic factors may not carry common sequence variants (Gorin 2012).

The central message of this section is that we have been somewhat limited in moving AMD genetics to clinical applications by our dependence on findings from studies designed to interrogate common sequence variants, characterized mainly as SNPs. Imputation and analyses conducted to place these common SNPs into plausible biologic pathways implicated in AMD-related pathology may better guide us toward finding functional DNA sequence variants (that have posttranscriptional and posttranslational effects) in coding or noncoding genomic regions. There is greater appreciation for examining the role of rare SNPs, variation in noncoding DNA linked to regulatory elements (microRNA, histone accessibility marks, DNase hypersensitivity clusters, and transcription factor binding sites), and structural variants (copy number variants, inversions, deletions, and insertions) in AMD. Clearly, in developing effective clinical applications of AMD genetics, we must turn to allied fields of biochemistry, biophysics, and cell biology to integrate evidence on AMD-associated exposures, pathogenesis, and pathophysiology in human cohorts and model systems.

KEY DISCOVERIES IN AMD GENETICS: PATHOGENESIS AND PATHOPHYSIOLOGY IN CONTEXT

Recently published works on the state of genomic science in AMD research (Miller 2013) and use of genetics-based findings for inference on AMD causality, risk, and therapeutics (Gorin 2012) provide valuable overviews on systems of genes that encode proteins implicated in AMD pathogenesis and pathophysiology. These systems include the alternative complement pathway, the innate immune response pathway, the chromosome 10q26 locus, extracellular matrix/cell adhesion complex genes, lipid metabolism/transport/signaling-related genes, the mitochondrial genome, vitamin D pathway genes, angiogenesis-related genes, iron metabolism genes, and cellular stress and toxicity genes. Reviews over the past decade have also addressed concepts of pathogenic mechanisms in the context of the human genome (Ambati et al. 2003; Haddad et al. 2006; Hageman et al. 2008; Bird 2010). Initially, family-based and GWA studies applied an empirical (data-driven) approach to identify and characterize mechanisms involved in AMD pathogenesis; hypothesis-driven research is now the mainstay, guided by or supported with evidence from model systems, epidemiologic studies, and clinical observations. There is general consensus that key mechanisms in AMD pathogenesis involve dysregulation of processes leading to (1) abnormal angiogenesis; (2) age-related deposition of amyloid, lipids, or lipofuscin; (3) apoptosis; and (4) activation or modulation of (a) cellular stress pathway constituents, (b) inflammatory-immune response, or (c) vascular resistance. Lists of AMD-associated genes that drive these processes are provided in recent reviews (Haddad et al. 2006; Gorin 2012; Miller 2013). Pathway and network enrichment analyses are now entering the evidence base (SanGiovanni and Mehta 2009; Silveira et al. 2010; Newman et al. 2012; Fritsche et al. 2013; SanGiovanni and Lee 2013) and may offer meaningful guidance on novel therapies. The majority of targeted therapies for AMD have been directed at inhibiting pathologic angiogenesis through perturbation of VEGF signaling or to alter activity of complement-based systems.

INTERPRETATION AND APPLICATION OF FINDINGS ON GENETICS-BASED CAUSALITY OF AMD

Successful efforts to develop effective clinic-based preventive, prognostic, and therapeutic applications for AMD will require integration of knowledge on AMD-associated genes and their encoded proteins with evidence from genetically modified model systems and epidemiologic, clinical, biochemical studies (Gorin 2012). In this section we discuss aspects of genetic findings essential for designing effective clinical applications (Manolio 2013), while providing commentary on these matters for applied research on interventions for AMD. Key factors influencing the interpretation and application of genetic findings for clinical use include: (1) variant frequency and effect magnitude (based partially on genotyping feature probe sets); (2) the nature of variation (based on genotyping feature probe sets); and (3) alternative explanations for findings (based on coinherited variants with capacity to alter gene activity or protein structure).

Variant Frequency and Effect Magnitude

There is an unmet need to assess the magnitude of disease-gene associations from variants with minor allele frequencies $<5\%$. Both common and rare variants have yielded useful information with the capacity for improving clinical care in AMD. It is likely that sets of common variants may act in aggregate to produce small but meaningful functional alterations in some people with AMD. The basis for this idea in complex disease etiology has been discussed in detail since the mid-1990s (Lander 1996; Manolio et al. 2009). Ward and Kellis (2012) have commented on works demonstrating the influence of common alleles contributing small but meaningful effects in traits or disease risk (Purcell et al. 2009); these loci, associated with complex traits at *P*-values far below those considered significant on a genome-wide level, have clustered across the genome within DNA sequence encoding constituents of biological pathways implicated in disease pathogenesis (Yang et al. 2010). A central premise is that inference based on a single locus may not elucidate important contributions of genetic variants both manifesting weak associations and the capacity to act together in alteration of disease risk (Lee et al. 2012; SanGiovanni and Lee 2013; Smoller et al. 2013). Robust findings have consistently emerged from the common variant approach to investigation, and such results have been successfully applied to identify systems acting in disease pathogenesis or pathophysiology (Manolio et al. 2009). As mentioned previously, the small proportion of trait heritability contributed by these common variants make them less than optimal for AMD risk prediction or classification (Jakobsdottir et al. 2009).

Disease-associated rare-frequency (minor allele frequency $<0.5\%$) and low-frequency variants (minor allele frequency 0.5%–5.0%) tend to have higher predictive value, and yield point estimates of higher magnitude than the common SNPs contained in most GWA gene chip probe feature sets. Stable estimates of effect (associations) for rare- and low-frequency variants require larger cohorts than those necessary for testing common variants. Efforts to identify rare variants have yielded promising results in AMD genetics (Raychaudhuri et al. 2011; Helgason et al. 2013; Seddon et al. 2013; Zhan et al. 2013). In some instances, high-impact rare causative variants may be resident in genes in which no common variants exist. If genes harboring common loci (likely detected with the GWA approach) are not proximal to those carrying rare variants, the process of detection is unlikely to be efficient. In this case, a pathway analysis may be useful to identify biologically plausible constituents for follow-up. Regions proximal to and within the 19 susceptibility loci reported by the AMD Genetics Consortium (Fritsche et al. 2013) are being evaluated with fine mapping and exome sequencing methods to expand knowledge on rare- and low-frequency variants associated with a doubling or more of AMD risk. Use of such variants in prediction models is expected to improve accuracy beyond levels explained by clinical, demographic, and lifestyle characteristics.

The Nature of Variation

A more sophisticated understanding of the structural nature of variation and nontranscribed DNA is a necessary condition for efficient translation of meaningful disease-variant findings that may not otherwise indicate obvious functional consequences. This process involves assessing the influence of genomic rearrangements and noncoding SNPs for their capacity to disrupt nontranscribed DNA involved in regulation of transcription. Structural variants and sites overlapping regulatory elements (transcription factor binding sites, DNase hypersensitivity clusters, microRNA-binding domains, and histone promoter or enhancer regions) are potentially important genomic elements in AMD susceptibility for which there is a lack of information. Many ($>80\%$) GWA-defined risk loci fall within noncoding regions of the genome—as these regions are enriched with transcription enhancer elements, it is important to conduct large-scale projects to determine capacity of variation in noncoding and intergenic sequence to induce functional change (e.g., nucleotide changes that alter processing or expression of the gene transcript or structural and functional alterations in integrity of the protein). The ENCODE Project is now archiving such annotations (see https://www.genome.gov/encode/) in a public access database.

Linkage Structure and Coinherited Variants of Functional Significance

We must thoroughly assess disease–SNP relationships for alternative explanations based on coinherited DNA variants—especially those with the capacity to influence gene transcription and protein structure. Disease–SNP relationships often are strongest for variants that have no apparent functional link to the encoded protein. Nonrandom cosegregation (coinheritance of DNA tracts in the genome) is one explanation for such observations—suggesting that the strongly associated SNP marks a susceptibility locus for a causative variant. Gains in accuracy of imputation (supported by the 1000 Genomes Project) and enhancements of annotation databases (supported by the ENCODE Project) have permitted an amplification of GWA study-derived signals with which to identify biologically meaningful findings. The application of whole-exome sequencing within loci identified through projects such as the AMD Gene Consortium (Fritsche et al. 2013) will target candidate functional variants.

The three factors discussed above are inextricably linked, and under certain circumstances may be used to: (1) increase discriminatory power for clinical risk assessment (through the application of predictive models); (2) distinguish clinical cohorts most likely to benefit from specific clinical interventions (through the application biomarkers with clinical information); and (3) assess genetic capacity for drug action and toxicity (through the applications of treatment response studies). We present overviews on these factors below.

Risk Prediction

AMD is a disease of public health significance, and early detection in the presence of an effective preventive intervention would alleviate a great burden of suffering. Most predictive models examining genetics-based causality of AMD are derived from measures of disease status (i.e., AMD prevalence). Gorin presents an astute commentary regarding the application of AMD genetics for risk prediction (Gorin 2012), stating that clinical applications leading to the most valuable preventive treatments should be informed by prospective studies assessing the genetic component of AMD incidence in people at moderate risk for developing advanced AMD. He notes that prevalent AMD can be predicted well in people carrying many or no susceptibility variants for the disease, but that existing models still lack sensitivity and specificity for the majority of people in the general population (most of whom carry a few risk variants). This point was initially elucidated by Jakobsdottir et al. (2009), who demonstrated that although accurate detection of 80% of AMD cases was possible with three strongly associated loci, prediction was poor for people without the disease (false-positive rates exceeded 40% at a sensitivity of 80%). The second key point is that, until an effective preventive intervention for advanced AMD is developed, risk prediction will offer only limited value in clinical care. AMD is a common disease in the elderly, and costs associated with universal screening are not likely to be supported. With the advent of effective and accessible treatments, positive predictive values may be increased through a screening process focused on people with family histories of AMD and high genetic risk prediction scores. A number of clinical characteristics and lifestyle practices have been identified with AMD risk, and these may be combined with genetic risk scores from common and rare SNPs and structural variants to more accurately predict likelihood of AMD in people who would otherwise show low risks based on demographic or behavioral factors alone.

Disease Classification and Subtyping

Outside of the AMD field, disease–gene relationships and molecular subtyping of disease phenotypes have led to enhanced discrimination of subpopulations likely to benefit from specific treatments (Manolio 2013). This molecular subtyping has elucidated biomarkers that may best be applied in conditions in which other prognostic indicators are less sensitive and more difficult or expensive to obtain. The value of biomarkers is highest for people in preclinical disease phases and for those at moderate risk for progressing to advanced stages of complex disease (Manolio and Green 2011). AMD may manifest as a number of phenotypes (see *AMD Phenotypes* section) that may not be accurately diagnosed in a clinical examination. The major clinical subtypes of advanced AMD (geographic atrophy and neovascular AMD) carry different risk factors and respond differently to a number of exposures (e.g., smoking) and therapies.

There is currently insufficient evidence to support the idea that the existing panel of serum biomarkers for AMD (C-reactive protein, complement component factors, VEGF, apo-lipoprotein B, antiretinal antibodies, sterol ester levels, anticarboxyethylpyrrole adducts and autoantibodies, and vitamin D) contains effective predictors of AMD incidence or progression (Gorin 2012). Biomarkers have been proposed to support assessment of intervention efficacy, and there is currently an unmet need to demonstrate that long-term alteration of a biomarker by a controlled preventive or therapeutic intervention for AMD will avert subsequent development of AMD. Gorin emphasizes the importance of determining whether a biomarker is constrained to represent the current state of disease (static marker) or whether it may reflect a dynamic response of causal processes to an intervention.

Genetic Basis of Drug Activity and Toxicity

Interventions Based on AMD-Associated Pathway Constituents. Findings from the field of AMD genetics have been integrated with those from biochemical assessments of pathologic specimens in people with moderate or advanced AMD to guide research on the etiologic role of the complement system. Troutbeck et al. (2012) present a background on the complement pathways and their influence on proteolytic cascades that produce the cytolytic membrane attack complex. Complement component inhibitors, antibody-based compounds, and receptor antagonists have been examined as targets for AMD interventions (Table 1). For neovascular AMD, molecular targets within the VEGF system have been proposed and tested on the basis of biochemical analyses and the existence of related angiogenic and neovascular lesions in numerous blinding retinal diseases. The *VEGFA* gene resides in a susceptibility locus on chromosome 6, and aggregates of genes encoding constituents of the extracellular matrix (altered in vascular remodeling) have supported the decision to target therapies at VEGF (Table 1 contains a list of drugs inhibiting the VEGF system). Details on AMD–VEGF findings from clinical trials are reviewed by Miller (2013).

Drug Development and Drug Safety. Disease–gene relationships have been aimed at identifying novel molecular targets and determining whether DNA sequence variants influence an individual's ability to (1) activate prodrugs and drug-related metabolic or catabolic enzymes, and (2) respond to therapy for the purposes adjusting dosage or switching to alternative agents of higher efficacy. Gorin (2012) has reviewed the AMD pharmacogenomic literature and concluded that there is currently little evidence to support the claim that any DNA sequence variant alters response to treatment with VEGF inhibitors or photodynamic therapy. He further remarks that relationships of susceptibility loci have been additive in nature (each contributing an exclusive aspect of risk); when identified, molecular targets are likely to be heterogeneous and best treated with combined therapies with pharmacologic and nonpharmacologic approaches. Gorin also stresses the point that accurate quantitation of AMD phenotype is paramount in classifying disease progression for drug response studies. A recently published position statement is expected to offer guidance on this matter (Ferris et al. 2013). Finally, regarding constraints to progress in AMD pharmacogenomics, there currently are no established biomarkers with which to monitor response to preventive interventions in AMD-free people at moderate risk for developing the disease. For studies on progression to neovascular AMD, in vivo imaging technologies have been used successfully to identify biomarkers effective for assessing response to anti-VEGF therapies.

The Comparison of AMD Treatments Trials research team recently reported their inves-

Table 1. Therapeutic agents evaluated for AMD treatment

Therapeutic agent	Target	Administration/comment
Complement System		
Terminal Components		
POT-4	C3	IVT/Inhibitory cyclic peptide
ARC1905	C5	IVT/Inhibitory anti-C5 aptamer
JSM-7717	C5a receptor	Antagonistic receptor peptidomimetic
JPE-1375	C5a receptor	Antagonistic receptor peptidomimetic
Eculizumab	C5	IV/MAb
CR2-fH	C3d/CFH	Recombinant CFH, animal models
Activation Components		
FCFD4514S	CFD	IVT/Inhibitory MAb
TA106	CFB	INH/Inhibitory MAb
VEGF System		
Pegaptanib (Macugen)	Heparin domain VEGF-A_{165}	IVT/Inhibitory anti-$VEGF_{165}$ aptamer
Ranibizumab (Lucentis)	All VEGF-A isomers	IVT/Inhibitory MAb fragment
Bevacizumab (Avastin)	All VEGF-A isomers	IVT/Inhibitory MAb
Aflibercept (VEGF Trap)	All VEGF isomers, PIGF	IVT/Fusion protein VEGFR1 + VEGFR2
Pazopanib	VEGF Receptors, PDGFR	Topical/tyrosine kinase inhibitor
AAV-sFLT1	VEGFR	Recombinant VEGFR
E10030	VEGF, PDGF	Anti-PDGF aptamer, used w/Lucentis
RetinoStat	Angiostatin, Endostatin	Lentivirus vector
ISONEP	Sphingosine-1-Phosphate	MAb
Sirolimus (Rapamycin)	mTOR/Akt	IVT/Inhibitory macrolide
OT-551	NF-κB constituents	Topical
AAV-PEDF	PEDF	IVT/SR, Recombinant PEDF, models

AAV, adeno-associated virus; C3, complement component 3; C5, complement component 5; CFB, complement factor B; CFD, complement factor D; CFH, complement factor H; INH, inhaled; IVT, intravitreal injection; IV, intravenous injection; Mab, monoclonal antibody; mTOR, mammalian target of rapamycin; PDGF, platelet-derived growth factor; PDGFR, PDGF receptor; PEDF, pigment epithelium-derived growth factor; PlGF, placental growth factor; SR, subretinal; VEGF, vascular endothelial growth factor; VEGFR, VEGF receptor.

tigations on common AMD-associated SNPs (rs1061170 [CFH], rs10490924 [ARMS2], rs11200638 [HTRA1], and rs2230199 [C3]) and response to treatment with ranibizumab or bevacizumab for neovascular AMD (Hagstrom 2013). In no instance did the tested SNPs predict response to the study regimen of anti-VEGF therapy at one year. Endpoints included mean visual acuity (VA), mean change in VA, 15-letter or more increase in VA, retinal thickness, mean change in total foveal thickness, presence of fluid on ocular coherence tomography (OCT), presence of leakage on fluorescein angiography (FA), mean change in lesion size, and mean number of injections administered.

CONCLUDING REMARKS

We have provided an overview on the state of science regarding the potential clinical value of genetic investigations for improving AMD-related risk prediction, disease classification, and the genetic basis of drug activity and toxicity. Research teams are now expanding and improving assessment of rare, structural, and noncoding DNA variants for the purposes of identifying genetic factors that might explain substantial proportions of variation in AMD outcomes. These findings will strengthen processes of prediction and classification. In 2013, an AMD phenotyping consortium published classification schemes that may be applied to assess changes in AMD associated with preventive and therapeutic interventions. Progress in developing effective clinical applications is dependent on successful integration of evidence from fields of molecular biology, biochemistry, biophysics, cell biology, and bioinformatics. A major constraint on risk prediction is the lack of information with which to characterize a genetics-based causality for AMD incidence and progression. Molecular subtyping of AMD phenotypes requires a set of dynamic biomarkers presenting prognostic value; although these have yet to be identified, the formation of multidisciplinary teams and their participation in large-scale consortia offers promise for a more efficient biomarker characterization. A number of drugs targeting complement and VEGF systems are under evaluation, and forthcoming work on the role of noncoding DNA in AMD pathogenesis will likely lead to the identification of biochemical pathways enriched with genes containing AMD-associated sequence variants. Pharmacologic targets in these pathways may inform a rational and effective therapeutic approach to preventing and treating this sight-threatening disease. In conclusion, while the evidence from studies of AMD genetics is now best suited for informing preclinical research, it is a useful resource that may be effectively applied to improving clinical care.

REFERENCES

Ambati J, Ambati BK, Yoo SH, Ianchulev S, Adamis AP. 2003. Age-related macular degeneration: Etiology, pathogenesis, and therapeutic strategies. *Surv Ophthalmol* **48:** 257–293.

Bindewald A, Schmitz-Valckenberg S, Jorzik JJ, Dolar-Szczasny J, Sieber H, Keilhauer C, Weinberger AW, Dithmar S, Pauleikhoff D, Mansmann U, et al. 2005. Classification of abnormal fundus autofluorescence patterns in the junctional zone of geographic atrophy in patients with age related macular degeneration. *Br J Ophthalmol* **89:** 874–878.

Bird AC. 2010. Therapeutic targets in age-related macular disease. *J Clin Invest* **120:** 3033–3041.

Cichon S, Craddock N, Daly M, Faraone SV, Gejman PV, Kelsoe J, Lehner T, Levinson DF, Moran A, Sklar P, et al. 2009. Genomewide association studies: History, rationale, and prospects for psychiatric disorders. *Am J Psychiatry* **166:** 540–556.

Ferris FL III, Wilkinson CP, Bird A, Chakravarthy U, Chew E, Csaky K, Sadda SR. 2013. Clinical classification of age-related macular degeneration. *Ophthalmology* **120:** 844–851.

Fritsche LG, Chen W, Schu M, Yaspan BL, Yu Y, Thorleifsson G, Zack DJ, Arakawa S, Cipriani V, Ripke S, et al. 2013. Seven new loci associated with age-related macular degeneration. *Nat Genet* **45:** 433–439.

Gorin MB. 2012. Genetic insights into age-related macular degeneration: Controversies addressing risk, causality, and therapeutics. *Mol Aspects Med* **33:** 467–486.

Haddad S, Chen CA, Santangelo SL, Seddon JM. 2006. The genetics of age-related macular degeneration: A review of progress to date. *Surv Ophthalmol* **51:** 316–363.

Hageman GS, Gehrs K, Johnson LV, Anderson D. 2008. Age-related Macular Degeneration (AMD). In *Webvision: The Organization of the Retina and Visual System* (ed. Kolb H, Nelson R, Fernandez E, Jones B) (source: http://webvision.med.utah.edu/)

Hagstrom SA, Ying G-S, Pauer GJ, Sturgill-Short GM, Huang J, Callanan DG, Kim IK, Klein ML, Maguire MG, Martin DF. 2013. Pharmacogenetics for genes associated with age-related macular degeneration in the comparison of AMD treatments. *Ophthalmology* **120:** 593–599.

Helgason H, Sulem P, Duvvari MR, Luo H, Thorleifsson G, Stefansson H, Jonsdottir I, Masson G, Gudbjartsson DF, Walters GB, et al. 2013. A rare nonsynonymous sequence variant in *C3* is associated with high risk of age-related macular degeneration. *Nat Genet* **45:** 1371–1374.

Jakobsdottir J, Gorin MB, Conley YP, Ferrell RE, Weeks DE. 2009. Interpretation of genetic association studies: Markers with replicated highly significant odds ratios may be poor classifiers. *PLoS Genet* **5:** e1000337.

Klaver CC, Wolfs RC, Assink JJ, van Duijn CM, Hofman A, de Jong PT. 1998. Genetic risk of age-related maculopathy. Population-based familial aggregation study. *Arch Ophthalmol* **116:** 1646–1651.

Klein RJ, Zeiss C, Chew EY, Tsai JY, Sackler RS, Haynes C, Henning AK, SanGiovanni JP, Mane SM, Mayne ST, et al. 2005. Complement factor H polymorphism in age-related macular degeneration. *Science* **308:** 385–389.

Lander ES. 1996. The new genomics: Global views of biology. *Science* **274:** 536–539.

Lee PH, O'Dushlaine C, Thomas B, Purcell SM. 2012. INRICH: Interval-based enrichment analysis for genome-wide association studies. *Bioinformatics* **28:** 1797–1799.

Lim LS, Mitchell P, Seddon JM, Holz FG, Wong TY. 2012. Age-related macular degeneration. *Lancet* **379:** 1728–1738.

Manolio TA. 2013. Bringing genome-wide association findings into clinical use. *Nat Rev Genet* **14:** 549–558.

Manolio TA, Green ED. 2011. Genomics reaches the clinic: From basic discoveries to clinical impact. *Cell* **147:** 14–16.

Manolio TA, Collins FS, Cox NJ, Goldstein DB, Hindorff LA, Hunter DJ, McCarthy MI, Ramos EM, Cardon LR, Chakravarti A, et al. 2009. Finding the missing heritability of complex diseases. *Nature* **461:** 747–753.

Manolio TA, Chisholm RL, Ozenberger B, Roden DM, Williams MS, Wilson R, Bick D, Bottinger EP, Brilliant MH, Eng C, et al. 2013. Implementing genomic medicine in the clinic: The future is here. *Genet Med* **15:** 258–267.

McCarthy MI, Abecasis GR, Cardon LR, Goldstein DB, Little J, Ioannidis JP, Hirschhorn JN. 2008. Genome-wide association studies for complex traits: Consensus, uncertainty and challenges. *Nat Rev Genet* **9:** 356–369.

Miller JW. 2013. Age-related macular degeneration revisited–piecing the puzzle: The LXIX Edward Jackson memorial lecture. *Am J Ophthalmol* **155:** 1–35, e13.

Newman AM, Gallo NB, Hancox LS, Miller NJ, Radeke CM, Maloney MA, Cooper JB, Hageman GS, Anderson DH, Johnson LV, et al. 2012. Systems-level analysis of age-related macular degeneration reveals global biomarkers and phenotype-specific functional networks. *Genome Med* **4:** 16.

Purcell SM, Wray NR, Stone JL, Visscher PM, O'Donovan MC, Sullivan PF, Sklar P. 2009. Common polygenic variation contributes to risk of schizophrenia and bipolar disorder. *Nature* **460:** 748–752.

Raychaudhuri S, Iartchouk O, Chin K, Tan PL, Tai AK, Ripke S, Gowrisankar S, Vemuri S, Montgomery K, Yu Y, et al. 2011. A rare penetrant mutation in *CFH* confers high risk of age-related macular degeneration. *Nat Genet* **43:** 1232–1236.

SanGiovanni JP, Lee PH. 2013. AMD-associated genes encoding stress-activated MAPK pathway constituents are identified by interval-based enrichment analysis. *PLoS ONE* **8:** e71239.

SanGiovanni JP, Mehta S. 2009. Variation in lipid-associated genes as they relate to risk of advanced age-related macular degeneration. *World Rev Nutr Diet* **99:** 105–158.

Seddon JM, Cote J, Page WF, Aggen SH, Neale MC. 2005. The US twin study of age-related macular degeneration: Relative roles of genetic and environmental influences. *Arch Ophthalmol* **123:** 321–327.

Seddon JM, Yu Y, Miller EC, Reynolds R, Tan PL, Gowrisankar S, Goldstein JI, Triebwasser M, Anderson HE, Zerbib J, et al. 2013. Rare variants in *CFI*, *C3* and *C9* are associated with high risk of advanced age-related macular degeneration. *Nat Genet* **45:** 1366–1370.

Silveira AC, Morrison MA, Ji F, Xu H, Reinecke JB, Adams SM, Arneberg TM, Janssian M, Lee JE, Yuan Y, et al. 2010. Convergence of linkage, gene expression and association data demonstrates the influence of the RAR-related orphan receptor α (*RORA*) gene on neovascular AMD: A systems biology based approach. *Vision Res* **50:** 698–715.

Smoller JW, Craddock N, Kendler K, Lee PH, Neale BM, Nurnberger JI, Ripke S, Santangelo S, Sullivan PF. 2013. Identification of risk loci with shared effects on five major psychiatric disorders: A genome-wide analysis. *Lancet* **381:** 1371–1379.

Troutbeck R, Al-Qureshi S, Guymer RH. 2012. Therapeutic targeting of the complement system in age-related macular degeneration: A review. *Clin Experiment Ophthalmol* **40:** 18–26.

Ward LD, Kellis M. 2012. Interpreting noncoding genetic variation in complex traits and human disease. *Nat Biotechnol* **30:** 1095–1106.

Yang J, Benyamin B, McEvoy BP, Gordon S, Henders AK, Nyholt DR, Madden PA, Heath AC, Martin NG, Montgomery GW, et al. 2010. Common SNPs explain a large proportion of the heritability for human height. *Nat Genet* **42:** 565–569.

Zhan X, Larson DE, Wang C, Koboldt DC, Sergeev YV, Fulton RS, Fulton LL, Fronick CC, Branham KE, Bragg-Gresham J, et al. 2013. Identification of a rare coding variant in complement 3 associated with age-related macular degeneration. *Nat Genet* **45:** 1375–1379.

Clinical Characteristics and Current Treatment of Glaucoma

Laura P. Cohen[1] and Louis R. Pasquale[1,2]

[1]Departments of Ophthalmology and Massachusetts Eye and Ear, Brigham and Women's Hospital, Harvard Medical School, Boston, Massachusetts 02114

[2]Channing Division of Network Medicine, Brigham and Women's Hospital, Harvard Medical School, Boston, Massachusetts 02114

Correspondence: louis_pasquale@meei.harvard.edu

Glaucoma is a neurodegenerative disorder in which degenerating retinal ganglion cells (RGC) produce significant visual disability. Clinically, glaucoma refers to an array of conditions associated with variably elevated intraocular pressure (IOP) that contributes to RGC loss via mechanical stress, vascular abnormalities, and other mechanisms, such as immune phenomena. The clinical diagnosis of glaucoma requires assessment of the ocular anterior segment with slit lamp biomicroscopy, which allows the clinician to recognize signs of conditions that can produce elevated IOP. After measurement of IOP, a specialized prismatic lens called a gonioscope is used to determine whether the angle is physically open or closed. The structural manifestation of RGC loss is optic nerve head atrophy and excavation of the neuroretinal rim tissue. Treatment is guided by addressing secondary causes for elevated IOP (such as inflammation, infection, and ischemia) whenever possible. Subsequently, a variety of medical, laser, and surgical options are used to achieve a target IOP.

Glaucoma refers to a heterogeneous group of diseases whose common clinical denominator is an excavation of neuroretinal rim tissue located in the intrascleral portion of the optic nerve. The optic nerve is a white matter tract with intrascleral, retrobulbar, intracanalicular, and intracranial segments. Only the intrascleral portion of the optic nerve is available for direct clinical inspection. Glaucomatous changes in the intrascleral portion of the optic nerve were appreciated soon after Hermann von Hemholtz invented the ophthalmoscope in 1850 and these changes seemed intuitively related to elevated intraocular pressure (IOP).

The typical course of chronic glaucoma progresses insidiously over decades (Fig. 1). Unless glaucoma is associated with markedly elevated IOP, it is not associated with pain; furthermore, visual symptoms do not develop until the disease is advanced. For most patients the disease is insidious in onset with a long and poorly defined preclinical phase. Visual symptoms attributable to glaucomatous optic neuropathy, such as difficulty reading a menu in a dimly lit

Cite this article as *Cold Spring Harb Perspect Med* doi: 10.1101/cshperspect.a017236

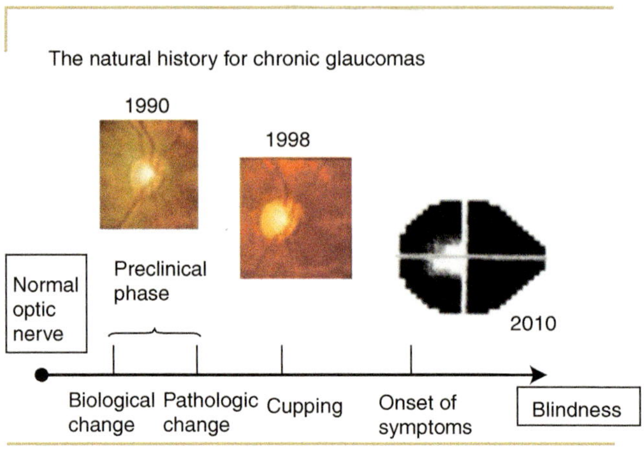

Figure 1. Natural history for chronic glaucomas. In the natural history of chronic glaucoma, there is a poorly defined preclinical phase that manifests here as enlargement of the vertical cup–disc ratio from 1990 to 1998. Symptoms typically develop late in the disease course, as depicted by the patient with advanced visual field loss in 2010.

restaurant, usually signify advanced disease. This symptom relates to impaired contrast sensitivity, which depends on the integrity of the optic nerve and deteriorates as the disease progresses (Abe et al. 1987). Glaucoma classically does not affect central vision first, but even when it does, the seeing portion of the fellow eye covers for the affected eye, and most patients are oblivious of the change.

Glaucoma can occur at any age, with developmental anomalies predominating as etiologic entities for young children. Trauma and inflammatory conditions produce the lion's share of glaucoma in young- and middle-aged adults. In the elderly, glaucoma usually presents as a chronic, complex disease of unclear etiology. It is estimated there will be 5.9 million people bilaterally blinded by open angle glaucoma (OAG) and 5.3 million people bilaterally blinded by angle closure glaucoma (ACG) by the year 2020 (Quigley and Broman 2006). The latter figure stems from the high prevalence of angle closure glaucoma in Asia. OAG and ACG have IOP-related optic neuropathy as a common endpoint, but in the former, the site of aqueous humor egress from the eye is physically open, whereas in the latter, it is mostly sealed off owing to a variety of pathologies. The two most common forms of OAG in the elderly are primary open angle glaucoma (POAG) and exfoliation glaucoma (XFG). In POAG, the anterior segment exam does not reveal any particular cause for elevated IOP. In XFG, on the other hand, the filtration apparatus remains physically open but is rendered dysfunctional by deposits of grayish-white material and pigment.

Etiologic causes for glaucoma include trauma, infection, inflammation, retinal ischemia, and intraocular tumors; these etiologies, along with illustrative examples and mechanisms, are summarized in Table 1, which is by no means an exhaustive list. Many drugs can trigger angle closure in patients who are anatomically predisposed to this condition, and a handful of drugs can produce bilateral angle closure glaucoma even if the patient does not have preexisting narrow outlets in the filtration apparatus. Aqueous humor continuously circulates from its site of production (the ciliary body) behind the iris around the pupil. This aqueous humor leaves the eye via a microporous structure housed within the filtration apparatus called the trabecular meshwork. Steroids might produce OAG by altering the hydraulic conductivity in the trabecular meshwork (Clark et al. 2005). Generally speaking, lifestyle and diet seem to play a minor role in glaucoma, although the discovery of the full complement of genes involved in the

 Cite this article as *Cold Spring Harb Perspect Med* doi: 10.1101/cshperspect.a017236

Table 1. Etiological entities known to produce glaucoma

Etiology	An example[a]	A mechanism[a]
Tumorigenic	Iris melanoma	Tumor seeding drainage angle
Traumatic	Angle recession	Direct angle contusion
Infectious	Herpes simplex	Trabeculitis
Inflammatory	Juvenile idiopathic arthritis	Scarring and inflammation in the outflow pathway
Degenerative	Primary open angle glaucoma	Multifactorial
Developmental	Congenital glaucoma	Incomplete angle development
Vascular	Neovascular glaucoma after diabetic retinopathy	Reduced outflow triggered by vascular endothelial growth factor diffusion into the anterior segment

[a]There are many examples and more than one mechanism involved in each etiological category.

disease process may clarify roles for lifestyle factors in this disorder.

CLINICAL FEATURES OF GLAUCOMA

Patient History

Because early to moderate glaucoma is generally asymptomatic, the initial question is whether there is a family history of glaucoma. A positive family history of glaucoma increases one's risk of disease by three- to fourfold (Tielsch et al. 1994; Wolfs et al. 1998; Kang et al. 2007).

For patients with known glaucoma who might present for a second opinion, it is best to ascertain when the glaucoma was first diagnosed from the patient's perspective. Patients who present with mild-stage glaucoma but claim a longer duration of disease may ultimately have a good prognosis, whereas patients with advanced disease (perhaps close to the symptomatic phase illustrated in Fig. 1) for a shorter duration may be less likely to retain vision. Acquire information regarding the highest known IOP to get a sense of the optic nerve's vulnerability to degeneration. Patients with advanced damage for whom the highest known IOP was measured in their mid-teens (which is normal for most patients) likely have optic nerves that are quite sensitive to damage. Finally, ask patients about prior intolerance to medical treatments for the glaucoma, so that patients are not rechallenged with medicines that previously caused allergy or significant side effects.

A systematic review of a patient's medical history is useful for determining the optimal IOP-lowering strategy in glaucoma. For example, it is best to avoid topical β-blocker in patients with asthma, as this treatment could exacerbate bronchospasm. Knowledge of specific medical conditions such as diabetes mellitus is important as well; when diabetic retinopathy leads to profound retinal ischemia, neovascular glaucoma can result.

Past ocular history might yield clues about potential causes of high IOP. A history of unilateral blunt ocular trauma may explain why IOP is high only in one eye. Prior ocular surgeries can occasionally lead to secondary damage to the filtration apparatus. For example, a retinal detachment repair requiring intraocular gas tamponade could result in forward rotation of the iris–lens diaphragm and closure of the trabecular meshwork. Thus, it is helpful to document prior ocular surgery and any known complications that ensued.

Some systemic medications used to treat nonophthalmic conditions elevate IOP whereas others may lower IOP and mask higher spontaneous ocular tension. Steroids administered by any route, including by dermatological application (Aggarwal et al. 1993) or nasal inhalation (Opatowsky et al. 1995), can lead to elevated IOP. On the other hand, systemic β-blockers used to treat systemic hypertension (Borthne 1976) and oral carbonic anhydrase inhibitors used to treat elevated intracranial pressure or seizure disorder can lower IOP and mask an otherwise higher spontaneous IOP. Of course, for patients with known glaucoma, it is important to document all topical ocular hypotensive medications currently in use.

Ophthalmic Examination

In glaucoma, Snellen acuity is preserved until the disease is advanced. In advanced disease, patients will read the chart more slowly or move their head in an attempt to see around the defect in the visual field. These details are not often documented when Snellen acuity is recorded. Red–green color vision, as recorded with Ishihara plates, is also well preserved until the disease is advanced. On the other hand, blue–yellow color vision, which is rarely recorded outside clinical research circles, has been reported to be depressed early in the disease process (Drance et al. 1981).

The optic nerve represents the afferent limb of the pupillary light reflex, whereas the efferent limb is carried by sympathetic and parasympathetic fibers to the pupil. This reflex is consensual, meaning that if the reflex is triggered in one eye, both pupils constrict owing to cross wiring of the pupillary light reflex in the midbrain. Thus unilateral or markedly asymmetric glaucoma does not alter pupil size but it will produce an afferent pupillary defect on a swinging flashlight test. (Schiefer et al. 2012; Chang et al. 2013). When light is placed in front of the healthier eye, both pupils constrict, but when the light swings over to the eye with more optic nerve disease, afferent conduction is slowed and the pupil exhibits a paradoxical dilatation. The relative pupillary light reflex should always be assessed during an evaluation for glaucoma.

An accurate diagnosis of glaucoma subtype requires meticulous assessment of the ocular anterior segment for pathological signs that are either a consequence of or an explanation for elevated IOP. Examples of a pathological change in the anterior segment resulting from elevated IOP are atrophy and blunting of the iris crypts caused by ischemic damage to the underlying longitudinal iris dilator muscle. An example of a sign that contributes to elevated IOP is the presence of exfoliation material in the ocular anterior segment. There are a myriad of anterior segment signs associated with the various forms of glaucoma. A detailed discussion of these signs is beyond the scope of this chapter, but some selected signs are summarized in Table 2.

Gonioscopy is an essential technique for stratifying the glaucomas into open-angle and closed-angle types. The "angle" refers to the tissues located at the internal junction of the peripheral cornea and peripheral iris. This junction houses the trabecular meshwork, which serves as the conduit of aqueous humor egress from the eye. The trabecular meshwork is not available for direct inspection because light emanating from this structure is internally reflected owing to refractive index differences between aqueous humor and air. A special prism applied to the anesthetized ocular surface, aided by slit lamp biomicroscopic magnification, couples the tear film to the cornea and affords a view of the angle structures. There is a myriad of pathologies that can be discovered by inspecting this region of the eye, as is beautifully illustrated at http://gonioscopy.org. If the angle is physically closed (i.e., the aqueous humor does not have access to the trabecular meshwork for egress), the IOP can be quite high. Measures must be taken to understand why this physical blockage exists so that therapeutic strategies can

Table 2. Selected anterior segment signs associated with glaucoma

Ocular region	Sign	Glaucoma diagnosis
Lids/adnexa	Nevus flameus	Sturge–Weber syndrome
Conjunctiva	Chemosis	Topiramate-induced, bilateral secondary angle closure glaucoma
Cornea	Haabs striae	Congenital glaucoma
Anterior chamber	Pigment release after pupil dilation	Pigmentary glaucoma
Iris	Melt holes and stretch holes	Iridocorneal endotheliopathy
Lens	Subluxation into the anterior chamber	Pupillary block glaucoma

be used to open it. Classically, a closed angle may result when there is abnormally high resistance to aqueous humor movement around the pupil and into the anterior chamber, a condition referred to as primary angle closure glaucoma. If this pupillary block is not responsible for physical closure of the angle, there are other mechanisms that include posterior pushing processes (for example, intraoperative choroidal hemorrhage from rupture of a posterior ciliary artery) or anterior pulling mechanisms (for example, epithelial downgrowth, a condition in which the epithelium of the ocular surface gains access to the intraocular space, proliferates and pulls the peripheral iris up against the trabecular meshwork). If the angle is open but the IOP is high, there may be clues that explain this phenomenon such as accumulation of excess pigment or angle contusion deformities from trauma. IOP can also be elevated when the trabecular meshwork appears normal. This is common in open angle glaucoma and suggests that subtle, as yet unknown biochemical and/or ultrastructural changes in the trabecular meshwork account for high IOP in these cases.

The Ocular Hypertension Treatment Study (OHTS) and European Glaucoma Prevention Study (EGPS) (Gordon et al. 2007) have shown that central corneal thickness (CCT) is an independent risk factor for the conversion from ocular hypertension to POAG. Thus measurement of CCT is an integral part of the glaucoma evaluation. The mean CCT is ~550 μm, but values between 420 μm and 640 μm can be measured in large populations. People of African descent have thinner CCT values than do their Caucasian counterparts (La Rosa et al. 2001). There is a positive correlation between CCT and IOP measured by Goldmann applanation tonometry (IOP measurements are discussed below) (Emara et al. 1998). Interestingly, in one tertiary glaucoma practice, glaucoma patients with thin CCT tended to have more advanced disease than did patients with thicker CCT. Furthermore, glaucoma patients with a known maximum IOP closer to the normal range had a thinner CCT compared to open angle glaucoma patients with a history of higher IOP (Kniestedt et al. 2006). Collectively, these data suggest that true IOP in eyes with thin CCT is higher than that measured with Goldman tonometry. Nonetheless, using different formulae to adjust IOP measured with Goldmann Tonometry for CCT did not improve prediction of risk for developing POAG, compared to the model in which nonadjusted IOP scores and CCT measurements were entered (Brandt et al. 2012). Furthermore, no nomograms are available that accurately correct Goldman-measured readings for CCT, when compared to gold-standard manometric IOP measurements.

Measurement of IOP is of central importance in glaucoma. All clinical methods to measure IOP are based on quantifying a force needed to deform the globe in some way. In Goldman tonometry, the standard method to assess IOP, the number of grams needed to flatten the 3.06 mm^2 of central corneal tissue is multiplied by 10 to arrive at the IOP in mm Hg. Thus, if 1.5 grams of force is needed to flatten the central corneal tissue, then the IOP is 15 mm Hg. When considering IOP levels the focus should not be on whether the value is inside or outside the normal range; rather, the IOP should be interpreted in the context of the CCT and overall health of the optic nerve. For example an IOP of 16 mm Hg, which may represent the statistical mean for a population, may be unacceptably high for an individual with a thin CCT (<500 μm) and advanced glaucomatous optic nerve degeneration. On the other hand, an IOP of 24 mm Hg may be entirely acceptable and not require treatment if the CCT is 600 μm and the optic nerve is healthy with no corresponding glaucomatous visual deficit. One must also be cognizant that any IOP measurement is a point estimate that is subject to considerable diurnal fluctuation. Thus, for some glaucoma patients who demonstrate rapid visual field deterioration, it can be helpful to obtain multiple IOP measurements throughout the course of a day.

Assessment of the optic nerve is critical in a glaucoma evaluation. The intrascleral portion of the optic nerve measures ~2.69 mm^2 (Jonas et al. 1988) and houses the confluence of ~1 million retinal ganglion cell (RGC) axons. Generally speaking, the optic nerve has only two clinically visible responses to pathologic insults:

swelling and atrophic change. In many instances, optic swelling is followed by atrophy. Glaucoma produces a specialized form of optic nerve atrophy that can be appreciated on neuroimaging (Kitsos et al. 2009) that results in excavation or undermining of the neuroretinal rim tissue. Evaluation of the optic nerve requires optical methods that produce optimum magnification and stereopsis so that excavation and erosion of the neuroretinal rim tissue can be observed. The direct ophthalmoscope provides 15× magnification but no stereopsis. Among the various methods that provide stereopsis, viewing the optic nerve with slit lamp biomicroscopy and a 60-diopter lens provides 11.5× magnification in a workable field of view.

Although the average optic nerve has a disc area of 2.69 mm^2, areas can range from 1 mm^2 to 5 mm^2 (Jonas et al. 1988). Smaller optic nerves will appear more crowded with a smaller central depression referred to as the cup. Larger optic nerves will have larger cups. We refer to the ratio of the central depression size to the total disc size as the cup–disc ratio (CDR). The most common way to quantify this value involves comparing the vertical extent of the cup to the vertical extent of the disc itself, and is termed the vertical CDR. Because glaucomatous optic nerve degeneration manifests as an erosion of the superior and inferior poles of the optic nerves, the vertical CDR can quickly convey the structural integrity of the optic nerve. RGC loss in glaucoma produces an increase in cup area that translates into an increased vertical CDR as illustrated in Figure 2A. Compared to the fellow eye illustrated in Figure 2B, there is erosion of the inferior neuroretinal rim tissue in the glaucomatous optic nerve. As the RGC axons disappear there are also attendant changes in the nerve fiber layer near its exit from the eye (the peripapillary nerve fiber layer). Thinning of the peripapillary nerve fiber layer results in increased visibility of the retinal arterial walls and the underlying retinal pigment epithelium; furthermore, choroidal tissue adjacent to the disc becomes more visible. Another important sign associated with glaucoma is the presence of disc hemorrhage. Disc hemorrhage was an independent risk factor for disease progression in three

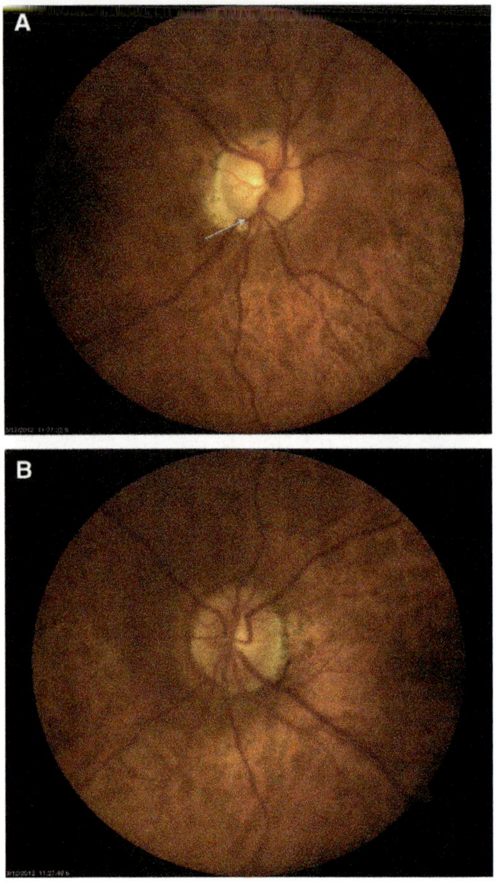

Figure 2. Erosion of rim tissue in glaucomatous optic nerve. (*A*) The fundus photo of this glaucomatous right eye shows vertical extension of the cup to the inferior margin of the disc (white arrow). The vertical cup–disc ratio is 0.7. (*B*) The fellow eye shows a disc with intact neuroretinal rims and a cup–disc ratio of 0.3.

randomized clinical trials: OHTS (Budenz et al. 2006), the Early Manifest Glaucoma Trial (EMGT) (Leske et al. 2004) and the Collaborative Normal Tension Glaucoma Study (CNTGS) (Drance et al. 2001). These trials suggest that the development of disc hemorrhage represents an IOP-independent mechanism of optic nerve deterioration in glaucoma. Understanding why disc hemorrhages develop represents fertile ground for future research in this field. The various optic nerve findings that occur in glaucoma are described at http://www.gone-project.com.

Because the intrascleral portion of the optic nerve represents a critical convergence of visual fibers into a small space, computerized optic nerve imaging is potentially useful to quantify structural features of the optic nerve such as disc size, CDR, and peripapillary nerve fiber layer thickness. Spectral domain optical coherence tomography (SD-OCT) has emerged as a modality that can provide quantitative structural information about the optic nerve and attendant nerve fiber layer tissue (Fig. 3). SD-OCT shows promise to reliably demonstrate disease progression (Wessel et al. 2013) before similar functional changes are manifest on visual field testing (Leung et al. 2012).

Although pathological cupping is a central sign in glaucoma, it is not pathognomonic for this condition. Other conditions that do not produce elevated IOP can also produce cupping, such as tumors that compress the anterior visual pathways (Bianchi-Marzoli et al. 1995). The cupping produced by chiasmal lesions can look similar to glaucomatous cupping, but these lesions also result in early onset red–green color vision deficits and ultimately visual field loss that respect the vertical meridian (in contrast, glaucomatous visual field loss respects the horizontal meridian). Other causes of nonglaucomatous cupping include arteritic anterior ischemic optic neuropathy, direct optic nerve trauma, methyl alcohol poisoning, and dominant optic atrophy. Careful history and physical exam that involves optic nerve head evaluation and visual field testing can readily differentiate these conditions from glaucoma.

Mapping of the island of vision is performed with manual or automated visual field tests. These tests provide an overview of the function of the entire visual pathway from the tear film to the occipital lobes of the brain. Defects on the visual field localize to one of 4 territories: anterior segment/retina/choroid, optic nerve, chiasm, or postchiasmal regions. The pattern of visual field loss for each region is distinct, although it may not be readily apparent when the defects are incomplete. Glaucoma produces visual field defects in the optic nerve territory that conform to the topology of the nerve fiber layer bundles. The fibers respect the horizontal raphe in the temporal retina and thus visual field defects tend to respect the horizontal meridian (Fig. 4). Visual field loss or progression has been an important outcome in several randomized clinical trials, for glaucoma, although structural changes in the optic nerve typically precede functional loss manifested on visual field tests in early glaucoma (Kerrigan-Baumrind et al. 2000). Nonetheless, as there are no parameters for IOP or optic nerve structure that define glaucoma in a highly sensitive and specific way, reproducible visual field loss on reliable tests represents the best way to definitively confirm glaucoma.

TREATMENT OF GLAUCOMA

In this section, we mostly discuss treatment of open angle glaucoma. A discussion of treatment for angle closure glaucoma is beyond the scope of this chapter.

No medical or surgical therapy to date stops or reverses optic nerve damage in glaucoma. Treatment strategies for OAG focus on delaying the disease progression by controlling IOP. One treatment strategy involves establishing a target IOP based on patient age, level of IOP that was associated RGC loss and disease severity. Because the target IOP treatment strategy is somewhat arbitrary, periodic reassessment of this goal is needed based on serial assessment of structural and functional optic nerve parameters. Lowering IOP with ocular hypotensive medicines, and/or surgical outflow procedures the main options for delaying disease progression.

Lowering of IOP in Different Patient Groups

In the OHTS study, patients with high IOP (IOP 24–32 mm Hg) experienced a 60% risk reduction for optic disc degeneration and/or visual field loss attributable to glaucoma when assigned to the treatment arm, which consisted of a $\geq$20% lowering of IOP (Kass et al. 2002). In a meta-analysis of randomized clinical trials, treating high IOP was associated with a significant reduction in glaucoma development (0.56 hazards ratio) for patients at high-risk of

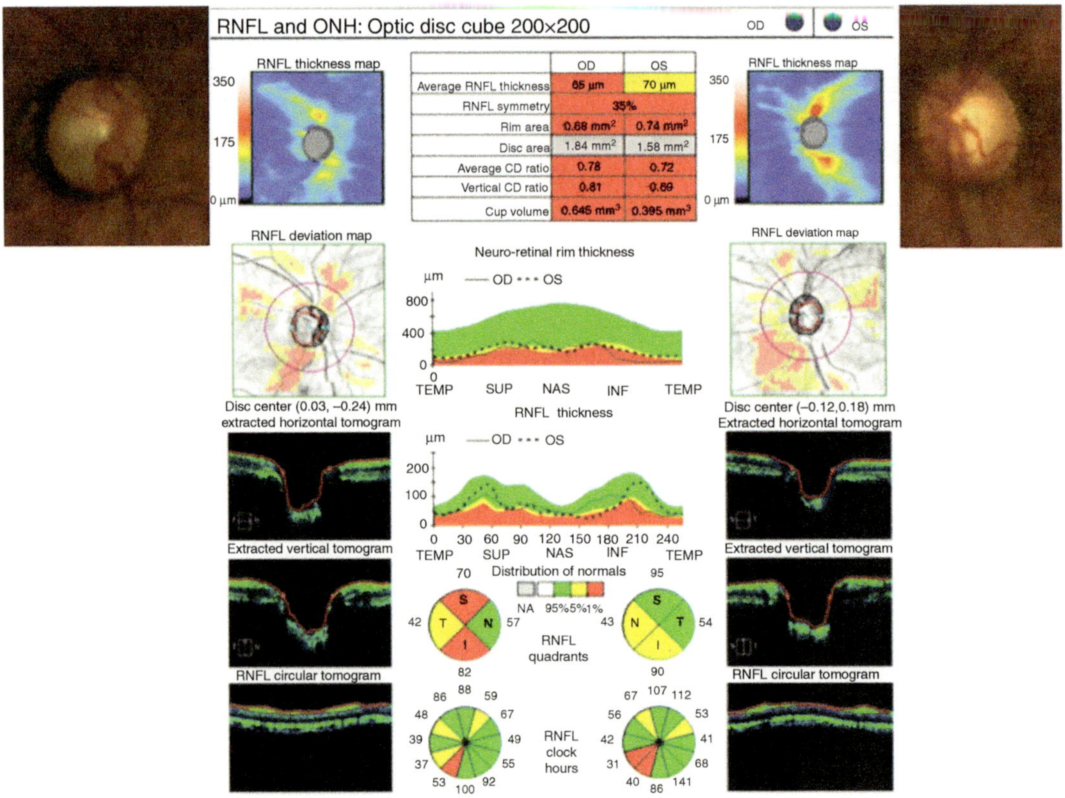

Figure 3. Quantitative structural information about the optic nerve and attendant nerve fiber layer tissue from SD-OCT. The *insets* on the *upper right* and *left* illustrate optic nerves with pathologic cupping. The spectral domain optical coherence tomogram (SD-OCT) assigned a vertical cup–disc ratio (CDR) of 0.81 for the *right* optic nerve and 0.69 for the *left* optic nerve. The SD-OCT also measures other optic nerve structural parameters such as rim area and cup volume. The rim area is abnormally low and the cup volume is abnormally large for both eyes compared to an age-matched control; hence they are highlighted in red. These abnormal values reflect loss of retinal ganglion cell axons. The SD-OCT also measures average retinal nerve fiber layer (RNFL) thickness in a swath of tissue around the optic nerve. It is significantly thinner in the *right* eye and borderline thinner in the *left* eye compared to an age-matched control. The nerve fiber layer thickness map assigns areas of thicker nerve fiber layer tissue with red and yellow colors and assigns areas where RNFL is thin with blue colors. Normally the nerve fiber layer is thickest at the superior and inferior pole and thinnest at 3 o'clock and 9 o'clock. Abnormal blue color adjacent to the inferior pole of the *right* eye corresponds to extension of the inferior cup to the neuroretinal rim on the optic nerve photo. The nerve fiber layer deviation map highlights regional areas where the nerve fiber layer is thin compared to an age matched control. Extracted horizontal and vertical tomograms provide cross-sectional views of the optic nerves, illustrating the abnormally large cup volume in both eyes. There is also an anatomical reconstruction of a circular swath of tissue around the optic nerve corresponding to the red circle drawn on the nerve fiber layer deviation map. The *middle* tile provides regional inter-eye comparisons as well as comparisons to a normative database for neuroretinal rim thickness and nerve fiber layer thickness. These graphs illustrate that nerve fiber layer loss is greater in the *right* optic nerve where the CDR is larger. Other abbreviations used: ONH, optic nerve head; T, temporal; N, nasal; S, superior; I, inferior; TEMP, temporal; SUP, superior; NAS, nasal; INF, inferior.

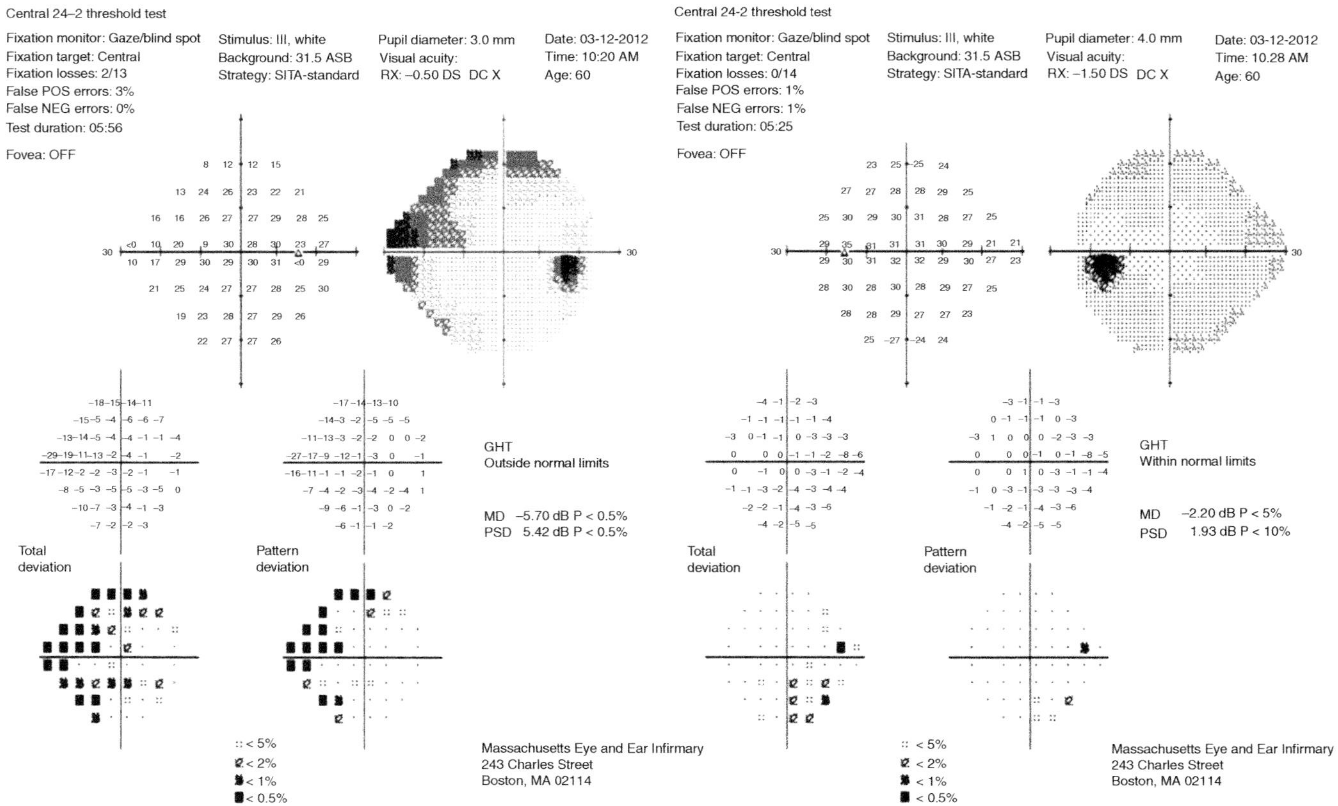

Figure 4. A Humphrey visual field for the patient illustrated in Figure 3 shows acceptable reliability parameters in both eyes (fixation loss ≤33%; false positive and false negative rates ≤20%). Raw retinal sensitivity data in decibels (converted from an apostilb scale ranging from 0 to 10,000 candela/m^2) are provided. The grayscale representation illustrates the blind spots corresponding to the optic nerves, where there are no light-sensitive cells. These raw data are compared to a normative database to generate a Total Deviation plot. For each point, the probability that the sensitivity difference versus an age-matched control is statistically different is provided. In the Pattern Deviation plot the general reduction in retinal sensitivity is factored out to yield focal defects in the visual field. The *right* eye shows superior and inferior nasal defects in the peripheral visual field. Interestingly the *left* eye, which showed structural loss, has minimal loss of visual field. Other abbreviations used: GHT, glaucoma hemifield test; MD, mean deviation; PSD, pattern standard deviation.

converting to POAG. Patients in the treatment arm of these trials did not progress to glaucoma diagnoses in 63%–91% of the cases (Maier et al. 2005). Overall, the results of OHTS and other trials suggest that IOP-lowering agents are effective in reducing disease progression for high IOP patients with moderate to high risk for developing POAG. Although the benefit of IOP lowering is well established for IOP >24 mm Hg associated with high-risk characteristics, treatment benefits remains unclear for patients with borderline pressure (21–24 mm Hg).

Lowering of IOP is known to delay disease progression for patients newly diagnosed with glaucoma. In the Early Manifest Glaucoma Trial (EMGT), lowering of IOP by 25% combined with betaxolol (a β-blocker) and argon laser trabeculoplasty (ALT) resulted in less disease progression (45% with treatment vs. 62% without treatment; $p < 0.007$) over a median follow-up period of 6 yr. Visual field or optic disc criteria defined disease progression. There was less benefit of IOP lowering for open-angle glaucoma with IOP <21 mm Hg versus IOP ≥21 mm Hg (Heijl et al. 2002).

The treatment benefits from lowering of IOP for normal-tension glaucoma patients are less clear-cut. Normal-tension glaucoma is defined by glaucomatous optic nerve changes developing in the context of normal anterior segment findings, open angles, and untreated IOP close to the statistical norm for the population and typically not higher than 21 mm Hg. In the CNTGS, there was no difference in visual field changes for normal-tension glaucoma patients in the treatment arm, although IOP was lowered by 25%–30% compared to the untreated arm. When patients with cataracts were excluded, however, lowering of IOP had a favorable effect on visual field changes in the treatment arm, with 60% of patients experiencing visual field changes at 3 yr compared to 80% of patients in the control (Anderson 2003).

The Low-Pressure Glaucoma Treatment Study (LoPGTS) compared two twice-daily topical therapies, brimonidine to timolol, for normal-tension glaucoma patients. Although the IOP-lowering effect was similar at all time points between the two treatment arms, there was significantly less progressive visual field loss in the brimonidine arm, with 9.1% of brimonidine-treated patients experiencing progressive visual field loss versus 39.2% of patients using timolol (Krupin et al. 2011). This result suggests that two drugs with equal efficacy in lowering IOP may have different effects on glaucoma progression.

Medical Therapies to Lower IOP

Five broad drug classes are commonly used to lower IOP in patients with glaucoma (Table 3): prostaglandin analogues, β-blockers, α-agonists, carbonic anhydrase inhibitors and cholinergic agents.

The goal of all therapy is to protect the optic nerve, yet only a few studies have been designed to determine whether pharmacological agents are neuroprotective. Those that investigated the efficacy of a single agent and used strict endpoints include the EGPS and the LoPGTS. The EGPS showed reductions in risk of glaucoma progression in moderate risk OHTN patients of 15% for 6 mo and 22% for 5 yr when using dorzolamide to lower IOP; however, compared to placebo, this result was not statistically significant (Miglior et al. 2005). The LoPGTS discussed above found brimonidine to be superior to timolol in terms of reducing progressive visual field loss in normal-tension glaucoma. Another study compared timolol to no timolol and found timolol to be significantly neuroprotective, with an adjusted risk ratio of 0.38 in OHTN patients (Epstein et al. 1989). More recently, the United Kingdom Glaucoma Prevention Study (UKGTS) assessed prostaglandins versus placebo using visual field loss over a 2-yr period as the primary end point (Garway-Heath et al. 2013); as of this writing, the results are pending.

Most clinical trials use lowering of IOP as a proxy for efficacy of glaucoma treatment. Head-to-head trials between β-blockers and prostaglandin analogues indicate that prostaglandin analogues are more effective than β-blockers in lowering IOP. In a pooled analysis of three randomized clinical trials, latanoprost, a prostaglandin analogue, lowered mean diurnal IOP

Table 3. Summary of drugs used to treat glaucoma

Drug class	Mechanism	Clinical use	Ocular side effects	Systemic side effects
Prostaglandin analogs –Latanoprost –Travoprost –Bimatoprost –Tafluprost	Increase aqueous humor outflow	Preferred first-line therapy (lowering of IOP by 6–7 mm Hg) Superior lowering of IOP; proof of neuroprotection pending	Blurred vision; lid changes; dry eyes; heterochromia; hypertrichosis; hyperemia	Uncommon
β-blockers –Timolol –Betaxolol –Levobunolol	Decrease aqueous humor production	Acceptable first line therapy (lowering of IOP by 5–6 mm Hg) Proof of neuropro-tection (Epstein et al. 1989)	Burning/stinging	Broncho-spasm; worsening heart failure; bradycardia; heart block; depression
α-agonists –Brimonidine	Increase aqueous humor outflow, decrease aqueous humor production	Appropriate first-line therapy (lowering of IOP by 3–4 mm Hg) Proof of neuroprotection (LoPGTS)	Hyperemia; allergic conjunctivitis	Somnolence (more common in children)
Carbonic anhydrase inhibitors –Dorzolamide –Brinzolamide	Decrease aqueous humor production	Appropriate first line therapy (lowering of IOP by 3–4 mm Hg) No proof of neuroprotection (EGPS 2005)	Burning; hyperemia; allergic conjunctivitis	Allergic reaction; angioedema (rare)

by 1.1 mm Hg more than timolol, a β-blocker. Among the prostaglandin analogues, bimatoprost was more effective than travoprost (Noecker et al. 2003) or latanoprost (Konstas et al. 2005, 2007) in some trials, although the effect differences were small and perhaps not clinically meaningful. Generic and branded latanoprost were equivalent in lowering IOP by 6–7 mm Hg (Hedman et al. 2003).

A meta-analysis of 28 randomized clinical trials assessed eight drugs compared to placebos. All of the drugs were more effective in lowering IOP than was the placebo. The rank order of effectiveness for lowering of peak IOP, from highest to lowest, was bimatoprost, travoprost and latanoprost, brimonidine, timolol, dorzolamide, betaxolol, followed by brinzolamide. For lowering of trough IOP, prostaglandin analogues remained the most effective and brimonidine dropped to the least effective with rankings as follows: bimatoprost, latanoprost, travoprost, timolol, betaxolol, dorzolamide, brinzolamide, brimonidine (van der Valk et al. 2009). Combined therapies (i.e., latanoprost/timolol and dorzolamide/timolol) were as efficacious and in some studies more potent in lowering IOP than were the individual components. However, physicians prefer to initiate treatment with monotherapy to avoid excessive side effects (Higginbotham et al. 2010).

A panel of 10 ophthalmologists reached consensus that prostaglandin analogues were the preferred first-line therapy for medical management of glaucoma (Singh et al. 2008). The Marshfield Eye Clinic in Wisconsin noted that β blockers were prescribed for a majority of patients until 2000, when prostaglandin analogues became more commonly used (McCarty et al. 2008). Although prostaglandin analogues are cited to be preferable for their lack of systemic side effects, the ocular side effects are significant. A cross-sectional observational study associated prostaglandin analogue use to an increased likelihood of upper lid ptosis, deepening of the upper lid sulcus, lower lid retraction, loss of periorbital fat, and levator muscle dysfunction (Shah et al. 2013).

β-Blockers are associated with systemic side effects including exacerbation of airway constriction, bradycardia, and heart failure. Thus these agents are contraindicated in asthmatics and patients with decompensated heart failure. α-Agonists are highly associated with allergic conjunctivitis, as are topical carbonic anhydrase inhibitors. When patients cannot tolerate these medications or fail medical therapy, lowering of IOP must be achieved with laser trabeculoplasty or incisional therapies.

Laser Therapies to Lower IOP

In laser trabeculoplasty, laser energy is delivered to the trabecular meshwork, typically using either an argon laser or frequency-doubled Q-switched Nd:YAG laser, with the goal of achieving lower IOP. The Glaucoma Laser Trial (GLT) established the long-term efficacy of argon laser trabeculoplasty (ALT). Initial IOP was lowered by 9 mm Hg versus 7 mm Hg in the laser and medical (timolol) groups, respectively. In the laser group, 34% experienced transient IOP increases and 30% developed peripheral anterior synechiae, although neither of these outcomes affected long-term visual acuity. This study used lowering of IOP as its endpoint and found ALT to be as effective as medical therapy in lowering IOP. There was less evidence to support repeat laser therapy; at one yr, repeat ALT had reported success rates of 21% to 70%. This effect decreased with longer follow-up, with success rates of 11% at 24 mo and 5% at 48 mo (The Glaucoma Research Group 1990).

Compared to ALT, selective laser trabeculoplasty targets melanin granules in the trabecular meshwork, which theoretically creates less collateral damage. Most trials suggest the two laser treatment modalities are equally effective in lowering IOP at 6 mo and 1 yr of follow-up. In a review of laser treatments, patients with persistently elevated IOP > 20 mm Hg after initial laser trabeculoplasty experienced greater improvement in IOP with selective laser trabeculoplasty than with ALT (6.24 mm Hg and 4.65 mm Hg, respectively). Diode laser, ALT, and selective laser trabeculoplasty had equivalent efficacy in most trials, and adverse events were equally likely for all types of laser treatment. The most common adverse event was a transient increase in IOP. The incidence of this event was 12% for an increase in IOP of >10 mm Hg and 34% for an increase in IOP of >5 mm Hg. Other adverse events included a low-grade iritis (Samples et al. 2011).

Surgical Treatments to Lower IOP

In trabeculectomy surgery, aqueous humor egress from the eye is facilitated via a partial thickness sclerostomy. Clinical trials from the Moorfields Eye Hospital indicated surgical trabeculectomy was the most effective IOP-lowering treatment. Trabeculectomy lowered IOP the most (by 60%), compared to laser trabeculoplasty (decrease of 38%) and medical therapy groups (decrease of 49%), but optic nerve integrity was not fully studied. Nonetheless, the nonsurgical groups had more deterioration in visual fields than did the trabeculectomy group (Rolim de Moura et al. 2007). In the 1990s, the Collaborative Initial Glaucoma Treatment Study (CIGTS) randomized newly diagnosed OAG patients to initial medical or surgical management. Both groups experienced successful lowering of IOP, although the average IOP for the surgical group was 2–3 mm Hg lower than that for the medical group. Ultimately, visual field and visual acuity outcomes were similar in both groups. Surgery was overall found to be more cataractogenic. On secondary analysis, patients with moderate disease had less visual field loss when treated with surgery first (Musch et al. 2011). Collectively, the findings of these surgical trials have not impacted glaucoma management.

The Advanced Glaucoma Intervention Study (AGIS) compared initial laser trabeculoplasty to trabeculectomy for patients with advanced glaucoma who failed medical therapy. Overall results indicated that either modality was effective as initial treatment. Subgroup

 Cite this article as *Cold Spring Harb Perspect Med* doi: 10.1101/cshperspect.a017236

Table 4. Summary of the randomized clinical trials in glaucoma along with their Likert impact scores

Study name (Likert score: 0–5)[a]	Study population	Treatment and control groups	Outcome	Clinical impact
OHTS (4.47)	Patients with ocular hypertension (no glaucoma)	T: IOP lowered by 20% (using any means) C: Observation	Neuroprotection when IOP was lowered (>24 mm Hg) in OHTN	Prophylactic lowering of IOP for OHTN patients; importance of CCT
EMGT (3.48)	Patients newly diagnosed with open-angle glaucoma	T: IOP lowered by 30% (using a β-blocker and ALT) C: Observation	A decrease in progression of glaucoma by 50% when IOP was lowered	Importance of IOP lowering in slowing disease progression
CNTGS (4.13)	Normal-tension glaucoma patients	T: IOP lowered by 30% C: Observation	No significant difference in glaucoma progression except when excluding cataract patients	Lowering of IOP not proven effective in normal-tension glaucoma patients
LoPGTS[b]	Normal-tension glaucoma patients	T: Brimonidine C: Timolol	Similar IOP lowering-results, but with brimonidine-treated subjects less likely to progress	Superior results with brimonidine in normal-tension glaucoma patients
EGPS (2.69)	Patients with moderate risk for glaucoma	T: Dorzolamide C: Placebo	No difference in glaucoma progression	Clinical impact lowest
GLT (3.39)	Newly diagnosed open-angle glaucoma patients	T: ALT (argon laser trabeculectomy) C: Timolol	No difference in IOP-lowering effect at 1yr	Established long-term efficacy of ALT
AGIS (3.78)	Advanced glaucoma patients with failed medical therapy	T: ATT (argon laser trabeculoplasty, trabeculectomy, trabeculectomy) C: TAT (trabeculectomy, argon laser trabeculoplasty, trabeculectomy)	Decreased failure rate (repeat intervention) for African Americans in the ATT arm	Trabeculectomy not necessarily superior to laser trabeculoplasty in advanced glaucoma
CIGTS (3.44)	Newly diagnosed open-angle glaucoma patients	T: Medical therapy C: Surgical trabeculectomy	Effective lowering of IOP for both, with more adverse effects associated with surgery	Confirmed conservative approach to surgical management

Abbreviations used: T, treatment arm; C, control arm; OHTS, Ocular Hypertension Treatment Study; EMGT, Early Manifest Glaucoma Trial; CNTGS, Collaborative Normal Tension Glaucoma Study; LoPGTS, Low-Pressure Glaucoma Treatment Study; EGPS, European Glaucoma Prevention Study; GLT, Glaucoma Laser Trial; AGIS, Advanced Glaucoma Intervention Study; CIGTS, Collaborative Initial Treatment Study; OHTN, ocular hypertension; CCT, central corneal thickness.

[a]The Likert scale is a psychosomatic scale that gauges responses to questionnaire data and quantifies the clinical impact of each randomized clinical trial.

[b]Likert score not available.

analysis results varied by race; African Americans experienced more success with initial ALT whereas Caucasians had better results with trabeculectomy as the first treatment. In both cases, failure rate was 50% by 10 yr of follow-up (Ederer et al. 2004). Approximately 50% of glaucoma doctors surveyed agree or strongly agree that this study has made race an important consideration when making treatment decisions (Panarelli et al. 2013).

A systematic review has demonstrated that surgical trabeculectomy decreases IOP more than do nonpenetrating surgeries. Furthermore, adjunctive use of the antimetabolites mitomycin C and 5-fluoruracil prevented scar tissue formation and helped lower IOP to a greater extent (by 4.5–5.5 mm Hg) than did trabeculectomy alone (Boland et al. 2013). In an early head-to-head study of eyes at high risk for surgical failure, mitomycin C was superior to 5-fluoruracil in terms of IOP-lowering ability (final IOP outcomes: 10.9 mm Hg and 14.2 mm Hg, respectively) and reduced corneal toxicity. Patients treated with mitomycin C also required fewer ocular hypotensive agents postsurgery (Skuta et al. 1992).

Prosthetic devices to enhance aqueous humor outflow during glaucoma filtration surgery experienced increased utilization in the 1990s (Ramulu et al. 2007). In the multicenter Tube versus Trabeculectomy (TVT) study, tube-shunt surgery had improved success at 3- and 5-yr follow-up periods compared to trabeculectomy with mitomycin C. Although tube-shunt surgery was associated with more adjunctive medical therapy and trabeculectomy associated with lower IOP in the short term, the two were equivalent in these measures at 3 yr. Trabeculectomy was associated with a greater number of postoperative complications, but visual field loss and cataract development were equal at 3 yr (Gedde et al. 2009). At the 5-yr follow-up, both modalities were associated with IOP in the 12–14 mm Hg range, but failure rates were lower in the tube group (29.8%) compared to the trabeculectomy group (46.9%). This resulted in 9% and 29% reoperation rates, respectively (Gedde et al. 2012). Trabeculectomy appears to be the most effective means to lower IOP when compared to laser and tube shunt surgery, but the long-term results are less clear, and the side effects and failure rate of surgical trabeculectomy are significant.

Summary of Major Glaucoma Treatment Trials

All randomized clinical trials do not have equal impact (Table 4). In a survey of 894 American Glaucoma Society members, OHTS was ranked as the most impactful glaucoma study to date. Not only did it suggest the possibility of glaucoma prevention for high risk patients, it also demonstrated the importance of assessing CCT in evaluating when to start treatment. Of the eight major glaucoma treatment trials addressed in this survey, those with results showing no difference in treatment outcomes (EGPS, GLT, CIGTS) had less reported impact than did those showing superiority of one treatment over another (OHTS, AGIS) (Panarelli et al. 2013).

CONCLUDING REMARKS

There are considerable differences in the pathophysiologies of the glaucoma subtypes and very few of these types are well understood at a molecular level. Nevertheless, advances in various bioinformatics disciplines are poised to increase this knowledge, as discussed elsewhere in this volume. A better understanding of glaucoma at the molecular level, will translate into more cost-effective treatments.

REFERENCES

Abe H, Hasegawa S, Iwata K. 1987. Contrast sensitivity and pattern visual evoked potential in patients with glaucoma. *Doc Ophthalmol* **65:** 65–70.

Aggarwal RK, Potamitis T, Chong NH, Guarro M, Shah P, Kheterpal S. 1993. Extensive visual loss with topical facial steroids. *Eye (Lond)* **7:** 664–666.

Anderson DR. 2003. Collaborative normal tension glaucoma study. *Curr Opin Ophthalmol* **14:** 86–90.

Bianchi-Marzoli S, Rizzo JF III, Brancato R, Lessell S. 1995. Quantitative analysis of optic disc cupping in compressive optic neuropathy. *Ophthalmology* **102:** 436–440.

Boland MV, Ervin AM, Friedman DS, Jampel HD, Hawkins BS, Vollenweider D, Chelladurai Y, Ward D, Suarez-Cuervo C, Robinson KA. 2013. Comparative effectiveness of treatments for open-angle glaucoma: A systematic review for the U.S. Preventive Services Task Force. *Ann Intern Med* **158:** 271–279.

Borthne A. 1976. The treatment of glaucoma with propranolol (Inderal). A clinical trial. *Acta Ophthalmol* **54:** 291–300.

Brandt JD, Gordon MO, Gao F, Beiser JA, Miller JP, Kass MA. 2012. Adjusting intraocular pressure for central corneal thickness does not improve prediction models for primary open-angle glaucoma. *Ophthalmology* **119:** 437–442.

Budenz DL, Anderson DR, Feuer WJ, Beiser JA, Schiffman J, Parrish RK II, Piltz-Seymour JR, Gordon MO, Kass MA. 2006. Detection and prognostic significance of optic disc hemorrhages during the ocular hypertension treatment study. *Ophthalmology* **113:** 2137–2143.

Chang DS, Xu L, Boland MV, Friedman DS. 2013. Accuracy of pupil assessment for the detection of glaucoma: A systematic review and meta-analysis. *Ophthalmology.*

Clark AF, Brotchie D, Read AT, Hellberg P, English-Wright S, Pang IH, Ethier CR, Grierson I. 2005. Dexamethasone alters F-actin architecture and promotes cross-linked actin network formation in human trabecular meshwork tissue. *Cell Motil Cytoskeleton* **60:** 83–95.

Drance SM, Lakowski R, Schulzer M, Douglas GR. 1981. Acquired color vision changes in glaucoma. Use of 100-hue test and Pickford anomaloscope as predictors of glaucomatous field change. *Arch Ophthalmol* **99:** 829–831.

Drance S, Anderson DR, Schulzer M. 2001. Risk factors for progression of visual field abnormalities in normal-tension glaucoma. *Am J Ophthalmol* **131:** 699–708.

Ederer F, Gaasterland DA, Dally LG, Kim J, VanVeldhuisen PC, Blackwell B, Prum B, Shafranov G, Allen RC, Beck A. 2004. The Advanced Glaucoma Intervention Study (AGIS): 13. Comparison of treatment outcomes within race: 10-year results. *Ophthalmology* **111:** 651–664.

Emara B, Probst LE, Tingey DP, Kennedy DW, Willms LJ, Machat J. 1998. Correlation of intraocular pressure and central corneal thickness in normal myopic eyes and after laser in situ keratomileusis. *J Cataract Refract Surg* **24:** 1320–1325.

Epstein DL, Krug JH Jr, Hertzmark E, Remis LL, Edelstein DJ. 1989. A long-term clinical trial of timolol therapy versus no treatment in the management of glaucoma suspects. *Ophthalmology* **96:** 1460–1467.

Garway-Heath DF, Lascaratos G, Bunce C, Crabb DP, Russell RA, Shah A. 2013. The United Kingdom Glaucoma Treatment Study: A multicenter, randomized, placebo-controlled clinical trial: Design and methodology. *Ophthalmology* **120:** 68–76.

Gedde SJ, Schiffman JC, Feuer WJ, Herndon LW, Brandt JD, Budenz DL. 2009. Three-year follow-up of the tube versus trabeculectomy study. *Am J Ophthalmol* **148:** 670–684.

Gedde SJ, Schiffman JC, Feuer WJ, Herndon LW, Brandt JD, Budenz DL. 2012. Treatment outcomes in the Tube Versus Trabeculectomy (TVT) study after five years of follow-up. *Am J Ophthalmol* **153:** 789–803, e782.

Gordon MO, Torri V, Miglior S, Beiser JA, Floriani I, Miller JP, Gao F, Adamsons I, Poli D, D'Agostino RB, et al. 2007. Validated prediction model for the development of primary open-angle glaucoma in individuals with ocular hypertension. *Ophthalmology* **114:** 10–19.

Hedman K, Alm A, Gross RL. 2003. Pooled-data analysis of three randomized, double-masked, six-month studies comparing intraocular pressure-reducing effects of latanoprost and timolol in patients with ocular hypertension. *J Glaucoma* **12:** 463–465.

Heijl A, Leske MC, Bengtsson B, Hyman L, Bengtsson B, Hussein M. 2002. Reduction of intraocular pressure and glaucoma progression: Results from the Early Manifest Glaucoma Trial. *Arch Ophthalmol* **120:** 1268–1279.

Higginbotham EJ, Olander KW, Kim EE, Grunden JW, Kwok KK, Tressler CS. 2010. Fixed combination of latanoprost and timolol vs individual components for primary open-angle glaucoma or ocular hypertension: A randomized, double-masked study. *Arch Ophthalmol* **128:** 165–172.

Jonas JB, Gusek GC, Naumann GO. 1988. Optic disc, cup and neuroretinal rim size, configuration and correlations in normal eyes. *Invest Ophthalmol Vis Sci* **29:** 1151–1158.

Kang JH, Willett WC, Rosner BA, Hankinson SE, Pasquale LR. 2007. Prospective study of alcohol consumption and the risk of primary open-angle glaucoma. *Ophthalmic Epidemiol* **14:** 141–147.

Kass MA, Heuer DK, Higginbotham EJ, Johnson CA, Keltner JL, Miller JP, Parrish RK II, Wilson MR, Gordon MO. 2002. The Ocular Hypertension Treatment Study: A randomized trial determines that topical ocular hypotensive medication delays or prevents the onset of primary open-angle glaucoma. *Arch Ophthalmol* **120:** 701–713; discussion 829–730.

Kerrigan-Baumrind LA, Quigley HA, Pease ME, Kerrigan DF, Mitchell RS. 2000. Number of ganglion cells in glaucoma eyes compared with threshold visual field tests in the same persons. *Invest Ophthalmol Vis Sci* **41:** 741–748.

Kitsos G, Zikou AK, Bagli E, Kosta P, Argyropoulou MI. 2009. Conventional MRI and magnetisation transfer imaging of the brain and optic pathway in primary open-angle glaucoma. *Br J Radiol* **82:** 896–900.

Kniestedt C, Lin S, Choe J, Nee M, Bostrom A, Sturmer J, Stamper RL. 2006. Correlation between intraocular pressure, central corneal thickness, stage of glaucoma, and demographic patient data: Prospective analysis of biophysical parameters in tertiary glaucoma practice populations. *J Glaucoma* **15:** 91–97.

Konstas AG, Katsimbris JM, Lallos N, Boukaras GP, Jenkins JN, Stewart WC. 2005. Latanoprost 0.005% versus bimatoprost 0.03% in primary open-angle glaucoma patients. *Ophthalmology* **112:** 262–266.

Konstas AG, Kozobolis VP, Katsimpris IE, Boboridis K, Koukoula S, Jenkins JN, Stewart WC. 2007. Efficacy and safety of latanoprost versus travoprost in exfoliative glaucoma patients. *Ophthalmology* **114:** 653–657.

Krupin T, Liebmann JM, Greenfield DS, Ritch R, Gardiner S. 2011. A randomized trial of brimonidine versus timolol in preserving visual function: Results from the Low-Pressure Glaucoma Treatment Study. *Am J Ophthalmol* **151:** 671–681.

La Rosa FA, Gross RL, Orengo-Nania S. 2001. Central corneal thickness of Caucasians and African Americans in glaucomatous and nonglaucomatous populations. *Arch Ophthalmol* **119:** 23–27.

Leske MC, Heijl A, Hyman L, Bengtsson B, Komaroff E. 2004. Factors for progression and glaucoma treatment: The Early Manifest Glaucoma Trial. *Curr Opin Ophthalmol* **15:** 102–106.

Leung CK, Yu M, Weinreb RN, Lai G, Xu G, Lam DS. 2012. Retinal nerve fiber layer imaging with spectral-domain optical coherence tomography: Patterns of retinal nerve fiber layer progression. *Ophthalmology* **119:** 1858–1866.

Maier PC, Funk J, Schwarzer G, Antes G, Falck-Ytter YT. 2005. Treatment of ocular hypertension and open angle glaucoma: Meta-analysis of randomised controlled trials. *BMJ* **331:** 134.

McCarty CA, Mukesh BN, Kitchner TE, Hubbard WC, Wilke RA, Burmester JK, Patchett RB. 2008. Intraocular pressure response to medication in a clinical setting: The Marshfield Clinic Personalized Medicine Research Project. *J Glaucoma* **17:** 372–377.

Miglior S, Zeyen T, Pfeiffer N, Cunha-Vaz J, Torri V, Adamsons I. 2005. Results of the European Glaucoma Prevention Study. *Ophthalmology* **112:** 366–375.

Musch DC, Gillespie BW, Niziol LM, Lichter PR, Varma R. 2011. Intraocular pressure control and long-term visual field loss in the Collaborative Initial Glaucoma Treatment Study. *Ophthalmology* **118:** 1766–1773.

Noecker RJ, Earl ML, Mundorf T, Peace J, Williams RD. 2003. Bimatoprost 0.03% versus travoprost 0.004% in black Americans with glaucoma or ocular hypertension. *Adv Ther* **20:** 121–128.

Opatowsky I, Feldman RM, Gross R, Feldman ST. 1995. Intraocular pressure elevation associated with inhalation and nasal corticosteroids. *Ophthalmology* **102:** 177–179.

Panarelli JF, Banitt MR, Sidoti PA, Budenz DL, Singh K. 2013. Clinical impact of 8 prospective, randomized, multicenter glaucoma trials. *J Glaucoma.*

Quigley HA, Broman AT. 2006. The number of people with glaucoma worldwide in 2010 and 2020. *Br J Ophthalmol* **90:** 262–267.

Ramulu PY, Corcoran KJ, Corcoran SL, Robin AL. 2007. Utilization of various glaucoma surgeries and procedures in Medicare beneficiaries from 1995 to 2004. *Ophthalmology* **114:** 2265–2270.

Rolim de Moura C, Paranhos A Jr, Wormald R. 2007. Laser trabeculoplasty for open angle glaucoma. *Cochrane Database Syst Rev*: CD003919.

Samples JR, Singh K, Lin SC, Francis BA, Hodapp E, Jampel HD, Smith SD. 2011. Laser trabeculoplasty for open-angle glaucoma: A report by the American academy of ophthalmology. *Ophthalmology* **118:** 2296–2302.

Schiefer U, Dietzsch J, Dietz K, Wilhelm B, Bruckmann A, Wilhelm H, Kitiratschky V, Januschowski K. 2012. Associating the magnitude of relative afferent pupillary defect (RAPD) with visual field indices in glaucoma patients. *Br J Ophthalmol* **96:** 629–633.

Shah M, Lee G, Lefebvre DR, Kronberg B, Loomis S, Brauner SC, Turalba A, Rhee DJ, Freitag SK, Pasquale LR. 2013. A cross-sectional survey of the association between bilateral topical prostaglandin analogue use and ocular adnexal features. *PLoS ONE* **8:** e61638.

Singh K, Lee BL, Wilson MR. 2008. A panel assessment of glaucoma management: Modification of existing RAND-like methodology for consensus in ophthalmology. Part II: Results and interpretation. *Am J Ophthalmol* **145:** 575–581.

Skuta GL, Beeson CC, Higginbotham EJ, Lichter PR, Musch DC, Bergstrom TJ, Klein TB, Falck FY Jr. 1992. Intraoperative mitomycin versus postoperative 5-fluorouracil in high-risk glaucoma filtering surgery. *Ophthalmology* **99:** 438–444.

Tielsch JM, Katz J, Sommer A, Quigley HA, Javitt JC. 1994. Family history and risk of primary open angle glaucoma. The Baltimore Eye Survey. *Arch Ophthalmol* **112:** 69–73.

The Glaucoma Research Group. 1990. The Glaucoma Laser Trial (GLT). 2. Results of argon laser trabeculoplasty versus topical medicines. *Ophthalmology* **97:** 1403–1413.

van der Valk R, Webers CA, Lumley T, Hendrikse F, Prins MH, Schouten JS. 2009. A network meta-analysis combined direct and indirect comparisons between glaucoma drugs to rank effectiveness in lowering intraocular pressure. *J Clin Epidemiol* **62:** 1279–1283.

Wessel JM, Horn FK, Tornow RP, Schmid M, Mardin CY, Kruse FE, Juenemann AG, Laemmer R. 2013. Longitudinal analysis of progression in glaucoma using spectral-domain optical coherence tomography. *Invest Ophthalmol Vis Sci* **54:** 3613–3620.

Wolfs RC, Klaver CC, Ramrattan RS, van Duijn CM, Hofman A, de Jong PT. 1998. Genetic risk of primary open-angle glaucoma. Population-based familial aggregation study. *Arch Ophthalmol* **116:** 1640–1645.

Common and Rare Genetic Risk Factors for Glaucoma

Ryan Wang and Janey L. Wiggs

Department of Ophthalmology, Harvard Medical School, Massachusetts Eye and Ear Infirmary, Boston, Massachusetts 02114

Correspondence: janey_wiggs@meei.harvard.edu

The characterization of genes responsible for glaucoma is the critical first step toward the development of gene-based diagnostic and screening tests, which could identify individuals at risk for disease before irreversible optic nerve damage occurs. Early-onset forms of glaucoma affecting children and young adults are typically inherited as Mendelian autosomal dominant or recessive traits whereas glaucoma affecting older adults has complex inheritance. In this report, we present a comprehensive overview of the genes and genomic regions contributing to inherited glaucoma.

RATIONALE FOR DISCOVERY OF GENES CONTRIBUTING TO GLAUCOMA

The characterization of genes responsible for glaucoma is the critical first step toward the development of gene-based diagnostic and screening tests, which could identify individuals at risk for disease before irreversible optic nerve damage occurs. Current glaucoma therapies are limited to reducing elevated intraocular pressure (IOP), a major risk factor for the disease. The discovery of disease-related genes could provide new insights into the underlying molecular mechanisms responsible for glaucoma that could form the basis of novel gene-based therapies, including strategies for neuroprotection. Understanding the role of the protein product in health and disease will also provide new insights into the underlying molecular mechanisms responsible for disease.

Glaucoma can affect individuals of all ages. Early-onset forms of glaucoma affecting children and young adults are typically inherited as Mendelian autosomal dominant or recessive traits whereas glaucoma affecting older adults has complex inheritance. Early-onset forms of glaucoma are rare whereas adult-onset forms are more common.

RARE VARIANTS CAUSING EARLY-ONSET GLAUCOMA WITH AUTOSOMAL DOMINANT OR AUTOSOMAL RECESSIVE INHERITANCE

Compared with adult-onset glaucoma, early-onset forms of glaucoma are rare with incidence ranging from 1/2500 to 1/20,000, depending on the condition and the population (Stoilov et al. 1997; Beijani et al. 2000; Chakrabarti et al. 2010). Genetic variants causing early-onset

Cite this article as *Cold Spring Harb Perspect Med* doi: 10.1101/cshperspect.a017244

glaucoma are highly penetrant, although variable expressivity may be observed. The genes currently known to cause early-onset glaucoma are listed in Table 1. All of these genes were initially identified using genetic linkage analyses of large, multigenerational families. These genes are responsible for congenital glaucoma (*CYP1B1* and *LTBP2*), developmental glaucoma (*PITX2*, *FOXC1*, *PAX6*, and *LMX1B*), juvenile-onset primary open angle glaucoma (*MYOC*), and familial normal-tension glaucoma (*OPTN* and *TBK1*).

Congenital Glaucoma

Congenital glaucoma (or infantile glaucoma) typically develops before three years of age (Aponte et al. 2010). The condition is primarily inherited as an autosomal recessive trait, although autosomal dominant families have been described (Sarfarazi et al. 2000). Genetic linkage studies have identified three loci likely to contain genes contributing to congenital glaucoma: GLC3A (2p21), GLC3B (1p36), and GLC3C (14q22) (Safarazi et al. 1995; Akarsu et al. 1996; Stoilov and Sarfarazi 2002). Two genes have been discovered: *CYP1B1*, encoding cytochrome P450 1B1 (GLC3A), and *LTBP2* (latent transforming growth factor binding protein 2) (Ali et al. 2009; Beijani et al. 2000). Mutations in both *CYP1B1* and *LTBP2* cause autosomal recessive disease.

CYP1B1 mutations are the most common cause of congenital glaucoma worldwide (Stoilov et al. 1997). Disease-causing mutations include missense mutations, nonsense mutations, frameshifts, and large-gene deletions (Stoilov et al. 1997; Sarfarazi 2000; Michels-Rautenstrauss et al. 2001). Although these mutations are highly penetrant, variable expressivity is a well-known feature of *CYP1B1*-related disease. Genotype–phenotype studies have suggested that mutations causing premature truncation of the protein (frameshifts, deletions, insertions, and nonsense mutations) cause more severe disease with earlier onset than disease caused by missense mutations. The gene product, cytochrome P450 1B1, metabolizes complex molecules such as polycyclic aromatic hydrocarbons and 17β-estradiol (Tokizane et al. 2005; Tsuchiya et al. 2005; Sowers et al. 2006). The role of the protein in congenital glaucoma is not clear; however, it has been hypothesized that cytochrome P450 1B1 activity is responsible for metabolism of compounds involved in ocular development (Choudhary et al. 2008; Choudhary et al. 2009).

LTBP2 (Latent transforming growth factor, TGF, β-binding protein 2) was initially identified as the causative gene in patients with early-onset glaucoma from Pakistan and in patients of Gypsy ethnicity (Ali et al. 2009; Narooie-Nejad et al. 2009). The gene is located 1.3 Mb from the GLC3C locus on 14q22; however, *LTBP2* mutations have not been identified in the family initially used to define the GLC3C locus, suggesting that a second congenital glaucoma gene is located in this region (Sharafieh et al. 2013).

Table 1. Genes responsible for early-onset glaucoma

Disease	Juvenile open-angle glaucoma	Anterior segment dysgenesis	Congenital glaucoma	Familial normal-tension glaucoma
Genes	*MYOC*	*PITX2, FOXC1, PAX6*	*CY1B1, LTBP2*	*OPTN, TBK1*
Protein function	Extracellular matrix	Developmental regulation of gene expression	Cytochrome P450 1B1 (*CYP1B1*); extracellular matrix (*LTBP2*)	TNF-α signaling, autophagy
Mutation	Endoplasmic reticulum stress	Abnormal ocular development	Abnormal ocular development	Increased rate retinal ganglion cell apoptosis
Reference(s)	Stone et al. 1997	Gould et al. 1997; Mears et al. 1998; Riise et al. 2001	Stoilov et al. 1997; Ali et al. 2009	Rezaie et al. 2002; Morton et al. 2008

The LTBP2 protein is located in the extracellular matrix, where it associates with micofibrils containing fibrillin-1 (Jelodari-Mamaghani et al. 2013). Interestingly, *LTBP2* mutations have been associated with Weill-Marchesani and Weill-Marchesani-like syndrome, a condition characterized by microspherophakia and abnormal ocular anterior segment development (Haji-Seyed-Javadi et al. 2012). *LTBP2* appears to be a rare cause of congenital glaucoma in ethnically diverse populations, such as in the United States (Lim et al. 2012).

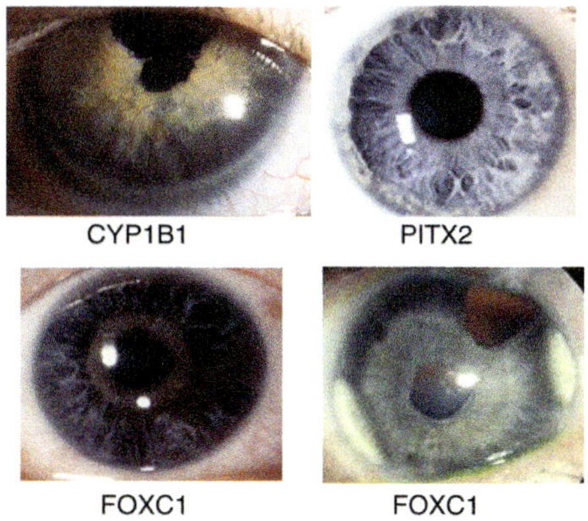

Figure 1. Anterior segment phenotypes in patients with developmental glaucoma. Anterior segment photographs taken with a camera attached to a slit-lamp are shown for four patients with mutations in genes associated with early-onset glaucoma. Notable features are peripheral corneal opacification (CYP1B1), irido-corneal adhesions (PITX2) and iris atrophy (FOXC1). In the patients with FOXC1 mutations the atrophic iris makes it possible to see the pupillary sphincter muscle, which is normally not visible because of overlying iris stroma.

Developmental Glaucoma

Abnormal development of the anterior segment can lead to dysgenesis of critical anterior segment structures involved in glaucoma, including the trabecular outflow pathways and Schlemn's canal. Developmental glaucoma may be syndromic (Axenfeld-Rieger syndrome and aniridia) or limited to only ocular involvement. Some patients with anterior segment dysgenesis never develop glaucoma, whereas others have very severe disease evident at birth (Gould and John 2002). Four genes coding for proteins involved in regulation of gene expression can contribute to developmental glaucoma (*PITX2*, *FOXC1*, *PAX6*, and *LMX1B*). Mutations in these genes cause autosomal dominant disease with high penetrance but variable expressivity both within and among affected families. The phenotypic features of disease caused by these genes, as well as those caused by *CYP1B1* and *LTBP2*, are similar, making it impossible to establish the genetic diagnosis through clinical examination alone (Fig. 1). Genetic testing can establish a molecular diagnosis as well as clarify the inheritance information necessary for accurate genetic counseling.

PITX2 and *LMX1B* cause syndromic forms of developmental glaucoma (Rieger syndrome and Nail-Patella syndrome, respectively). Approximately 50% of patients with *PITX2* mutations develop glaucoma (Reis et al. 2012). Recently, mutations involving a genomic region distal to *PITX2* have been identified as disease causing (Volkmann et al. 2011). Patients with *LMX1B* mutations are affected by Nail-Patella syndrome, which can involve the eye, causing a variety of glaucoma-related features (Chen et al. 1998; Dreyer et al. 1998; Mimiwati et al. 2006). Mutations in *PAX6* cause abnormal development of stem cells in the iris and corneal limbus, resulting in a broad range of clinical features, from agenesis of the iris to corneal opacification caused by a deficiency of limbal stem cells (Hingorani et al. 2009). *FOXC1* was initially identified as a gene responsible for iris hypoplasia (Mears et al. 1998). Subsequent studies have identified cardiac abnormalities and possibly other systemic features in patients with mutations in these genes (Gould et al. 1997; Swiderski et al. 1999; Winnier et al. 1999).

Juvenile-Onset Primary Open-Angle Glaucoma

Patients affected by open-angle glaucoma have disease despite normal anatomic structures.

Adult-onset primary open-angle glaucoma (POAG) develops after 50 years of age, whereas juvenile-onset (or early-onset) open-angle glaucoma affects children and young adults, with onset typically between the ages of 3 and 20. Juvenile open-angle glaucoma is inherited as an autosomal dominant trait (Wiggs et al. 1998) and is characterized by very high IOP (Wiggs et al. 1995; Johnson et al. 1996). Linkage studies using large families have identified a number of juvenile open-angle glaucoma loci: GLC1A (1q24.3-q25.2) (Sheffield et al. 1993), GLC1J (9q22) (Wiggs et al. 2004), GLC1K (20p12) (Wiggs et al. 2004), GLC1M (5q22.1-q32) (Wang et al. 2004; Pang et al. 2006; Fan et al. 2007), and GLC1N (15q22-q24) (Wang et al. 2006). Among these loci only one gene, *MYOC*, coding for myocilin, has been identified (Kubota et al. 1997; Stone et al. 1997). Missense changes in the protein account for 10% of the cases of juvenile open-angle glaucoma and also 3%–5% of the cases of adult-onset POAG (Wiggs et al. 1998; Fingert et al. 1999). Disease-causing mutations are primarily located in the protein's olfactomedin domain (Fig. 2) (Adam et al. 1997; Stone et al. 1997; Fingert et al. 1999). Myocilin is an extracellular protein of unknown function, and loss of the protein function does not result in glaucoma (Wiggs and Vollrath 2001; Kim et al. 2001), suggesting that the underlying genetic mechanism is likely to be a gain-of-function or dominant-negative effect. Additionally, a common nonsense variant located in exon 1 (Fig. 2) is a benign polymorphism and does not cause glaucoma or any other phenotype (Lam et al. 2000). Disease-causing mutations reduce the solubility of the protein, leading to protein misfolding and subsequent protein aggregation in the endoplasmic reticulum (Aroca-Aguilar et al. 2010). The misfolded protein response may lead to a loss of trabecular meshwork cells, resulting in high IOP (Joe et al. 2003). Interestingly, limiting protein aggregation using the small molecule phenyl butyrate (PBA) causes reduction in IOP both in vitro and in vivo, possibly pointing to novel gene-based therapy for patients with myocilin mutations (Yam et al. 2007; Zode et al. 2011, 2012). Recently, common variants in genes coding for multiplexin collagens XV and XVIII have been shown to modify the severity of myocilin-related glau-

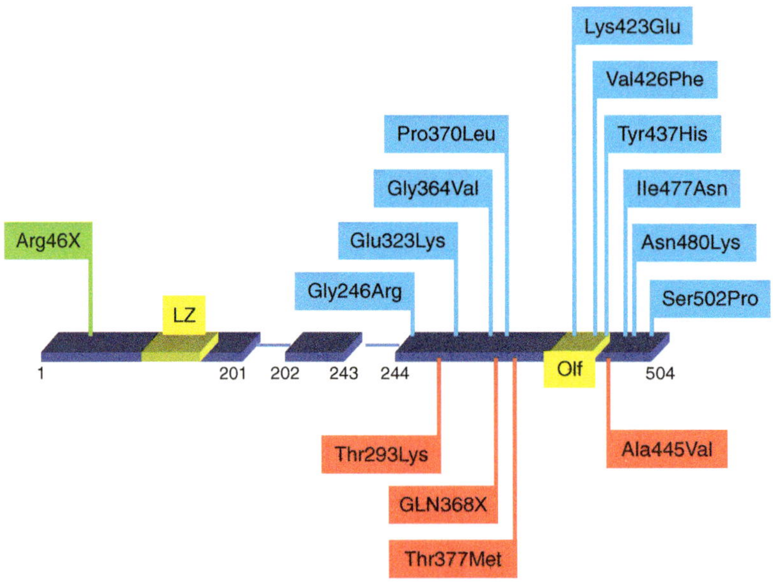

Figure 2. *MYOC* mutations causing glaucoma. The gene location of selected *MYOC* mutations known to cause glaucoma are shown. Exon 1 extends from codon 1–201, exon 2 from codon 202–243, and exon 3 from codon 244–504. Exon 1 contains a leucine zipper (LZ) and exon 3 contains the Olfactomedin domain (Olf). Mutations causing early-onset glaucoma are shown in blue, adult-onset glaucoma in red, and a nonsense mutation known to be a benign polymorphism in green.

coma, suggesting that myocilin may interact with these protein in the extracellular matrix and/or in maintaining the integrity of the trabecular outflow pathways (Liton et al. 2005; Wiggs et al. 2013b).

Familial Normal-Tension Glaucoma

Normal-tension glaucoma (NTG) is a type of open-angle glaucoma characterized by optic nerve degeneration despite normal IOP. Most NTG patients have adult-onset disease; however, rarely, the disease can have early onset with autosomal dominant inheritance. Two genes have been associated with familial NTG: *OPTN* and *TBK1* (Rezaie et al. 2002; Morton et al. 2008; Fingert et al. 2011).

Rare missense mutations in *OPTN*, which encodes optineurin and particularly the E50K mutation, cause a severe early-onset familial form of NTG. (Aung et al. 2005; Morton et al. 2008). Optineurin is involved in basic cellular functions including protein trafficking, maintenance of the Golgi apparatus, as well as the NF-κB pathway, antiviral responses, and antibacterial signaling (Ying 2012). Of interest, optineurin interacts with Tank1 (*TBK1*), which has also been implicated in familial NTG (Morton et al. 2008). The optineurin E50K mutation causes the protein to become inactive and/or insoluble (Minegeshi et al. 2013). This mutation also enhances the interaction of optineurin with Tank1 (Fingert et al. 2011).

COMMON VARIANTS CONTRIBUTING TO ADULT-ONSET GLAUCOMA WITH COMPLEX INHERITANCE

POAG, adult-onset NTG, pseudoexfoliation glaucoma, and primary angle-closure glaucoma are common traits with complex inheritance. Genetic variants contributing to these conditions have been identified using genome-wide association approaches (Thorleifsson et al. 2007, 2010; Burdon et al. 2011; Vithana et al. 2012; Wiggs et al. 2012, 2013a). Generally, variants contributing to common complex traits such as adult-onset glaucoma have small individual effects on disease development. Aggregated effects from multiple risk factors, including environmental risk factors, can have a larger impact. Robust genetic associations have been observed for POAG (*CDKN2BAS* [Burdon et al. 2011; Wiggs et al. 2012], *SIX1/SIX6* [Wiggs et al. 2012], *CAV1/CAV2* [Thorliefsson et al. 2010; Wiggs et al. 2011], *TMCO1* [Burdon et al. 2011]), NTG (*CDKN2BAS* [Wiggs et al. 2012] and a regulatory region on 8q22 [Wiggs et al. 2012]), pseudoexfoliation (*LOXL1* [Thorleifsson et al. 2007]), and primary angle-closure glaucoma (*PLEKHA7* and *COL11A1* [Vithana et al. 2012]) (Table 2). Additionally, genetic variants associated with quantitative ocular traits that are risk factors for common forms of glaucoma have also been identified. These include IOP (van Koolwijk et al. 2012), central corneal thickness (CCT) (Vithana et al. 2011; Lu et al. 2013), and optic nerve parameters including

Table 2. Genes/loci contributing to adult-onset glaucoma

Gene	Disease	Function	Reference(s)
CDKN2BAS	POAG, NTG	Cell cycle regulation, TGF-β signaling	Burdon et al. 2011; Wiggs et al. 2012
TMCO1	POAG	Unknown	Burdon et al. 2011
SIX1/SIX6	POAG	Optic nerve development	Fan et al. 2011; Ramdas et al. 2011
8q22 enhancer	NTG	Regulation of fluid production in ciliary body and choroid plexus	Wiggs et al. 2012
CAV1/CAV2	POAG	Endothelial membranes	Thorleifsson et al. 2010
LOXL1	Pseudoexfoliation	Elastinogenesis and maintenance	Thorleifsson et al. 2007
PLEKHA7	Angle-closure glaucoma	Adherens junction protein	Vithana et al. 2012
COL11A1	Angle-closure glaucoma	Sclera development	Vithana et al. 2012

cup-to-disc ratio and optic nerve area (Ramdas et al. 2010; Macgregor et al. 2010; Axenovich et al. 2011) (Table 3).

The clinical features of POAG generally include both elevated IOP and optic nerve degeneration. Patients with optic nerve disease without elevation of IOP are referred to as the NTG subgroup. Large genome-wide association studies (GWAS) have been completed for POAG in the Icelandic population (Thorleifsson et al. 2010), Australian population (Burdon et al. 2011), and in the United States (Wiggs et al. 2012). The Icelandic study identified a significant association between genetic variants located in the *CAV1/CAV2* genomic region and POAG. This finding has been replicated in a case-control sample from the US (Wiggs et al. 2011) and recently, *CAV1/CAV2* variants have been shown to be preferentially associated with patients who have loss of the central visual field early in the disease (Loomis et al. 2014). Both the Australian and the US studies identified significant associations with *CDKN2BAS*, a long noncoding antisense RNA that inhibits the expression of CDKN2B, an inhibitor of CDK4, a protein involved in promoting cell division (Burdon et al. 2011; Wiggs et al. 2012). The Australian study showed significant association with variants in the *TMCO1* genomic region, a gene that also appears to be associated with elevated IOP (see below). The US study identified significant association with variants in the *SIX1/SIX6* genomic region; these are also associated with the cup-to disc ratio, a quantitative optic nerve parameter (Ramdas et al. 2010; Wiggs et al. 2012).

NTG

Optic nerve degeneration without IOP elevation (<21 mmHg) is the defining clinical feature of NTG. Identifying the genetic factors that contribute to this condition could provide important insights into neuroprotective therapies for glaucoma. An analysis of the NTG subgroup in a large genome-wide association study of POAG using a United States case-control sample identified common variants in the *CDKN2BAS* region and a novel regulatory region on chromosome 8q22 as significant risk factors (Wiggs et al. 2012). The 8q22 region is a DNaseI hypersensitivity site that has high activity in the choroid plexus, which is responsible for the production of cerebrospinal fluid, and the ciliary body, which is responsible for the production of aqueous humor. Interestingly, recent hypotheses suggest that the translaminar pressure across the lamina cribrosa may be a risk factor for optic nerve damage, and this pressure gradient is defined by the difference between the IOP and cerebrospinal fluid pressure (Jonas and Wang 2013).

Pseudoexfoliation Syndrome

Pseudoexfoliation syndrome is a generalized disorder of extracellular matrix that results in a chronic deposition of fibrillar aggregates throughout the ocular anterior segment. Accumulation of the fibrillar material in the trabecular meshwork is thought to contribute to the development of glaucoma associated with this condition (Schlötzer-Schrehardt et al. 1995;

Table 3. Selected genes/loci contributing to quantitative ocular traits related to glaucoma

Gene	Trait	Function	Reference(s)
CDKN2BAS	Cup-to-disc-ratio	Cell cyle regulation, TGF-β signaling	Fan et al. 2011; Ramdas et al. 2011
SIX1/SIX6	Cup-to-disc-ratio	Developmental protein	Fan et al. 2011
ATOH7	Optic nerve area	Developmental protein	Macgregor et al. 2010
TMCO1	IOP	Unknown function	van Koolwijk et al. 2012
GAS7	IOP	Unknown function	van Koolwijk et al. 2012
ZNF469	CCT	Regulates expression of extracellular matrix components	Abu et al. 2008
COL5A1	CCT	Extracellular matrix	Lu et al. 2013
COL8A2	CCT	Extracellular matrix	Vithana et al. 2011

Naumann et al. 1998). A genome-wide association study conducted in the Icelandic population first identified common variants in the *LOXL1* gene as significant risk factors (Thorleifsson et al. 2007). Subsequently, association between *LOXL1* gene variants and pseudoexfoliation has been replicated in populations worldwide (Fan et al. 2011). LOXL1 (lysyl-oxidale like 1) is necessary for formation and maintenance of elastin. It is not yet known how LOXL1 variants influence development of pseudoexfoliation; however, recent evidence suggests that the variants associated with disease cause a decrease in gene expression, possibly resulting in reduced enzyme activity (Schlotzer-Schrehardt 2009). The *LOXL1* risk alleles are very common in pseudoexfoliation cases (95%–99%) but are also common in the normal population (60%–80%) suggesting that the gene variants are necessary but not sufficient for disease development (Fan et al. 2011). Recently, residence in northern latitudes has been identified as an environmental risk factor for this condition (Stein et al. 2011; Kang et al. 2012).

Primary Angle-Closure Glaucoma

Primary angle-closure glaucoma is common in Asian countries. A recent genome-wide association study using five independent Asian case-control samples identified three genomic regions statistically associated with POAG: rs3753841 (*COL11A1*), rs1015213 (located between *PCMTD1* and *ST18*), and rs11024102 (*PLEKHA7*) (Vithana et al. 2012). All of these single-nucleotide polymorphisms were also replicated in a combined Australian-Nepalese case-control sample (Awadalla et al. 2013). *COL11A1* is expressed in the sclera, and mutations in *COL11A1* are known to cause Stickler's syndrome, a condition that includes myopia, among other ocular features (Richards et al. 1996). As primary angle-closure glaucoma can be related to hyperopia, the genome-wide association study results may point to a role for *COL111A1* in development of refractive errors, possibly because of abnormal scleral development.

Quantitative Ocular Traits that Are Risk Factors for Glaucoma

For traits with complex inheritance, it can be useful to identify genetic factors influencing the underlying individual traits, such as IOP, optic nerve parameters, and CCT, that contribute to the overall disease (Charlesworth et al. 2010). These traits are quantitative, highly heritable, and show substantial variation in human populations. IOP is the only modifiable risk factor for glaucoma. Recent genome-wide analyses using normal populations have identified two genes significantly associated with IOP, *GAS7* and *TMCO1* (van Koolwijk et al. 2012). Similar analyses for optic nerve parameters associated with glaucoma risk have identified *CDKN2BAS* and *SIX1SIX6* as genetic risk factors contributing to cup-to-disc-ratio (Ramdas et al. 2010; Fan et al. 2011) and *ATOH7* as an important determinant of optic nerve size (Macgregor et al. 2010). Populations from around the world have been used to identify genetic factors contributing to CCT, one of the most heritable of the quantitative ocular traits (Toh et al. 2005). A recent study from the International Glaucoma Genetics Consortium (IGGC) identified 16 loci significantly associated with CCT (Fig. 3) (Lu et al. 2013). Pathway analyses suggested that collagen and extracellular matrix pathways are important regulators of CCT (Lu et al. 2013).

COMPLEX INTERACTIONS: GENE–ENVIRONMENT, GENE–GENE INTERACTIONS, AND EPIGENETIC EFFECTS

Complex genetic and gene–environment interactions are expected to contribute to the genetic architecture of common adult-onset disorders. Nutritional factors, such as dietary fat, antioxidant intake, and other lifestyle factors including smoking and postmenopausal hormone use may influence the development of POAG (Pasquale and Kang 2009). A gene–environment interaction involving hormone replacement therapy and *NOS3* (the gene coding for nitric oxide synthase 3) has been identified as a risk

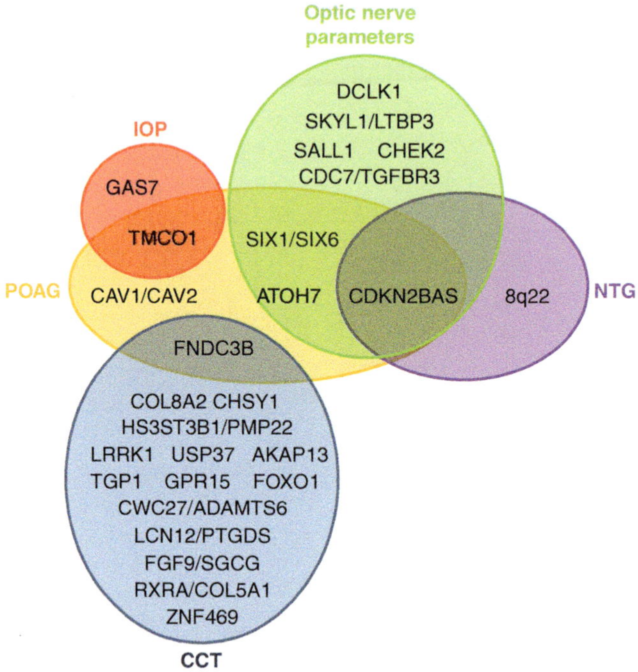

Figure 3. Gene and genomic regions with common variants that contribute to glaucoma and glaucoma-related ocular quantitative traits. Variants contributing to both primary open-angle glaucoma and normal tension glaucoma as well as selected ocular quantitative traits (CCT, IOP, and optic nerve parameters) are shown. Gene names are presented in dark font. Genes contributing to POAG are contained in the orange ellipse, NTG in the purple ellipse, CCT in the blue ellipse, IOP in the red ellipse, and optic nerve parameters in the green ellipse. Genes that contribute to more than one trait are indicated by their placement in the overlapping regions. For example, *CDKN2BAS* contributes to NTG, POAG, and to optic nerve parameters.

factor for POAG (Kang et al. 2010). The estrogen metabolism pathway is also associated with POAG in women (Pasquale et al. 2013). Gene–gene interactions contributing to POAG have been suggested for *WDR36* and *p53* (both influencing apoptosis) (Blanco-Marchite et al. 2011) and for genetic variants in *ATOH7* and *SIX1/SIX6* (Fan et al. 2011).

BIOLOGICAL PATHWAYS AND PROCESSES SUGGESTED BY GENETIC VARIANTS CONTRIBUTING TO GLAUCOMA

Genome-wide association studies have identified multiple genes potentially involved in glaucoma pathogenesis; however, the stringent correction for multiple testing and type I error identifies only variants with the largest main effects as statistically significant (Manolio et al. 2008). Many biologically meaningful associations of smaller effect size may go undetected; including variants with smaller effect size in systematic groups could reveal novel biological pathways or systems underlying disease susceptibility. Pathway-based analysis groups gene variants into biologically meaningful entities to distinguish the actual from the false-positive associations. In short, this type of analysis can be used to uncover additional genotype–phenotype associations that the single-allele genome-wide association analysis may have missed. Hypothesis-independent pathway analyses suggest that the underlying molecular pathogenesis of POAG involves a broad range of biological processes, including cell adhesion, immune responsiveness, energy metabolism, and neurotransmission (Cooke Bailey et al. 2013). Identification of genes contributing to both early-onset and adult-onset forms of glaucoma are also highlighting biological pathways and processes of importance to glaucoma pathogenesis. Several of these are discussed below.

Extracellular Matrix Metabolism

Maintenance of extracellular matrix is emerging as an important theme in glaucoma pathogenesis (Acott et al. 2008; Crawford Downs et al. 2011). Several of the genes contributing to early-onset glaucoma (*MYOC, LTBP2, COL18A1*) and adult-onset glaucoma (*LOXL1*) have important roles in extracellular matrix (Ueda et al. 2002; Ali et al. 2009; Sethi et al. 2011; Wiggs et al. 2013b), and three important genes related to CCT impact extracellular matrix (Lu et al. 2013). Further investigation of genes shown to contribute to extracellular processes in ocular tissues relevant to glaucoma could be of interest.

Transforming Growth Factor β (TGF-β) Signaling

TGF-β I and TGF-β II appear to have important roles in optic nerve degeneration (Zode et al. 2009; Fuchshofer 2011) as well as trabecular meshwork function (Sethi et al. 2011; Fuchshofer 2012). *LTPB2* (associated with congenital glaucoma and anterior segment dysgenesis) and *CDKN2BAS* (associated with POAG, NTG) are part of the overall TGF-β signaling pathway. Additionally, NTG pathway analysis showed significant association with the TGF-β signaling pathway overall (Wiggs et al. 2012).

Tumor Necrosis Factor α (TNF-α) Signaling

Both genes contributing to familial NTG (*OPTN, TBK1*) can impact TNF-α signaling (Fingert et al. 2011). Blocking of the TNF-α receptor in an animal model of glaucoma appears to be neuroprotective (Roh et al. 2012). These results suggest that TNF-α signaling can have an important role in ganglion cell apoptosis in glaucoma. Higher levels of soluble TNF-α have been identified in women before the development of NTG (Kang et al. 2013), a finding consistent with this hypothesis.

Estrogen Metabolism

The hormone 17β-estradiol can regulate expression of both *CAV1* and *NOS3* (both associated with POAG), and loss of caveolin-1 function can cause increased expression of *NOS3* (Zhou et al. 2009; Sud et al. 2010), suggesting an interaction between these proteins. Additionally, P450 1B1 (*CYP1B1*, associated with congenital glaucoma) is an important factor in estrogen metabolism (Hanna et al. 2000). Gender effects in glaucoma have also been suggested by studies showing that estrogen receptors are expressed on the retinal ganglion cells of the optic nerve (Munaut et al. 2001), and that estrogen may have a neuroprotective effect in animal models of glaucoma (Zhou et al. 2007; Russo et al. 2008). Further studies examining gender effects in POAG, and gender interactions with genes contributing to this disorder will be of interest.

CONCLUDING REMARKS

Genes responsible for both early-onset and adult-onset glaucoma have been identified using genetic and genomic technologies and approaches. Family-based genetic linkage analyses have yielded disease-causing genes for early-onset glaucoma, whereas genome-wide association studies have identified genes and genomic regions contributing to adult-onset forms of the disease. Biological pathways contributing to glaucoma and other complex interactions (gene–gene and gene–environment) are emerging. Future directions for new gene discovery include whole exome sequencing and other next generation sequencing technologies, genome-wide association studies using larger numbers of cases and controls and including rare variant analyses, and further evaluation of the contributions of biological pathways, gene–gene and gene–environment interactions.

REFERENCES

Abu A, Frydman M, Marek D, Pras E, Nir U, Reznik-Wolf H, Pras E. 2008. Deleterious mutations in the Zinc-Finger 469 gene cause brittle cornea syndrome. *Am J Hum Genet* **82:** 1217–1222.

Acott TS, Kelley MJ. 2008. Extracellular matrix in the trabecular meshwork. *Exp Eye Res* **86:** 543–561.

Adam MF, Belmouden A, Binisti P, Brézin AP, Valtot F, Béchetoille A, Dascotte JC, Copin B, Gomez L, Chaventré A, et al. 1997. Recurrent mutations in a single exon encoding the evolutionarily conserved olfactomedin-homology domain of TIGR in familial open-angle glaucoma. *Hum Mol Genet* **6.12:** 2091–2097.

Akarsu A, Nurten M, Erol Turacli S, Gulderen Aktan, Magda Barsoum-Homsy, Line Chevrette, B, Sitki Sayli, Mansoor Sarfarazi. 1996. A second locus (*GLC3B*) for primary congenital glaucoma (Buphthalmos) maps to the 1p36 region. *Hum Mol Genet* **5:** 1199–1203.

Ali M, McKibbin M, Booth A, Parry DA, Jain P, Riazuddin SA, Hejtmancik JF, Khan SN, Firasat S, Shires M, et al. 2009. Null mutations in *LTBP2* cause primary congenital glaucoma. *Am J Hum Genet* **84:** 664–671.

Aponte EP, Diehl N, Mohney BG. 2010. Incidence and clinical characteristics of childhood glaucoma: A population-based study. *Arch Ophthalmol* **128:** 478–482.

Aroca-Aguilar JD, Martínez-Redondo F, Sánchez-Sánchez F, Coca-Prados M, Escribano J. 2010. Functional role of proteolytic processing of recombinant myocilin in self-aggregation. *Invest Ophthalmol Vis Sci* **51:** 72–78.

Aung T, Rezaie T, Okada K, Viswanathan AC, Child AH, Brice G, Bhattacharya SS, Lehmann OJ, Sarfarazi M, Hitchings RA. 2005. Clinical features and course of patients with glaucoma with the E50K mutation in the optineurin gene. *Invest Ophthalmol Vis Sci* **46:** 2816–2822.

Awadalla MS, Thapa SS, Hewitt AW, Burdon KP, Craig JE. 2013. Association of genetic variants with primary angle closure glaucoma in two different populations. *PLoS ONE* **8:** e67903.

Axenovich T, Zorkoltseva I, Belonogova N, van Koolwijk LM, Borodin P, Kirichenko A, Babenko V, Ramdas WD, Amin N, Despriet DD, et al. 2011. Linkage and association analyses of glaucoma related traits in a large pedigree from a Dutch genetically isolated population. *J Med Genet* **48:** 802–809.

Bejjani BA, Stockton DW, Lewis RA, Tomey KF, Dueker DK, Jabak M, Astle WF, Lupski JR. 2000. Multiple *CYP1B1* mutations and incomplete penetrance in an inbred population segregating primary congenital glaucoma suggest frequent de novo events and a dominant modifier locus. *Hum Mol Genet* **9:** 367–374.

Blanco-Marchite C, Sánchez-Sánchez F, López-Garrido MP, Iñigez-de-Onzoño M, López-Martínez F, López-Sánchez E, Alvarez L, Rodríguez-Calvo PP, Méndez-Hernández C, Fernández-Vega L, et al. 2011. *WDR36* and *P53* gene variants and susceptibility to primary open-angle glaucoma: Analysis of gene-gene interactions. *Invest Ophthalmol Vis Sci* **52:** 8467–8478.

Burdon KP, Macgregor S, Hewitt AW, Sharma S, Chidlow G, Mills RA, Danoy P, Casson R, Viswanathan AC, Liu JZ, et al. 2011. Genome-wide association study identifies susceptibility loci for open angle glaucoma at *TMCO1* and *CDKN2B-AS1*. *Nat Genet* **43:** 574–578.

Chakrabarti S, Ghanekar Y, Kaur K, Kaur I, Mandal AK, Rao KN, Parikh RS, Thomas R, Majumder PP. 2010. A polymorphism in the *CYP1B1* promoter is functionally associated with primary congenital glaucoma. *Hum Mol Genet* **19:** 4083–4090.

Charlesworth J, Kramer PL, Dyer T, Diego V, Samples JR, Craig JE, Mackey DA, Hewitt AW, Blangero J, Wirtz MK. 2010. The path to open-angle glaucoma gene discovery: Endophenotypic status of intraocular pressure, cup-to-disc ratio, and central corneal thickness. *Invest Ophthalmol Vis Sci* **51:** 3509–3514.

Chen H, Lun Y, Ovchinnikov D, Kokubo H, Oberg KC, Pepicelli CV, Can L, Lee B, Johnson RL. 1998. Limb and kidney defects in *Lmx1b* mutant mice suggest an involvement of *LMX1B* in human nail patella syndrome. *Nat Genet* **19:** 51–55.

Choudhary D, Jansson I, Sarfarazi M, Schenkman JB. 2008. Characterization of the biochemical and structural phenotypes of four *CYP1B1* mutations observed in individuals with primary congenital glaucoma. *Pharmacogenet Genomics* **18:** 665–676.

Choudhary D, Jansson I, Schenkman JB. 2009. *CYP1B1*, a developmental gene with a potential role in glaucoma therapy. *Xenobiotica* **39:** 606–615.

Cooke Bailey JN, Sobrin L, Pericak-Vance MA, Haines JL, Hammond CJ, Wiggs JL. 2013. Advances in the genomics of common eye diseases. *Hum Mol Genet* **22:** R59–R65.

Crawford Downs J, Roberts MD, Sigal IA. 2011. Glaucomatous cupping of the lamina cribrosa: A review of the evidence for active progressive remodeling as a mechanism. *Exp Eye Res* **93:** 133–140.

Dreyer SD, Zhou G, Baldini A, Winterpacht A, Zabel B, Cole W, Johnson RL, Lee B. 1998. Mutations in *LMX1B* cause abnormal skeletal patterning and renal dysplasia in nail patella syndrome. *Nat Genet* **19:** 47–50.

Fan BJ, Ko WC, Wang DY, Canlas O, Ritch R, Lam DS, Pang CP. 2007. Fine mapping of new glaucoma locus *GLC1M* and exclusion of neuregulin 2 as the causative gene. *Mol Vis* **13:** 779–784.

Fan BJ, Wang DY, Pasquale LR, Haines JL, Wiggs JL. 2011. Genetic variants associated with optic nerve vertical cup-to-disc ratio are risk factors for primary open angle glaucoma in a US Caucasian population. *Invest Ophthalmol Vis Sci* **52:** 1788–1792.

Fingert JH, Héon E, Liebmann JM, Yamamoto T, Craig JE, Rait J, Kawase K, Hoh ST, Buys YM, Dickinson J, et al. 1999. Analysis of myocilin mutations in 1703 glaucoma patients from five different populations. *Hum Mol Genet* **8:** 899–905.

Fingert JH, Robin AL, Stone JL, Roos BR, Davis LK, Scheetz TE, Bennett SR, Wassink TH, Kwon YH, Alward WL, et al. 2011. Copy number variations on chromosome 12q14 in patients with normal tension glaucoma. *Hum Mol Genet* **20:** 2482–2494.

Fuchshofer R. 2011. The pathogenic role of transforming growth factor-β2 in glaucomatous damage to the optic nerve head. *Exp Eye Res* **93:** 165–169.

Fuchshofer R, Tamm ER. 2012. The role of TGF-β in the pathogenesis of primary open-angle glaucoma. *Cell Tissue Res* **347:** 279–290.

Gould DB, John SW. 2002. Anterior segment dysgenesis and the developmental glaucomas are complex traits. *Hum Mol Genet* **11:** 1185–1193.

Gould DB, Mears AJ, Pearce WG, Walter MA. 1997. Autosomal dominant Axenfeld-Rieger anomaly maps to 6p25. *Am J Hum Genet* **61:** 765–768.

Haji-Seyed-Javadi R, Jelodari-Mamaghani S, Paylakhi SH, Yazdani S, Nilforushan N, Fan JB, Klotzle B, Mahmoudi MJ, Ebrahimian MJ, Chelich N, et al. 2012. *LTBP2* mutations cause Weill-Marchesani and Weill-Marchesani-like syndrome and affect disruptions in the extracellular matrix. *Hum Mutat* **33:** 1182–1187.

Hanna IH, Dawling S, Roodi N, Guengerich FP, Parl FF. 2000. Cytochrome P450 *1B1* (*CYP1B1*) pharmacogenetics: Association of polymorphisms with functional differences in estrogen hydroxylation activity. *Cancer Res* **60:** 3440–3444.

Hingorani M, Williamson KA, Moore AT, Van Heyningen V. 2009. Detailed ophthalmologic evaluation of 43 individuals with *PAX6* mutations. *Invest Ophthalmol Vis Sci* **14:** 2581–2590.

Jelodari-Mamaghani S, Haji-Seyed-Javadi R, Suri F, Nilforushan N, Yazdani S, Kamyab K, Elahi E. 2013. Contribution of the latent transforming growth factor-β binding protein 2 gene to etiology of primary open angle glaucoma and pseudoexfoliation syndrome. *Mol Vis* **19:** 333–347.

Joe MK, Sohn S, Hur W, Moon Y, Choi YR, Kee C. 2003. Accumulation of mutant myocilins in ER leads to ER stress and potential cytotoxicity in human trabecular meshwork cells. *Biochem Biophys Res Commun* **312:** 592–600.

Johnson AT, Richards JE, Boehnke M, Stringham HM, Herman SB, Wong DJ, Lichter PR. 1996. Clinical phenotype of juvenile-onset primary open-angle glaucoma linked to chromosome 1q. *Ophthalmology* **103:** 808–814.

Jonas JB, Wang N. 2013. Cerebrospinal fluid pressure and glaucoma. *J Ophthalmic Vis Res* **8:** 257–263.

Kang JH, Wiggs JL, Rosner BA, Hankinson SE, Abdrabou W, Fan BJ, Haines J, Pasquale LR. 2010. Endothelial nitric oxide synthase gene variants and primary open-angle glaucoma: Interactions with sex and postmenopausal hormone use. *Invest Ophthalmol Vis Sci* **51:** 971–979.

Kang JH, Loomis S, Wiggs JL, Stein JD, Pasquale LR. 2012. Demographic and geographic features of exfoliation glaucoma in 2 United States-based prospective cohorts. *Ophthalmology* **119:** 27–35.

Kang JH, Wiggs JL, Pasquale LR. 2013. A nested case control study of plasma ICAM-1, E-selectin and TNF receptor 2 levels, and incident primary open-angle glaucoma. *Invest Ophthalmol Vis Sci* **54:** 1797–1804.

Kim BS, Savinova OV, Reedy MV, Martin J, Lun Y, Gan L, Smith RS, Tomarev SI, John SW, Johnson RL. 2001. Targeted disruption of the myocilin gene (*Myoc*) suggests that human glaucoma-causing mutations are gain of function. *Mol Cell Biol* **21:** 7707–7713.

Kubota R, Noda S, Wang Y, Minoshima S, Asakawa S, Kudoh J, Mashima Y, Oguchi Y, Shimizu N. 1997. A novel myosin-like protein (myocilin) expressed in the connecting cilium of the photoreceptor: Molecular cloning, tissue expression, and chromosomal mapping. *Genomics* **41:** 360–369.

Lam DS, Leung YF, Chua JK, Baum L, Fan DS, Choy KW, Pang CP. 2000. Truncations in the *TIGR* gene in individuals with and without primary open-angle glaucoma. *Invest Ophthalmol Vis Sci* **41:** 1386–1391.

Lim SH, Tran-Viet KN, Yanovitch TL, Freedman SF, Klemm T, Call W, Powell C, Ravichandran A, Metlapally R, Nading EB, et al. 2013. *CYP1B1*, *MYOC*, and *LTBP2* mutations in primary congenital glaucoma patients in the United States. *Am J Ophthalmol* **155:** 508–517.

Liton PB, Liu X, Stamer WD, Challa P, Epstein DL, Gonzalez P. 2005. Specific targeting of gene expression to a subset of human trabecular meshwork cells using the chitinase 3-like 1 promoter. *Invest Ophthalmol Vis Sci* **46:** 183–190.

Loomis SJ, Kang JH, Weinreb RN, Yaspan BL, Cooke Bailey JN, Gaasterland D, Gaasterland T, Lee RK, Lichter PR, Budenz DL, Liu Y, et al. 2014. Association of CAV1/CAV2 genomic variants with primary open-angle glaucoma overall and by gender and pattern of visual field loss. *Ophthalmology* **121:** 508–516.

Lu Y, Vitart V, Burdon KP, Khor CC, Bykhovskaya Y, Mirshahi A, Hewitt AW, Koehn D, Hysi PG, Ramdas WD, et al. 2013. Genome-wide association analyses identify multiple loci associated with central corneal thickness and keratoconus. *Nat Genet* **45:** 155–163.

Macgregor S, Hewitt AW, Hysi PG, Ruddle JB, Medland SE, Henders AK, Gordon SD, Andrew T, McEvoy B, Sanfilippo PG, et al. 2010. Genome-wide association identifies *ATOH7* as a major gene determining human optic disc size. *Hum Mol Genet* **19:** 2716–2724.

Manolio TA, Brooks LD, Collins FS. 2008. A HapMap harvest of insights into the genetics of common disease. *J Clin Invest* **118:** 1590–1605.

Mears AJ, Jordan T, Mirzayans F, Dubois S, Kume T, Parlee M, Ritch R, Koop B, Kuo WL, Collins C, et al. 1998. Mutations of the Forkhead/Winged-Helix gene, *FKHL7*, in patients with Axenfeld-Rieger anomaly. *Am J Hum Genet* **63:** 1316–1328.

Michels-Rautenstrauss KG, Mardin CY, Zenker M, Jordan N, Gusek-Schneider GC, Rautenstrauss BW. 2001. Primary congenital glaucoma: Three case reports on novel mutations and combinations of mutations in the GLC3A (*CYP1B1*) gene. *J Glaucoma* **10:** 354–357.

Mimiwati Z, Mackey DA, Craig JE, Mackinnon JR, Rait JL, Liebelt JE, Ayala-Lugo R, Vollrath D, Richards JE. 2006. Nail-patella syndrome and its association with glaucoma: A review of eight families. *Br J Ophthalmol* **90:** 1505–1509.

Minegishi Y, Iejima D, Kobayashi H, Chi ZL, Kawase K, Yamamoto T, Seki T, Yuasa S, Fukuda K, Iwata T. 2013. Enhanced optineurin E50K–TBK1 interaction evokes protein insolubility and initiates familial primary open-angle glaucoma. *Hum Mol Genet* **22:** 3559–3567.

Morton S, Hesson L, Peggie M, Cohen P. 2008. Enhanced binding of TBK1 by an optineurin mutant that causes a familial form of primary open angle glaucoma. *FEBS Lett* **582:** 997–1002.

Munaut C, Lambert V, Noël A, Frankenne F, Deprez M, Foidart JM, Rakic JM. 2001. Presence of oestrogen receptor type β in human retina. *Br J Ophthalmol* **85:** 877–882.

Narooie-Nejad M, Paylakhi SH, Shojaee S, Fazlali Z, Kanavi MR, Nilforushan N, Yazdani S, Babrzadeh F, Suri F, Ronaghi M, et al. 2009. Loss of function mutations in the gene encoding latent transforming growth factor β binding protein 2, *LTBP2*, cause primary congenital glaucoma. *Hum Mol Genet* **18:** 3969–3977.

Naumann GO, Schlötzer-Schrehardt U, Küchle M. 1998. Pseudoexfoliation syndrome for the comprehensive ophthalmologist: Intraocular and systemic manifestations. *Ophthalmology* **105:** 951–968.

Pang CP, Fan BJ, Canlas O, Wang DY, Dubois S, Tam PO, Lam DS, Raymond V, Ritch R. 2006. A genome-wide scan maps a novel juvenile-onset primary open angle glaucoma locus to chromosome 5q. *Mol Vis* **12:** 85–92.

Pasquale LR, Kang JH. 2009. Lifestyle, nutrition and glaucoma. *J Glaucoma* **18:** 423.

Pasquale LR, Loomis SJ, Weinreb RN, Kang JH, Yaspan BL, Bailey JC, Gaasterland D, Gaasterland T, Lee RK, Scott WK, et al. 2013. Estrogen pathway polymorphisms in relation to primary open angle glaucoma: An analysis accounting for gender from the United States. *Mol Vis* **19:** 1471–1481.

Ramdas WD, van Koolwijk LM, Ikram MK, Jansonius NM, de Jong PT, Bergen AA, Isaacs A, Amin N, Aulchenko YS, Wolfs RC, et al.. 2010. A genome-wide association study of optic disc parameters. *PLoS Genet* **6:** e1000978.

Ramdas WD, van Koolwijk LM, Ikram MK, Jansonius NM, de Jong PT, Bergen AA, Isaacs A, Amin N, Aulchenko YS, Wolfs RC, et al. 2011. Common genetic variants associated with open-angle glaucoma. *Hum Mol Genet* **20:** 2464–2471.

Reis LM, Tyler RC, Volkmann Kloss BA, Schilter KF, Levin AV, Lowry RB, Zwijnenburg PJ, Stroh E, Broeckel U, Murray JC, et al. 2012. *PITX2* and *FOXC1* spectrum of mutations in ocular syndromes. *Eur J Hum Genet* **20:** 1224–1233.

Rezaie T, Child A, Hitchings R, Brice G, Miller L, Coca-Prados M, Héon E, Krupin T, Ritch R, Kreutzer D, et al. 2002. Adult-onset primary open-angle glaucoma caused by mutations in optineurin. *Science* **295:** 1077–1079.

Richards AJ, Yates JR, Williams R, Payne SJ, Pope FM, Scott JD, Snead MP. 1996. A family with Stickler syndrome type 2 has a mutation in the *COL11A1* gene resulting in the substitution of glycine 97 by valine in a1(XI) collagen. *Hum Mol Genet* **5:** 1339–1343.

Riise R, Storhaug K, Brøndum-Nielsen K. 2001. Rieger syndrome is associated with PAX6 deletion. *Acta Ophthalmol Scand* **79:** 201–203.

Roh M, Zhang Y, Murakami Y, Thanos A, Lee SC, Vavvas DG, Benowitz LI, Miller JW. 2012. Etanercept, a widely used inhibitor of tumor necrosis factor-α (TNF-α), prevents retinal ganglion cell loss in a rat model of glaucoma. *PLoS ONE* **7:** e40065.

Russo R, Cavaliere F, Watanabe C, Nucci C, Bagetta G, Corasaniti MT, Sakurada S, Morrone LA. 2008. 17β-Estradiol prevents retinal ganglion cell loss induced by acute rise of intraocular pressure in rat. *Prog Brain Res* **173:** 583–590.

Sarfarazi M, Stoilov I. 2000. Molecular genetics of primary congenital glaucoma. *Eye* **14:** 422–428.

Sarfarazi M, Akarsu NA, Hossain A, Turacli EM, Aktan GS, Barsoum-Homsy M, Chevrette L, Sayli SB. 1995. Assignment of a locus (GLC3A) for primary congenital glaucoma (Buphthalmos) to 2p21 and evidence for genetic heterogeneity. *Genomics* **30:** 2171–2177.

Schlötzer-Schrehardt U. 2009. Molecular pathology of pseudoexfoliation syndrome/glaucoma—New insights from *LOXL1* gene associations. *Exp Eye Res* **88:** 776–785.

Schlötzer-Schrehardt U, Naumann GO. 1995. Trabecular meshwork in pseudoexfoliation syndrome with and without open-angle glaucoma. A morphometric, ultrastructural study. *Invest Ophthalmol Vis Sci* **36:** 1750–1764.

Sethi A, Mao W, Wordinger RJ, Clark AF. 2011. Transforming growth factor–β induces extracellular matrix protein cross-linking lysyl oxidase (*LOX*) genes in human trabecular meshwork cells. *Invest Ophthalmol Vis Sci* **52:** 5240–5250.

Sharafieh R, Child AH, Khaw PT, Fleck B, Sarfarazi M. 2013. *LTBP2* gene analysis in the *GLC3C*-linked family and 94 *CYP1B1*-negative cases with primary congenital glaucoma. *Ophthalmic Genet* **34:** 14–20.

Sheffield VC, Stone EM, Alward WL, Drack AV, Johnson AT, Streb LM, Nichols BE. 1993. Genetic linkage of familial open angle glaucoma to chromosome 1q21-q31. *Nat Genet* **4:** 47–50.

Sowers MR, Wilson AL, Kardia SR, Chu J, McConnell DS. 2006. *CYP1A1* and *CYP1B1* polymorphisms and their association with estradiol and estrogen metabolites in women who are premenopausal and perimenopausal. *Am J Med* **119:** S44–S51.

Stein JD, Pasquale LR, Talwar N, Kim DS, Reed DM, Nan B, Kang JH, Wiggs JL, Richards JE. 2011. Geographic and climatic factors associated with exfoliation syndrome. *Arch Ophthalmol* **129:** 1053–1060.

Stoilov I, Akarsu AN, Sarfarazi M. 1997. Identification of three different truncating mutations in cytochrome P4501B1 (*CYP1B1*) as the principal cause of primary congenital glaucoma (Buphthalmos) in families linked to the GLC3A locus on chromosome 2p21. *Hum Mol Genet* **6:** 641–647.

Stoilov IR, Sarfarazi M. 2002. The third genetic locus (GLC3C) for primary congenital glaucoma (PCG) maps to chromosome 14q24.3. *Invest Ophthalmol Vis Sci* **43:** E3015.

Stone EM, Fingert JH, Alward WL, Nguyen TD, Polansky JR, Sunden SL, Nishimura D, Clark AF, Nystuen A, Nichols BE, et al. 1997. Identification of a gene that causes primary open angle glaucoma. *Science* **275:** 668–670.

Sud N, Wiseman DA, Black SM. 2010. Caveolin 1 is required for the activation of endothelial nitric oxide synthase in response to 17β-estradiol. *Mol Endocrinol* **24:** 1637–1649.

Swiderski RE, Reiter RS, Nishimura DY, Alward WL, Kalenak JW, Searby CS, Stone EM, Sheffield VC, Lin JJ. 1999. Expression of the *Mf1* gene in developing mouse hearts: Implication in the development of human congenital heart defects. *Dev Dyn* **216:** 16–27.

Thorleifsson G, Magnusson KP, Sulem P, Walters GB, Gudbjartsson DF, Stefansson H, Jonsson T, Jonasdottir A, Jonasdottir A, Stefansdottir G, et al. 2007. Common sequence variants in the *LOXL1* gene confer susceptibility to exfoliation glaucoma. *Science* **317:** 1397–1400.

Thorleifsson G, Walters GB, Hewitt AW, Masson G, Helgason A, DeWan A, Sigurdsson A, Jonasdottir A, Gudjonsson SA, Magnusson KP, et al. 2010. Common variants near *CAV1* and *CAV2* are associated with primary open-angle glaucoma. *Nat Genet* **42:** 906–909.

Toh T, Liew SH, MacKinnon JR, Hewitt AW, Poulsen JL, Spector TD, Gilbert CE, Craig JE, Hammond CJ, Mackey DA. 2005. Central corneal thickness is highly heritable:

The twin eye studies. *Invest Ophthalmol Vis Sci* **46:** 3718–3722.

Tokizane T, Shiina H, Igawa M, Enokida H, Urakami S, Kawakami T, Ogishima T, Okino ST, Li LC, Tanaka Y, et al. 2005. Cytochrome *P*450 1B1 is overexpressed and regulated by hypomethylation in prostate cancer. *Clin Cancer Res* **11:** 5793–5801.

Tsuchiya Y, Nakajima M, Yokoi T. 2005. Cytochrome P450-mediated metabolism of estrogens and its regulation in human. *Cancer Lett* **227:** 115–124.

Ueda J, Wentz-Hunter K, Yue BY. 2002. Distribution of myocilin and extracellular matrix components in the juxtacanalicular tissue of human eyes. *Invest Ophthalmol Vis Sci* **43:** 1068–1076.

van Koolwijk LM, Ramdas WD, Ikram MK, Jansonius NM, Pasutto F, Hysi PG, Macgregor S, Janssen SF, Hewitt AW, Viswanathan AC, et al. 2012. Common genetic determinants of intraocular pressure and primary open-angle glaucoma. *PLoS Genet* **8:** e1002611.

Vithana EN, Aung T, Khor CC, Cornes BK, Tay WT, Sim X, Lavanya R, Wu R, Zheng Y, Hibberd ML, et al. 2011. Collagen-related genes influence the glaucoma risk factor, central corneal thickness. *Hum Mol Genet* **20:** 649–658.

Vithana EN, Khor CC, Qiao C, Nongpiur ME, George R, Chen LJ, Do T, Abu-Amero K, Huang CK, Low S, et al. 2012. Genome-wide association analyses identify three new susceptibility loci for primary angle closure glaucoma. *Nat Genet* **44:** 1142–1146.

Volkmann BA, Zinkevich NS, Mustonen A, Schilter KF, Bosenko DV, Reis LM, Broeckel U, Link BA, Semina EV. 2011. Potential novel mechanism for Axenfeld-Rieger syndrome: Deletion of a distant region containing regulatory elements of *PITX2*. *Invest Ophthalmol Vis Sci* **52:** 1450–1459.

Wang DY, Fan BJ, Canlas O, Tam PO, Ritch R, Lam DS, Fan DS, Pang CP. 2004. Absence of myocilin and optineurin mutations in a large Philippine family with juvenile onset primary open angle glaucoma. *Mol Vis* **10:** 851–856.

Wang DY, Fan BJ, Chua JK, Tam PO, Leung CK, Lam DS, Pang CP. 2006. A genome-wide scan maps a novel juvenile-onset primary open-angle glaucoma locus to 15q. *Invest Ophthalmol Vis Sci* **47:** 5315–5321.

Wiggs JL, Vollrath D. 2001. Molecular and clinical evaluation of a patient hemizygous for *TIGR/MYOC*. *Arch Ophthalmol* **119:** 1674–1678.

Wiggs JL, Del Bono EA, Schuman JS, Hutchinson BT, Walton DS. 1995. Clinical features of five pedigrees genetically linked to the juvenile glaucoma locus on chromosome 1q21-q31. *Ophthalmology* **102:** 1782–1789.

Wiggs JL, Allingham RR, Vollrath D, Jones KH, De La Paz M, Kern J, Patterson K, Babb VL, Del Bono EA, Broomer BW, et al. 1998. Prevalence of mutations in TIGR/Myocilin in patients with adult and juvenile primary open-angle glaucoma. *Am J Hum Genet* **63:** 1549–1552.

Wiggs JL, Lynch S, Ynagi G, Maselli M, Auguste J, Del Bono EA, Olson LM, Haines JL. 2004. A genomewide scan identifies novel early-onset primary open-angle glaucoma loci on 9q22 and 20p12. *Am J Hum Genet* **74:** 1314–1320.

Wiggs JL, Kang JH, Yaspan BL, Mirel DB, Laurie C, Crenshaw A, Brodeur W, Gogarten S, Olson LM, Abdrabou W, et al. 2011. Common variants near CAV1 and CAV2 are associated with primary open-angle glaucoma in Caucasians from the USA. *Hum Mol Genet* **20:** 4707–4713.

Wiggs JL, Kang JH, Yaspan BL, Mirel DB, Laurie C, Crenshaw A, Brodeur W, Gogarten S, Olson LM, Abdrabou W, et al. 2012. Common variants at 9p21 and 8q22 are associated with increased susceptibility to optic nerve degeneration in glaucoma. *PLoS Genet* **8:** e1002654.

Wiggs JL, Hauser MA, Abdrabou W, Allingham RR, Budenz DL, Delbono E, Friedman DS, Kang JH, Gaasterland D, Gaasterland T, et al. 2013a. The NEIGHBOR Consortium primary open-angle glaucoma genome-wide association study: Rationale, study design, and clinical variables. *J Glaucoma* **22:** 517–525.

Wiggs JL, Howell GR, Linkroum K, Abdrabou W, Hodges E, Braine CE, Pasquale LR, Hannon GJ, Haines JL, John SW. 2013b. Variations in *COL15A1* and *COL18A1* influence age of onset of primary open angle glaucoma. *Clin Genet* **84:** 167–174.

Winnier GE, Kume T, Deng K, Rogers R, Bundy J, Raines C, Walter MA, Hogan BL, Conway SJ. 1999. Roles for the winged helix transcription factors MF1 and MFH1 in cardiovascular development revealed by nonallelic noncomplementation of null alleles. *Dev Biol* **213:** 418–431.

Yam GH, Gaplovska-Kysela K, Zuber C, Roth J. 2007. Sodium 4-phenylbutyrate acts as a chemical chaperone on misfolded myocilin to rescue cells from endoplasmic reticulum stress and apoptosis. *Invest Ophthalmol Vis Sci* **48:** 1683–1690.

Ying H, Yue BY. 2012. Cellular and molecular biology of optineurin. *Int Rev Cell Mol Biol* **294:** 223–258.

Zhou X, Li F, Ge J, Sarkisian SR, Tomita H, Zaharia A, Chodosh J, Cao W. 2007. Retinal ganglion cell protection by 17-β-estradiol in a mouse model of inherited glaucoma. *Dev Neurobiol* **67:** 603–616.

Zhou YY, Zhao Y, Mirza MK, Huang JH, Potula HHSK, Vogel SM, Brovkovych V, Yuan JXJ, Wharton J, Malik AB. 2009. Persistent eNOS activation secondary to caveolin-1 deficiency induces pulmonary hypertension in mice and humans through PKG nitration. *J Clin Invest* **119:** 2009–2018.

Zode GS, Clark AF, Wordinger RJ. 2009. Bone morphogenetic protein 4 inhibits TGF-β2 stimulation of extracellular matrix proteins in optic nerve head cells: Role of gremlin in ECM modulation. *Glia* **57:** 755–766.

Zode GS, Kuehn MH, Nishimura DY, Searby CC, Mohan K, Grozdanic SD, Bugge K, Anderson MG, Clark AF, Stone EM, et al. 2011. Reduction of ER stress via a chemical chaperone prevents disease phenotypes in a mouse model of primary open angle glaucoma. *J Clin Invest* **121:** 3542–3553.

Zode GS, Bugge KE, Mohan K, Grozdanic SD, Peters JC, Koehn DR, Anderson MG, Kardon RH, Stone EM, Sheffield VC. 2012. Topical ocular sodium 4-phenylbutyrate rescues glaucoma in a myocilin mouse model of primary open-angle glaucoma. *Invest Ophthalmol Vis Sci* **53:** 1557–1565.

Differential Gene Expression in Glaucoma

Tatjana C. Jakobs

Department of Ophthalmology, Massachusetts Eye and Ear Infirmary, Harvard Medical School, Boston, Massachusetts 02114

Correspondence: tatjana_jakobs@meei.harvard.edu

In glaucoma, regardless of its etiology, retinal ganglion cells degenerate and eventually die. Although age and elevated intraocular pressure (IOP) are the main risk factors, there are still many mysteries in the pathogenesis of glaucoma. The advent of genome-wide microarray expression screening together with the availability of animal models of the disease has allowed analysis of differential gene expression in all parts of the eye in glaucoma. This review will outline the findings of recent genome-wide expression studies and discuss their commonalities and differences. A common finding was the differential regulation of genes involved in inflammation and immunity, including the complement system and the cytokines transforming growth factor β (TGF-β) and tumor necrosis factor α (TNF-α). Other genes of interest have roles in the extracellular matrix, cell–matrix interactions and adhesion, the cell cycle, and the endothelin system.

The term glaucoma refers to a group of diseases that lead to the degeneration and eventual death of ganglion cells, the retina's projection neurons. There is wide agreement that elevated IOP and age are the most important risk factors (Quigley 2011), and that the ganglion cells die by apoptosis (Quigley et al. 1995; Qu et al. 2010). However, the exact sequence of events that leads to ganglion cell degeneration is not fully understood.

Although it is the loss of ganglion cells that leads to visual impairment, pathological changes in glaucoma have been demonstrated in most structures of the eye. In the anterior chamber, the major structures regulating production and outflow of aqueous humor, including the ciliary body, the trabecular meshwork, and Schlemm's canal, can be affected (Johnson 2006; Coca-Prados and Escribano 2007; Tamm 2009). The retina and, in particular, the ganglion cells themselves (Danias et al. 2003; Jakobs et al. 2005; Schlamp et al. 2006; Morgan 2012) are affected. Finally, the optic nerve head (ONH), including the lamina cribrosa (Hernandez 2000; Hernandez et al. 2008; Roberts et al. 2009; Burgoyne 2011), the optic nerve proper (Nakazawa et al. 2006), and the central projection targets of the ganglion cells in the lateral geniculate body and the superior colliculus (Gupta et al. 2007; Liu et al. 2011) all can display pathological changes in glaucoma.

The advent of animal models for glaucoma and the wide availability of genome-wide expression analysis techniques have led to a considerable number of recent studies that address gene expression changes associated with glauco-

Cite this article as *Cold Spring Harb Perspect Med* doi: 10.1101/cshperspect.a020636

ma (Yang and Zack 2011). Transcriptome-wide expression studies are generally better at generating hypotheses than at elucidating mechanisms, and the differences in animal models and expression profiling methods have introduced a lot of experimental variation. However, several common themes have emerged. This review will summarize recent advances in gene expression profiling studies of glaucoma, considering each anatomical location in turn.

DIFFERENTIAL GENE EXPRESSION IN STRUCTURES OF THE ANTERIOR EYE

The production and outflow of aqueous humor has a direct relation to IOP, and pharmacological interventions to lower IOP are still the first-line treatment for glaucoma. Aqueous humor is produced by the ciliary epithelium. Although there is at present no published study which specifically compares ciliary epithelia from glaucomatous and nonglaucomatous eyes, gene expression profiling of the normal epithelium or the whole ciliary body has been carried out (Coca-Prados et al. 1999; Janssen et al. 2012; Wagner et al. 2013). It has been demonstrated that the ciliary epithelium is a source of proteins in the aqueous humor (Escribano et al. 1995; Escribano and Coca-Prados 2002), and that several glaucoma-related genes are expressed in this tissue, most notably myocilin and CYP1B1 (Coca-Prados and Escribano 2007; Janssen et al. 2012). In addition, the ciliary epithelium produces a variety of neuroendocrine factors, such as natriuretic peptides, neurotensin, and somatostatin (Coca-Prados and Escribano 2007). Their potential role in regulating the production of aqueous humor and their influence on outflow resistance is an intriguing topic for further research.

The trabecular meshwork and the wall of Schlemm's canal are major points of resistance for the outflow of aqueous humor (Tamm 2009), and morphological changes of the trabecular meshwork in glaucoma are apparent using both light and electron microscopy (Lutjen-Drecoll et al. 1981; Rohen et al. 1981; Tektas and Lutjen-Drecoll 2009; Tektas et al. 2010). Microarray studies of gene expression have been conducted using isolated trabecular meshwork cells, organ cultures, and fresh tissue from a variety of animal models and humans (Gonzalez et al. 2000; Ishibashi et al. 2002; Lo et al. 2003; Vittitow and Borras 2004; Zhao et al. 2004; Diskin et al. 2006; Liton et al. 2006; Rozsa et al. 2006; Fan et al. 2008; Wang et al. 2008a; Danias et al. 2011; Liu et al. 2013). The conditions assayed in these studies were primary open angle glaucoma, elevated pressure, and treatment of trabecular meshwork cells with steroids or TGF-β. Because of the differences in experimental models and microarray platforms used in these studies, the results have varied considerably. For instance, myocilin was found to be induced by dexamethasone treatment of cultured human trabecular meshwork cells (Ishibashi et al. 2002; Lo et al. 2003; Fan et al. 2008), confirming other studies (Polansky et al. 1997; Nguyen et al. 1998), but was not observed in the bovine trabecular meshwork after steroid treatment (Danias et al. 2011). Several studies identified mediators of inflammation or immunity in the trabecular meshwork, such as up-regulation of interleukin (IL) 6 by elevated IOP (Gonzalez et al. 2000), up-regulation of the IL6 receptor in glaucoma (Diskin et al. 2006), and up-regulation of IL8 in response to steroid treatment (Lo et al. 2003). One study, which investigated differential regulation at the mRNA and protein level after treatment of human trabecular meshwork cells with TGF-β1 and TGF-β2, found that the classes of genes most up-regulated by TGF-β encoded extracellular matrix proteins and other extracellular proteins, including versican (Zhao et al. 2004). In glaucoma, TGF-β2 levels in the aqueous humor are elevated compared to controls (Inatani et al. 2001; Picht et al. 2001), and TGF-β2 is also involved in the regulation of some matricellular proteins like secreted protein, acidic and rich in cystein (SPARC) (Kang et al. 2013). The up-regulation of extracellular proteins in response to TGF-β is an interesting mechanical link between high IOP and increased outflow resistance.

DIFFERENTIAL GENE EXPRESSION IN THE GLAUCOMATOUS RETINA

As retinal ganglion cells are the main cell type vulnerable to glaucomatous degeneration, many

 Cite this article as *Cold Spring Harb Perspect Med* doi: 10.1101/cshperspect.a020636

studies have been undertaken to find the underlying molecular causes of their vulnerability and the processes that are responsible for their eventual death. In these studies, several different models and species have been employed. In one model, usually used in rats but more recently also in mice, elevated IOP results from obliteration of the episcleral veins caused by an injection of hypertonic saline solution (Morrison et al. 1997; Walsh et al. 2009). Translimbal laser photocoagulation of the trabecular meshwork has also been used to increase the IOP in one eye of rats and monkeys (Miyahara et al. 2003; Yang et al. 2007). Retinal ganglion cells degenerate reproducibly after axotomy (Berkelaar et al. 1994). Although not models of glaucoma per se, optic nerve crush and optic nerve transection have been used to induce ganglion cell death (Yang et al. 2007; Agudo et al. 2008). Finally, the mouse strain DBA/2J develops glaucoma secondary to iris stroma disease caused by two mutations in the genes *Gpnmb* and *Tyrp1* (Anderson et al. 2002). These mice develop an increase in IOP at ~6 mo of age, followed by a sectorial degeneration of retinal ganglion cells (Danias et al. 2003; Jakobs et al. 2005; Libby et al. 2005; Schlamp et al. 2006). Among the studies that used an ocular hypertension model, some have assayed differential gene expression in the whole retina (Miyahara et al. 2003; Ahmed et al. 2004; Walsh et al. 2009), and others have analyzed cells isolated from the ganglion cell layer by laser capture microdissection (Guo et al. 2010, 2011; Wang et al. 2010). For microarray analysis in the inherited glaucoma models in mice (DBA/2J) and rats (RCS-rdy$^-$), whole retinas were used (Naskar and Thanos 2006; Steele et al. 2006; Panagis et al. 2010, 2011; Howell et al. 2011). This is an important consideration because the retina is a complex tissue, and ganglion cells make up only 1% of the neurons in the retina (Jeon et al. 1998). In addition to the neuronal cells, there are also macroglia (Mueller cells and astrocytes), microglia, and vascular cell types.

Despite these differences in models and sample preparation, the studies share many common findings. One of them is the prominent up-regulation of genes involved in the inflammatory and immune response. For instance, several studies reported up-regulation of lipocalin 2, both after an increase of IOP and in DBA/2J mice (Ahmed et al. 2004; Steele et al. 2006; Yang et al. 2007; Guo et al. 2010, 2011; Howell et al. 2011). Lipocalin 2 is a general marker of tissue response to injury and is up-regulated among others by IL1β, IL17, and TNF-α (Li and Chan 2011). It has also emerged as a marker of astrocyte reactivity in the brain (Zamanian et al. 2012). Other immune response genes found to be up-regulated in glaucoma models include α-2-macroglobulin, MHC class II RT1.u-D-α chain, Interferon-induced transmembrane protein 1 (Ifitm3/Fgls), and Chemokine (C-C motif) ligand 12 (Ahmed et al. 2004; Steele et al. 2006; Guo et al. 2010). Of particular interest among the immune response genes are members of the complement cascade. Most studies identified at least one member of the complement cascade as significantly up-regulated (Miyahara et al. 2003; Ahmed et al. 2004; Piri et al. 2006; Steele et al. 2006; Yang et al. 2007; Panagis et al. 2010; Wang et al. 2010; Howell et al. 2011). Importantly, complement up-regulation seems to precede morphological signs of ganglion cell degeneration in the DBA/2J model (Howell et al. 2011). The complement system was recently found to mediate synapse elimination in the CNS (Stevens et al. 2007). Synapses are decorated with complement and stripped off the dendrites by microglia (Schafer et al. 2012). This mechanism, physiological during CNS maturation, may be pathologically reactivated in the glaucomatous retina and lead to synapse loss followed by dendritic remodeling (Stephan et al. 2012). Members of the complement cascade are expressed at the mRNA and protein levels in several models of glaucoma, as well as in other types of retinal insult, such as a direct tear injury (Vazquez-Chona et al. 2004; Kuehn et al. 2006, 2008; Stasi et al. 2006). Finally, genetic disruption of the complement cascade is highly protective of ganglion cells in the DBA/2J model of glaucoma (Howell et al. 2011).

Ganglion cells die by apoptosis in glaucoma and after axotomy (Garcia-Valenzuela et al. 1994, 1995; Quigley et al. 1995; Qu et al. 2010). In retinal ganglion cells isolated after induction of elevated IOP, genes involved in apoptosis and response to oxidative stress (such as Angptl4, Ednrb, and Pnkp) were among the most up-regulated, whereas genes involved in neuronal development and function (including Gja1, Snap25, and Gabrg2) were down-regulated (Wang et al. 2010). The same study found that several prosurvival genes were significantly down-regulated, but the prosurvival gene STAT3 was up-regulated at the mRNA, and protein levels and glaucomatous retinas showed increased labeling for the phosphorylated, active form of STAT3 (Wang et al. 2010). The up-regulation of STAT3 seems to be relatively specific for glaucomatous damage, as it was not observed after optic nerve transection or ischemia/reperfusion injury (Yoshimura et al. 2003; Yang et al. 2007). A simultaneous up-regulation of proapoptotic and antiapoptotic genes (like the caspase inhibitor IAP1) was also observed in a rat model of increased IOP and optic nerve transection (Levkovitch-Verbin et al. 2006b). This suggests that there is a balance between protective and detrimental processes when the ganglion cells are threatened by injury. Conceivably, this balance could be tilted in favor of the protective side by timely therapeutic intervention. As an example of such a strategy, minocycline, an anti-inflammatory and neuroprotective second-generation tetracycline, was found to delay retinal ganglion cell death in a rat model of glaucoma (Levkovitch-Verbin et al. 2006a). Both ocular hypertension and optic nerve transection lead to up-regulation of immediate early response genes. C-Jun, Junb, and Atf3 (activating transcription factor 3) were up-regulated in both models (Yang et al. 2007; Guo et al. 2010). These factors are downstream from JNK, and the phosphorylated, active form of JNK is present at increased levels in glaucoma (Kwong and Caprioli 2006; Levkovitch-Verbin et al. 2007). Therefore, blocking the activation of the JNK pathway may also be of therapeutic benefit in glaucoma. In an attempt to identify other pathways that are involved in ganglion cell degeneration and death and that may be amenable to drug treatment, Welsbie and coworkers recently identified dual leucine zipper kinase (DLK) via RNAi-based screening (Welsbie et al. 2013). DLK inhibition promotes ganglion cell survival in in vitro cultures and in vivo after optic nerve injury. Importantly, a small molecule inhibitor of DLK, tozasertib, administered intraocularly with drug-eluting microspheres, protected ganglion cells after optic nerve transection (Welsbie et al. 2013).

Another pathway that was differentially regulated in several studies is the endothelin/endothelin receptor system (Ahmed et al. 2004; Yang et al. 2007; Panagis et al. 2010; Howell et al. 2011). Endothelin 2 (Edn2) up-regulation occurs in the retina and the ONH before morphological signs of glaucomatous damage are observed in DBA/2J mice (Howell et al. 2011). Endothelins exist in three isoforms and exert their effects through two types of receptors (Davenport 2002). They are potent vasoconstrictors and have been found to be elevated in the aqueous humor of glaucoma patients (Noske et al. 1997; Tezel et al. 1997). Intraocular administration of endothelin 1 leads to acute blockage of axonal transport (Taniguchi et al. 2006; Wang et al. 2008b), optic neuropathy, and ganglion cell loss (Chauhan et al. 2004; Sasaoka et al. 2006). It was recently shown that endothelin 2, which binds to the same receptors as endothelin 1, also causes ganglion cell loss and optic nerve damage (Howell et al. 2011). In DBA/2J mice, endothelin 2 is expressed by retinal microglia, and administration of bosentan, an inhibitor of both types of endothelin receptors, protects ganglion cells in this model (Howell et al. 2011).

Microglial activation in the retina and the ONH are among the earliest changes in the DBA/2J mouse model of glaucoma (Bosco et al. 2008, 2011). Consistent with this, an up-regulation of Aif1 was observed in retinas after elevation of IOP (Ahmed et al. 2004). In a mouse model of ocular hypertension that assayed gene expression before the onset of retinal cell apoptosis, serum amyloid A (SAA), too, was found to be up-regulated in retinal microglia (Walsh et al. 2009). It is interesting in this context that SAA is also up-regulated in the glaucomatous trabecular meshwork (Wang et al. 2008a). Microglial activation may be detrimental to ganglion cell survival. A possible mechanism involves TNF-α, whose levels are elevated in the retina and ONH of glaucoma patients (Yan et al. 2000; Yuan and Neufeld 2000, 2001; Sawada et al. 2010). In a mouse model of glaucoma, TNF-α was found to mediate the cytotoxic effects of elevated IOP on ganglion cells, and injection of TNF-α led to ganglion cell death and optic neuropathy (Nakazawa et al. 2006). The source of the TNF-α in the retina seems to be a population of microglia that resides around the ONH and becomes activated in ocular hypertension (Roh et al. 2012). Importantly, the TNF-α-decoy receptor etanercept prevents ganglion cell loss and optic nerve pathology in this model (Roh et al. 2012).

GENE EXPRESSION IN THE ONH IN GLAUCOMA

Experimental evidence points to the ONH as the site of initial insult to retinal ganglion cell axons in glaucoma. Most importantly, the topology of ganglion cell loss in glaucoma and the resulting visual field defects (radial in humans, sectorial in rodents), is difficult to explain without reference to the ONH because there the ganglion cell axons run in bundles with topological relationship to the retina (Danias et al. 2003; Jakobs et al. 2005; Schlamp et al. 2006; Howell et al. 2007; Soto et al. 2011; Nickells et al. 2012). In humans this region contains the lamina cribrosa, a stack of collagenous plates with pores through which the ganglion cells' axons pass (Quigley and Addicks 1981). An increase in IOP leads to increased pressure across the lamina cribrosa and mechanical strain within it (Burgoyne 2011). This may cause direct mechanical injury to the axons, as they are compressed against this rigid structure. Indeed, blockage of axonal transport has been identified in the region of the lamina cribrosa (Quigley and Addicks 1980; Quigley et al. 1981; Johansson 1983, 1988; Balaratnasingam et al. 2007). This may lead to an interruption of retrograde transport of neurotrophic factors, such as brain-derived neurotrophic factor (BDNF), to the ganglion cell body, followed by degeneration of the cell (Pease et al. 2000; Quigley et al. 2000). However, a rigid lamina cribrosa is not necessary to develop glaucoma. Rodents are susceptible to the disease, yet mice do not show staining for any collagen other than collagen 4 associated with blood vessels, and the ONH of rats contains only sparse collagenous septa (Morrison et al. 1995; May and Lutjen-Drecoll 2002; Sun et al. 2009). A commonality between ONH of humans and all other species, including rodents, is that this region contains an abundance of astrocytes that line the pores of the lamina cribrosa and ensheath the axons, or, in rodents, form glial tubes around axon bundles that visually resemble a lamina cribrosa so much that they are referred to as the "glial lamina" (Morcos and Chan-Ling 2000; Howell et al. 2007; Sun et al. 2009). In addition to astrocytes, the human laminar region contains lamina cribrosa cells (Hernandez et al. 1988). Although negative for the astrocyte marker glial fibrillary acidic protein (GFAP), lamina cribrosa cells have many similarities to ONH astrocytes, and may be a subtype of astrocyte (Lambert et al. 2001; Zode et al. 2007; Nickells et al. 2012). The ONH also contains microglia/macrophages and endothelial cells. Given the importance of the ONH in glaucoma, several studies have addressed differential gene expression in this tissue. Cultured astrocytes and lamina cribrosa cells and whole tissues from a variety of models, including ocular hypertension following episcleral vein injection, the DBA/2J mouse, and human glaucoma, have been used.

In reaction to injury to the CNS, astrocytes become reactive. Originally, astrocyte reactivity was described as an up-regulation of GFAP and cellular hypertrophy, but it has become clear that astrocyte reactivity is a complex process that involves differential gene expression and morphological changes (Sofroniew 2005; Sofroniew and Vinters 2010; Sun and Jakobs 2012). In glaucoma, too, ONH astrocytes show signs of reactivity (Hernandez and Pena 1997; Hernandez 2000; Lye-Barthel et al. 2013). To characterize astrocyte reactivity in glaucoma, Hernandez and coworkers (2002) cultured astrocytes from normal human eyes and from donors with primary open angle glaucoma and subjected them to microarray screening. They found an up-regulation of genes involved in cell motility and migration, including gelsolin, periplakin, and LIM binding protein 1, and a down-regulation of genes associated with attachment, such as several integrins and chondroitin sulfate proteoglycan 4. Astrocytes from glaucomatous donors did indeed migrate faster than did normal astrocytes in an in vitro assay of migration. In glaucomatous astrocytes there is also evidence for increased signaling by insulin-like growth factor II and the TGF-β receptor (Hernandez et al. 2002). More recently, microarray screening and pathway analysis was applied to immunopurified ONH astrocytes from normal and glaucomatous donors (Nikolskaya et al. 2009). Processes that were up-regulated in glaucoma were the complement system, signal transduction (e.g., NF-κB, SP1, VDR, AP-1, STAT5), the inflammatory and immune response, nervous system development, and cell adhesion. Fewer pathways were down-regulated; among them were platelet-derived growth factor signaling, membrane trafficking, and signal transduction via G-α1. Some of these changes could be interpreted as being neuroprotective, such as the up-regulation of VDR and AP-1, whereas others, namely the activation of NF-κB and complement, may contribute to a neurotoxic activity of ONH astrocytes toward the axons of ganglion cell (Nikolskaya et al. 2009). A different approach, also making use of astrocytes cultured from human donors, was taken in a recent study that compared the transcriptome of normal astrocytes from African American versus Caucasian American donors (Miao et al. 2008). As African Americans are affected by primary open angle glaucoma more often than are Caucasians (Leske 2007), this study aimed at finding underlying differences in the astrocytes of these populations. Astrocytes from African American donors showed higher expression of genes that are associated with cAMP signaling (adenylatecylase 3 and 9), intracellular vesicular transport, G protein signaling (such as regulator of G protein signaling 5, RGS5), and protein phosphatases. Astrocytes from African Americans also showed decreased cell adhesion and increased cell migration, and expressed significantly more elastin. Finally, glutathione-metabolizing enzymes were up-regulated in astrocytes from African American donors, and glutathione levels were lower, which may hint at a compromised antioxidant response in these cells (Miao et al. 2008). Although these results do not fully explain the higher vulnerability of African Americans to primary open angle glaucoma, it is possible that in this population the ONH astrocytes exhibit an increased tendency to become reactive, which may be associated with higher cell mobility in the ONH, and are less able to withstand oxidative stress and protect ganglion cell axons from threatened injury.

One of the characteristics of primary open angle glaucoma is a remodeling of the ONH accompanied by deposition of fibrotic material (Hernandez and Ye 1993), including collagens I, IV, and VI, and the disruption of normal elastin fibers (Morrison et al. 1990; Quigley et al. 1991a,b; Fukuchi et al. 1992; Hernandez 1992; Hernandez et al. 1994; Hernandez and Pena 1997). Lamina cribrosa cells synthesize extracellular matrix in the human ONH. In a recent study, Kirwan and coworkers (2009) performed microarray screening on lamina cribrosa cells cultured from normal and glaucomatous human optic nerves. Among the functional categories most significantly up-regulated were extracellular matrix, collagen, and extracellular space. The most highly regulated gene was periostin, a secreted protein involved in adhesion and differentiation that is up-regulated under conditions of tissue stress such as myocardial pressure overload (Litvin et al. 2005). Other genes up-regulated in glaucomatous lamina cribrosa cells included dystrophin, cartilage linking protein, SPARC, thrombospondin 1, TGF-β1, and collagens I, V, and XI; in contrast, fibulin 1, decorin, and collagen VIII were down-regulated (Kirwan et al. 2009). These results are indicative of a profibrotic state of the glaucomatous lamina cribrosa cells. Recently, the same data set was used in a graph-clustering approach that identified three clusters of differentially regulated genes, including genes involved in axon guidance (such as BDNF), the basal cell carcinoma pathway (such as frizzled family receptor 2 and 7), and cell adhesion (such as versican and integrin α4) (Luo et al. 2013).

Cell cultures from ONH astrocytes have the advantage that they contain only one defined cell population. On the other hand, cells in culture tend to undergo changes in their gene expression profile. Several studies have therefore used whole ONH tissue for analysis. Although the majority of the cells in the ONH are astrocytes, microglia, and endothelial cells, axons are also present; and each of them contribute to the total RNA being analyzed. Johnson and coworkers (2007, 2011) used unilateral injection of hypertonic saline into the episcleral veins in rats to induce ocular hypertension and compared the transcriptome of the experimental eye with the control eye. Biological processes that were significantly regulated in the ocular hypertension group included cell proliferation (cyclin D1 was up-regulated 3.5-fold), immune response (including all members of the complement 1 complex, F_C receptor, and β2 microglobulin), ribosomal and lysosomal genes, and extracellular matrix (including periostin and tenascin C). The isoforms of TGF-β were differentially regulated: expression of TGF-β 1 increased while that of TGF-β 2 decreased slightly with elevated IOP. The up-regulation of cell proliferation genes corresponded to an increase in cellularity of the ONH (Johnson et al. 2007). In an attempt to characterize early changes in response to ocular hypertension, Johnson and coworkers used microarray analysis of ONHs with only minimal axon damage (Johnson et al. 2011). Cell cycle genes displayed the greatest up-regulation, followed by cytoskeletal genes and immune process genes. Several cytokines were among the most highly up-regulated genes, for example, leukemia inhibitory factor (LIF), Clcf1, and IL6. The up-regulation of these IL6-like cytokines could have a variety of effects on the ONH: all three can induce astrocytic differentiation from precursor cells (Klein et al. 1997; Uemura et al. 2002) and they may be neuroprotective (Leibinger et al. 2009; Suzuki et al. 2009). LIF has recently been shown to mediate the neuroprotective effect of preconditioning with moderate oxidative stress in the retina (Chollangi et al. 2009). The expression of IL6-like cytokines in the early phase of ocular hypertension may therefore be indicative of a protective role of the ONH glia. Whole ONHs were also used for microarray screening in a recent study that made use of the ocular laser-induced hypertension model in cynomolgus macaques (Kompass et al. 2008). The most important finding was that early in the course of the disease, before the appearance of visual field defects, retinal ganglion cells make an attempt at regeneration as evidenced by the appearance of $GAP43^+$ and $pNEFH^+$ growth cones. Astrocytes apparently facilitated this attempt by expressing neuroprotective factors such as apolipoprotein E, cellular retinol binding protein 1, and pigment epithelium—derived factor (Kompass et al. 2008).

Using the DBA/2J inherited mouse model of glaucoma, Howell and coworkers (2011, 2012) characterized the early stages of molecular changes in the ONH. Before the onset of morphological signs of axon degeneration, over 400 genes were differentially expressed compared to a control strain that does not develop glaucoma (D2-$Gpnmb^+$). Pathways that were up-regulated early in the disease process involved the immune response, chemotaxis, and leukocyte activation. Cell–matrix interaction genes were up-regulated at a slightly later stage in the disease; these included tenascin C, which has also been identified in the glaucomatous optic nerve by immunohistochemistry (Pena et al. 1999), as well as various integrins, fibronectin 1, Timp 1 and 2, and several collagens. Up-regulation of endothelin 2 and several members of the complement cascade was observed at early stages in the optic nerve as well as in the retina (Howell et al. 2011). A pathway that is activated very early in the optic nerve of DBA/2J mice compared to nonglaucomatous controls is the leukocyte transendothelial migration pathway, characterized, e.g., by the genes for P- and E-selectins (Howell et al. 2012). It was shown recently that whole-body irradiation protects ganglion cells from glaucomatous degeneration (Anderson et al. 2005). In an extension of this study, Howell and coworkers (2012) found that irradiation of the eye was equally protective, and that in irradiated eyes the up-regulation of P-selectin and monocyte entry into the eye did not occur. Irradiation also had a mitigating effect on microglial activation in the ONH while having minimal effect on the astrocytes (Bosco et al. 2012). These important results underscore the implication of neuroinflammatory events in the pathogenesis of glaucoma.

The crush model of damage to the optic nerve has the advantage that the onset of the injury is clearly defined and it lends itself to time-course studies. Astrocyte reactivity after optic nerve crush follows a biphasic temporal pattern: in the first phase (lasting days) after the injury, astrocytes reduce their special coverage, retract processes and become "amoeboid" in shape; in a second phase ($>$14 d after injury), they re-extend long processes and resume a more normal appearance (Sun et al. 2010). Analysis of differentially expressed genes after optic nerve crush revealed that the changes occur in three partially overlapping waves: a first wave of genes involved in inflammation and immunity (1–7 d), a second wave of genes involved in cell cycle and proliferation (3–7 d), followed by a slower wave of genes involved in extracellular matrix restructuring, cell–matrix interaction, and debris removal. By 3 mo after the optic nerve crush, the tissue reached a stationary phase that reflects structural changes in the axons (Qu and Jakobs 2013). Cell labeling with BrdU revealed that it was primarily the microglial population that proliferated rather than the astrocytes in this model (Qu and Jakobs 2013).

GENE EXPRESSION IN THE OPTIC NERVE PROPER

In contrast to the glial lamina, in which astrocytes ensheath the unmyelinated axons, the optic nerve proper contains myelinating oligodendrocytes in addition to astrocytes, microglia, and NG2-cells. Oligodendrocyte death may be an early event in optic nerve damage caused by increased IOP. In a mouse model of laser-induced ocular hypertension, TNF-α levels were increased in the retina followed by oligodendrocyte loss in the optic nerve that preceded ganglion cell death (Nakazawa et al. 2006). Although no study so far has compared gene expression in the optic nerve proper with that of the glial lamina in glaucoma, in some studies parts of the myelinated optic nerve were analyzed together with the glial lamina (Johnson et al. 2007; Qu and Jakobs 2013). Not surprisingly, optic nerve damage is accompanied by down-regulation of oligodendrocyte-specific genes. For example, among the genes that were permanently down-regulated after optic nerve crush was oligodendrocyte transcription factor 1, myelin-associated oligodendrocytic basic protein, and myelin basic protein (Qu and Jakobs 2013). Recently, Nguyen and coworkers identified a novel function of astrocytes in the myelination transition zone behind the glial lamina. These astrocytes express the phagocytic marker Mac-2. The astrocytes up-regulate this protein in glaucoma, and they engulf and internalize evulsed material from the ganglion cell axons (Nguyen et al. 2011). Astrocytes have been shown to be phagocytically active in vitro and in vivo (Kalmar et al. 2001; Ito et al. 2007), and constitutively express several genes involved in phagocytosis (Cahoy et al. 2008). Thus, dysregulated phagocytosis of axonal material may play a role in glaucomatous neuropathy.

GENE EXPRESSION IN THE CENTRAL PROJECTING TARGETS OF THE GANGLION CELLS

At present, no transcriptome-wide expression study has targeted the superior colliculus or the lateral geniculate nucleus in glaucoma. Although dendritic changes in the lateral geniculate nucleus have been described in glaucoma, their molecular mechanisms remain unclear (Liu et al. 2011). The lateral geniculate nucleus of monkeys with experimental glaucoma also shows signs of reactive gliosis, as GFAP and S100β expression was increased (Dai et al. 2012).

CONCLUDING REMARKS

Despite the experimental differences, a number of common themes have emerged. A consistent finding is the involvement of immune and inflammatory pathways in all tissues of the eye in glaucoma. An example of this is the up-regulation of members of the complement cascade in retina and ONH. Up-regulation of complement is of course not specific for glaucoma. Complement factors have been identified as constituents of drusen in age-related macular degeneration, and several genetic studies have associated variants of complement factor genes with this disease (Anderson et al. 2010). Complement up-regulation is also a factor in Alzheimer's disease and many other neurodegenerative diseases (Stephan et al. 2012). As complement has been shown to play a role in synapse elimination, its up-regulation in the glaucomatous retina may mediate synapse elimination followed by remodeling of ganglion cell dendrites (Stevens et al. 2007). Complement factors are also up-regulated in the glaucomatous ONH, although its role there is presently unclear (Howell et al. 2011). Another common finding is the up-regulation of proinflammatory cytokines, most notably TNF-α and TGF-β, and of genes regulated by them. This is of importance for new treatment approaches to glaucoma. A TNF-α antagonist has already been used in animal studies to ameliorate ganglion cell loss caused by ocular hypertension (Roh et al. 2012). As TNF-α antagonists are already approved for therapy of rheumatoid arthritis, these drugs could have a place in glaucoma therapy as well. Another pathway that has been implicated in the pathogenesis of glaucoma by several studies is the endothelin/endothelin receptor system. This pathway, too, is a potential target for therapeutic intervention.

There is much evidence that glial reactivity, both of astrocytes and microglia, is a feature of the glaucomatous optic nerve, but it is less clear whether glial reactivity is a helpful or a deleterious response. Astrocytes produce TNF-α as a response to elevated IOP (Tezel and Wax 2000), which may in turn stimulate the production of nitric oxide (Neufeld 1999; Shareef et al. 1999; Yuan and Neufeld 2000). This has led to the concept of "misbehaving glia" in glaucoma (Neufeld and Liu 2003). The mechanism of ganglion cell damage through up-regulation of nitric oxide synthetase is still controversial, however, as other studies have found no evidence of enhanced nitric oxide production (Pang et al. 2005; Libby et al. 2007). On the other hand, reactive astrocytes have been shown to exert beneficial effects on neurons (Bush et al. 1999; Faulkner et al. 2004; Myer et al. 2006; Okada et al. 2006), and astrocyte reactivity per se is not immediately harmful to ganglion cell axons (Sun et al. 2013). It is possible that the initial reaction of astrocytes to elevated IOP is indeed neuroprotective and only if this response is overwhelmed, as is the case in severe or prolonged insult, do the astrocytes react by forming a permanent glial scar.

Genome-wide microarray expression screening has unearthed a wealth of information about the reactions of different tissues of the eye to increased IOP and glaucoma. Several new leads to novel therapeutic approaches to the disease have been identified and the coming years may see some of them come into clinical practice.

ACKNOWLEDGMENTS

The author would like to thank Drs. Richard Masland, Daniel Sun, Hee Joo Choi, and Ms. Elizabeth Zawidzka for critically reading the manuscript.

REFERENCES

Agudo M, Perez-Marin MC, Lonngren U, Sobrado P, Conesa A, Canovas I, Salinas-Navarro M, Miralles-Imperial J, Hallbook F, Vidal-Sanz M. 2008. Time course profiling of the retinal transcriptome after optic nerve transection and optic nerve crush. *Mol Vis* **14:** 1050–1063.

Ahmed F, Brown KM, Stephan DA, Morrison JC, Johnson EC, Tomarev SI. 2004. Microarray analysis of changes in mRNA levels in the rat retina after experimental elevation of intraocular pressure. *Invest Ophthalmol Vis Sci* **45:** 1247–1258.

Anderson MG, Smith RS, Hawes NL, Zabaleta A, Chang B, Wiggs JL, John SW. 2002. Mutations in genes encoding melanosomal proteins cause pigmentary glaucoma in DBA/2J mice. *Nat Genet* **30:** 81–85.

Anderson MG, Libby RT, Gould DB, Smith RS, John SW. 2005. High-dose radiation with bone marrow transfer prevents neurodegeneration in an inherited glaucoma. *Proc Natl Acad Sci* **102:** 4566–4571.

Anderson DH, Radeke MJ, Gallo NB, Chapin EA, Johnson PT, Curletti CR, Hancox LS, Hu J, Ebright JN, Malek G, et al. 2010. The pivotal role of the complement system in aging and age-related macular degeneration: Hypothesis re-visited. *Prog Retin Eye Res* **29:** 95–112.

Balaratnasingam C, Morgan WH, Bass L, Matich G, Cringle SJ, Yu DY. 2007. Axonal transport and cytoskeletal changes in the laminar regions after elevated intraocular pressure. *Invest Ophthalmol Vis Sci* **48:** 3632–3644.

Berkelaar M, Clarke DB, Wang YC, Bray GM, Aguayo AJ. 1994. Axotomy results in delayed death and apoptosis of retinal ganglion cells in adult rats. *J Neurosci* **14:** 4368–4374.

Bosco A, Inman DM, Steele MR, Wu G, Soto I, Marsh-Armstrong N, Hubbard WC, Calkins DJ, Horner PJ, Vetter ML. 2008. Reduced retina microglial activation and improved optic nerve integrity with minocycline treatment in the DBA/2J mouse model of glaucoma. *Invest Ophthalmol Vis Sci* **49:** 1437–1446.

Bosco A, Steele MR, Vetter ML. 2011. Early microglia activation in a mouse model of chronic glaucoma. *J Comp Neurol* **519:** 599–620.

Bosco A, Crish SD, Steele MR, Romero CO, Inman DM, Horner PJ, Calkins DJ, Vetter ML. 2012. Early reduction of microglia activation by irradiation in a model of chronic glaucoma. *PLoS ONE* **7:** e43602.

Burgoyne CF. 2011. A biomechanical paradigm for axonal insult within the optic nerve head in aging and glaucoma. *Exp Eye Res* **93:** 120–132.

Bush TG, Puvanachandra N, Horner CH, Polito A, Ostenfeld T, Svendsen CN, Mucke L, Johnson MH, Sofroniew MV. 1999. Leukocyte infiltration, neuronal degeneration, and neurite outgrowth after ablation of scar-forming, reactive astrocytes in adult transgenic mice. *Neuron* **23:** 297–308.

Cahoy JD, Emery B, Kaushal A, Foo LC, Zamanian JL, Christopherson KS, Xing Y, Lubischer JL, Krieg PA, Krupenko SA, et al. 2008. A transcriptome database for astrocytes, neurons, and oligodendrocytes: A new resource for understanding brain development and function. *J Neurosci* **28:** 264–278.

Chauhan BC, LeVatte TL, Jollimore CA, Yu PK, Reitsamer HA, Kelly ME, Yu DY, Tremblay F, Archibald ML. 2004. Model of endothelin-1-induced chronic optic neuropathy in rat. *Invest Ophthalmol Vis Sci* **45:** 144–152.

Chollangi S, Wang J, Martin A, Quinn J, Ash JD. 2009. Preconditioning-induced protection from oxidative injury is mediated by leukemia inhibitory factor receptor (LIFR) and its ligands in the retina. *Neurobiol Dis* **34:** 535–544.

Coca-Prados M, Escribano J. 2007. New perspectives in aqueous humor secretion and in glaucoma: The ciliary body as a multifunctional neuroendocrine gland. *Prog Retin Eye Res* **26:** 239–262.

Coca-Prados M, Escribano J, Ortego J. 1999. Differential gene expression in the human ciliary epithelium. *Prog Retin Eye Res* **18:** 403–429.

Dai Y, Sun X, Yu X, Guo W, Yu D. 2012. Astrocytic responses in the lateral geniculate nucleus of monkeys with experimental glaucoma. *Vet Ophthalmol* **15:** 23–30.

Danias J, Lee KC, Zamora MF, Chen B, Shen F, Filippopoulos T, Su Y, Goldblum D, Podos SM, Mittag T. 2003. Quantitative analysis of retinal ganglion cell (RGC) loss in aging DBA/2NNia glaucomatous mice: Comparison with RGC loss in aging C57/BL6 mice. *Invest Ophthalmol Vis Sci* **44:** 5151–5162.

Danias J, Gerometta R, Ge Y, Ren L, Panagis L, Mittag TW, Candia OA, Podos SM. 2011. Gene expression changes in steroid-induced IOP elevation in bovine trabecular meshwork. *Invest Ophthalmol Vis Sci* **52:** 8636–8645.

Davenport AP. 2002. International Union of Pharmacology. XXIX. Update on endothelin receptor nomenclature. *Pharmacol Rev* **54:** 219–226.

Diskin S, Kumar J, Cao Z, Schuman JS, Gilmartin T, Head SR, Panjwani N. 2006. Detection of differentially expressed glycogenes in trabecular meshwork of eyes with primary open-angle glaucoma. *Invest Ophthalmol Vis Sci* **47:** 1491–1499.

Escribano J, Coca-Prados M. 2002. Bioinformatics and reanalysis of subtracted expressed sequence tags from the human ciliary body: Identification of novel biological functions. *Mol Vis* **8:** 315–332.

Escribano J, Ortego J, Coca-Prados M. 1995. Isolation and characterization of cell-specific cDNA clones from a subtractive library of the ocular ciliary body of a single normal human donor: Transcription and synthesis of plasma proteins. *J Biochem* **118:** 921–931.

Fan BJ, Wang DY, Tham CC, Lam DS, Pang CP. 2008. Gene expression profiles of human trabecular meshwork cells induced by triamcinolone and dexamethasone. *Invest Ophthalmol Vis Sci* **49:** 1886–1897.

Faulkner JR, Herrmann JE, Woo MJ, Tansey KE, Doan NB, Sofroniew MV. 2004. Reactive astrocytes protect tissue and preserve function after spinal cord injury. *J Neurosci* **24:** 2143–2155.

Fukuchi T, Sawaguchi S, Hara H, Shirakashi M, Iwata K. 1992. Extracellular matrix changes of the optic nerve lamina cribrosa in monkey eyes with experimentally chronic glaucoma. *Graefes Arch Clin Exp Ophthalmol* **230:** 421–427.

Garcia-Valenzuela E, Gorczyca W, Darzynkiewicz Z, Sharma SC. 1994. Apoptosis in adult retinal ganglion cells after axotomy. *J Neurobiol* **25:** 431–438.

Garcia-Valenzuela E, Shareef S, Walsh J, Sharma SC. 1995. Programmed cell death of retinal ganglion cells during experimental glaucoma. *Exp Eye Res* **61:** 33–44.

Gonzalez P, Epstein DL, Borras T. 2000. Genes upregulated in the human trabecular meshwork in response to elevated intraocular pressure. *Invest Ophthalmol Vis Sci* **41:** 352–361.

Guo Y, Cepurna WO, Dyck JA, Doser TA, Johnson EC, Morrison JC. 2010. Retinal cell responses to elevated intraocular pressure: A gene array comparison between the whole retina and retinal ganglion cell layer. *Invest Ophthalmol Vis Sci* **51:** 3003–3018.

Guo Y, Johnson EC, Cepurna WO, Dyck JA, Doser T, Morrison JC. 2011. Early gene expression changes in the retinal ganglion cell layer of a rat glaucoma model. *Invest Ophthalmol Vis Sci* **52:** 1460–1473.

Gupta N, Ly T, Zhang Q, Kaufman PL, Weinreb RN, Yucel YH. 2007. Chronic ocular hypertension induces dendrite pathology in the lateral geniculate nucleus of the brain. *Exp Eye Res* **84:** 176–184.

Hernandez MR. 1992. Ultrastructural immunocytochemical analysis of elastin in the human lamina cribrosa. Changes in elastic fibers in primary open-angle glaucoma. *Invest Ophthalmol Vis Sci* **33:** 2891–2903.

Hernandez MR. 2000. The optic nerve head in glaucoma: Role of astrocytes in tissue remodeling. *Prog Retin Eye Res* **19:** 297–321.

Hernandez MR, Pena JD. 1997. The optic nerve head in glaucomatous optic neuropathy. *Arch Ophthalmol* **115:** 389–395.

Hernandez MR, Ye H. 1993. Glaucoma: Changes in extracellular matrix in the optic nerve head. *Ann Med* **25:** 309–315.

Hernandez MR, Igoe F, Neufeld AH. 1988. Cell culture of the human lamina cribrosa. *Invest Ophthalmol Vis Sci* **29:** 78–89.

Hernandez MR, Ye H, Roy S. 1994. Collagen type IV gene expression in human optic nerve heads with primary open angle glaucoma. *Exp Eye Res* **59:** 41–51.

Hernandez MR, Agapova OA, Yang P, Salvador-Silva M, Ricard CS, Aoi S. 2002. Differential gene expression in astrocytes from human normal and glaucomatous optic nerve head analyzed by cDNA microarray. *Glia* **38:** 45–64.

Hernandez MR, Miao H, Lukas T. 2008. Astrocytes in glaucomatous optic neuropathy. *Prog Brain Res* **173:** 353–373.

Howell GR, Libby RT, Jakobs TC, Smith RS, Phalan FC, Barter JW, Barbay JM, Marchant JK, Mahesh N, Porciatti V, et al. 2007. Axons of retinal ganglion cells are insulted in the optic nerve early in DBA/2J glaucoma. *J Cell Biol* **179:** 1523–1537.

Howell GR, Macalinao DG, Sousa GL, Walden M, Soto I, Kneeland SC, Barbay JM, King BL, Marchant JK, Hibbs M, et al. 2011. Molecular clustering identifies complement and endothelin induction as early events in a mouse model of glaucoma. *J Clin Invest* **121:** 1429–1444.

Howell GR, Soto I, Zhu X, Ryan M, Macalinao DG, Sousa GL, Caddle LB, MacNicoll KH, Barbay JM, Porciatti V, et al. 2012. Radiation treatment inhibits monocyte entry into the optic nerve head and prevents neuronal damage in a mouse model of glaucoma. *J Clin Invest* **122:** 1246–1261.

Inatani M, Tanihara H, Katsuta H, Honjo M, Kido N, Honda Y. 2001. Transforming growth factor-β 2 levels in aqueous humor of glaucomatous eyes. *Graefes Arch Clin Exp Ophthalmol* **239:** 109–113.

Ishibashi T, Takagi Y, Mori K, Naruse S, Nishino H, Yue BY, Kinoshita S. 2002. cDNA microarray analysis of gene expression changes induced by dexamethasone in cultured human trabecular meshwork cells. *Invest Ophthalmol Vis Sci* **43:** 3691–3697.

Ito U, Nagasao J, Kawakami E, Oyanagi K. 2007. Fate of disseminated dead neurons in the cortical ischemic penumbra: Ultrastructure indicating a novel scavenger mechanism of microglia and astrocytes. *Stroke* **38:** 2577–2583.

Jakobs TC, Libby RT, Ben Y, John SW, Masland RH. 2005. Retinal ganglion cell degeneration is topological but not cell type specific in DBA/2J mice. *J Cell Biol* **171:** 313–325.

Janssen SF, Gorgels TG, Bossers K, Ten Brink JB, Essing AH, Nagtegaal M, van der Spek PJ, Jansonius NM, Bergen AA. 2012. Gene expression and functional annotation of the human ciliary body epithelia. *PLoS ONE* **7:** e44973.

Jeon CJ, Strettoi E, Masland RH. 1998. The major cell populations of the mouse retina. *J Neurosci* **21:** 8936–8946.

Johansson JO. 1983. Inhibition of retrograde axoplasmic transport in rat optic nerve by increased IOP in vitro. *Invest Ophthalmol Vis Sci* **24:** 1552–1558.

Johansson JO. 1988. Inhibition and recovery of retrograde axoplasmic transport in rat optic nerve during and after elevated IOP in vivo. *Exp Eye Res* **46:** 223–227.

Johnson M. 2006. What controls aqueous humour outflow resistance?. *Exp Eye Res* **82:** 545–557.

Johnson EC, Jia L, Cepurna WO, Doser TA, Morrison JC. 2007. Global changes in optic nerve head gene expression after exposure to elevated intraocular pressure in a rat glaucoma model. *Invest Ophthalmol Vis Sci* **48:** 3161–3177.

Johnson EC, Doser TA, Cepurna WO, Dyck JA, Jia L, Guo Y, Lambert WS, Morrison JC. 2011. Cell proliferation and interleukin-6-type cytokine signaling are implicated by gene expression responses in early optic nerve head injury in rat glaucoma. *Invest Ophthalmol Vis Sci* **52:** 504–518.

Kalmar B, Kittel A, Lemmens R, Kornyei Z, Madarasz E. 2001. Cultured astrocytes react to LPS with increased cyclooxygenase activity and phagocytosis. *Neurochem Int* **38:** 453–461.

Kang MH, Oh DJ, Kang JH, Rhee DJ. 2013. Regulation of SPARC by transforming growth factor β2 in human trabecular meshwork. *Invest Ophthalmol Vis Sci* **54:** 2523–2532.

Kirwan RP, Wordinger RJ, Clark AF, O'Brien CJ. 2009. Differential global and extra-cellular matrix focused gene expression patterns between normal and glaucomatous human lamina cribrosa cells. *Mol Vis* **15:** 76–88.

Klein MA, Moller JC, Jones LL, Bluethmann H, Kreutzberg GW, Raivich G. 1997. Impaired neuroglial activation in interleukin-6 deficient mice. *Glia* **19:** 227–233.

Kompass KS, Agapova OA, Li W, Kaufman PL, Rasmussen CA, Hernandez MR. 2008. Bioinformatic and statistical analysis of the optic nerve head in a primate model of ocular hypertension. *BMC Neurosci* **9:** 93.

Kuehn MH, Kim CY, Ostojic J, Bellin M, Alward WL, Stone EM, Sakaguchi DS, Grozdanic SD, Kwon YH. 2006. Retinal synthesis and deposition of complement components induced by ocular hypertension. *Exp Eye Res* **83:** 620–628.

Kuehn MH, Kim CY, Jiang B, Dumitrescu AV, Kwon YH. 2008. Disruption of the complement cascade delays retinal ganglion cell death following retinal ischemia-reperfusion. *Exp Eye Res* **87:** 89–95.

Kwong JM, Caprioli J. 2006. Expression of phosphorylated c-Jun N-terminal protein kinase (JNK) in experimental glaucoma in rats. *Exp Eye Res* **82:** 576–582.

Lambert W, Agarwal R, Howe W, Clark AF, Wordinger RJ. 2001. Neurotrophin and neurotrophin receptor expression by cells of the human lamina cribrosa. *Invest Ophthalmol Vis Sci* **42:** 2315–2323.

Leibinger M, Muller A, Andreadaki A, Hauk TG, Kirsch M, Fischer D. 2009. Neuroprotective and axon growth-promoting effects following inflammatory stimulation on mature retinal ganglion cells in mice depend on ciliary neurotrophic factor and leukemia inhibitory factor. *J Neurosci* **29:** 14334–14341.

Leske MC. 2007. Open-angle glaucoma—An epidemiologic overview. *Ophthalmic Epidemiol* **14:** 166–172.

Levkovitch-Verbin H, Kalev-Landoy M, Habot-Wilner Z, Melamed S. 2006a. Minocycline delays death of retinal ganglion cells in experimental glaucoma and after optic nerve transection. *Arch Ophthalmol* **124:** 520–526.

Levkovitch-Verbin H, Dardik R, Vander S, Nisgav Y, Kalev-Landoy M, Melamed S. 2006b. Experimental glaucoma and optic nerve transection induce simultaneous up-regulation of proapoptotic and prosurvival genes. *Invest Ophthalmol Vis Sci* **47:** 2491–2497.

Levkovitch-Verbin H, Harizman N, Dardik R, Nisgav Y, Vander S, Melamed S. 2007. Regulation of cell death and survival pathways in experimental glaucoma. *Exp Eye Res* **85:** 250–258.

Li C, Chan YR. 2011. Lipocalin 2 regulation and its complex role in inflammation and cancer. *Cytokine* **56:** 435–441.

Libby RT, Anderson MG, Pang IH, Robinson ZH, Savinova OV, Cosma IM, Snow A, Wilson LA, Smith RS, Clark AF, et al. 2005. Inherited glaucoma in DBA/2J mice: Pertinent disease features for studying the neurodegeneration. *Vis Neurosci* **22:** 637–648.

Libby RT, Howell GR, Pang IH, Savinova OV, Mehalow AK, Barter JW, Smith RS, Clark AF, John SW. 2007. Inducible nitric oxide synthase, *Nos2*, does not mediate optic neuropathy and retinopathy in the DBA/2J glaucoma model. *BMC Neurosci* **8:** 108.

Liton PB, Luna C, Challa P, Epstein DL, Gonzalez P. 2006. Genome-wide expression profile of human trabecular meshwork cultured cells, nonglaucomatous and primary open angle glaucoma tissue. *Mol Vis* **12:** 774–790.

Litvin J, Zhu S, Norris R, Markwald R. 2005. Periostin family of proteins: Therapeutic targets for heart disease. *Anat Rec A Discov Mol Cell Evol Biol* **287:** 1205–1212.

Liu M, Duggan J, Salt TE, Cordeiro MF. 2011. Dendritic changes in visual pathways in glaucoma and other neurodegenerative conditions. *Exp Eye Res* **92:** 244–250.

Liu Y, Allingham RR, Qin X, Layfield D, Dellinger AE, Gibson JR, Wheeler J, Ashley-Koch AE, Stamer WD, Hauser MA. 2013. Gene expression profile in human trabecular meshwork with primary open angle glaucoma. *Invest Ophthalmol Vis Sci* **54:** 6382–6389.

Lo WR, Rowlette LL, Caballero M, Yang P, Hernandez MR, Borras T. 2003. Tissue differential microarray analysis of dexamethasone induction reveals potential mechanisms of steroid glaucoma. *Invest Ophthalmol Vis Sci* **44:** 473–485.

Luo D, Liu K, Zhu B, Xu X. 2013. Expression profiling in glaucomatous human lamina cribrosa cells based on graph-clustering approach. *Curr Eye Res* **38:** 767–773.

Lutjen-Drecoll E, Futa R, Rohen JW. 1981. Ultrahistochemical studies on tangential sections of the trabecular meshwork in normal and glaucomatous eyes. *Invest Ophthalmol Vis Sci* **21:** 563–573.

Lye-Barthel M, Sun D, Jakobs TC. 2013. Morphology of astrocytes in a glaucomatous optic nerve. *Invest Ophthalmol Vis Sci* **54:** 909–917.

May CA, Lutjen-Drecoll E. 2002. Morphology of the murine optic nerve. *Invest Ophthalmol Vis Sci* **43:** 2206–2212.

Miao H, Chen L, Riordan SM, Li W, Juarez S, Crabb AM, Lukas TJ, Du P, Lin SM, Wise A, et al. 2008. Gene expression and functional studies of the optic nerve head astrocyte transcriptome from normal African Americans and Caucasian Americans donors. *PLoS ONE* **3:** e2847.

Miyahara T, Kikuchi T, Akimoto M, Kurokawa T, Shibuki H, Yoshimura N. 2003. Gene microarray analysis of experimental glaucomatous retina from cynomologous monkey. *Invest Ophthalmol Vis Sci* **44:** 4347–4356.

Morcos Y, Chan-Ling T. 2000. Concentration of astrocytic filaments at the retinal optic nerve junction is coincident with the absence of intra-retinal myelination: Comparative and developmental evidence. *J Neurocytol* **29:** 665–678.

Morgan JE. 2012. Retina ganglion cell degeneration in glaucoma: An opportunity missed? A review. *Clin Experiment Ophthalmol* **40:** 364–368.

Morrison JC, Dorman-Pease ME, Dunkelberger GR, Quigley HA. 1990. Optic nerve head extracellular matrix in primary optic atrophy and experimental glaucoma. *Arch Ophthalmol* **108:** 1020–1024.

Morrison J, Farrell S, Johnson E, Deppmeier L, Moore CG, Grossmann E. 1995. Structure and composition of the rodent lamina cribrosa. *Exp Eye Res* **60:** 127–135.

Morrison JC, Moore CG, Deppmeier LM, Gold BG, Meshul CK, Johnson EC. 1997. A rat model of chronic pressure-induced optic nerve damage. *Exp Eye Res* **64:** 85–96.

Myer DJ, Gurkoff GG, Lee SM, Hovda DA, Sofroniew MV. 2006. Essential protective roles of reactive astrocytes in traumatic brain injury. *Brain* **129:** 2761–2772.

Nakazawa T, Nakazawa C, Matsubara A, Noda K, Hisatomi T, She H, Michaud N, Hafezi-Moghadam A, Miller JW, Benowitz LI. 2006. Tumor necrosis factor-α mediates oligodendrocyte death and delayed retinal ganglion cell loss in a mouse model of glaucoma. *J Neurosci* **26:** 12633–12641.

Naskar R, Thanos S. 2006. Retinal gene profiling in a hereditary rodent model of elevated intraocular pressure. *Mol Vis* **12:** 1199–1210.

Neufeld AH. 1999. Nitric oxide: A potential mediator of retinal ganglion cell damage in glaucoma. *Surv Ophthalmol* **43:** S129–135.

Neufeld AH, Liu B. 2003. Glaucomatous optic neuropathy: When glia misbehave. *Neuroscientist* **9:** 485–495.

Nguyen TD, Chen P, Huang WD, Chen H, Johnson D, Polansky JR. 1998. Gene structure and properties of TIGR, an olfactomedin-related glycoprotein cloned from glucocorticoid-induced trabecular meshwork cells. *J Biol Chem* **273:** 6341–6350.

Nguyen JV, Soto I, Kim KY, Bushong EA, Oglesby E, Valiente-Soriano FJ, Yang Z, Davis CH, Bedont JL, Son JL, et al. 2011. Myelination transition zone astrocytes are constitutively phagocytic and have synuclein dependent reactivity in glaucoma. *Proc Natl Acad Sci* **108:** 1176–1181.

Nickells RW, Howell GR, Soto I, John SW. 2012. Under pressure: Cellular and molecular responses during glaucoma, a common neurodegeneration with axonopathy. *Annu Rev Neurosci* **35:** 153–179.

Nikolskaya T, Nikolsky Y, Serebryiskaya T, Zvereva S, Sviridov E, Dezso Z, Rahkmatulin E, Brennan RJ, Yankovsky N, Bhattacharya SK, et al. 2009. Network analysis of human glaucomatous optic nerve head astrocytes. *BMC Med Genomics* **2:** 24.

Noske W, Hensen J, Wiederholt M. 1997. Endothelin-like immunoreactivity in aqueous humor of patients with primary open-angle glaucoma and cataract. *Graefes Arch Clin Exp Ophthalmol* **235:** 551–552.

Okada S, Nakamura M, Katoh H, Miyao T, Shimazaki T, Ishii K, Yamane J, Yoshimura A, Iwamoto Y, Toyama Y, et al. 2006. Conditional ablation of Stat3 or Socs3 discloses a dual role for reactive astrocytes after spinal cord injury. *Nat Med* **12:** 829–834.

Panagis L, Zhao X, Ge Y, Ren L, Mittag TW, Danias J. 2010. Gene expression changes in areas of focal loss of retinal ganglion cells in the retina of DBA/2J mice. *Invest Ophthalmol Vis Sci* **51:** 2024–2034.

Panagis L, Zhao X, Ge Y, Ren L, Mittag TW, Danias J. 2011. Retinal gene expression changes related to IOP exposure and axonal loss in DBA/2J mice. *Invest Ophthalmol Vis Sci* **52:** 7807–7816.

Pang IH, Johnson EC, Jia L, Cepurna WO, Shepard AR, Hellberg MR, Clark AF, Morrison JC. 2005. Evaluation of inducible nitric oxide synthase in glaucomatous optic neuropathy and pressure-induced optic nerve damage. *Invest Ophthalmol Vis Sci* **46:** 1313–1321.

Pease ME, McKinnon SJ, Quigley HA, Kerrigan-Baumrind LA, Zack DJ. 2000. Obstructed axonal transport of BDNF and its receptor TrkB in experimental glaucoma. *Invest Ophthalmol Vis Sci* **41:** 764–774.

Pena JD, Varela HJ, Ricard CS, Hernandez MR. 1999. Enhanced tenascin expression associated with reactive astrocytes in human optic nerve heads with primary open angle glaucoma. *Exp Eye Res* **68:** 29–40.

Picht G, Welge-Luessen U, Grehn F, Lutjen-Drecoll E. 2001. Transforming growth factor β2 levels in the aqueous humor in different types of glaucoma and the relation to filtering bleb development. *Graefes Arch Clin Exp Ophthalmol* **239:** 199–207.

Piri N, Kwong JM, Song M, Elashoff D, Caprioli J. 2006. Gene expression changes in the retina following optic nerve transection. *Mol Vis* **12:** 1660–1673.

Polansky JR, Fauss DJ, Chen P, Chen H, Lutjen-Drecoll E, Johnson D, Kurtz RM, Ma ZD, Bloom E, Nguyen TD. 1997. Cellular pharmacology and molecular biology of the trabecular meshwork inducible glucocorticoid response gene product. *Ophthalmologica* **211:** 126–139.

Qu J, Jakobs TC. 2013. The time course of gene expression during reactive gliosis in the optic nerve. *PLoS ONE* **8:** e67094.

Qu J, Wang D, Grosskreutz CL. 2010. Mechanisms of retinal ganglion cell injury and defense in glaucoma. *Exp Eye Res* **91:** 48–53.

Quigley HA. 2011. Glaucoma. *Lancet* **377:** 1367–1377.

Quigley HA, Addicks EM. 1980. Chronic experimental glaucoma in primates. II. Effect of extended intraocular pressure elevation on optic nerve head and axonal transport. *Invest Ophthalmol Vis Sci* **19:** 137–152.

Quigley HA, Addicks EM. 1981. Regional differences in the structure of the lamina cribrosa and their relation to glaucomatous optic nerve damage. *Arch Ophthalmol* **99:** 137–143.

Quigley HA, Addicks EM, Green WR, Maumenee AE. 1981. Optic nerve damage in human glaucoma. II. The site of injury and susceptibility to damage. *Arch Ophthalmol* **99:** 635–649.

Quigley HA, Brown A, Dorman-Pease ME. 1991a. Alterations in elastin of the optic nerve head in human and experimental glaucoma. *Br J Ophthalmol* **75:** 552–557.

Quigley HA, Dorman-Pease ME, Brown AE. 1991b. Quantitative study of collagen and elastin of the optic nerve head and sclera in human and experimental monkey glaucoma. *Curr Eye Res* **10:** 877–888.

Quigley HA, Nickells RW, Kerrigan LA, Pease ME, Thibault DJ, Zack DJ. 1995. Retinal ganglion cell death in experimental glaucoma and after axotomy occurs by apoptosis. *Invest Ophthalmol Vis Sci* **36:** 774–786.

Quigley HA, McKinnon SJ, Zack DJ, Pease ME, Kerrigan-Baumrind LA, Kerrigan DF, Mitchell RS. 2000. Retrograde axonal transport of BDNF in retinal ganglion cells is blocked by acute IOP elevation in rats. *Invest Ophthalmol Vis Sci* **41:** 3460–3466.

Roberts MD, Grau V, Grimm J, Reynaud J, Bellezza AJ, Burgoyne CF, Downs JC. 2009. Remodeling of the connective tissue microarchitecture of the lamina cribrosa in early experimental glaucoma. *Invest Ophthalmol Vis Sci* **50:** 681–690.

Roh M, Zhang Y, Murakami Y, Thanos A, Lee SC, Vavvas DG, Benowitz LI, Miller JW. 2012. Etanercept, a widely used inhibitor of tumor necrosis factor-α (TNF-α), prevents retinal ganglion cell loss in a rat model of glaucoma. *PLoS ONE* **7:** e40065.

Rohen JW, Futa R, Lutjen-Drecoll E. 1981. The fine structure of the cribriform meshwork in normal and glaucomatous eyes as seen in tangential sections. *Invest Ophthalmol Vis Sci* **21:** 574–585.

Rozsa FW, Reed DM, Scott KM, Pawar H, Moroi SE, Kijek TG, Krafchak CM, Othman MI, Vollrath D, Elner VM, et al. 2006. Gene expression profile of human trabecular meshwork cells in response to long-term dexamethasone exposure. *Mol Vis* **12:** 125–141.

Sasaoka M, Taniguchi T, Shimazawa M, Ishida N, Shimazaki A, Hara H. 2006. Intravitreal injection of endothelin-1 caused optic nerve damage following to ocular hypoperfusion in rabbits. *Exp Eye Res* **83:** 629–637.

Sawada H, Fukuchi T, Tanaka T, Abe H. 2010. Tumor necrosis factor-α concentrations in the aqueous humor of patients with glaucoma. *Invest Ophthalmol Vis Sci* **51:** 903–906.

Schafer DP, Lehrman EK, Kautzman AG, Koyama R, Mardinly AR, Yamasaki R, Ransohoff RM, Greenberg ME, Barres BA, Stevens B. 2012. Microglia sculpt postnatal neural circuits in an activity and complement-dependent manner. *Neuron* **74:** 691–705.

Schlamp CL, Li Y, Dietz JA, Janssen KT, Nickells RW. 2006. Progressive ganglion cell loss and optic nerve degeneration in DBA/2J mice is variable and asymmetric. *BMC Neurosci* **7:** 66.

Shareef S, Sawada A, Neufeld AH. 1999. Isoforms of nitric oxide synthase in the optic nerves of rat eyes with chronic moderately elevated intraocular pressure. *Invest Ophthalmol Vis Sci* **40:** 2884–2891.

Sofroniew MV. 2005. Reactive astrocytes in neural repair and protection. *Neuroscientist* **11:** 400–407.

Sofroniew MV, Vinters HV. 2010. Astrocytes: Biology and pathology. *Acta Neuropathol* **119:** 7–35.

Soto I, Pease ME, Son JL, Shi X, Quigley HA, Marsh-Armstrong N. 2011. Retinal ganglion cell loss in a rat ocular hypertension model is sectorial and involves early optic nerve axon loss. *Invest Ophthalmol Vis Sci* **52:** 434–441.

Stasi K, Nagel D, Yang X, Wang RF, Ren L, Podos SM, Mittag T, Danias J. 2006. Complement component 1Q (C1Q) upregulation in retina of murine, primate, and human glaucomatous eyes. *Invest Ophthalmol Vis Sci* **47:** 1024–1029.

Steele MR, Inman DM, Calkins DJ, Horner PJ, Vetter ML. 2006. Microarray analysis of retinal gene expression in the DBA/2J model of glaucoma. *Invest Ophthalmol Vis Sci* **47:** 977–985.

Stephan AH, Barres BA, Stevens B. 2012. The complement system: An unexpected role in synaptic pruning during development and disease. *Annu Rev Neurosci* **35:** 369–389.

Stevens B, Allen NJ, Vazquez LE, Howell GR, Christopherson KS, Nouri N, Micheva KD, Mehalow AK, Huberman AD, Stafford B, et al. 2007. The classical complement cascade mediates CNS synapse elimination. *Cell* **131:** 1164–1178.

Sun D, Jakobs TC. 2012. Structural remodeling of astrocytes in the injured CNS. *Neuroscientist* **18:** 567–588.

Sun D, Lye-Barthel M, Masland RH, Jakobs TC. 2009. The morphology and spatial arrangement of astrocytes in the optic nerve head of the mouse. *J Comp Neurol* **516:** 1–19.

Sun D, Lye-Barthel M, Masland RH, Jakobs TC. 2010. Structural remodeling of fibrous astrocytes after axonal injury. *J Neurosci* **30:** 14008–14019.

Sun D, Qu J, Jakobs TC. 2013. Reversible reactivity by optic nerve astrocytes. *Glia* **61:** 1218–1235.

Suzuki S, Tanaka K, Suzuki N. 2009. Ambivalent aspects of interleukin-6 in cerebral ischemia: Inflammatory versus neurotrophic aspects. *J Cereb Blood Flow Metab* **29:** 464–479.

Tamm ER. 2009. The trabecular meshwork outflow pathways: Structural and functional aspects. *Exp Eye Res* **88:** 648–655.

Taniguchi T, Shimazawa M, Sasaoka M, Shimazaki A, Hara H. 2006. Endothelin-1 impairs retrograde axonal transport and leads to axonal injury in rat optic nerve. *Curr Neurovasc Res* **3:** 81–88.

Tektas OY, Lutjen-Drecoll E. 2009. Structural changes of the trabecular meshwork in different kinds of glaucoma. *Exp Eye Res* **88:** 769–775.

Tektas OY, Hammer CM, Danias J, Candia O, Gerometta R, Podos SM, Lutjen-Drecoll E. 2010. Morphologic changes in the outflow pathways of bovine eyes treated with corticosteroids. *Invest Ophthalmol Vis Sci* **51:** 4060–4066.

Tezel G, Wax MB. 2000. Increased production of tumor necrosis factor-α by glial cells exposed to simulated ischemia or elevated hydrostatic pressure induces apoptosis in cocultured retinal ganglion cells. *J Neurosci* **20:** 8693–8700.

Tezel G, Kass MA, Kolker AE, Becker B, Wax MB. 1997. Plasma and aqueous humor endothelin levels in primary open-angle glaucoma. *J Glaucoma* **6:** 83–89.

Uemura A, Takizawa T, Ochiai W, Yanagisawa M, Nakashima K, Taga T. 2002. Cardiotrophin-like cytokine induces astrocyte differentiation of fetal neuroepithelial cells via activation of STAT3. *Cytokine* **18:** 1–7.

Vazquez-Chona F, Song BK, Geisert EE Jr. 2004. Temporal changes in gene expression after injury in the rat retina. *Invest Ophthalmol Vis Sci* **45:** 2737–2746.

Vittitow J, Borras T. 2004. Genes expressed in the human trabecular meshwork during pressure-induced homeostatic response. *J Cell Physiol* **201:** 126–137.

Wagner AH, Anand VN, Wang WH, Chatterton JE, Sun D, Shepard AR, Jacobson N, Pang IH, Deluca AP, Casavant TL, et al. 2013. Exon-level expression profiling of ocular tissues. *Exp Eye Res* **111:** 105–111.

Walsh MM, Yi H, Friedman J, Cho KI, Tserentsoodol N, McKinnon S, Searle K, Yeh A, Ferreira PA. 2009. Gene and protein expression pilot profiling and biomarkers in an experimental mouse model of hypertensive glaucoma. *Exp Biol Med (Maywood)* **234:** 918–930.

Wang WH, McNatt LG, Pang IH, Hellberg PE, Fingert JH, McCartney MD, Clark AF. 2008a. Increased expression of serum amyloid A in glaucoma and its effect on intraocular pressure. *Invest Ophthalmol Vis Sci* **49:** 1916–1923.

Wang X, Baldridge WH, Chauhan BC. 2008b. Acute endothelin-1 application induces reversible fast axonal transport blockade in adult rat optic nerve. *Invest Ophthalmol Vis Sci* **49:** 961–967.

Wang DY, Ray A, Rodgers K, Ergorul C, Hyman BT, Huang W, Grosskreutz CL. 2010. Global gene expression changes in rat retinal ganglion cells in experimental glaucoma. *Invest Ophthalmol Vis Sci* **51:** 4084–4095.

Welsbie DS, Yang Z, Ge Y, Mitchell KL, Zhou X, Martin SE, Berlinicke CA, Hackler L Jr, Fuller J, Fu J, et al. 2013. Functional genomic screening identifies dual leucine zipper kinase as a key mediator of retinal ganglion cell death. *Proc Natl Acad Sci* **110:** 4045–4050.

Yan X, Tezel G, Wax MB, Edward DP. 2000. Matrix metalloproteinases and tumor necrosis factor α in glaucomatous optic nerve head. *Arch Ophthalmol* **118:** 666–673.

Yang Z, Zack DJ. 2011. What has gene expression profiling taught us about glaucoma? *Exp Eye Res* **93:** 191–195.

Yang Z, Quigley HA, Pease ME, Yang Y, Qian J, Valenta D, Zack DJ. 2007. Changes in gene expression in experimental glaucoma and optic nerve transection: The equilibrium between protective and detrimental mechanisms. *Invest Ophthalmol Vis Sci* **48:** 5539–5548.

Yoshimura N, Kikuchi T, Kuroiwa S, Gaun S. 2003. Differential temporal and spatial expression of immediate early genes in retinal neurons after ischemia-reperfusion injury. *Invest Ophthalmol Vis Sci* **44:** 2211–2220.

Yuan L, Neufeld AH. 2000. Tumor necrosis factor-α: A potentially neurodestructive cytokine produced by glia in the human glaucomatous optic nerve head. *Glia* **32:** 42–50.

Yuan L, Neufeld AH. 2001. Activated microglia in the human glaucomatous optic nerve head. *J Neurosci Res* **64:** 523–532.

Zamanian JL, Xu L, Foo LC, Nouri N, Zhou L, Giffard RG, Barres BA. 2012. Genomic analysis of reactive astrogliosis. *J Neurosci* **32:** 6391–6410.

Zhao X, Ramsey KE, Stephan DA, Russell P. 2004. Gene and protein expression changes in human trabecular meshwork cells treated with transforming growth factor-β. *Invest Ophthalmol Vis Sci* **45:** 4023–4034.

Zode GS, Clark AF, Wordinger RJ. 2007. Activation of the BMP canonical signaling pathway in human optic nerve head tissue and isolated optic nerve head astrocytes and lamina cribrosa cells. *Invest Ophthalmol Vis Sci* **48:** 5058–5067.

The Complex Role of Neuroinflammation in Glaucoma

Ileana Soto[1] and Gareth R. Howell[1,2]

[1]The Jackson Laboratory, Bar Harbor, Maine 04609
[2]School of Medicine, Tufts University, Boston, Massachusetts 02111
Correspondence: gareth.howell@jax.org

Glaucoma is a multifactorial neurodegenerative disorder affecting 80 million people worldwide. Loss of retinal ganglion cells and degeneration of their axons in the optic nerve are the major pathological hallmarks. Neuroinflammatory processes, inflammatory processes in the central nervous system, have been identified in human glaucoma and in experimental models of the disease. Furthermore, neuroinflammatory responses occur at early stages of experimental glaucoma, and inhibition of certain proinflammatory pathways appears neuroprotective. Here, we summarize the current understanding of neuroinflammation in the central nervous system, with emphasis on events at the optic nerve head during early stages of glaucoma.

Glaucoma is a complex neurodegenerative disease that results in the degeneration of retinal ganglion cells (RGCs) and their axons in the optic nerve. Age and elevation of intraocular pressure (IOP) over baseline are major risk factors for glaucoma (Quigley 1993, 2011). Strong evidence suggests that an early insult occurs to RGC axons at the optic nerve head (ONH) (Jakobs et al. 2005; Schlamp et al. 2006; Howell et al. 2007; Soto et al. 2008; Burgoyne 2011; Quigley 2011; Nickells et al. 2012). The exact mechanisms by which RGC axons are insulted and ultimately degenerate are not clear, although early neuroinflammatory responses by astrocytes, microglia, and other blood-derived immune cells are observed in the ONH, suggesting a primary role of inflammation in glaucoma (Howell et al. 2012; Nickells et al. 2012; Tezel 2013). Furthermore, some evidence suggests that other RGC compartments, such as dendrites, synapses, and soma, are impacted early in the disease and that these events may also involve, even be mediated by, inflammatory responses in the retina (Howell et al. 2011a; Nickells et al. 2012; Tezel 2013). Therefore, the role of inflammation in glaucomatous neurodegeneration is currently of great interest.

In this review we focus on the role of inflammation in glaucomatous RGC loss (referred to as neuroinflammation). In particular, we discuss the proposed roles of astrocytes, resident microglia and other monocyte-derived cells in early stages of glaucoma in the optic nerve head. Evidence is suggesting these cell types are criti-

Cite this article as *Cold Spring Harb Perspect Med* doi: 10.1101/cshperspect.a017269

cal players in the early neuroinflammatory responses in glaucoma.

NEUROINFLAMMATORY RESPONSES IN THE CNS RELEVANT TO GLAUCOMA

Although there is still much to be explored, neuroinflammatory responses identified to date in glaucoma show some hallmarks of classic inflammatory responses to disease, injury or infection in the central nervous system (CNS). Therefore, we can learn from what has been studied in other diseases, particularly neurodegenerative diseases. The CNS, which includes the brain, retina, and optic nerve, is an immune privileged tissue (Glass et al. 2010; Lampron et al. 2013); in contrast to other tissues, communication between the CNS and the systemic immune system is relatively limited (Glass et al. 2010; Ransohoff and Brown 2012; Lampron et al. 2013). Therefore, immune responses in the CNS are generally mediated by a limited number of cell types.

Major Players in CNS Immune Responses

The CNS includes resident astrocytes and microglial cells (collectively termed glial cells) that perform immune surveillance and mediate primary inflammatory responses to infection, disease, or injury. Astrocytes are glial cells that are in contact with neurons, blood vessels and other glial cells to provide an array of functions including metabolic support, modulation of synaptic activity, regulation of extracellular ion concentrations, and maintenance of the blood–brain barrier (Ullian et al. 2001; Simard and Nedergaard 2004; Iadecola and Nedergaard 2007; Pellerin et al. 2007; Rouach et al. 2008). Microglial cells, myeloid-derived cells that reside in the CNS, are generated from the yolk sac before vascularization and possess phagocytic and antigen-presenting capabilities, although these are more limited than those of peripheral antigen-presenting cells (Ginhoux et al. 2010; Glass et al. 2010; Ransohoff and Brown 2012; Lampron et al. 2013). Blood-derived monocytes, dendritic cells and other immune cells are generally excluded from the CNS parenchyma under healthy conditions (Ransohoff and Brown 2012; Ransohoff and Engelhardt 2012). However, following proinflammatory stimulation, glial cells are activated and produce cytokines and chemokines to recruit infiltrating blood-derived immune cells to amplify the inflammatory response in the CNS (Ransohoff et al. 2003; Callahan and Ransohoff 2004).

Triggering Inflammatory Responses: PAMPs, DAMPs, and Their Sensors

The main role of astrocytes and microglia is to recognize and respond to perturbations in the environment. Perturbations can arise from two major sources: invading microbial pathogens and age- or disease-related stress or injury. Astrocytes and microglial cells possess signaling mechanisms for host defense that are activated by the recognition of structural characteristics found in pathogens, known as pathogen-associated molecular patterns (PAMPs) (Glass et al. 2010; Lampron et al. 2013). Astrocytes and microglial cells also recognize signals released from damaged or stressed cells, known as damage-associated molecular patterns (DAMPs) (Rifkin et al. 2005; Yu et al. 2010; Zhang et al. 2010; Zhu et al. 2011). It has been hypothesized that DAMPs are preexisting intracellular adjuvants that are released when necrotic cell death occurs or when apoptotic cells are not rapidly cleared (Kono and Rock 2008). These DAMPs can also be delivered to the cell surface of damaged cells after injury (Zhu et al. 2011). Molecules identified as bona fide DAMPs include heat shock proteins (HSPs), uric acid, high-mobility group box-1 protein and double stranded DNA (Kono and Rock 2008). The existence of additional DAMPs cannot be ruled out, and efforts are ongoing to identify them. Both PAMPs and DAMPs are recognized by pattern recognition receptors (PRRs) on astrocytes and/or microglia that trigger and mediate the inflammatory response (Fig. 1).

An important class of pattern recognition receptors is the toll-like receptors (TLRs) (Gorina et al. 2009; Downes and Crack 2010; Lehnardt 2010). TLRs can recognize a diverse group of pathogenic molecules that are not present

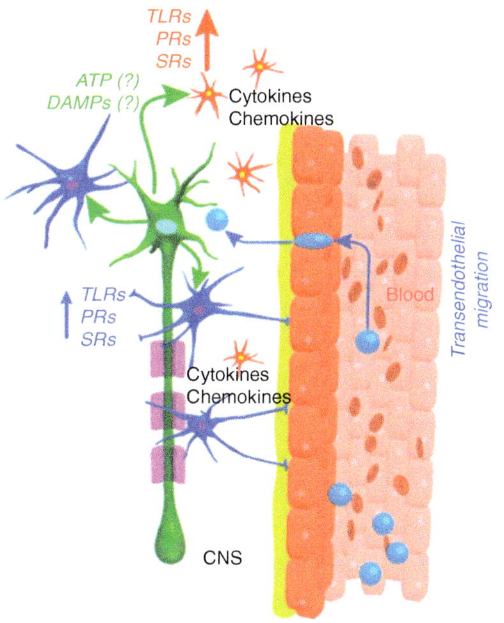

Figure 1. Inflammatory responses in the CNS are mediated by resident astrocytes and microglia. The neurovascular unit comprises neurons (green), astrocytes (blue, with processes) and components of the blood–brain barrier such as endothelial cells (red, vessel). In addition, microglia (red, with processes) sense environmental changes. Glial cells (astrocytes and microglia) express pattern recognition receptors (PRRs) such as toll-like receptors (TLRs), purinergic receptors (PRs) and scavenger receptors (SRs) to respond to DAMPs released by cells during injury or disease. The activation of these receptors promotes proinflammatory signaling that leads to the production of cytokines and chemokines. These cytokines and chemokines induce changes in the endothelial cells and blood–brain barrier integrity, resulting in recruitment of blood-derived immune cells (blue) and amplification of the innate immune response.

in the host (e.g., lipopolysaccharide and viral RNA), but are also able to recognize endogenously derived molecules that are released from injured or dying cells such as HSP60, HSP70 and αB-crystallin (Takeuchi and Akira 2010; Zhang et al. 2010; Ransohoff and Engelhardt 2012). Whereas all thirteen TLRs are expressed on microglial cells, only TLR2, TLR3, TLR4, TLR5, and TLR9 are expressed on astrocytes (Farina et al. 2007). On activation, TLRs recruit the downstream signal adaptor proteins MyD88 and TRIF, which lead to the activation of kinases IκB and MAPK and their downstream group of transcription factors that include members of the NF-κB, AP-1 and interferon regulator factor families resulting in the transcription of several amplifiers and effectors (Glass et al. 2010; Takeuchi and Akira 2010). Among these amplifiers and effectors are cytokines, such as tumor necrosis factor (TNF)-α, interleukin (IL)-1β, and IL-6, as well as an array of chemokines (e.g., CCL2, CXCL1, CXCL10).

A second class of pattern recognition receptor is the NOD-like receptors, specifically the NALP family, which are components of the multiprotein complexes termed the "inflammasome" that can modulate the inflammatory response (Takeuchi and Akira 2010; Ransohoff and Brown 2012). Cooperative interactions between TLRs and the inflammasome lead to the maturation and secretion of cytokines such as IL-1β and IL-18. Other types of pattern recognition receptors include the mannose receptor, scavenger receptor, and the ionic purinergic receptor. The mannose receptor is a C-type lectin that recognizes surfaces that are glycosylated with a mannose moiety (Gazi and Martinez-Pomares 2009) and can trigger immune responses including the activation of the complement cascade (Kerrigan and Brown 2009). Scavenger receptors are involved in the recognition and uptake of oxidized proteins and lipids released by damaged cells (Husemann et al. 2002). The ionic purinergic receptors (such as P2X7R) are activated by ATP released from damaged cells and facilitate formation of the inflammasome (Takeuchi and Akira 2010; Ransohoff and Brown 2012).

Under conditions of injury or disease, astrocytes and microglia become reactive and their PRRs are activated, leading to the generation of innate inflammatory mediators that include members of the complement pathway, cytokines, and several chemokines (such as those listed above). Certainly these proinflammatory molecules affect neuronal function and amplify the inflammatory response of microglial cells during pathological conditions (Glass et al. 2010). Activation of proinflammatory mediators by microglia can result in a cascade of events, including proliferation, migration, expression of adhesion molecules on endothelial cells, and the promotion of leukocyte infiltration into the CNS parenchyma through the blood-brain barrier (Ransohoff and Brown 2012).

Transendothelial Migration in the CNS

Migration (or infiltration) of leukocytes (immune cells) into the CNS is a highly regulated process involving interactions between circulating leukocytes and endothelial cells (Fig. 2) (Ransohoff et al. 2003). Transendothelial migration of leukocytes is a multistep process and involves: (1) tethering and rolling of leukocytes on the endothelial cells; (2) activation of key molecules on both endothelial cells and leukocytes; and finally (3) paracellular or transcellular migration of leukocytes into the CNS. Leukocyte infiltration is a common event in CNS disease and injury, and is thought to occur after chronic stress (Ransohoff et al. 2003; Callahan and Ransohoff 2004; Ransohoff and Brown 2012). Leukocyte infiltration is commonly initiated by the release of cytokines and chemokines from glial cells (Carson et al. 2006; Ifergan et al. 2008). Studies using intravital microscopy found that activation of leukocytes was not sufficient to promote interaction of endothelial cells and leukocytes. However, leukocyte tethering was observed when endothelial cells were activated with lipopolysaccharide or TNF-α (Piccio et al. 2002). It is thought that after cytokine stimulation, tethering and rolling occurs as a result of the up-regulation of selectins (e.g., P-selectin) and integrin ligands (e.g., VCAM-1 and ICAM-1) on the lumen of endothelial cells that are sensed by selectin ligands (e.g., PSGL1) and integrins (e.g., LFA1) present on the surface of circulating leukocytes (Lampron et al. 2013). These signaling processes between endothelial cells and leukocytes promote the loosening of the tight junctions between the endothelial cells, facilitating migration of leukocytes into the CNS (Ransohoff et al. 2003; Lampron et al. 2013).

The cellular and molecular mechanisms by which transendothelial migration occurs in the CNS during injury and disease are complex and still not completely understood. More research is needed to elucidate the identity and role of these infiltrating cells during neurodegenerative diseases.

The Complement Cascade Modulates Inflammatory Responses

The complement cascade was originally named as it "complements" immune responses. How-

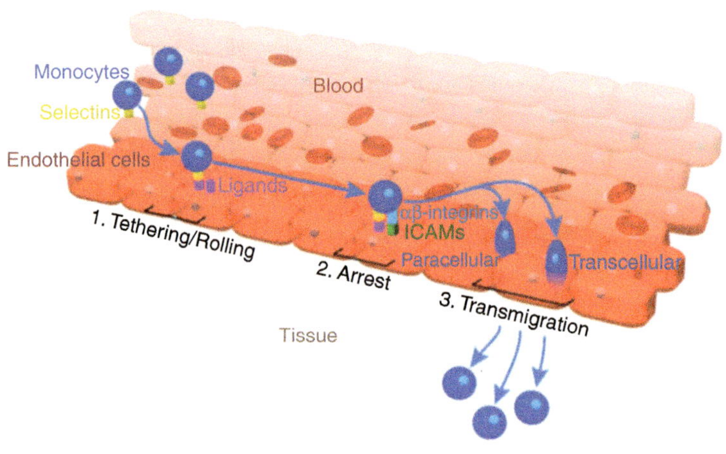

Figure 2. Transendothelial migration in the CNS. Schematic representation of the different steps involved in leukocyte extravasation. Selectin ligands and molecular adhesion molecules that are up-regulated in endothelial cells at the ONH interact with selectins and integrins present at the cell surface of leukocytes, leading to leukocyte infiltration.

ever, recent and emerging evidence suggests it plays a much more complex role in the CNS in health and disease. Components of the complement cascade play a significant role in immune surveillance and inflammatory processes, both peripherally and in the CNS (Janeway et al. 2001). In addition to its involvement in pathogen targeting and elimination, the complement system is also involved in synapse elimination and clearance of potential mediators of damage or injury (Ricklin et al. 2010; Rosen and Stevens 2010).

The complement system is a cascade of three separate pathways known as the classical, alternative, and lectin pathways (Ricklin et al. 2010). A strong complement response includes opsonization of the foreign pathogen or apoptotic cell/cellular compartment by complement fragments, induction of proinflammatory signaling by anaphylatoxins that recruit macrophages, and enable phagocytosis and the formation of the membrane attack complex (MAC), which leads to the lysis of the targeted cell (Ricklin et al. 2010). The classical pathway is initiated by the C1 complex that recognizes pathogens or DAMPs, leading to the formation of the C3 convertase that cleaves the C3 protein to generate the active fragments C3a and C3b. C3a induces proinflammatory signaling and C3b deposition induces cleavage of the C5 protein to C5a and C5b by C5 convertases. C5a is a potent anaphylatoxin, whereas C5b is a fundamental member of the MAC, a cell lysis-inducing channel. Other complement factors in the MAC are C6, C7, C8, and C9. The C3 convertase is also activated by the alternative and lectin pathways, and all three pathways can result in the activation of the MAC (Ricklin et al. 2010). Activation of the complement system has been observed in the CNS after injury and in neurodegenerative diseases such as Alzheimer's disease, Parkinson's disease, and glaucoma (Bonifati and Kishore 2007).

Beneficial and Damaging Effects of the Immune Response in the CNS

As described above, the immune response is a complex series of events involving resident glial cells (e.g., astrocytes and microglia), components of the blood–brain barrier (e.g., endothelial cells), and infiltrating blood-derived cells (e.g., monocytes). The early immune responses are likely the body's natural attempts to minimize damage after an initial injury or insult in chronic and age-related CNS diseases. Later immune responses, as the disease enters a chronic phase, are likely more detrimental. In some cases, these beneficial and detrimental events involve molecules in the same pathway, such as the complement cascade. Therefore, when considering therapies, it is important to fully understand the beneficial and detrimental natures of inflammatory processes in CNS injury and disease.

NEUROINFLAMMATORY RESPONSES IN GLAUCOMA

So far, we have described immune responses as they relate generally to the CNS in response to infection, injury, or disease. We now describe what is known about the role of the immune system in glaucoma, and highlight areas for further investigation.

Activation of Astrocytes and Microglia in the Optic Nerve Head in Early Stages of Glaucoma

Retinal cells and glial cells in the ONH respond rapidly and early to glaucomatous insults, including elevation of IOP. Changes in astrocyte morphology, such as enlargement of the cell body and processes, as well as up-regulation of cytoskeletal and extracellular matrix proteins, have been observed in the retina and ONH in human glaucoma (Wang et al. 2002; Inman and Horner 2007; Hernandez et al. 2008; Kompass et al. 2008; Nikolskaya et al. 2009). Several studies have demonstrated that this reactivity and remodeling of astrocytes, and the increased deposition of extracellular matrix occur in early stages of experimental glaucoma (Johnson and Morrison 2009; Howell et al. 2011a; Johnson et al. 2011; Lye-Barthel et al. 2013; Qu and Jakobs 2013). In fact, just a short term elevation of IOP induces rapid and reversible morphological changes in astrocytes of the ONH that include hypertrophy, process retraction, and simplification of the shape without changing gene expression (Sun et al. 2013). Furthermore, changes in gene expression in astrocytes are observed at early stages of experimental glaucoma before RGC axon damage (Johnson et al. 2000, 2011; Howell et al. 2011a; Qu and Jakobs 2013). This early up-regulation of extracellular matrix in astrocytes of the ONH may function to repair or prevent damage to the blood–brain barrier in response to high IOP. This has been shown in other settings (Sofroniew and Vinters 2010). For instance, inhibition of reactive astrogliosis by the conditional deletion of the STAT3 protein in models of spinal cord injury promotes massive infiltration of blood-derived leukocytes and increased neurodegeneration, suggesting that astrocyte reactivity is a protective response in CNS injury (Okada et al. 2006; Herrmann et al. 2008). Consistent with this idea is the observation that components of the basement membrane of the blood–brain barrier, such as collagen, are up-regulated in the ONH in human glaucoma and in experimental models of the disease (Hernandez et al. 1990, 1994; Morrison et al. 1990; Johnson et al. 2011). On the other hand, the overexpression of cell adhesion proteins, including several integrins, by astrocytes in glaucoma could also promote the adhesion and migration of immune cells into damaged areas of the ONH (Howell et al. 2011a; Johnson et al. 2011; Tanigami et al. 2012). Furthermore, ONH astrocytes in human glaucoma and experimental models up-regulate tenascin-C (Pena et al. 1999; Howell et al. 2011a; Johnson et al. 2011), an extracellular matrix glycoprotein that supports proinflammatory responses through TLR4 signaling (Midwood et al. 2009), suggesting a proinflammatory role of astrocytes in glaucoma.

Activation of microglial cells in the ONH and retina has also been observed in experimental models of glaucoma (Neufeld 1999; Yuan and Neufeld 2001; Johnson and Morrison 2009; Ebneter et al. 2010; Bosco et al. 2011; Taylor et al. 2011). This microglial reactivity is characterized by increased proliferation, increased phagocytic activity (revealed by an increase in the phagocytosis-related protein CD68), changes in morphology, and expression of proinflammatory molecules, such as members of the complement cascade, major histocompatibility complex class I, and major histocompatibility complex class II (Ebneter et al. 2010; Howell et al. 2011a; Bosco et al. 2012). Although the role of microglia in glaucoma progression is not clear, it is notable that the extent of microglia activation is closely related to axonal degeneration in the ONH. In fact, reduction in microglial number is evident when axonal degeneration (but not high IOP) is prevented by radiation treatment of the eye or head in a mouse model of glaucoma (Howell et al. 2012; Bosco et al. 2012).

What Triggers Inflammatory Responses in Glaucoma?

Early neuroinflammatory responses by astrocytes and microglia occur in glaucoma, but it is not known which stresses or damage-associated molecules trigger the responses. One possibility is that DAMPs are released or presented by stressed or damaged RGC axons in the ONH. In glaucoma, heat shock proteins, a type of DAMP, are up-regulated in response to elevation in IOP (Tezel et al. 2004; Tezel 2011), and levels of a variety of heat shock proteins were also increased in human glaucomatous retinas (Luo et al. 2010). A second possibility is that astrocytes and/or microglia produce DAMPs independent of or before changes in RGCs. One candidate for this is tenascin-C, which is up-regulated in astrocytes of the glaucomatous ONH (Pena et al. 1999; Howell et al. 2011a; Johnson et al. 2011). Tenascin-C is an endogenous activator of the TLR4 in inflammation associated with arthritis (Midwood et al. 2009). Identification of initiator(s) of inflammatory events is a key area of study in glaucoma research.

Inflammatory Signaling Pathways in Glaucoma

Although the specific triggers for inflammatory responses in glaucoma remain poorly defined, inflammatory processes, mediated in part by astrocytes and resident microglia, clearly play a crucial role in glaucoma. Several studies using transcriptional profiling have identified early up-regulation of genes associated with inflammatory pathways in the retina and ONH in experimental models of glaucoma (Ahmed et al. 2004; Johnson et al. 2007, 2011; Yang et al. 2007; Kompass et al. 2008; Nikolskaya et al. 2009; Panagis et al. 2010; Howell et al. 2011a, 2012). Collectively, these studies showed an up-regulation of inflammatory inducers/sensors (PRRs, e.g., TLRs), transducers (e.g., *Mapk*, *Trif*, *MyD88*) and amplifiers (e.g., *Il1*, *Il6*, *Tnf*, *Ccl2*) in human glaucoma (Luo et al. 2010; Yang et al. 2011; Tezel et al. 2012) and in early stages of experimental glaucoma (Howell et al. 2011a; Johnson et al. 2011). In our study using DBA/2J mice, an inherited model of glaucoma, we were able to define early molecular changes that occur before detectable loss of RGCs and axons (Howell et al. 2011a). Gene ontology analysis revealed that genes associated with "immune response," "leukocyte activation," and "chemotaxis" were among the genes up-regulated earliest in mice with high IOP but no detectable loss of axons.

Evidence from both human glaucoma patients and animal models of glaucoma suggest that immune responses are mediated, at least in part, by TLRs. For instance, proteomic analysis of glaucomatous human retinas revealed up-regulation of TLR signaling (Luo et al. 2010). Expression of TLR2, TLR3, and TLR4 was observed in microglia and astrocytes from glaucomatous retinas. In early stages of DBAJ glaucoma, 11 of the 13 TLRs were up-regulated in the ONH at early stages of DBA/2J glaucoma (Howell et al. 2011a,b). These included *Tlr3*, *Tlr7*, and *Tlr9*, whose proteins detect nucleic acids released from damaged cells, and *Tlr2* and *Tlr4*, whose gene products sense host cell HSPs (Rifkin et al. 2005; Yu et al. 2010; Zhang et al. 2010). The TLR adaptor protein MyD88 and members of the MAPK pathway were also up-regulated in retinas from glaucoma patients and in the ONH of DBA/2J mice (Luo et al. 2010; Howell et al. 2011a,b).

As mentioned previously, engagement of TLRs by DAMPs can lead to the activation of NF-κB. Not surprisingly, proteomic analysis of glaucomatous retinas from humans and rats found increased expression of kinases such as RIPK, NIK, and IκK that are involved in the activation of the NF-κB pathway (Yang et al. 2011; Tezel et al. 2012). Activation of NF-κB results in the transcription of genes from the IL-1 cytokine family. Secretion of these cytokines can promote production of a secondary cascade of inflammatory cytokines in microglia (e.g., TNF-α) and astrocytes (e.g., IL-6) that amplifies the immune response by recruiting other cells to the site of damage. In support of this sequence of events, members of the IL-1 family were found to be up-regulated in the ONH at early stages of DBA/2J glaucoma (Howell et al. 2011a,b).

Studies have also suggested an important role for tumor necrosis factor (TNF) family members in the pathogenesis of glaucoma. Increased levels of TNF-α have been found in the aqueous humor, retina, and optic nerve microglia and optic nerve astrocytes from glaucoma patients (Yan et al. 2000; Yuan and Neufeld 2000, 2001; Tezel et al. 2001; Sawada et al. 2010). Activation of the signaling pathway downstream from TNF-α in glaucomatous human retinas has also been reported (Yang et al. 2011). Several ligands and receptors of the TNF family were overexpressed at early stages of DBA/2J glaucoma, although not as early as was observed for the *Il1*-related cytokines (Howell et al. 2011a,b). Genetic and pharmaceutical inhibition of TNF-α activity in experimental models of glaucoma can prevent microglia activation, axonal degeneration and RGC loss (Fig. 3) (Nakazawa et al. 2006; Roh et al. 2012). Another member of the TNF family implicated in glaucoma pathogenesis is the proapoptotic protein Fas ligand, which was found to be damaging to RGCs in DBA/2J glaucoma (Gregory et al. 2011). Inhibition of Fas ligand activity prevented death of RGCs after intraocular injection of TNF-α, indicating that Fas ligand mediates TNF-α cytotoxicity in RGCs (Gregory et al. 2011).

In summary, it has been clearly demonstrated that proinflammatory pathways (likely activated by DAMPs) are important contributors to the early progression of glaucoma. Further

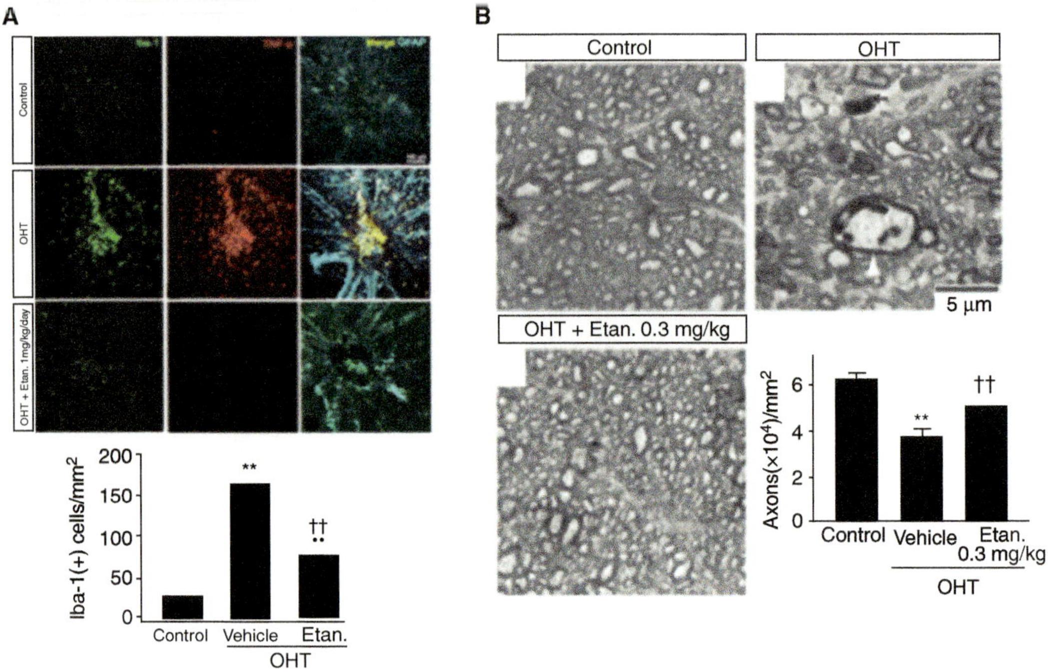

Figure 3. Inhibition of TNF-α activity reduces microglial activation and axonal degeneration in the optic nerve after ocular hypertension. (*A*) Ocular hypertension (OHT) increased the number of Iba-1-positive microglial cells in the ONH and induced TNF-α expression in these cells. Treatment with the TNF-α inhibitor Etanercept (Etan.) significantly reduced the number of microglia and the expression of TNF-α. (*B*) Axonal degeneration in the optic nerve is reduced by Etanercept treatment in ocular hypertension (Roh et al. 2012). Mann-Whitney U test, ** $P < 0.01$ comparing control vs. Etanercept treated ocular hypertension; †† $P < 0.01$ comparing vehicle vs. Etanercept treated OHT. (Adapted from data in Roh et al. 2012.)

studies are needed to identify the precise roles of the different cell types at different stages of disease, keeping in mind that inflammatory molecules can mediate both damaging and beneficial responses.

Transendothelial Migration of Leukocytes in Glaucoma

One of the earliest processes to be significantly up-regulated in our transcriptional profiling of DBA/2J mice was transendothelial migration of leukocytes (Howell et al. 2012). In DBA/2J glaucoma, up-regulation of selectins (e.g., P-selectin), adhesion molecules (e.g. VCAM-1) and chemokines (e.g., CCL2) was observed at early stages of disease (Howell et al. 2012). Flow cytometry experiments confirmed the entry of monocyte-derived cells into the ONH (Fig. 4A) (Howell et al. 2012). No other type of immune cell (including B cells or T cells) was found in DBA/2J glaucomatous tissue, although one study has shown B cells in human glaucomatous retinas (Gramlich et al. 2013). Monocyte infiltration was apparently blocked by DBA/2J mice treated with radiation (Fig. 4B) indicating that monocyte infiltration could be an important mediator of RGC and axonal damage in glaucoma (Howell et al. 2012). In support of this, a second study using a different experimental mouse model of glaucoma found that deletion of CD11b prevented the activation of monocyte-derived cells and loss of RGCs after induction of high IOP (Nakazawa et al. 2006). However, this study was not able to distinguish between resident microglia and infiltrating monocytes. The mechanism(s) by which monocytes affect RGCs in glaucoma has not been

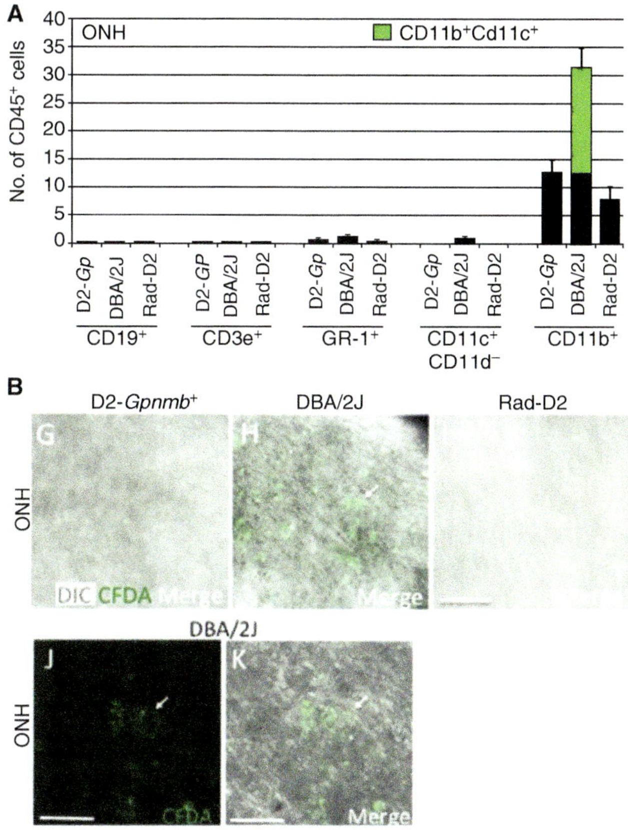

Figure 4. Monocyte infiltration occurs early in DBA/2J glaucoma. (*A*) Flow cytometry revealed that the major blood-derived immune cell detected in the ONH of DBA/2J glaucomatous mice was the CD11b$^+$Cd11c$^+$ monocyte. These cells were completely absent in radiation-treated DBA/2J eyes (Rad-D2) or control (D2-Gp) eyes. (*B*) Cell infiltration was also assessed using the injection of a fluorescent tracer into the spleen (CFDA, green). Spleen-derived CFDA$^+$ cells entered the optic nerves of untreated DBA/2J eyes but not Rad-D2 eyes or control eyes (Howell et al. 2012). (From Howell et al. 2013; adapted, with permission, from the authors.)

elucidated and further studies are needed to define the contribution of these infiltrating monocytes in glaucoma progression.

The Complement Cascade in Glaucoma

Components of the complement cascade are induced in human and animal models of glaucoma, suggesting a key role for this system in progression of the disease (Ahmed et al. 2004; Kuehn et al. 2006, 2008; Stasi et al. 2006; Steele et al. 2006; Stevens et al. 2007; Ren and Danias 2010; Tezel et al. 2010; Howell et al. 2011a). In experimental models of glaucoma, induction of complement components in the retina and ONH was one of the earliest signaling responses to high IOP (Howell et al. 2011a; Johnson et al. 2011). Up-regulation of *C1qa*, a member of the C1 complex that triggers activation of the classical pathway, was observed in microglial cells in the ONH before detection of axonal damage in DBA/2J glaucomatous mice (Howell et al. 2011a). Deposition of C1QA protein was also observed in RGC dendrites in glaucomatous DBA/2J retinas as well as in primate and human glaucomatous retinas (Fig. 5A) (Kuehn et al. 2006; Stasi et al. 2006; Stevens et al. 2007; Tezel et al. 2010), suggesting an involvement of the complement cascade in pathological synapse elimination and/or dendrite remodeling in

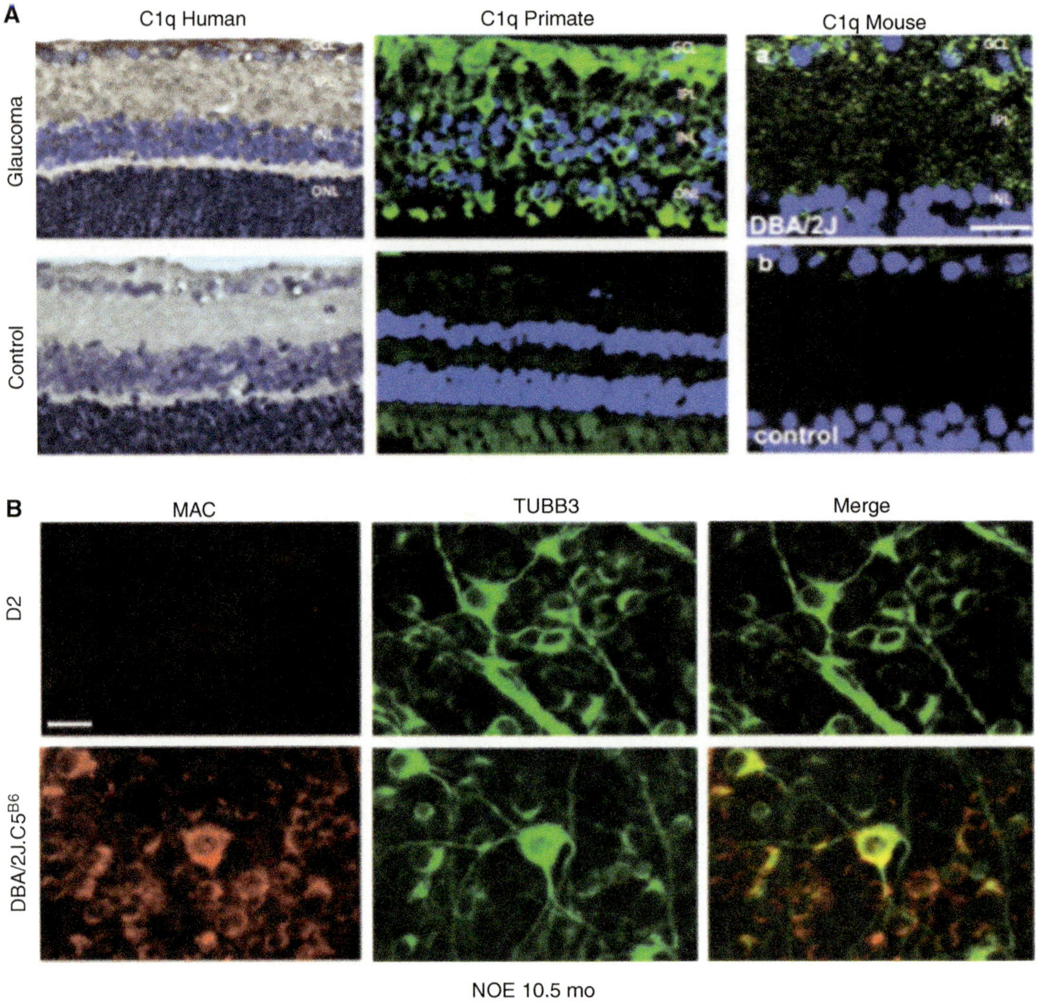

Figure 5. The complement system is activated in human and animal models of glaucoma. (*A*) C1Q protein is increased in RGCs and in the inner plexiform layer of human (Tezel et al. 2010), primate (Stasi et al. 2006), and mouse (Howell et al. 2011a) retinas in response to high IOP. (*B*) MAC deposition is found in RGCs from C5-sufficient glaucomatous DBA/2J.C5^{B6} mice (Howell et al. 2013). TUBB3, tubulin β-3; NOE, normal or early.

glaucoma. Importantly, DBA/2J mice deficient in C1QA were protected from glaucomatous RGC loss, demonstrating an important and damaging contribution for *C1qa* in glaucoma (Howell et al. 2011a).

A second component of the complement cascade that likely plays a damaging role in glaucoma is complement component C5, a necessary component in generation of the MAC. Significant deposition of MAC was found in glaucomatous RGCs in human eyes and in experimental models of glaucoma (Kuehn et al. 2006; Jha et al. 2011; Howell et al. 2013). Drug inhibition of complement activation reduced MAC deposition and apoptosis of RGCs in a rat model of glaucoma (Jha et al. 2011). Furthermore, C5-deficient DBA/2J mice showed reduced neurodegeneration compared with C5-sufficient DBA/2J mice (Howell et al. 2013). Although it is not clear how C5 contributes to glaucoma, significant deposition of MACs was observed in RGCs and in dystrophic neurites in the optic

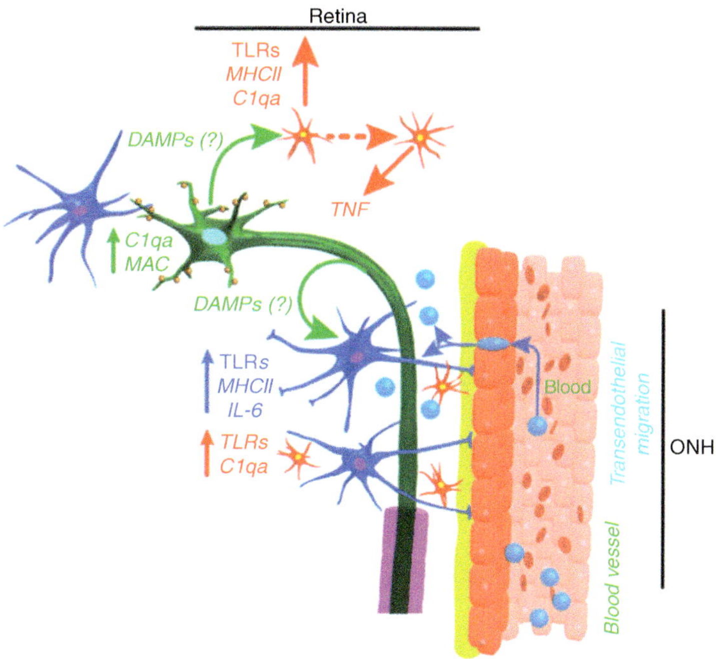

Figure 6. A model of early neuroinflammatory responses in glaucoma. We hypothesize that initiation of these immune responses occurs after the release of DAMPs from RGCs, glial cells or both. The TLRs expressed in glial cells activate the production and secretion of cytokines such as those of the IL-1 family. A secondary expression of cytokines, such as TNF-α in microglia and IL-6 in astrocytes, is induced, leading to an amplified inflammatory response. These neuroinflammatory responses are likely modulated by complement proteins, such as *C1qa*, in the ONH. In addition, intrinsic up-regulation of complement molecules in RGCs (such as *C1qa* and *C3*) occurs early and mediates synaptic dysfunction. The cell types shown here are described in the legend for Figure 1.

nerve (Fig. 5B), suggesting a detrimental contribution of C5b to glaucoma progression.

Much work is being done (in our laboratory, the Danias laboratory, and others) regarding the role of the complement cascade in glaucoma. Areas of active research include assessment of other key components of the cascade such as C3 and C4. Complement proteins are expressed in multiple cell types and it will be important to understand the cell-specific roles of complement components in glaucoma.

CONCLUDING REMARKS

In recent years a critical role for neuroinflammatory processes mediated by astrocytes, microglia, endothelial cells, infiltrating monocytes and other cell types in the pathogenesis of glaucoma has been demonstrated (Fig. 6). However, many challenges remain. The potential for beneficial and detrimental inflammatory processes occurring at different stages of glaucoma make developing therapies that target these processes a complex but, in our view, solvable problem. Furthermore, these cells do not function in isolation, and understanding the changes to the neurovascular unit as a whole will also be critical. Development of a detailed spatial and temporal understanding of these neuroinflammatory events in humans and in multiple animal models is critical as we move toward new neuroprotective treatments for human glaucoma.

ACKNOWLEDGMENTS

The authors thank Pete Williams and Jeffrey Harder for critical comments. This work was supported by The Glaucoma Foundation (GRH) and EY021525 (GRH).

REFERENCES

Ahmed F, Brown KM, Stephan DA, Morrison JC, Johnson EC, Tomarev SI. 2004. Microarray analysis of changes in mRNA levels in the rat retina after experimental elevation of intraocular pressure. *Invest Ophthalmol Vis Sci* **45:** 1247–1258.

Bonifati DM, Kishore U. 2007. Role of complement in neurodegeneration and neuroinflammation. *Mol Immunol* **44:** 999–1010.

Bosco A, Steele MR, Vetter ML. 2011. Early microglia activation in a mouse model of chronic glaucoma. *J Comp Neurol* **519:** 599–620.

Bosco A, Crish SD, Steele MR, Romero CO, Inman DM, Horner PJ, Calkins DJ, Vetter ML. 2012. Early reduction of microglia activation by irradiation in a model of chronic glaucoma. *PLoS ONE* **7:** e43602.

Burgoyne CF. 2011. A biomechanical paradigm for axonal insult within the optic nerve head in aging and glaucoma. *Exp Eye Res* **93:** 120–132.

Callahan MK, Ransohoff RM. 2004. Analysis of leukocyte extravasation across the blood-brain barrier: Conceptual and technical aspects. *Curr Allergy Asthma Rep* **4:** 65–73.

Carson MJ, Doose JM, Melchior B, Schmid CD, Ploix CC. 2006. CNS immune privilege: Hiding in plain sight. *Immunol Rev* **213:** 48–65.

Downes CE, Crack PJ. 2010. Neural injury following stroke: Are Toll-like receptors the link between the immune system and the CNS? *Br J Pharmacol* **160:** 1872–1888.

Ebneter A, Casson RJ, Wood JP, Chidlow G. 2010. Microglial activation in the visual pathway in experimental glaucoma: Spatiotemporal characterization and correlation with axonal injury. *Invest Ophthalmol Vis Sci* **51:** 6448–6460.

Farina C, Aloisi F, Meinl E. 2007. Astrocytes are active players in cerebral innate immunity. *Trends Immunol* **28:** 138–145.

Gazi U, Martinez-Pomares L. 2009. Influence of the mannose receptor in host immune responses. *Immunobiology* **214:** 554–561.

Ginhoux F, Greter M, Leboeuf M, Nandi S, See P, Gokhan S, Mehler MF, Conway SJ, Ng LG, Stanley ER, et al. 2010. Fate mapping analysis reveals that adult microglia derive from primitive macrophages. *Science* **330:** 841–845.

Glass CK, Saijo K, Winner B, Marchetto MC, Gage FH. 2010. Mechanisms underlying inflammation in neurodegeneration. *Cell* **140:** 918–934.

Gorina R, Santalucia T, Petegnief V, Ejarque-Ortiz A, Saura J, Planas AM. 2009. Astrocytes are very sensitive to develop innate immune responses to lipid-carried short interfering RNA. *Glia* **57:** 93–107.

Gramlich OW, Beck S, von Thun Und Hohenstein-Blaul N, Boehm N, Ziegler A, Vetter JM, Pfeiffer N, Grus FH. 2013. Enhanced insight into the autoimmune component of glaucoma: IgG autoantibody accumulation and pro-inflammatory conditions in human glaucomatous retina. *PloS ONE* **8:** e57557.

Gregory MS, Hackett CG, Abernathy EF, Lee KS, Saff RR, Hohlbaum AM, Moody KS, Hobson MW, Jones A, Kolovou P, et al. 2011. Opposing roles for membrane bound and soluble Fas ligand in glaucoma-associated retinal ganglion cell death. *PLoS ONE* **6:** e17659.

Hernandez MR, Andrzejewska WM, Neufeld AH. 1990. Changes in the extracellular matrix of the human optic nerve head in primary open-angle glaucoma. *Am J Ophthalmol* **109:** 180–188.

Hernandez MR, Ye H, Roy S. 1994. Collagen type IV gene expression in human optic nerve heads with primary open angle glaucoma. *Exp Eye Res* **59:** 41–51.

Hernandez MR, Miao H, Lukas T. 2008. Astrocytes in glaucomatous optic neuropathy. *Prog Brain Res* **173:** 353–373.

Herrmann JE, Imura T, Song B, Qi J, Ao Y, Nguyen TK, Korsak RA, Takeda K, Akira S, Sofroniew MV. 2008. STAT3 is a critical regulator of astrogliosis and scar formation after spinal cord injury. *J Neurosci* **28:** 7231–7243.

Howell GR, Libby RT, Jakobs TC, Smith RS, Phalan FC, Barter JW, Barbay JM, Marchant JK, Mahesh N, Porciatti V, et al. 2007. Axons of retinal ganglion cells are insulted in the optic nerve early in DBA/2J glaucoma. *J Cell Biol* **179:** 1523–1537.

Howell GR, Macalinao DG, Sousa GL, Walden M, Soto I, Kneeland SC, Barbay JM, King BL, Marchant JK, Hibbs M, et al. 2011a. Molecular clustering identifies complement and endothelin induction as early events in a mouse model of glaucoma. *J Clin Invest* **121:** 1429–1444.

Howell GR, Walton DO, King BL, Libby RT, John SW. 2011b. Datgan, a reusable software system for facile interrogation and visualization of complex transcription profiling data. *BMC Genomics* **12:** 429.

Howell GR, Soto I, Zhu X, Ryan M, Macalinao DG, Sousa GL, Caddle LB, MacNicoll KH, Barbay JM, Porciatti V, et al. 2012. Radiation treatment inhibits monocyte entry into the optic nerve head and prevents neuronal damage in a mouse model of glaucoma. *J Clin Invest* **122:** 1246–1261.

Howell GR, Soto I, Ryan M, Graham LC, Smith RS, John SW. 2013. Deficiency of complement component 5 ameliorates glaucoma in DBA/2J mice. *J Neuroinflammation* **10:** 76.

Husemann J, Loike JD, Anankov R, Febbraio M, Silverstein SC. 2002. Scavenger receptors in neurobiology and neuropathology: Their role on microglia and other cells of the nervous system. *Glia* **40:** 195–205.

Iadecola C, Nedergaard M. 2007. Glial regulation of the cerebral microvasculature. *Nat Neurosci* **10:** 1369–1376.

Ifergan I, Kebir H, Bernard M, Wosik K, Dodelet-Devillers A, Cayrol R, Arbour N, Prat A. 2008. The blood-brain barrier induces differentiation of migrating monocytes into Th17-polarizing dendritic cells. *Brain* **131:** 785–799.

Inman DM, Horner PJ. 2007. Reactive nonproliferative gliosis predominates in a chronic mouse model of glaucoma. *Glia* **55:** 942–953.

Jakobs TC, Libby RT, Ben Y, John SWM, Masland RH. 2005. Retinal ganglion cell degeneration is topological but not cell type specific in DBA/2J mice. *J Cell Biol* **171:** 313–325.

Janeway CA, Travers P, Walport M, Shlomchik M. 2001. *Immunobiology: The Immune System in Health and Disease* 5th edition. Garland Science, New York.

Jha P, Banda H, Tytarenko R, Bora PS, Bora NS. 2011. Complement mediated apoptosis leads to the loss of retinal ganglion cells in animal model of glaucoma. *Mol Immunol* **48:** 2151–2158.

Johnson EC, Deppmeier LM, Wentzien SK, Hsu I, Morrison JC. 2000. Chronology of optic nerve head and retinal responses to elevated intraocular pressure. *Invest Ophthalmol Vis Sci* **41:** 431–442.

Johnson EC, Doser TA, Cepurna WA, Dyck JA, Jia L, Guo Y, Lambert WS, Morrison JC. 2011. Cell proliferation and interleukin-6-type cytokine signaling are implicated by gene expression responses in early optic nerve head injury in rat glaucoma. *Invest Ophthalmol Vis Sci* **52:** 504–518.

Johnson EC, Jia L, Cepurna WA, Doser TA, Morrison JC. 2007. Global changes in optic nerve head gene expression after exposure to elevated intraocular pressure in a rat glaucoma model. *Invest Ophthalmol Vis Sci* **48:** 3161–3177.

Johnson EC, Morrison JC. 2009. Friend or foe? Resolving the impact of glial responses in glaucoma. *J Glaucoma* **18:** 341–353.

Kerrigan AM, Brown GD. 2009. C-type lectins and phagocytosis. *Immunobiology* **214:** 562–575.

Kompass KS, Agapova OA, Li W, Kaufman PL, Rasmussen CA, Hernandez MR. 2008. Bioinformatic and statistical analysis of the optic nerve head in a primate model of ocular hypertension. *BMC Neurosci* **9:** 93.

Kono H, Rock KL. 2008. How dying cells alert the immune system to danger. *Nat Rev Immunol* **8:** 279–289.

Kuehn MH, Kim CY, Ostojic J, Bellin M, Alward WL, Stone EM, Sakaguchi DS, Grozdanic SD, Kwon YH. 2006. Retinal synthesis and deposition of complement components induced by ocular hypertension. *Exp Eye Res* **83:** 620–628.

Kuehn MH, Kim CY, Jiang B, Dumitrescu AV, Kwon YH. 2008. Disruption of the complement cascade delays retinal ganglion cell death following retinal ischemia-reperfusion. *Exp Eye Res* **87:** 89–95.

Lampron A, Elali A, Rivest S. 2013. Innate immunity in the CNS: Redefining the relationship between the CNS and its environment. *Neuron* **78:** 214–232.

Lehnardt S. 2010. Innate immunity and neuroinflammation in the CNS: The role of microglia in Toll-like receptor-mediated neuronal injury. *Glia* **58:** 253–263.

Luo C, Yang X, Kain AD, Powell DW, Kuehn MH, Tezel G. 2010. Glaucomatous tissue stress and the regulation of immune response through glial Toll-like receptor signaling. *Invest Ophthalmol Vis Sci* **51:** 5697–5707.

Lye-Barthel M, Sun D, Jakobs TC. 2013. Morphology of astrocytes in a glaucomatous optic nerve. *Invest Ophthalmol Vis Sci* **54:** 909–917.

Midwood K, Sacre S, Piccinini AM, Inglis J, Trebaul A, Chan E, Drexler S, Sofat N, Kashiwagi M, Orend G, et al. 2009. Tenascin-C is an endogenous activator of Toll-like receptor 4 that is essential for maintaining inflammation in arthritic joint disease. *Nat Med* **15:** 774–780.

Morrison JC, Dorman-Pease ME, Dunkelberger GR, Quigley HA. 1990. Optic nerve head extracellular matrix in primary optic atrophy and experimental glaucoma. *Arch Ophthalmol* **108:** 1020–1024.

Nakazawa T, Nakazawa C, Matsubara A, Noda K, Hisatomi T, She H, Michaud N, Hafezi-Moghadam A, Miller JW, Benowitz LI. 2006. Tumor necrosis factor-α mediates oligodendrocyte death and delayed retinal ganglion cell loss in a mouse model of glaucoma. *J Neurosci* **26:** 12633–12641.

Neufeld AH. 1999. Microglia in the optic nerve head and the region of parapapillary chorioretinal atrophy in glaucoma. *Arch Ophthalmol* **117:** 1050–1056.

Nickells RW, Howell GR, Soto I, John SW. 2012. Under pressure: Cellular and molecular responses during glaucoma, a common neurodegeneration with axonopathy. *Annu Rev Neurosci* **35:** 153–179.

Nikolskaya T, Nikolsky Y, Serebryiskaya T, Zvereva S, Sviridov E, Dezso Z, Rahkmatulin E, Brennan RJ, Yankovsky N, Bhattacharya SK, et al. 2009. Network analysis of human glaucomatous optic nerve head astrocytes. *BMC Med Genomics* **2:** 24.

Okada S, Nakamura M, Katoh H, Miyao T, Shimazaki T, Ishii K, Yamane J, Yoshimura A, Iwamoto Y, Toyama Y, et al. 2006. Conditional ablation of Stat3 or Socs3 discloses a dual role for reactive astrocytes after spinal cord injury. *Nat Med* **12:** 829–834.

Panagis L, Zhao X, Ge Y, Ren L, Mittag TW, Danias J. 2010. Gene expression changes in areas of focal loss of retinal ganglion cells in the retina of DBA/2J mice. *Invest Ophthalmol Vis Sci* **51:** 2024–2034.

Pellerin L, Bouzier-Sore AK, Aubert A, Serres S, Merle M, Costalat R, Magistretti PJ. 2007. Activity-dependent regulation of energy metabolism by astrocytes: An update. *Glia* **55:** 1251–1262.

Pena JD, Varela HJ, Ricard CS, Hernandez MR. 1999. Enhanced tenascin expression associated with reactive astrocytes in human optic nerve heads with primary open angle glaucoma. *Exp Eye Res* **68:** 29–40.

Piccio L, Rossi B, Scarpini E, Laudanna C, Giagulli C, Issekutz AC, Vestweber D, Butcher EC, Constantin G. 2002. Molecular mechanisms involved in lymphocyte recruitment in inflamed brain microvessels: Critical roles for P-selectin glycoprotein ligand-1 and heterotrimeric G_i-linked receptors. *J Immunol* **168:** 1940–1949.

Qu J, Jakobs TC. 2013. The time course of gene expression during reactive gliosis in the optic nerve. *PloS ONE* **8:** e67094.

Quigley HA. 1993. Open-angle glaucoma. *New Engl J Med* **328:** 1097–1106.

Quigley HA. 2011. Glaucoma. *Lancet* **377:** 1367–1377.

Ransohoff RM, Brown MA. 2012. Innate immunity in the central nervous system. *J Clin Invest* **122:** 1164–1171.

Ransohoff RM, Engelhardt B. 2012. The anatomical and cellular basis of immune surveillance in the central nervous system. *Nat Rev Immunol* **12:** 623–635.

Ransohoff RM, Kivisakk P, Kidd G. 2003. Three or more routes for leukocyte migration into the central nervous system. *Nat Rev Immunol* **3:** 569–581.

Ren L, Danias J. 2010. A role for complement in glaucoma? *Adv Exp Med Biol* **703:** 95–104.

Ricklin D, Hajishengallis G, Yang K, Lambris JD. 2010. Complement: A key system for immune surveillance and homeostasis. *Nat Immunol* **11:** 785–797.

Rifkin IR, Leadbetter EA, Busconi L, Viglianti G, Marshak-Rothstein A. 2005. Toll-like receptors, endogenous ligands, and systemic autoimmune disease. *Immunol Rev* **204:** 27–42.

Roh M, Zhang Y, Murakami Y, Thanos A, Lee SC, Vavvas DG, Benowitz LI, Miller JW. 2012. Etanercept, a widely used inhibitor of tumor necrosis factor-α (TNF-α), prevents retinal ganglion cell loss in a rat model of glaucoma. *PloS ONE* **7:** e40065.

Rosen AM, Stevens B. 2010. The role of the classical complement cascade in synapse loss during development and glaucoma. *Adv Exp Med Biol* **703:** 75–93.

Rouach N, Koulakoff A, Abudara V, Willecke K, Giaume C. 2008. Astroglial metabolic networks sustain hippocampal synaptic transmission. *Science* **322:** 1551–1555.

Sawada H, Fukuchi T, Tanaka T, Abe H. 2010. Tumor necrosis factor-α concentrations in the aqueous humor of patients with glaucoma. *Invest Ophthalmol Vis Sci* **51:** 903–906.

Schlamp CL, Li Y, Dietz JA, Janssen KT, Nickells RW. 2006. Progressive ganglion cell loss and optic nerve degeneration in DBA/2J mice is variable and asymmetric. *BMC Neurosci* **7:** 66.

Simard M, Nedergaard M. 2004. The neurobiology of glia in the context of water and ion homeostasis. *Neuroscience* **129:** 877–896.

Sofroniew MV, Vinters HV. 2010. Astrocytes: Biology and pathology. *Acta Neuropathol* **119:** 7–35.

Soto I, Oglesby E, Buckingham BP, Son JL, Roberson EDO, Steele MR, Inman DM, Vetter ML, Horner PJ, Marsh-Armstrong N. 2008. Retinal ganglion cells downregulate gene expression and lose their axons within the optic nerve head in a mouse glaucoma model. *J Neurosci* **28:** 548–561.

Stasi K, Nagel D, Yang X, Wang RF, Ren L, Podos SM, Mittag T, Danias J. 2006. Complement component 1Q (C1Q) upregulation in retina of murine, primate, and human glaucomatous eyes. *Invest Ophthalmol Vis Sci* **47:** 1024–1029.

Steele MR, Inman DM, Calkins DJ, Horner PJ, Vetter ML. 2006. Microarray analysis of retinal gene expression in the DBA/2J model of glaucoma. *Invest Ophthalmol Vis Sci* **47:** 977–985.

Stevens B, Allen NJ, Vazquez LE, Howell GR, Christopherson KS, Nouri N, Micheva KD, Mehalow AK, Huberman AD, Stafford B, et al. 2007. The classical complement cascade mediates CNS synapse elimination. *Cell* **131:** 1164–1178.

Sun D, Qu J, Jakobs TC. 2013. Reversible reactivity by optic nerve astrocytes. *Glia* **61:** 1218–1235.

Takeuchi O, Akira S. 2010. Pattern recognition receptors and inflammation. *Cell* **140:** 805–820.

Tanigami H, Okamoto T, Yasue Y, Shimaoka M. 2012. Astroglial integrins in the development and regulation of neurovascular units. *Pain Res Treat* **2012:** 964652.

Taylor S, Calder CJ, Albon J, Erichsen JT, Boulton ME, Morgan JE. 2011. Involvement of the CD200 receptor complex in microglia activation in experimental glaucoma. *Exp Eye Res* **92:** 338–343.

Tezel G. 2011. The immune response in glaucoma: A perspective on the roles of oxidative stress. *Exp Eye Res* **93:** 178–186.

Tezel G. 2013. Immune regulation toward immunomodulation for neuroprotection in glaucoma. *Curr Opin Pharmacol* **13:** 23–31.

Tezel G, Li LY, Patil RV, Wax MB. 2001. TNF-α and TNF-α receptor-1 in the retina of normal and glaucomatous eyes. *Invest Ophthalmol Vis Sci* **42:** 1787–1794.

Tezel G, Yang J, Wax MB. 2004. Heat shock proteins, immunity and glaucoma. *Brain Res Bull* **62:** 473–480.

Tezel G, Yang X, Luo C, Kain AD, Powell DW, Kuehn MH, Kaplan HJ. 2010. Oxidative stress and the regulation of complement activation in human glaucoma. *Invest Ophthalmol Vis Sci* **51:** 5071–5082.

Tezel G, Yang X, Luo C, Cai J, Powell DW. 2012. An astrocyte-specific proteomic approach to inflammatory responses in experimental rat glaucoma. *Invest Ophthalmol Vis Sci* **53:** 4220–4233.

Ullian EM, Sapperstein SK, Christopherson KS, Barres BA. 2001. Control of synapse number by glia. *Science* **291:** 657–661.

Wang L, Cioffi GA, Cull G, Dong J, Fortune B. 2002. Immunohistologic evidence for retinal glial cell changes in human glaucoma. *Invest Ophthalmol Vis Sci* **43:** 1088–1094.

Yan X, Tezel G, Wax MB, Edward DP. 2000. Matrix metalloproteinases and tumor necrosis factor α in glaucomatous optic nerve head. *Arch Ophthalmol* **118:** 666–673.

Yang Z, Quigley HA, Pease ME, Yang Y, Qian J, Valenta D, Zack DJ. 2007. Changes in gene expression in experimental glaucoma and optic nerve transection: The equilibrium between protective and detrimental mechanisms. *Invest Ophthalmol Vis Sci* **48:** 5539–5548.

Yang X, Luo C, Cai J, Powell DW, Yu D, Kuehn MH, Tezel G. 2011. Neurodegenerative and inflammatory pathway components linked to TNF-α/TNFR1 signaling in the glaucomatous human retina. *Invest Ophthalmol Vis Sci* **52:** 8442–8454.

Yuan L, Neufeld AH. 2000. Tumor necrosis factor-α: A potentially neurodestructive cytokine produced by glia in the human glaucomatous optic nerve head. *Glia* **32:** 42–50.

Yuan L, Neufeld AH. 2001. Activated microglia in the human glaucomatous optic nerve head. *J Neurosci Res* **64:** 523–532.

Yu L, Wang L, Chen S. 2010. Endogenous toll-like receptor ligands and their biological significance. *J Cell Mol Med* **14:** 2592–2603.

Zhang Q, Raoof M, Chen Y, Sumi Y, Sursal T, Junger W, Brohi K, Itagaki K, Hauser CJ. 2010. Circulating mitochondrial DAMPs cause inflammatory responses to injury. *Nature* **464:** 104–107.

Zhu H, Wang L, Ruan Y, Zhou L, Zhang D, Min Z, Xie J, Yu M, Gu J. 2011. An efficient delivery of DAMPs on the cell surface by the unconventional secretion pathway. *Biochem Biophys Res Commun* **404:** 790–795.

Genetics of Primary Inherited Disorders of the Optic Nerve: Clinical Applications

Keri F. Allen, Eric D. Gaier, and Janey L. Wiggs

Harvard Medical School, Massachusetts Eye and Ear Infirmary, Boston, Massachusetts 02114
Correspondence: janey_wiggs@meei.harvard.edu

Inherited disorders of the optic nerve significantly impact vision in children and adults. The optic nerve disorders most commonly encountered clinically are glaucoma and primary optic neuropathy including Leber's hereditary optic neuropathy (LHON) and autosomal dominant or Kjer's optic atrophy. Current knowledge of the genetics of optic neuropathy and glaucoma makes it possible to test for mutations in disease-causing genes allowing for presymptomatic testing and risk assessment, and recent advances have revealed important disease mechanisms that may suggest potential therapeutic targets. In this perspective, we describe the current approaches and limitations to genetic testing for these disorders and provide an update on the development of gene-based therapies.

Inherited diseases of the optic nerve, including glaucoma and optic neuropathy, are important causes of blindness in children and adults. The inherited optic neuropathies most frequently encountered clinically are Leber's hereditary optic neuropathy (LHON) and autosomal dominant (or Kjer) optic neuropathy (Neuhann and Rautenstrauss 2013).

Glaucoma is a complex disorder that includes neurodegeneration of the optic nerve as a defining clinical feature. Elevated intraocular pressure (IOP) is an important risk factor for glaucomatous optic nerve degeneration, however, ~33% of affected individuals have normal tension glaucoma (NTG) defined by progressive retinal ganglion cell loss despite IOP measurements in the normal range (<21 mmHg) (Fan and Wiggs 2010). Phenotypically, NTG can share clinical features with the inherited optic neuropathies. Glaucoma with onset before age 40 (early-onset) can be inherited as Mendelian autosomal recessive or autosomal dominant traits, whereas adult onset disease has complex inheritance (Wang and Wiggs 2014).

Current knowledge of the genetics of optic neuropathy and glaucoma makes it possible to test for mutations in disease-causing genes allowing for presymptomatic testing and risk assessment. Recent advances have revealed important disease mechanisms that may suggest potential therapeutic targets. In this perspective, we review the current recommendations, approaches, and limitations of genetic testing for glaucoma and optic neuropathy, and summarize progress toward novel gene-based and neuroprotective therapies.

Cite this article as *Cold Spring Harb Perspect Med* doi: 10.1101/cshperspect.a017277

GENETIC TESTING FOR GLAUCOMA

For many glaucoma patients reducing IOP through medical or surgical treatment can slow disease progression. Genetic testing can identify patients at risk for glaucoma so that presymptomatic surveillance and treatment plans can be developed. Currently, glaucoma genetic testing is most beneficial for patients with disease onset before age 40 (early-onset glaucoma). Mutations causing early-onset glaucoma are rare and have large biological effects, whereas DNA variants contributing to adult-onset glaucoma are common and individually have small effects (Fig. 1). Types of early-onset glaucoma caused by rare mutations with large effects are congenital glaucoma, developmental glaucoma, juvenile open-angle glaucoma, and familial normal tension glaucoma. Common variants with small individual effect sizes contribute to adult-onset primary open angle glaucoma, angle closure glaucoma, and exfoliation glaucoma.

Early-Onset Glaucoma Genetic Testing

Eight genes are currently known to cause early-onset (before age 40) glaucoma with autosomal recessive (AR) or autosomal dominant (AD) inheritance (Wang and Wiggs 2014). Approximately 20% of patients ascertained with early-onset glaucoma through tertiary care facilities will have mutations in one of the genes known to cause early-onset glaucoma (Fig. 2) (Sena et al. 2004; Lim et al. 2013). Of these, mutations in *FOXC1* are most common followed by *MYOC*, *CYP1B1*, *PAX6*, and *PITX2*. Mutations are rarely identified in *OPTN*, *TBK1* or *LTBP2*, even in the tertiary care setting (Hauser et al. 2006; Huang et al. 2014; Ritch et al. 2014). Although the overall clinical sensitivity for genetic testing for this group of genes is ~20%, testing for disease-causing mutations in patients and family members has several important benefits including: informed genetic counseling; presymptomatic risk assessment; and development of appropriate treatment and surveillance plans. Each of these will be discussed in the sections below.

Informed Genetic Counseling

Mutations in early-onset glaucoma genes can cause AD or AR disease: *CYP1B1* and *LTBP2* cause AR disease, whereas mutations in *FOXC1*, *PITX2*, *PAX6*, *MYOC*, and *OPTN* all cause glaucoma inherited as a dominant trait (Wang and Wiggs 2014). Phenotypically, disease caused by mutations in these genes can have similar clinical features making it difficult to make a genetic diagnosis by clinical examination alone. For example, patients with *CYP1B1* mutations can present with severe glaucoma that develops during the first three years of life (congenital glaucoma); however, recent studies have shown that some *CYP1B1* mutations cause disease that is not clinically evident until the second decade of life (juvenile glaucoma) (Abu-Amero et al. 2013; Millá et al. 2013). The

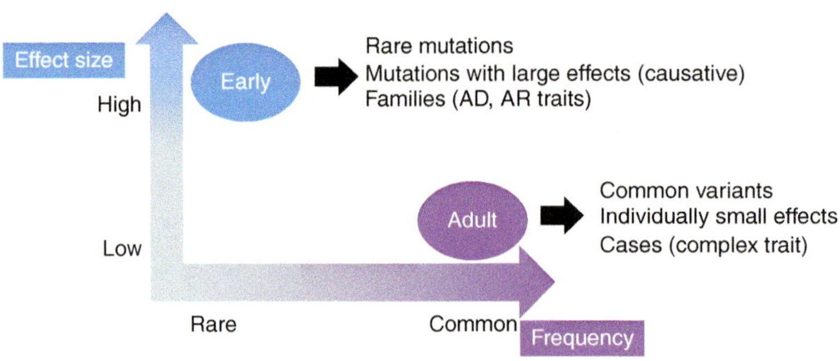

Figure 1. Characteristics of mutations causing early-onset glaucoma compared with genetic variants associated with adult-onset glaucoma. The frequency of the variant is listed on the x-axis and the magnitude of the biological effect (i.e., odds ratio or relative risk) is represented by the values on the y-axis.

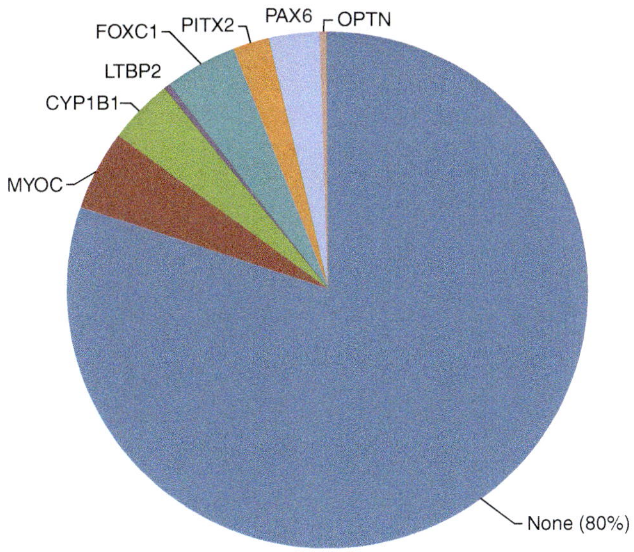

Figure 2. Distribution of mutations in early-onset glaucoma genes in a cohort of glaucoma patients with onset before age 40. Mutations in early-onset glaucoma genes are presented as a fraction of 220 patients evaluated through the genetic testing service at the Massachusetts Eye and Ear Infirmary. Eighty percent of patients with early-onset glaucoma do not have a mutation in a known gene.

CYP1B1-related juvenile glaucoma is inherited as a recessive trait and clinically may not be distinguished from dominantly inherited juvenile or developmental glaucoma caused by mutations in *MYOC*, *FOXC1*, *PITX2*, or *PAX6*. Establishing the molecular diagnosis for these patients will clarify the inheritance pattern making informed genetic counseling and risk assessment possible.

Mutations in both *LTBP2* and *CYP1B1* can cause autosomal recessive congenital glaucoma (onset before the age of 3). In the United States, the incidence of congenital glaucoma is estimated to be approximately 1/10,000 (Fung et al. 2013). *CYP1B1* mutations are found in ~20% of patients, whereas *LTBP2* mutations are very rare (Lim et al. 2013). Interestingly, in the United States the *CYP1B1* mutation carrier frequency is three to five times higher than the incidence of congenital glaucoma would predict using Hardy-Weinberg distribution (Wiggs et al. 2014). The most prevalent *CYP1B1* mutations in the United States carriers are missense alleles which may contribute to less severe early-onset disease (Wiggs et al. 2014). These results suggest that CYP1B1-related glaucoma may be more common than expected and that patients with juvenile and developmental glaucoma should be tested for *CYP1B1* mutations, in addition to patients with severe congenital glaucoma.

Presymptomatic Risk Assessment

A family history of glaucoma is an important risk factor for disease development (Kooner et al. 2014), however, risk assessment based on family history alone is not precise. Genetic testing makes it possible to accurately identify mutation carriers with significantly increased risk for disease because of the high penetrance of mutations in early-onset glaucoma genes. The identification of individuals at risk for glaucoma makes it possible to begin treatment before the onset of irreversible optic nerve disease, thus providing the best opportunity to maintain useful sight.

Surveillance and Treatment Plans

For patients identified as early-onset glaucoma mutation carriers, defining the molecular diagnosis can impact therapeutic decisions. For example, several *MYOC* mutations (Pro370Leu, Tyr437His) (Liu and Vollrath 2004) cause severe early-onset disease that usually requires surgery for treatment, whereas the most common *MYOC* mutation (GLN368X) can cause much milder disease that can be managed with topical medications (Allingham et al. 1998; Hogewind et al. 2010). Patients with less severe *MYOC* mutations can have earlier onset of disease if they also carry common modifying variants in *COL15A1* and *COL18A1* (Wiggs et al. 2013), suggesting that testing should be performed for both the primary mutations as well as modifier alleles.

Additionally, several early-onset glaucoma gene mutations can also cause systemic manifestations requiring further clinical attention. Patients with early-onset glaucoma related to Anridia caused by deletion of *PAX6* may also be at risk for Wilm's tumor and should have a screening renal ultrasound (Hingorani et al. 2012). Patients with mutations in *FOXC1* or *PITX2* can also have cardiac abnormalities (Gripp et al. 2013; Wang et al. 2013) and hearing loss (D'haene et al. 2011).

GENETIC TESTING FOR ADULT-ONSET GLAUCOMA

Nine genes have been statistically associated with adult-onset glaucoma (disease onset after the age of 40) (Wang and Wiggs 2014). Although these associations are robust, genetic testing for adult-onset disease has several challenges. First, individual variants have a small effect on the overall disease risk and likely do not have a significant clinical impact unless they are in the context of other genetic and/or environmental risk factors. Second, the variants currently associated with adult onset disease are common and although the distribution among affected and unaffected individuals is significant, individually the sensitivity and specificity is not sufficient for a clinically useful test. For example, variants in the *LOXL1* genomic region are significantly associated with pseudoexfoliation glaucoma and are found in ~99% of affected patients, however, they are also found in 60%–80% of unaffected individuals (Fan et al. 2011). The development of gene panels, single nucleotide polymorphism (SNP) scores, and combinations of gene and environmental risk factors may yield useful gene-based tests for adult-onset glaucomas, however, these tests need to be validated in the clinical setting and should be correlated with clinical outcomes.

CURRENT RECOMMENDATIONS FOR GLAUCOMA GENETIC TESTING

Genetic testing is clinically useful for glaucoma patients with disease onset before age 40. Up to 20% of these patients will have a mutation in one of the genes currently known to cause early-onset disease. This recommendation is consistent with the policy advocated by the Genetic Testing Task Force for the American Academy of Ophthalmology (Stone et al. 2012). If a mutation in the affected patient is found, further testing of members can be performed. In one study of Australian patients, testing of individuals with a family history of glaucoma and with onset up to age 50 was useful if the disease was advanced (Souzeau et al. 2013). Testing for patients with onset after age 50 is not currently useful clinically, but as more genetic and environmental risk factors are discovered comprehensive risk panel tests can be developed and validated.

GENETIC TESTING FOR PRIMARY OPTIC NEUROPATHY

Approximately 30%–50% of patients with primary optic atrophy will have mutations in *OPA1* or mitochondrial DNA (LHON) (Fig. 3) (Yu-Wai-Man et al. 2011). *OPA1* mutations cause dominantly inherited optic atrophy that usually is bilateral and develops during the first or second decade of life. Three point mutations in the mitochondrial ND4 gene are responsible for ~90% of LHON (Mackey et al. 1996). These mutations are maternally inherited and can have an asymmetric presentation. The mitochondrial DNA haplogroup appears to contribute to disease pathogenicity with haplogroup J of particular importance (Howell et al. 2003; Sadun et al. 2004). Rarely, mutations in *OPA3*

 Cite this article as *Cold Spring Harb Perspect Med* doi: 10.1101/cshperspect.a017277

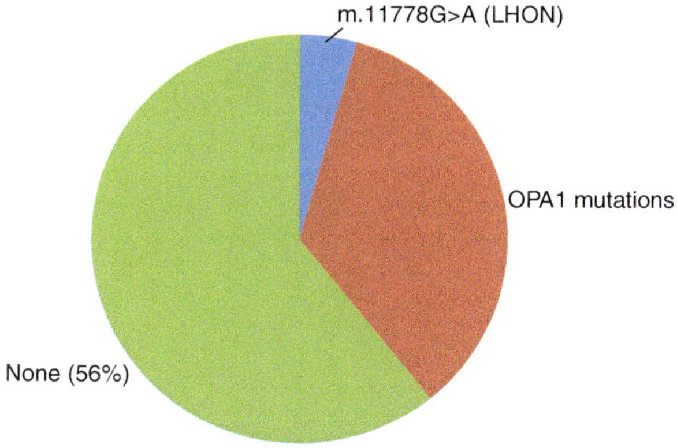

Figure 3. Distribution of mutation in mitochondrial DNA or *OPA1* in a cohort of primary optic atrophy patients. Mutations in mitochondrial DNA or *OPA1* are presented as a fraction of 64 patients evaluated through the genetic testing service at the Massachusetts Eye and Ear Infirmary. Fifty-six percent of patients with primary optic atrophy do not have a mutation in mitochondrial DNA, *OPA1*, or *OPA3*.

cause recessive optic atrophy that is commonly associated with cataracts and other neurological abnormalities (Ferré et al. 2009). Genetic testing for mutations in *OPA1*, *OPA3*, and mitochondrial DNA has important benefits for patients and family members including informed genetic counseling and risk assessment, avoidance of environmental exposures that may contribute to disease severity and identification of individuals who could be eligible for emerging gene-based clinical therapy.

Informed Genetic Counseling and Risk Assessment

The clinical features of the primary optic neuropathies are sufficiently similar that clinical examination cannot reliably differentiate individuals with dominantly inherited disease caused by mutations in *OPA1*, maternally inherited disease caused by mitochondrial DNA mutations, or recessively inherited disease in patients with *OPA3* mutations. By identifying the disease-causing mutation, genetic testing can accurately define the inheritance pattern and subsequent disease risk for family members. In addition, genetic testing can measure mitochondrial heteroplasmy, which is an important feature of mitochondrial disease pathogenicity (Wallace and Chalkia 2013).

Avoidance of Environmental Risk Factors

Studies have suggested that patients with mitochondrial DNA mutations causing LHON may have worse disease if exposed to excessive alcohol consumption, smoking, or have poor nutrition (Sadun et al. 2003; Kirkman et al. 2009). Patients carrying disease-causing mitochondrial DNA mutations may benefit from avoiding these risk factors. Additionally, there is some evidence to suggest that males with LHON may develop more severe disease than females owing to a putative protective effect of the X chromosome (Shankar et al. 2008).

Identify Individuals with Mitochondrial DNA Mutations Who May be Eligible for Gene-Based Clinical Therapy

Patients with selected mitochondrial DNA mutations may be eligible for gene-based therapies. A clinical trial evaluating the safety of adeno-associated virus (AAV) delivery of mitochondrial DNA to patients with Leber's hereditary optic atrophy is underway (Cwerman-Thibault et al. 2014; Koilkonda et al. 2014; Lam et al. 2014). Future gene-based therapies may be available for patients with mitochondrial DNA mutations as well as other genetic forms of primary optic atrophy.

APPROACHES TO GENETIC TESTING FOR OPTIC ATROPHY (GLAUCOMA AND PRIMARY OPTIC NEUROPATHY)

The group of genes currently known to cause early-onset glaucoma and primary optic atrophy could be tested by sequentially screening individual genes, however, because of the extensive phenotypic overlap among these conditions a panel test that simultaneously tests for mutations in all known genes is preferred. Because the primary open angle glaucoma normal-tension subgroup can have a clinical presentation similar to patients with primary optic atrophy, it is useful to include *OPA1*, *OPA3*, and the mitochondrial genome as well as the eight genes known to cause early-onset forms of glaucoma in the test. Panel testing can be accomplished using selective exon capture for all coding/ genomic regions of interest followed by next generation sequencing. A streamlined bioinformatic analysis is necessary to rapidly identify disease-causing mutations. Bioinformatic approaches are also required to identify the mitochondrial DNA heteroplasmy as well as the underlying mitochondrial DNA haplogroup that can impact the disease pathogenicity (Bannwarth et al. 2013). Another benefit of the gene panel approach is the opportunity to discover combinations of disease-causing mutations that may be overlooked using sequential screening.

Evaluation of copy number variation (CNVs, large genomic deletions and duplications) is necessary for comprehensive genetic testing. For the glaucoma and optic atrophy genes, genomic deletions and duplications, which would not be identified by DNA sequencing methods, are known to cause disease. In particular, both deletions and duplications of *FOXC1* and *OPA1* are relatively common disease-causing mutations (Chanda et al. 2008; Fuhrmann et al. 2009; Almind et al. 2011). Deletions and duplications may also impact regulatory elements that would not be targeted as part of the sequencing approaches (McBride et al. 2011; Volkmann et al. 2011). CNVs can be detected using a variety of approaches, including MLPA (Multiplex ligation-dependent probe amplification) (Redeker et al. 2008), array CGH (array Comparative Genomic Hybridization) (Delahaye et al. 2012), and quantitative PCR (Wang et al. 2001).

LIMITATIONS FOR GENETIC TESTING FOR OPTIC NEUROPATHIES (EARLY-ONSET GLAUCOMA AND PRIMARY OPTIC ATROPHY)

The low clinical sensitivity is a major limitation of current genetic testing for early-onset glaucoma and primary optic atrophy (20% and 50%, respectively). The discovery of more disease-causing genes will improve the overall sensitivity of genetic testing for these disorders. Recent advances in genomic technologies, including whole exome and whole genome sequencing are making it possible to efficiently identify novel disease genes.

Another important limitation is the lack of clinical correlations and outcomes for disease-related mutations and variants. Early-onset glaucoma and primary optic atrophy can show considerable variable expressivity, both within and among affected families, which can complicate the clinical utility of the genetic diagnostic test. More research is needed to understand the molecular events that contribute to the spectrum of disease caused by early-onset glaucoma and primary optic atrophy genes.

For adult-onset glaucomas, clinical correlations and outcomes associated with specific genetic variants are also lacking. More complete risk panels (including both genetic and environmental factors) need to be developed and tested for disease risk prediction. Additionally, for adult-onset disease, specific risk factors could be correlated with selected clinical features such as IOP level, optic nerve disease susceptibility, and other glaucoma-related clinical features such as thin central corneal thickness.

OPPORTUNITIES FOR NOVEL THERAPIES

The identification of disease-causing genes is an important first step toward the development of gene-based therapies, which may involve gene replacement, gene inactivation or may use small molecules or other chemicals to modulate the mutation pathogenicity. Some opportunities for gene-based therapies for selected early-onset glaucoma and optic neuropathy genes are discussed in the following sections.

MYOC

Compelling evidence suggests that *MYOC* mutations cause a misfolded protein response that leads to endoplasmic reticulum stress and subsequent cellular dysfunction (Anholt and Carbone 2013). Interestingly, sodium phenyl butrate, a small molecule known to modulate the misfolded protein response can reduce IOP in a transgenic mouse with the *MYOC* mutation (Zode et al. 2011, 2012). This result supports the hypothesis that the misfolded protein response contributes to disease development and suggests that treatment approaches could involve reducing *MYOC* expression, inactivating the mutant mRNA using siRNA or other approaches such as CRISPR.

CYP1B1

Loss of CYP1B1 function results in early onset glaucoma. Patients with *CYP1B1*-related disease can show variable expressivity resulting in a range of disease phenotypes extending from severe congenital glaucoma to disease onset in later teenage years (Suri et al. 2009). In general, null alleles cause the most severe disease, whereas missense alleles can result in milder disease with later onset (López-Garrido et al. 2013). Phenotypically, CYP1B1-related glaucoma is caused, at least in part, by abnormal development of critical structures in the ocular anterior segment (Hollander et al. 2006). However, in patients with later onset disease ocular development may not be severely impaired and other processes related to reduced protein activity may be responsible for disease. For these patients, gene-based therapies could restore sufficient protein function that glaucoma development could be delayed and even eliminated.

ND4 Leber's Hereditary Optic Neuropathy (LHON)

More than 90% of patients affected by LHON have a point mutation in the mitochondrial ND4 gene that codes for a critical subunit of respiratory chain complex I (Farrar et al. 2013). A gene-based treatment trial is currently in progress to test the safety and efficacy of delivery of a nuclear ND4 gene that could restore this critical protein to impaired mitochondria (Cwerman-Thibault et al. 2014; Lam et al. 2014). Mitochondrial defects may also be a factor in the development of adult-onset glaucoma (Jeoung et al. 2014) and the development of mitochondrial DNA therapies could potentially be beneficial for selected glaucoma patients. Additionally, gene-based therapies could be targeted in the future to other mitochondrial DNA mutations affecting other genes can also cause and/or contribute to optic neuropathies.

Neuroprotective Therapies

Therapies capable of protecting or repairing optic nerve function will provide the best opportunities to maintain and preserve sight in patients affected with inherited optic neuropathies. Genes associated with common forms of glaucoma, and especially the subgroup of primary open angle glaucoma with optic nerve degeneration without elevation of IOP (normal-tension glaucoma) could be targets for gene-based neuroprotective therapies. For example, *CDKN2BAS* has been associated with primary open angle glaucoma (POAG), normal-tension glaucoma (NTG), and optic nerve CDR (Wiggs et al. 2012). This gene codes for an antisense RNA that regulates the expression of other proteins involved in cell cycle progression. The robust association between *CDKN2BAS* variants and optic nerve disease in glaucoma suggests that modulating *CDKN2BAS* expression, perhaps through a gene-based approach, could be neuroprotective.

Cell-based therapies, particularly the use of glial cells and mesenchymal stem cells, could protect against neurodegeneration and may also be capable of repairing optic nerve damage (Johnson and Martin 2013). Stem cells produce a variety of nerve growth factors that may have the ability to preserve and repair ganglion cell function. A clinical trial evaluating delivery of ciliary neurotrophic factor (CNTF), a nerve growth factor that may have neuroprotective effects in glaucoma (Pease et al. 2009; Johnson et al. 2011), is currently ongoing (NCT014 08472). The results of these and other studies could lead to the development of novel therapies capable of preventing optic nerve degeneration in both glaucoma and primary optic atrophy.

CONCLUDING REMARKS

Glaucoma and primary optic atrophy are the most common inherited optic neuropathies encountered in a clinical setting and are important causes of blindness throughout the world. Genetic studies have revealed important genes responsible for these conditions and genetic testing for mutations in known genes can be beneficial. For early-onset glaucoma, genetic testing is most useful for patients with disease onset before age 40. The overall clinical sensitivity of genetic testing for both early-onset glaucoma and primary optic atrophy will improve as new genes responsible for these conditions are discovered. For some optic nerve disorders, genetic information is defining approaches to novel gene-based therapies. Cell-based therapies and replacement of neurotrophic factors may also lead to novel neuroprotective treatment.

REFERENCES

**Reference is also in this subject collection.*

Abu-Amero KK, Morales J, Aljasim LA, Edward DP. 2013. *CYP1B1* mutations are a major contributor to juvenile-onset open angle glaucoma in Saudi Arabia. *Ophthalmic Genet* doi: 10.3109/13816810.2013.841961.

Allingham RR, Wiggs JL, De La Paz MA, Vollrath D, Tallett DA, Broomer B, Jones KH, Del Bono EA, Kern J, Patterson K, et al. 1998. *Gln368STOP* myocilin mutation in families with late-onset primary open-angle glaucoma. *Invest Ophthalmol Vis Sci* **39:** 2288–2295.

Almind GJ, Grønskov K, Milea D, Larsen M, Brøndum-Nielsen K, Ek J. 2011. Genomic deletions in *OPA1* in Danish patients with autosomal dominant optic atrophy. *BMC Med Genet* **12:** 49.

Anholt RR, Carbone MA. 2013. A molecular mechanism for glaucoma: Endoplasmic reticulum stress and the unfolded protein response. *Trends Mol Med* **19:** 586–593.

Bannwarth S, Procaccio V, Lebre AS, Jardel C, Chaussenot A, Hoarau C, Maoulida H, Charrier N, Gai X, Xie HM, et al. 2013. Prevalence of rare mitochondrial DNA mutations in mitochondrial disorders. *J Med Genet* **50:** 704–714.

Chanda B, Asai-Coakwell M, Ye M, Mungall AJ, Barrow M, Dobyns WB, Behesti H, Sowden JC, Carter NP, Walter MA, et al. 2008. A novel mechanistic spectrum underlies glaucoma-associated chromosome 6p25 copy number variation. *Hum Mol Genet* **17:** 3446–3458.

Cwerman-Thibault H, Augustin S, Ellouze S, Sahel JA, Corral-Debrinski M. 2014. Gene therapy for mitochondrial diseases: Leber hereditary optic neuropathy as the first candidate for a clinical trial. *C R Biol* **337:** 193–206.

D'haene B, Meire F, Claerhout I, Kroes HY, Plomp A, Arens YH, de Ravel T, Casteels I, De Jaegere S, Hooghe S, et al. 2011. Expanding the spectrum of *FOXC1* and *PITX2* mutations and copy number changes in patients with anterior segment malformations. *Invest Ophthalmol Vis Sci* **52:** 324–333.

Delahaye A, Bitoun P, Drunat S, Gérard-Blanluet M, Chassaing N, Toutain A, Verloes A, Gatelais F, Legendre M, Faivre L, et al. 2012. Genomic imbalances detected by array-CGH in patients with syndromal ocular developmental anomalies. *Eur J Hum Genet* **20:** 527–533.

Fan BJ, Wiggs JL. 2010. Glaucoma: Genes, phenotypes, and new directions for therapy. *J Clin Invest* **120:** 3064–3072.

Fan BJ, Pasquale LR, Rhee D, Li T, Haines JL, Wiggs JL. 2011. *LOXL1* promoter haplotypes are associated with exfoliation syndrome in a U.S. Caucasian population. *Invest Ophthalmol Vis Sci* **52:** 2372–2378.

Farrar GJ, Chadderton N, Kenna PF, Millington-Ward S. 2013. Mitochondrial disorders: Aetiologies, models systems, and candidate therapies. *Trends Genet* **29:** 488–497.

Ferré M, Bonneau D, Milea D, Chevrollier A, Verny C, Dollfus H, Ayuso C, Defoort S, Vignal C, Zanlonghi X, et al. 2009. Molecular screening of 980 cases of suspected hereditary optic neuropathy with a report on 77 novel *OPA1* mutations. *Hum Mutat* **30:** E692–E705.

Fuhrmann N, Alavi MV, Bitoun P, Woernle S, Auburger G, Leo-Kottler B, Yu-Wai-Man P, Chinnery P, Wissinger B. 2009. Genomic rearrangements in *OPA1* are frequent in patients with autosomal dominant optic atrophy. *J Med Genet* **46:** 136–144.

Fung DS, Roensch MA, Kooner KS, Cavanagh HD, Whitson JT. 2013. Epidemiology and characteristics of childhood glaucoma: Results from the Dallas Glaucoma Registry. *Clin Ophthalmol* **7:** 1739–1746.

Gripp KW, Hopkins E, Jenny K, Thacker D, Salvin J. 2013. Cardiac anomalies in Axenfeld-Rieger syndrome due to a novel *FOXC1* mutation. *Am J Med Genet A* **161A:** 114–119.

Hauser MA, Sena DF, Flor J, Walter J, Auguste J, Larocque-Abramson K, Graham F, Delbono E, Haines JL, Pericak-Vance MA, et al. 2006. Distribution of optineurin sequence variations in an ethnically diverse population of low-tension glaucoma patients from the United States. *J Glaucoma* **15:** 358–363.

Hingorani M, Hanson I, van Heyningen V. 2012. Aniridia. *Eur J Hum Genet* **20:** 1011–1017.

Hogewind BF, Mukhopadhyay A, Theelen T, Hollander AI, Hoyng CB. 2010. Variable clinical spectrum of the myocilin *Gln368X* mutation in a Dutch family with primary open angle glaucoma. *Curr Eye Res* **35:** 31–36.

Hollander DA, Sarfarazi M, Stoilov I, Wood IS, Fredrick DR, Alvarado JA. 2006. Genotype and phenotype correlations in congenital glaucoma: *CYP1B1* mutations, goniodysgenesis, and clinical characteristics. *Am J Ophthalmol* **142:** 993–1004.

Howell N, Herrnstadt C, Shults C, Mackey DA. 2003. Low penetrance of the 14484 LHON mutation when it arises in a non-haplogroup J mtDNA background. *Am J Med Genet A* **119A:** 147–151.

Huang X, Li M, Guo X, Li S, Xiao X, Jia X, Liu X, Zhang Q. 2014. Mutation analysis of seven known glaucoma-associated genes in Chinese patients with glaucoma. *Invest Ophthalmol Vis Sci* **55:** 3594–3602.

Jeoung JW, Seong MW, Park SS, Kim DM, Kim SH, Park KH. 2014. Mitochondrial DNA variant discovery in normal-tension glaucoma patients by next-generation sequencing. *Invest Ophthalmol Vis Sci* **55:** 986–992.

Johnson TV, Martin KR. 2013. Cell transplantation approaches to retinal ganglion cell neuroprotection in glaucoma. *Curr Opin Pharmacol* **13:** 78–82.

Johnson TV, Bull ND, Martin KR. 2011. Neurotrophic factor delivery as a protective treatment for glaucoma. *Exp Eye Res* **93:** 196–203.

Kirkman MA, Yu-Wai-Man P, Korsten A, Leonhardt M, Dimitriadis K, De Coo IF, Klopstock T, Chinnery PF. 2009. Gene-environment interactions in Leber hereditary optic neuropathy. *Brain* **132:** 2317–2326.

Koilkonda RD, Yu H, Chou TH, Feuer WJ, Ruggeri M, Porciatti V, Tse D, Hauswirth WW, Chiodo V, Boye SL, et al. 2014. Safety and effects of the vector for the Leber hereditary optic neuropathy gene therapy clinical trial. *JAMA Ophthalmol* **132:** 409–420.

Kooner K, Harrison M, Prasla Z, Albdour M, Adams-Huet B. 2014. Pediatric glaucoma suspects. *Clin Ophthalmol* **8:** 1139–1145.

Lam BL, Feuer WJ, Schiffman JC, Porciatti V, Vandenbroucke R, Rosa PR, Gregori G, Guy J. 2014. Trial end points and natural history in patients with G11778A Leber hereditary optic neuropathy: Preparation for gene therapy clinical trial. *JAMA Ophthalmol* **132:** 428–436.

Lim SH, Tran-Viet KN, Yanovitch TL, Freedman SF, Klemm T, Call W, Powell C, Ravichandran A, Metlapally R, Nading EB, et al. 2013. *CYP1B1*, *MYOC*, and *LTBP2* mutations in primary congenital glaucoma patients in the United States. *Am J Ophthalmol* **155:** 508–517.e5.

Liu Y, Vollrath D. 2004. Reversal of mutant myocilin non-secretion and cell killing: Implications for glaucoma. *Hum Mol Genet* **13:** 1193–1204.

López-Garrido MP, Medina-Trillo C, Morales-Fernandez L, Garcia-Feijoo J, Martínez-de-la-Casa JM, García-Antón M, Escribano J. 2013. Null *CYP1B1* genotypes in primary congenital and nondominant juvenile glaucoma. *Ophthalmology* **120:** 716–723.

Mackey DA, Oostra RJ, Rosenberg T, Nikoskelainen E, Bronte-Stewart J, Poulton J, Harding AE, Govan G, Bolhuis PA, Norby S. 1996. Primary pathogenic mtDNA mutations in multigeneration pedigrees with Leber hereditary optic neuropathy. *Am J Hum Genet* **59:** 481–485.

McBride DJ, Buckle A, van Heyningen V, Kleinjan DA. 2011. DNaseI hypersensitivity and ultraconservation reveal novel, interdependent long-range enhancers at the complex Pax6 *cis*-regulatory region. *PLoS ONE* **6:** e28616.

Millá E, Mañé B, Duch S, Hernan I, Borràs E, Planas E, Dias Mde S, Carballo M, Gamundi MJ, Spanish Multicenter Glaucoma Group-Estudio Multicéntrico Español de Investigación Genética del Glaucoma, EMEIGG. 2013. Survey of familial glaucoma shows a high incidence of cytochrome P450, family 1, subfamily B, polypeptide 1 (*CYP1B1*) mutations in non-consanguineous congenital forms in a Spanish population. *Mol Vis* **19:** 1707–1722.

Neuhann T, Rautenstrauss B. 2013. Genetic and phenotypic variability of optic neuropathies. *Expert Rev Neurother* **13:** 357–367.

Pease ME, Zack DJ, Berlinicke C, Bloom K, Cone F, Wang Y, Klein RL, Hauswirth WW, Quigley HA. 2009. Effect of CNTF on retinal ganglion cell survival in experimental glaucoma. *Invest Ophthalmol Vis Sci* **50:** 2194–2200.

Redeker EJ, de Visser AS, Bergen AA, Mannens MM. 2008. Multiplex ligation-dependent probe amplification (MLPA) enhances the molecular diagnosis of aniridia and related disorders. *Mol Vis* **14:** 836–840.

Ritch R, Darbro B, Menon G, Khanna CL, Solivan-Timpe F, Roos BR, Sarfarzi M, Kawase K, Yamamoto T, Robin AL, et al. 2014. *TBK1* gene duplication and normal-tension glaucoma. *JAMA Ophthalmol* **132:** 544–548.

Sadun AA, Carelli V, Salomao SR, Berezovsky A, Quiros PA, Sadun F, DeNegri AM, Andrade R, Moraes M, Passos A, et al. 2003. Extensive investigation of a large Brazilian pedigree of 11778/haplogroup J Leber hereditary optic neuropathy. *Am J Ophthalmol* **136:** 231–238.

Sadun F, De Negri AM, Carelli V, Salomao SR, Berezovsky A, Andrade R, Moraes M, Passos A, Belfort R, da Rosa AB, et al. 2004. Ophthalmologic findings in a large pedigree of 11778/Haplogroup J Leber hereditary optic neuropathy. *Am J Ophthalmol* **137:** 271–277.

Sena DF, Finzi S, Rodgers K, Del Bono E, Haines JL, Wiggs JL. 2004. Founder mutations of *CYP1B1* gene in patients with congenital glaucoma from the United States and Brazil. *J Med Genet* **41:** e6.

Shankar SP, Fingert JH, Carelli V, Valentino ML, King TM, Daiger SP, Salomao SR, Berezovsky A, Belfort R Jr, Braun TA, et al. 2008. Evidence for a novel X-linked modifier locus for Leber hereditary optic neuropathy. *Ophthalmic Genet* **29:** 17–24.

Souzeau E, Burdon KP, Dubowsky A, Grist S, Usher B, Fitzgerald JT, Crawford A, Hewitt AW, Goldberg I, Mills RA, et al. 2013. Higher prevalence of *myocilin* mutations in advanced glaucoma in comparison with less advanced disease in an Australasian disease registry. *Ophthalmology* **120:** 1135–1143.

Stone EM, Aldave AJ, Drack AV, Maccumber MW, Sheffield VC, Traboulsi E, Weleber RG. 2012. Recommendations for genetic testing of inherited eye diseases: Report of the American Academy of Ophthalmology task force on genetic testing. *Ophthalmology* **119:** 2408–2410.

Suri F, Yazdani S, Narooie-Nejhad M, Zargar SJ, Paylakhi SH, Zeinali S, Pakravan M, Elahi E. 2009. Variable expressivity and high penetrance of *CYP1B1* mutations associated with primary congenital glaucoma. *Ophthalmology* **116:** 2101–2109.

Volkmann BA, Zinkevich NS, Mustonen A, Schilter KF, Bosenko DV, Reis LM, Broeckel U, Link BA, Semina EV. 2011. Potential novel mechanism for Axenfeld-Rieger syndrome: Deletion of a distant region containing regulatory elements of *PITX2*. *Invest Ophthalmol Vis Sci* **52:** 1450–1459.

Wallace DC, Chalkia D. 2013. Mitochondrial DNA genetics and the heteroplasmy conundrum in evolution and disease. *Cold Spring Harb Perspect Med* **3:** a021220.

* Wang R, Wiggs JL. 2014. Common and rare genetic risk factors for glaucoma. *Cold Spring Harb Perspect Biol* **4:** a017244.

Wang WH, McNatt LG, Shepard AR, Jacobson N, Nishimura DY, Stone EM, Sheffield VC, Clark AF. 2001. Optimal procedure for extracting RNA from human ocular tissues and expression profiling of the congenital glaucoma gene *FOXC1* using quantitative RT-PCR. *Mol Vis* **7:** 89–94.

Wang J, Xin YF, Xu WJ, Liu ZM, Qiu XB, Qu XK, Xu L, Li X, Yang YQ. 2013. Prevalence and spectrum of PITX2c mutations associated with congenital heart disease. *DNA Cell Biol* **32:** 708–716.

Wiggs JL, Yaspan BL, Hauser MA, Kang JH, Allingham RR, Olson LM, Abdrabou W, Fan BJ, Wang DY, Brodeur W, et al. 2012. Common variants at 9p21 and 8q22 are associated with increased susceptibility to optic nerve degeneration in glaucoma. *PLoS Genet* **8:** e1002654.

Wiggs JL, Howell GR, Linkroum K, Abdrabou W, Hodges E, Braine CE, Pasquale LR, Hannon GJ, Haines JL, John SW. 2013. Variations in *COL15A1* and *COL18A1* influence age of onset of primary open angle glaucoma. *Clin Genet* **84:** 167–174.

Wiggs JL, Langguth AM, Allen KF. 2014. Carrier Frequency of CYP1B1 Mutations in the United States. *Trans Am Ophthalmol Soc* (*in press*).

Yu-Wai-Man P, Shankar SP, Biousse V, Miller NR, Bean LJ, Coffee B, Hegde M, Newman NJ. 2011. Genetic screening for *OPA1* and *OPA3* mutations in patients with suspected inherited optic neuropathies. *Ophthalmology* **118:** 558–563.

Zode GS, Kuehn MH, Nishimura DY, Searby CC, Mohan K, Grozdanic SD, Bugge K, Anderson MG, Clark AF, Stone EM, et al. 2011. Reduction of ER stress via a chemical chaperone prevents disease phenotypes in a mouse model of primary open angle glaucoma. *J Clin Invest* **121:** 3542–3553.

Zode GS, Bugge KE, Mohan K, Grozdanic SD, Peters JC, Koehn DR, Anderson MG, Kardon RH, Stone EM, Sheffield VC. 2012. Topical ocular sodium 4-phenylbutyrate rescues glaucoma in a myocilin mouse model of primary open-angle glaucoma. *Invest Ophthalmol Vis Sci* **53:** 1557–1565.

The Status of *RPE65* Gene Therapy Trials: Safety and Efficacy

Eric A. Pierce[1] and Jean Bennett[2]

[1]Department of Ophthalmology, Ocular Genomics Institute, Massachusetts Eye and Ear Infirmary and Harvard Medical School, Boston, Massachusetts 02114

[2]Department of Ophthalmology, Center for Advanced Retinal and Ophthalmic Therapeutics, F.M. Kirby Center for Molecular Ophthalmology, University of Pennsylvania School of Medicine, Philadelphia, Pennsylvania 19104

Correspondence: eric_pierce@meei.harvard.edu; jebennet@mail.med.upenn.edu

Several groups have reported the results of clinical trials of gene augmentation therapy for Leber congenital amaurosis (LCA) because of mutations in the *RPE65* gene. These studies have used subretinal injection of adeno-associated virus (AAV) vectors to deliver the human *RPE65* cDNA to the retinal pigment epithelial (RPE) cells of the treated eyes. In all of the studies reported to date, this approach has been shown to be both safe and effective. The successful clinical trials of gene augmentation therapy for retinal degeneration caused by mutations in the *RPE65* gene sets the stage for broad application of gene therapy to treat retinal degenerative disorders.

Inherited retinal degenerations (IRDs) are important causes of blindness that are characterized by progressive dysfunction and death of rod and cone photoreceptor cells leading to vision loss (Berger et al. 2010). Several types of IRD, such as Leber congenital amaurosis (LCA), cause vision loss in infancy or childhood (Weleber 2002; Michaelides et al. 2006; Chung and Traboulsi 2009). More than 200 different types of IRDs have been identified across all age groups by clinical and genetic studies, making IRDs one of the most genetically diverse groups of inherited disorders (Hsiau et al. 2007; RetNet 2014). This includes 19 genes initially reported to be associated with LCA (RetNet 2014). LCA is usually diagnosed in infancy, based on the presence of poor vision, nystagmus, abnormal electroretinography responses, and pupillary light reflexes (Perrault et al. 1999; Lorenz et al. 2000; Aleman et al. 2004; Simonelli et al. 2007). Most patients with LCA have severe visual impairment throughout childhood; vision deteriorates over time and patients often have total blindness by the third or fourth decade of life (Perrault et al. 1999). Despite the notable progress made in identifying the genetic causes for IRDs, the specific genetic cause remains elusive for up to half of IRD patients (Hartong et al. 2006; Daiger et al. 2007; Stone 2007; den Hollander et al. 2010; Audo et al. 2012; Neveling et al. 2012; Shanks et al. 2013).

Research on gene therapy for IRDs is now in a translational phase, following the reports of the success of Phase I clinical trials of gene ther-

Cite this article as *Cold Spring Harb Perspect Med* doi: 10.1101/cshperspect.a017285

apy for *RPE65* LCA, choroideremia, X-linked adrenoleukodystrophy, and hemophilia (Bainbridge et al. 2008; Cideciyan et al. 2008; Maguire et al. 2008, 2009; Cartier et al. 2009; Nathwani et al. 2011; Bennett et al. 2012; Jacobson et al. 2012; MacLaren et al. 2014). As a follow-up to these initial proof-of-concept trials, clinical trials of gene therapy for four other genetic forms of IRD are currently in progress (Table 1). Further, gene therapy studies in animal models have reported efficacy for multiple additional genetic types of IRD (Ali et al. 2000; Min et al. 2005; Alexander et al. 2007; Pang et al. 2008, 2012; Tam et al. 2008; Boye et al. 2010; Cai et al. 2010; Komaromy et al. 2010; Pawlyk et al. 2010; Sun et al. 2010; Mao et al. 2011; Mihelec et al. 2011; Simons et al. 2011; Beltran et al. 2012; Han et al. 2012). There is thus an unprecedented opportunity to translate research progress into sight preserving and/or restoring treatment for patients with IRDs.

Much of the optimism about the use of gene therapy to treat IRDs comes from the success of the initial trials of gene augmentation therapy for *RPE65*-associated LCA. The goal of this article is to briefly review the results of the Phase I and Phase II clinical trials of gene therapy for *RPE65* LCA and discuss the importance of these reports.

RPE65

Mutations in the *RPE65* gene were first identified to cause LCA in 1997 (Gu et al. 1997; Marlhens et al. 1997b). The *RPE65* gene encodes the enzyme that catalyzes the isomerization of all-*trans* retinyl esters into the chromophore 11-*cis* retinal (Redmond et al. 1998, 2005; Jin et al. 2005; Moiseyev et al. 2006). Lack or reduction of this enzyme activity limits response of photoreceptors and thus vision and subsequently results in degeneration of the retinal pigment epithelial (RPE) cells and neural retina (Jacobson et al. 2005; Travis et al. 2007).

Dogs with retinal degeneration, caused by a mutation in the RPE65 gene, were identified in 1999 (Veske et al. 1999), shortly after the first *RPE65* mutations were identified in humans with LCA (Gu et al. 1997; Marlhens et al. 1997a). The phenotype of the *RPE65* mutant dog had already been characterized (Narfstrom et al. 1989). The parallels of the animal model to the human counterpart led to tests of adeno-associated virus (AAV) mediated gene augmentation therapy for the *RPE65*-associated retinal degeneration in these dogs beginning in 2000. Subretinal injection of an adeno-associated virus serotype 2 (AAV2) vector delivering the canine wild-type *RPE65* cDNA resulted in rapid development of visual function, which was sustained over many years and more than a decade in a dog followed the longest (Acland et al. 2001, 2005; Cideciyan et al. 2013). Successful restoration of vision in the treated dogs was an important step toward clinical trials of gene augmentation therapy for *RPE65*-associated disease in humans (Acland et al. 2001; Narfstrom et al. 2003). Further studies in affected dogs compared effects of dose, vector capsid, species of origin of the cDNA, volume, and age of intervention. Optimal results were found in juvenile animals (Acland et al. 2005; Bennicelli et al. 2008). Several groups also reported successful treatment of (young) *Rpe65*-deficient mice with AAV-mediated gene therapy (Dejneka et al. 2004; Lai et al. 2004; Chen et al. 2006; Pang et al. 2006; Bennicelli et al. 2008).

PHASE I/II CLINICAL TRIALS

Initial Results from Phase I/II Trials

Based on preclinical studies performed in dogs and mice, clinical trials of gene augmentation therapy for *RPE65* LCA were initiated in 2007. The initial reports of the results of these trials were published in 2008.

Before the initiation of human clinical trials, safety studies of AAV-RPE65 therapy were performed in affected dogs and unaffected nonhuman primates (NHPs) (Jacobson et al. 2006b). Several of the groups used AAV2 and a cytomegalovirus promoter and chicken beta-actin enhancer (CMV-CBA) to drive expression (Table 1), although the constructs were not identical. Another group used AAV serotype 1 and drove expression with an *RPE65* promoter (Table 1). For the preclinical toxicity studies that were

Table 1. Clinical trials that have been initiated for gene therapy of IRDs

Disease target	Vector name (serotype or envelope)	Surgical administration site[a]	Phase	Target enrollment	Approximate start date	ClinicalTrials.gov identifier	Publications
LCA2	AAV2-hRPE65v2	Consortium of CHOP, UPENN, TIGEM, and SUN	I/II	12	October 2007	NCT00516477	Maguire et al. 2008, 2009; Simonelli et al. 2010; Testa et al. 2013
LCA2	AAV2-CBSB-hRPE65	UFL,UPENN	I	15	October 2007	NCT00481546	Cideciyan et al. 2008, 2009a,b, 2013; Hauswirth et al. 2008; Jacobson et al. 2012
LCA2	AAV2-CB-hRPE65 (contained a longer CMV sequence than AAV2-CBSB-hRPE65)	Hadassah Hospital, Jerusalem, Israel	I	10	January 2009	NCT00821340	Banin et al. 2010
LCA2	AAV2-CB-hRPE65	OHSU, UPort, UMass	I/II	12	December 2008	NCT00749957	
LCA2	rAAV2/4.hRPE65	Nantes University, France	I/II	9	November 2011	NCT01496040	
LCA2	rAAV2/2.hRPE65p.hRPE65	Moorefields, UCL, London, UK	I/II	12	2007	NCT00643747	Bainbridge et al. 2008
LCA2	AAV2-hRPE65v2	CHOP, UPENN	I/II Follow on	12 (same subjects as above)	September 2010	NCT01208389	Bennett et al. 2012
LCA2	AAV2-hRPE65v2	CHOP, UPENN, UIowa	III	24	November 2013	NCT00999609	
Stargardt	StarGen (recombinant lentivirus based in equine infectious anemia virus [EIAV])	OHSU, UPort, Paris, France	I/IIa	28		NCT01367444	
Usher IB	UshStat (recombinant lentivirus based in equine infectious anemia virus (EIAV)	OHSU, UPort and Paris, France	Ib	18	January 2012	NCT01505062	

Continued

Table 1. *Continued*

Disease target	Vector name (serotype or envelope)	Surgical administration site[a]	Phase	Target enrollment	Approximate start date	ClinicalTrials.gov identifier	Publications
RP-MERTK	rAAV2-VMD2-hMERTK	Riyadh, Saudi Arabia	I	6	September 2011	NCT01482195	
CHM	rAAV2.REP1	Oxford, Southampton, Manchester, UK	I	9	October 2011	NCT01461213	Maclaren et al. 2014

The trials targeting LCA2 used different vectors. Although all trials using AAV2 used a chicken beta enhancer with a CMV promoter, the CHOP group also incorporated a Kozak sequence and a splice donor-acceptor sequence and the proviral plasmid included a long stuffer sequence than prevented reverse packaging (i.e., packaging of empty virus capsids).

The groups at CHOP, UIowa, and Oxford used a surfactant in the excipient to minimize binding of vector to inert surfaces (Maguire et al. 2008, 2009; Maclaren et al. 2014).

[a]CHOP, Children's Hospital of Philadelphia; TIGEM, Telethon Institute of Genetics and Medicine; SUN, Second University of Naples; UFL, University of Florida; OHSU, Oregon Health Sciences University; UIowa, University of Iowa, Iowa City, IA; UPort, University of Portland, Portland, OR; UMass, University of Massachusetts, Worcester, MA.

Cite this article as *Cold Spring Harb Perspect Med* doi: 10.1101/cshperspect.a017285

published, affected dogs were injected subretinally with AAV2.RPE65 with doses ranging from 1.5E8 to 4.5E12 vector genomes (vg) in 100–150 μL (Jacobson et al. 2006a). Additional affected dogs were injected with 8.25E10 vg AAV2.RPE65 (Bennicelli et al. 2008).

Normal cynomolgus monkeys were injected subretinally with a single dose/volume of AAV-2/2.RPE65. There were no serious adverse effects of vector injection on retinal structure or function, as tested at 3 wk, 3 mo posttreatment. Healed retinotomy sites from subretinal injections were noted, as were subtle abnormalities in foveal architecture in a subset of eyes injected with vector or vehicle (Jacobson et al. 2006b).

The first results of clinical trials of gene augmentation therapy for *RPE65*-LCA were reported by two groups in 2008 (Table 1). The group from University College London reported treatment of three subjects with an AAV 2/2 vector containing the human *RPE65* cDNA, with expression driven by the human *RPE65* promoter (ClinicalTrials.gov number NCT00643747). The vector was delivered by subretinal injection using 1 mL volume, with detachment of approximately one-third of the retina, including the macula. There were no serious adverse events. There were also no clinically significant changes in visual acuity or in peripheral visual fields detected in any of the three patients. One of the treated subjects did have significant improvement in visual function on microperimetry and on dark-adapted perimetry. This subject also showed improvement in a subjective test of visual mobility (Bainbridge et al. 2008).

The consortium led by Children's Hospital of Philadelphia (CHOP) and including the Telethon Institute of Genetics and Medicine (TIGEM), University of Pennsylvania (UPENN), and the Second University of Naples (SUN) also reported the results from treatment of three subjects with AAV2.hRPE65v2 (Table 1) (Maguire et al. 2008). In this study, the vector solution contained a surfactant to prevent the loss of the vector to the surfaces of the syringe and injection tubing. Treatment was also via subretinal injection, in this case with 1.5×10^{10} vg in 150 μL volume. Resolution of the subretinal bleb produced by the injection was noted within 14 h. All three subjects had an acceptable local and systemic adverse event profile after delivery of AAV2.hRPE65v2. In one patient, an asymptomatic macular hole developed, and although the occurrence was considered to be an adverse event, the patient had some return of retinal function. The macular hole was thought to be caused by the presence of an epiretinal membrane, which was not removed before subretinal injection. Pupillary light responses improved notably in the injected eyes of each subject. Consistent with this, all three subjects reported improved vision in dim light starting 2 wk after surgery. Visual acuity also improved significantly, and there was a trend toward enlarged visual field areas (Maguire et al. 2008). These improvements in vision were noted by 6 wk; there was slower improvement in visual function after that time.

Several months later, a group from UPENN and the University of Florida (UFL) also reported similar results in two publications (Table 1) (Cideciyan et al. 2008; Hauswirth et al. 2008). In that study, three subjects were treated with subretinal injections of AAV2-CB^{SB}-h*RPE65* (Jacobson et al. 2006b). Injections contained 6×10^{10} vg in 150 μL, and were delivered to regions outside the macula in two of the three subjects; the injection involved the macula and fovea in the third subject. No serious adverse events or evidence of systemic toxicity was reported. Visual acuity did not improve compared with baseline. Dark adapted full field threshold sensitivities increased significantly in all three treated eyes and subjects reported improved visual sensitivity in their treated eye (Hauswirth et al. 2008). In the regions of the retinas treated with gene therapy, cone and rod sensitivities were recorded to be increased significantly. The investigators estimated that treatment was able to restore almost normal light sensitivity in the treated regions of retina, although the recovery time of the rods in the treated portions of retina were slow compared with normal (Cideciyan et al. 2008).

Although the follow-up periods for these three studies were short, and normal vision was not achieved, these studies provided the basis for further gene therapy studies in patients with *RPE65*-LCA.

Complete Results from Phase I/II Trials

More complete results from the Phase I/II trials were published beginning in 2009. The results from all trials reported showed improvements in vision in treated subjects. In aggregate, the reported results suggest that the response to treatment is at least in part age dependent.

The CHOP/TIGEM/UPENN/SUN group reported the retinal and visual function in 12 patients (aged 8–44 yr) with *RPE65*-associated LCA treated with a subretinal injection of the AAV2-hRPE65v2 vector (NCT00516477). Doses given were 1.5×10^{10} (low), 4.8×10^{10} (medium), and 1.5×10^{11} (high) vg delivered in 150 or 300 μL. These data included the first three subjects reported on in 2008, and nine additional subjects. The surgical procedure was altered after the first three subjects to include removal of epiretinal membranes when present, and use of perfluorooctane liquid to tamponade the fovea during the subretinal injections (Maguire et al. 2009). The follow-up period ranged from 3 mo to 2 yr. As in the initial report, the AAV2-hRPE65v2 treatment was well tolerated and all patients showed sustained improvement in subjective and objective measurements of vision. For example, all subjects had at least a 2 log unit increase in pupillary light responses and corresponding increases in full-field threshold sensitivities. Seven of the 12 subjects had improvement in visual acuity. The greatest improvements in visual function were noted in children, all of who gained ambulatory vision. One 8-yr-old subject had nearly the same level of light sensitivity as that in age-matched normal-sighted individuals. Four children also had substantial improvement in their ability to navigate a standardized obstacle course, especially in dim light (Maguire et al. 2009).

Additional reports regarding the sustained benefit observed in these subjects have been published, with follow-up periods of up to 3 yr. Analyses show that the maximum improvement in vision was achieved within 6 mo after treatment and the improvements in vision observed in the initial report have been stable (Simonelli et al. 2010; Testa et al. 2013). Further, fMRI (functional MRI) measurements, performed after they already had their initial eye injected, showed restoration of the neural circuitry connecting the retina and the visual cortex in individuals who had been deprived of vision for up to 35 yr (Ashtari et al. 2011). The subjects were able to see dim and low contrast stimuli with their treated eyes—targets that had been invisible to them before treatment. The areas of activation correlated closely with the areas of retina that had been treated. It had been previously thought that the brain would not be able to interpret signal delivered from the retina if retinal function were to be restored beyond early childhood. The data thus suggest that there may be more plasticity in the visual pathways than previously thought (Ashtari et al. 2011). Although not quantified in publications, the changes in visual function in the treated subjects has enabled many of them to do activities which they were not able to perform before treatment. This includes riding a bicycle without assistance, reading books, and being able to see faces during a candlelight dinner. Based on the improvements in vision obtained, some of the treated no longer meet the definition of "legally blind."

The UPENN/UFL group also reported longer-term results from their clinical trial (Cideciyan et al. 2009a; Jacobson et al. 2012). In these publications, the investigators report their results from treatment of 15 subjects who were 11–30 yr of age with the AAV2-CB^{SB}-h*RPE65* vector. Four different dose levels and two injection strategies were evaluated. The first three cohorts received single subretinal injections of 150 or 300 μL of vector. Cohorts 4 and 5 had two injections of 225 μL each, some involving the fovea and some not. Total vector doses ranged from 6×10^{10} to 18×10^{10} vg. The only adverse events reported were related to surgery, with retinal detachment requiring additional surgery in one subject and persistent choroidal effusions in another subject. All study eyes were reported to have recovered completely. There was no evidence of systemic toxicity. Visual function improved in all subjects, although to different degrees. Cone and rod sensitivities improved significantly in the treated regions of retina and the improvements reported initially at 3 mo were sustained through 3 yr. Some improvement in visual acuity was reported, and this was largest in eyes with the lowest entry acuities. It was suggested that some subjects with better foveal structure may have experienced decreases in retinal thickness and acuity following subfoveal injections (Jacobson et al. 2012).

Although more than half a dozen Phase I clinical trials for LCA-RPE65 have been initiated (Table 1), there is only one additional peer-reviewed publication describing results in one subject treated in Israel. This describes the short-term results of one subject who received injection of a vector that was slightly different than that injected in the UPENN/UFL study (Table 1). In that subject, there was an increase in vision present in the treated area as early as 15 d after the intervention (Banin et al. 2010).

PHASE II CLINICAL TRIAL

The success of the unilateral injections in the Phase I/II studies described above begged the question of whether further benefit would result from injection of the second eye. Before evaluating the safety of AAV2-hRPE65v2 in humans, the concern was that the initial injection of AAV might have served as a vaccination. An immune response resulting from exposure of the first eye might not only prevent benefit in the second eye but might also cause damage to the initially injected eye through inflammatory response.

The readministration studies in the human clinical trial subjects was preceded by testing readministration in large animal models (Amado et al. 2010). Sequential subretinal readministration of high dose (1.5E11 vg) AAV2-hRPE65v2 was tested in both Briard (affected) dogs as well as unaffected NHPs that had been previously exposed systemically to AAV (Amado et al. 2010). There were no safety concerns with respect to readministration in either the initially injected eye or the second (contralateral) eye (Amado et al. 2010). An additional preclinical toxicology study examined the effects of readministration in unaffected NHPs of doses that were two to five times higher than the highest dose of the Phase I human trial and at CHOP. Again, there was no indication of ocular toxicity and there were no test article-related clinical signs of systemic toxicity, paving the way to initiate a human readministration clinical trial (Amado et al. 2010).

In the human clinical trial, oldest individuals (least likely to benefit from the intervention) were enrolled first. Subjects were evaluated on a weekly basis and there was a 3-mo stagger between enrollments of each of these individuals (Bennett et al. 2012). The data showed that not only was readministration to the second eye safe, but also it was efficacious. Administration of AAV2-hRPE65v2 to the contralateral eye was well tolerated. There were no cytotoxic T-cell responses to either vector (AAV2) or transgene product (RPE65) in any of the subjects. Neutralizing antibody (NAb) responses to AAV2 and RPE65 protein remained at or close to baseline in the postoperative period (Bennett et al. 2012). Equally important, each of the subjects showed improved pupillary light reflexes and light sensitivity, and two of the three subjects became able to navigate the mobility course (Bennett et al. 2012). Results from fMRI testing showed that the visual cortex responded to the newly treated retina in a manner reflecting the region of retina exposed to vector and the corresponding known neuro-anatomic pathways (Bennett et al. 2012). The remaining eligible subjects have been enrolled and injected and long-term follow-up data will soon be available.

PHASE III CLINICAL TRIAL

Based on the results of the Phase I and II trials described above, a Phase III ("pivotal") trial for *RPE65* gene augmentation therapy is now in progress at CHOP and University of Iowa (NCT00999609). Enrollment is expected to be completed in late 2014, leading to potential registration of this as a therapy in 2015.

The Phase III study involves bilateral subretinal delivery of AAV2.hRPE65v2 at 1.5E11 vg in eligible individuals ages 3 yr and older. To obtain additional natural history data, the study includes a control arm. Subjects are randomized 2:1 to the intervention or control group, respectively. Individuals in the control arm are evaluated at the same time intervals as the intervention subjects for 1 yr, and then they cross to the intervention group. Efforts are taken to assure that the individuals grading the primary endpoints are masked as to the study visit and as to whether the subjects had been assigned to the control or the intervention arm of the study. Every step of the protocol is monitored, starting with the informed consent/assent process. All of the data are processed by an outside data/statistical analysis organization, Westat (Rockville, MD).

Enrollment in the Phase III study is time-consuming for the subjects and their families. After a screening visit, they undergo baseline testing. The testing is noninvasive and is designed such that it is appropriate for individuals in the wide age range enrolled in the study. After baseline testing, randomization to the intervention or the control arm is made by the outside data organization. Subjects assigned to the intervention arm of the study who do not live in the area typically stay near the Center for 3.5 wk at the time of the surgical administration. There are then at least five follow-up visits in year 1 for both intervention and control subjects. Although the number and frequency of follow-up visits tapers after year 1, the follow-up visits will continue for another 14 yr, as the U.S. (FDA) mandates 15 yr of follow-up for gene therapy trial subjects.

True to the reiterative nature of translational research, there will likely be additional studies in the future relating to development of this particular therapeutic. One question is, will it be safe to readminister the reagent to a different part of the previously injected retina? Initial studies in two affected dogs indicated that this approach can be safe and effective (J Bennett, F Mingozzi, AM Maguire, unpubl.), however, the potential for an adverse immune response should be further explored before moving to humans.

CONTROVERSIES IN THE FIELD

Will Gene Augmentation Therapy Prevent Further Degeneration of the Retina?

This is an important question in the neurodegeneration field in general as the ultimate gene therapy would not only restore function, but also prevent any further deterioration. Either effect alone would be meaningful to a patient with neurodegeneration. We know the answer for the retina with respect to the question regarding restoration of function (see above), however, we do not yet know the answer to the question—can we halt the disease in its tracks?

There are several challenges to answering this question: (1) It likely takes ~5–10 yr to observe progression of retinal degeneration in these slowly progressive IRDs. How reliably will we be able to measure this after only a few years have passed? Loss-of-function may potentially be used to monitor progression of retinal degeneration. So far, these have not been reported. Structural studies can also be used to quantify retinal cell structure and density now that sensitive equipment is available (this was not available when LCA2—LCA caused by *RPE65* mutations—trials were initiated in 2007). (2) As in most Phase I (safety) clinical trials in orphan diseases, there are a huge amount of variables to negotiate and only a small number of subjects to study. Variables include type of vector, the dose and volume of the vector, the location of subretinal injection and whether there were one or two injections made in the retina, the region of the retina that is analyzed (i.e., exposed to vector or not exposed to vector; macular vs. peripheral), the age of the subject and the corresponding amount of disease progression, the type of mutation in each subject, whether or not there were complications associated with the surgery, which subjects were included in the measurements, and given that nystagmus is a common finding in LCA2, the fixation/concentration abilities of the subject, and the effects therein on the precision of measurements of retinal thickness and structure (Wojno et al. 2013).

With respect to the first challenge, the slow nature of the disease progression, Cideciyan et al. 2013 used a creative and unconventional statistical modeling approach. They generated their own model of disease progression by taking multiple measures within a small set of samples and then related multiple measurements within their experimental samples to this model. Their answer to this question in studies of patients aged 11–30 yr old was that, although function was recovered, degeneration continues (Wojno et al. 2013). Notably, when Cideciyan et al. 2013 studied an affected dog that had been injected at age 4 mo and then evaluated 11 yr later, they showed that degenerative changes in the injected portion of the retina were minimal. If there was indeed a halting of disease progression after injection in an affected puppy, but not in the humans, is the difference because of the young age at treatment in the dog model, the mutation, the lack of complications, or one of the other variables (see above)? It will be interesting to see, in future studies, whether similar conclusions are drawn using data from subjects injected with similar injection techniques, with the same dose and volume, in similar retinal locations, and in the same age groups.

It may indeed be that treatment beyond a certain age/stage of disease does not prevent degeneration, but it may require longer studies in a larger cohort of (young) subjects treated with the same dose and volume of vector to be sure. What should not be dismissed is that the results of the Phase I interventions achieved the goals of the studies—a safe, stable, and long-term improvement in retinal function (Wojno et al. 2013).

Is it Safe to Deliver Gene Therapy through Subretinal Injection?

Subretinal delivery of AAV2, lentivirus (and the majority of other recombinant and nonviral vectors) is required to transduce photoreceptors and RPE cells efficiently and safely (Fig. 1). Because, normally photoreceptors and RPE cells are tightly apposed, subretinal injection causes a localized disruption of the outer retinal architecture. The retina usually reattaches within hours leaving a minimal amount of histologic damage. Given that primate photoreceptors normally renew their outer segments within a 2 mo time period (Young and Bok 1969) and that after experimental retinal detachment, primate outer segments reform quickly (Guerin et al. 1993), the normal configuration is thought to return close to normal within 1 to 2 mo. This knowledge forms the foundation for use of subretinal surgery techniques, such as those used by retinal surgeons to remove neovascular membranes (Cooper and Thomas 2000). Subretinal surgery in IRDs carries an added risk of physical stress of the injection damaging the fovea, the most vulnerable area of the retina, because the disease can make this already thin region even thinner. The major concern with respect to outcomes is that the fovea is the region which confers best visual acuity. A reason to target the

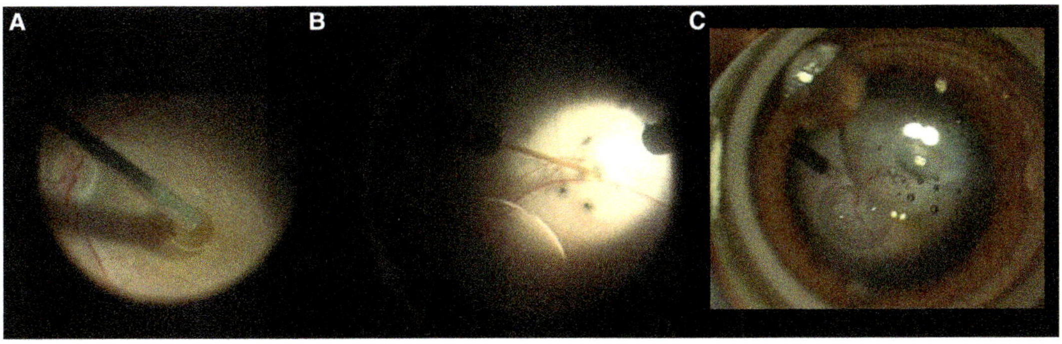

Figure 1. Frames from an intraoperative video of surgical delivery of AAV2-hRPE65.v2 in a Phase I/II clinical trial at CHOP. (*A*) A drop of dense Perfluoron liquid is layered onto the fovea to buttress it during the retinal detachment. (*B*) The subretinal injection cannula is opposed to the neural retina. Injection of the excipient (containing the AAV) causes a separation between the neural retina and the underlying retinal pigment epithelium (i.e., a localized retinal detachment). (*C*) A view of the detached region of the retina at lower magnification. The optic disk is visible and the detachment includes the superior arcade and extends through the fovea. A few small bubbles, introduced with the AAV, are now visible in the subretinal space.

fovea, however, is that this is also the region that, if rescued, could provide the most meaningful visual improvements (Fig. 1). The risk-benefit ratio of subfoveal injection thus can vary depending on the level of baseline function of this region. An accumulation of data relating to the effects of subretinal injection of foveal thickness and function is therefore of great interest. Jacobson et al. (2012) reported that subretinal injections, even outside of the fovea, could cause a decrease in foveal thickness. However, it was not clear whether these changes had any effect on visual acuity as one individual with a foveal injection and decreased foveal thickness showed improved visual acuity (Wojno et al. 2013; Jacobson et al. 2012). More recently, MacLaren et al. (2014) published the first set of results of a gene therapy trial for choroideremia. In that study, the goal was to deliver AAV.hCHM to the central macula, as this was the only viable tissue in those adults with choroideremia. The foveas of five of the six subjects were exposed to the vector. Notably, all six patients recovered their baseline acuity and two of the patients who had received foveal injections showed large gains in acuity, with one patient gaining more than three lines on the eye chart (i.e., significant improvement) (Maclaren et al. 2014). Thus, AAV can be delivered safely to the human fovea through subretinal injection.

Nevertheless, there can be complications as with any surgery, and in the case of subretinal delivery, these can include those that have been reported in the various LCA2 clinical trials, including macular hole (Maguire et al. 2008; Simonelli et al. 2010), unresolved retinal detachment requiring surgical repair, choroidal effusions, hypotonia, and retinal tears (Hauswirth et al. 2008; Jacobson et al. 2012) (see above). Further, the ideal anesthesia for subretinal injection is general anesthesia, which carries its own risks and requires an operating room. Therefore, there is a great deal of interest in developing vectors that can target the outer retina after intravitreal injection, which can be performed as an office procedure.

The more "traditional" AAV vectors do not target the outer retina efficiently after intravitreal injection (Bennett et al. 2000; Lebherz et al. 2008; Vandenberghe et al. 2011; Yin et al. 2011). It is thus exciting that experiments using either directed evolution or generating specific capsid mutations have led to vectors that can target the outer retina after intravitreal injection (Dalkara et al. 2013; Kay et al. 2013). Initial proof-of-concept studies using these vectors were performed in rodent models. It will be interesting to see whether the data can be extrapolated to large animal models and using doses that are safe.

What Outcome Measures Should Be Used in Retinal Gene Therapy Trials?

At present, there are only two outcome measures that have been used successfully to approve new drugs for retinal applications and these are based on measures that reflect improvements in day-to-day life: visual acuity (the ability to resolve high contrast visual angles) and, in one case, visual fields using an automated threshold perimeter (see Briefing document: FDA Cellular, Tissue, and Gene Therapies Advisory Committee; CTGTAC Meeting #52; Cellular and Gene Therapies for Retinal Disorders; available at http://www.fda.gov/downloads/advisor.../ucm259087.pdf). For many forms of IRD, these outcome measures are irrelevant. There can be a loss of sensitivity in patients with either end of the visual acuity range (very good or poor visual acuity) that would make it difficult to achieve a 15 letter change. Many patients with IRD have such poor vision or fixation that visual field testing cannot be performed reliably. Thus, there is a great need for development of additional outcome measures. Although it is now possible to obtain reliable imaging data, imaging data can only be supportive as it is not deemed "clinically meaningful." The current Phase III clinical trial for LCA2 uses a primary outcome measure based on an improvement in the ability to navigate accurately. If these data show improvement, the mobility test endpoint could be used to monitor efficacy in future clinical trials. It will be important to develop additional endpoints that could be used to assess efficacy of gene-based treatments for other IRDs.

CHALLENGES THAT LIE AHEAD

LCA2 is likely one of the easiest targets for gene augmentation therapy. There are both real and theoretical challenges in developing gene therapy for other retinal degenerative conditions. The details that made LCA2 "easy," include: (1) a slow degenerative component of the disease; (2) the *RPE65* transgene cassette fits within the limited confines of the AAV cargo hold; (3) RPE cells are the targets, and they are efficiently transduced by AAV2; (4) because each RPE cell subserves ~20–40 photoreceptor cells in the primate retina (Snodderly et al. 2002), the effect of intervention is amplified; and (5) the RPE65 defect is enzymatic in nature and it appears that as long as there is a critical amount of enzyme delivered, the disease can be corrected. The presence of excess RPE65 protein does not appear to be harmful.

Some forms of LCA, for example, LCA caused by *AIPL1* or *CRX* mutations, will be challenging to target as there is an early onset degenerative component or even a component which may prevent the retina from developing appropriately. In such forms, a gene augmentation intervention would need to be applied very early in life and perhaps even in utero. In utero or early postnatal delivery would entail both ethical and practical challenges.

For diseases such as autosomal recessive Stargardt disease and LCA caused by *CEP290* mutations, the cDNA is too large to fit into AAV. Nonviral vectors are appealing in that there are no size limits, but so far none have been tested in humans with blinding diseases. For use of AAV, there may be complementation mediated by the infected cell after coinfection with virus particles carrying different portions of the gene cassette (Colella et al. 2014; Puppo et al. 2014; Trapani et al. 2014). Other viral or nonviral vectors may also be useful for those conditions (Kong et al. 2008; Puppo et al. 2014). Alternative strategies, such as use of a truncated cDNA, trans-splicing, gene correction, or delivery of antisense nucleic acids may be effective (Lai et al. 2008; Collin et al. 2012; Drivas et al. 2013).

Whereas RPE cells are the target for LCA2, photoreceptors are the primary cell targets for the majority of retinal degenerative diseases. AAV2 transduces photoreceptors, but is not as efficient at photoreceptor transduction as other, more recently identified vectors. Higher doses of AAV2 would have to be used compared with AAV8, for example, to achieve similar levels of transduction (Vandenberghe et al. 2011). The most efficient transduction will be required in photoreceptor diseases because there will be no amplification of effect inherent in the system, such as that mediated by transduction of one RPE cell that then contacts up to fourfold photoreceptor cells (see above). Use of higher doses of vector may increase the risk of toxicity or harmful immune response. In some cases, the selection of vector capsid may not be scientific but may be based on business principles. For example, while AAV2 is in the common domain, there is intellectual property on most other vectors which would require negotiations/licensing fees should there ultimately be a product that is sold.

Finally, in many retinal degenerative conditions, such as diseases involving protein trafficking or cilia function deficits, the cell may only tolerate a particular amount of protein product. An upset in variables affecting protein trafficking parameters could potentially exacerbate disease.

With the great progress in development of proof-of-principle in animal models and in personalized cell models of human retinal disease, we are now at a stage in which strategies aimed to deliver corrective genes/proteins to photoreceptors can be tested directly in humans. Indeed, there are already two different disease targets for which studies testing the safety and efficacy of lentivirus-mediated gene augmentation therapy for primary photoreceptor disease in humans are in progress (Table 1).

SUMMARY AND VISION

The results of multiple clinical trials of gene augmentation therapy for *RPE65*-associated retinal degeneration show that this approach is both safe and effective. These landmark studies thus provide the basis for testing gene augmentation therapy in other genetic forms of inherited retinal degeneration (IRD). The recently reported results from a clinical trial of gene augmentation therapy for choroideremia support this conclusion, as do reports of successful preclinical studies of gene therapy for multiple other genetic forms of IRD.

REFERENCES

Acland GM, Aguirre GD, Ray J, Zhang Q, Aleman TS, Cideciyan AV, Pearce-Kelling SE, Anand V, Zeng Y, Maguire AM, et al. 2001. Gene therapy restores vision in a canine model of childhood blindness. *Nat Genet* **28:** 92–95.

Acland GM, Aguirre GD, Bennett J, Aleman TS, Cideciyan AV, Bennicelli J, Dejneka NS, Pearce-Kelling SE, Maguire AM, Palczewski K, et al. 2005. Long-term restoration of rod and cone vision by single dose rAAV-mediated gene transfer to the retina in a canine model of childhood blindness. *Mol Ther* **12:** 1072–1082.

Aleman TS, Jacobson SG, Chico JD, Scott ML, Cheung AY, Windsor EA, Furushima M, Redmond TM, Bennett J, Palczewski K, et al. 2004. Impairment of the transient pupillary light reflex in Rpe65$^{-/-}$ mice and humans with Leber congenital amaurosis. *Invest Ophthalmol Vis Sci* **45:** 1259–1271.

Alexander JJ, Umino Y, Everhart D, Chang B, Min SH, Li Q, Timmers AM, Hawes NL, Pang JJ, Barlow RB, et al. 2007. Restoration of cone vision in a mouse model of achromatopsia. *Nat Med* **13:** 685–687.

Ali RR, Sarra GM, Stephens C, Alwis MD, Bainbridge JW, Munro PM, Fauser S, Reichel MB, Kinnon C, Hunt DM, et al. 2000. Restoration of photoreceptor ultrastructure and function in retinal degeneration slow mice by gene therapy. *Nat Genet* **25:** 306–310.

Amado D, Mingozzi F, Hui D, Bennicelli J, Wei Z, Chen Y, Bote E, Grant R, Golden J, Narfstrom K, et al. 2010. Safety and efficacy of subretinal readministration of an AAV2 vector in large animal models: Implications for studies in humans. *Sci Transl Med* **2:** 21ra16.

Ashtari M, Cyckowski LL, Monroe JF, Marshall KA, Chung DC, Auricchio A, Simonelli F, Leroy BP, Maguire AM, Shindler KS, et al. 2011. The human visual cortex responds to gene therapy-mediated recovery of retinal function. *J Clin Invest* **121:** 2160–2168.

Audo I, Bujakowska KM, Leveillard T, Mohand-Said S, Lancelot ME, Germain A, Antonio A, Michiels C, Saraiva JP, Letexier M, et al. 2012. Development and application of a next-generation-sequencing (NGS) approach to detect known and novel gene defects underlying retinal diseases. *Orphanet J Rare Dis* **7:** 8.

Bainbridge JW, Smith AJ, Barker SS, Robbie S, Henderson R, Balaggan K, Viswanathan A, Holder GE, Stockman A, Tyler N, et al. 2008. Effect of gene therapy on visual function in Leber's congenital amaurosis. *N Engl J Med* **358:** 2231–2239.

Banin E, Bandah-Rozenfeld D, Obolensky A, Cideciyan AV, Aleman TS, Marks-Ohana D, Sela M, Boye S, Sumaroka A, Roman AJ, et al. 2010. Molecular anthropology meets genetic medicine to treat blindness in the North African Jewish population: Human gene therapy initiated in Israel. *Hum Gene Ther* **21:** 1749–1757.

Beltran WA, Cideciyan AV, Lewin AS, Iwabe S, Khanna H, Sumaroka A, Chiodo VA, Fajardo DS, Roman AJ, Deng WT, et al. 2012. Gene therapy rescues photoreceptor blindness in dogs and paves the way for treating human X-linked retinitis pigmentosa. *Proc Natl Acad Sci* **109:** 2132–2137.

Bennett J, Anand V, Acland GM, Maguire AM. 2000. Cross-species comparison of in vivo reporter gene expression after recombinant adeno-associated virus-mediated retinal transduction. *Methods Enzymol* **316:** 777–789.

Bennett J, Ashtari M, Wellman J, Marshall KA, Cyckowski LL, Chung DC, McCague S, Pierce EA, Chen Y, Bennicelli JL, et al. 2012. AAV2 gene therapy readministration in three adults with congenital blindness. *Sci Transl Med* **4:** 120ra115.

Bennicelli J, Wright JF, Komaromy A, Jacobs JB, Hauck B, Zelenaia O, Mingozzi F, Hui D, Chung D, Rex TS, et al. 2008. Reversal of blindness in animal models of Leber congenital amaurosis using optimized AAV2-mediated gene transfer. *Mol Ther* **16:** 458–465.

Berger W, Kloeckener-Gruissem B, Neidhardt J. 2010. The molecular basis of human retinal and vitreoretinal diseases. *Prog Retin Eye Res* **29:** 335–375.

Boye SE, Boye SL, Pang J, Ryals R, Everhart D, Umino Y, Neeley AW, Besharse J, Barlow R, Hauswirth WW. 2010. Functional and behavioral restoration of vision by gene therapy in the guanylate cyclase-1 (GC1) knockout mouse. *PLoS ONE* **5:** e11306.

Cai X, Conley SM, Nash Z, Fliesler SJ, Cooper MJ, Naash MI. 2010. Gene delivery to mitotic and postmitotic photoreceptors via compacted DNA nanoparticles results in improved phenotype in a mouse model of retinitis pigmentosa. *FASEB J* **24:** 1178–1191.

Cartier N, Hacein-Bey-Abina S, Bartholomae CC, Veres G, Schmidt M, Kutschera I, Vidaud M, Abel U, Dal-Cortivo L, Caccavelli L, et al. 2009. Hematopoietic stem cell gene therapy with a lentiviral vector in X-linked adrenoleukodystrophy. *Science* **326:** 818–823.

Chen Y, Moiseyev G, Takahashi Y, Ma JX. 2006. RPE65 gene delivery restores isomerohydrolase activity and prevents early cone loss in Rpe65$^{-/-}$ mice. *Invest Ophthalmol Vis Sci* **47(3):** 1177–1184.

Chung DC, Traboulsi EI. 2009. Leber congenital amaurosis: Clinical correlations with genotypes, gene therapy trials update, and future directions. *J AAPOS* **13:** 587–592.

Cideciyan AV, Aleman TS, Boye SL, Schwartz SB, Kaushal S, Roman AJ, Pang JJ, Sumaroka A, Windsor EA, Wilson JM, et al. 2008. Human gene therapy for RPE65 isomerase deficiency activates the retinoid cycle of vision but with slow rod kinetics. *Proc Natl Acad Sci* **105:** 15112–15117.

Cideciyan AV, Hauswirth WW, Aleman TS, Kaushal S, Schwartz SB, Boye SL, Windsor EA, Conlon TJ, Sumaroka A, Pang JJ, et al. 2009a. Human *RPE65* gene therapy for Leber congenital amaurosis: Persistence of early visual improvements and safety at 1 year. *Hum Gene Ther* **20:** 999–1004.

Cideciyan AV, Hauswirth WW, Aleman TS, Kaushal S, Schwartz SB, Boye SL, Windsor EA, Conlon TJ, Sumaroka A, Roman AJ, et al. 2009b. Vision 1 year after gene therapy for Leber's congenital amaurosis. *N Engl J Med* **361:** 725–727.

Cideciyan AV, Jacobson SG, Beltran WA, Sumaroka A, Swider M, Iwabe S, Roman AJ, Olivares MB, Schwartz SB, Komaromy AM, et al. 2013. Human retinal gene therapy for Leber congenital amaurosis shows advancing retinal degeneration despite enduring visual improvement. *Proc Natl Acad Sci* **110:** E517–E525.

Colella P, Trapani I, Cesi G, Sommella A, Manfredi A, Puppo A, Iodice C, Rossi S, Simonelli F, Giunti M, et al. 2014. Efficient gene delivery to the cone-enriched pig retina by dual AAV vectors. *Gene Ther* **21:** 450–456.

Collin RW, den Hollander AI, van der Velde-Visser SD, Bennicelli J, Bennett J, Cremers FP. 2012. Antisense oligonucleotide (AON)-based therapy for Leber congenital amaurosis caused by a frequent mutation in *CEP290*. *Mol Ther Nucleic Acids* **1:** e14.

Cooper BA, Thomas MA. 2000. Submacular surgery to remove choroidal neovascularization associated with central serous chorioretinopathy. *Am J Ophthalmol* **130:** 187–191.

Daiger SP, Bowne SJ, Sullivan LS. 2007. Perspective on genes and mutations causing retinitis pigmentosa. *Arch Ophthalmol* **125:** 151–158.

Dalkara D, Byrne LC, Klimczak RR, Visel M, Yin L, Merigan WH, Flannery JG, Schaffer DV. 2013. In vivo-directed evolution of a new adeno-associated virus for therapeutic outer retinal gene delivery from the vitreous. *Sci Transl Med* **5:** 189ra176.

Dejneka NS, Surace EM, Aleman TS, Cideciyan AV, Lyubarsky A, Savchenko A, Redmond TM, Tang W, Wei Z, Rex TS, et al. 2004. In utero gene therapy rescues vision in a murine model of congenital blindness. *Mol Ther* **9(2):** 182–188.

den Hollander AI, Black A, Bennett J, Cremers FP. 2010. Lighting a candle in the dark: Advances in genetics and gene therapy of recessive retinal dystrophies. *J Clin Invest* **120:** 3042–3053.

Drivas TG, Holzbaur ELF, Bennett J. 2013. Disruption of CEP290 microtubule/membrane-binding domains causes retinal degeneration. *J Clin Invest* **123:** 4525–4539.

Gu SM, Thompson DA, Srikumari CR, Lorenz B, Finckh U, Nicoletti A, Murthy KR, Rathmann M, Kumaramanickavel G, Denton MJ, et al. 1997. Mutations in *RPE65* cause autosomal recessive childhood-onset severe retinal dystrophy. *Nat Genet* **17:** 194–197.

Guerin CJ, Lewis GP, Fisher SK, Anderson DH. 1993. Recovery of photoreceptor outer segment length and analysis of membrane assembly rates in regenerating primate photoreceptor outer segments. *Invest Ophthalmol Vis Sci* **34:** 175–183.

Han Z, Conley SM, Makkia RS, Cooper MJ, Naash MI. 2012. DNA nanoparticle-mediated *ABCA4* delivery rescues Stargardt dystrophy in mice. *J Clin Invest* **122:** 3221–3226.

Hartong DT, Berson EL, Dryja TP. 2006. Retinitis pigmentosa. *Lancet* **368:** 1795–1809.

Hauswirth WW, Aleman TS, Kaushal S, Cideciyan AV, Schwartz SB, Wang L, Conlon TJ, Boye SL, Flotte TR, Byrne BJ, et al. 2008. Treatment of Leber congenital amaurosis due to *RPE65* mutations by ocular subretinal injection of adeno-associated virus gene vector: Short-term results of a phase I trial. *Hum Gene Ther* **19:** 979–990.

Hsiau TH, Diaconu C, Myers CA, Lee J, Cepko CL, Corbo JC. 2007. The *cis*-regulatory logic of the mammalian photoreceptor transcriptional network. *PLoS ONE* **2:** e643.

Jacobson SG, Aleman TS, Cideciyan AV, Sumaroka A, Schwartz SB, Windsor EA, Traboulsi EI, Heon E, Pittler SJ, Milam AH, et al. 2005. Identifying photoreceptors in blind eyes caused by *RPE65* mutations: Prerequisite for human gene therapy success. *Proc Natl Acad Sci* **102:** 6177–6182.

Jacobson SG, Acland GM, Aguirre GD, Aleman TS, Schwartz SB, Cideciyan AV, Zeiss CJ, Komaromy AM, Kaushal S, Roman AJ, et al. 2006a. Safety of recombinant adeno-associated virus type 2-*RPE65* vector delivered by ocular subretinal injection. *Mol Ther* **13:** 1074–1084.

Jacobson SG, Boye SL, Aleman TS, Conlon TJ, Zeiss CJ, Roman AJ, Cideciyan AV, Schwartz SB, Komaromy AM, Doobrajh M, et al. 2006b. Safety in nonhuman primates of ocular AAV2-*RPE65*, a candidate treatment for blindness in Leber congenital amaurosis. *Hum Gene Ther* **17:** 845–858.

Jacobson SG, Cideciyan AV, Ratnakaram R, Heon E, Schwartz SB, Roman AJ, Peden MC, Aleman TS, Boye SL, Sumaroka A, et al. 2012. Gene therapy for Leber congenital amaurosis caused by *RPE65* mutations: Safety and efficacy in 15 children and adults followed up to 3 years. *Arch Ophthalmol* **130:** 9–24.

Jin M, Li S, Moghrabi WN, Sun H, Travis GH. 2005. Rpe65 is the retinoid isomerase in bovine retinal pigment epithelium. *Cell* **122:** 449–459.

Kay CN, Ryals RC, Aslanidi GV, Min SH, Ruan Q, Sun J, Dyka FM, Kasuga D, Ayala AE, Van Vliet K, et al. 2013. Targeting photoreceptors via intravitreal delivery using novel, capsid-mutated AAV vectors. *PLoS ONE* **8:** e62097.

Komaromy AM, Alexander JJ, Rowlan JS, Garcia MM, Chiodo VA, Kaya A, Tanaka JC, Acland GM, Hauswirth WW, Aguirre GD. 2010. Gene therapy rescues cone function in congenital achromatopsia. *Hum Mol Genet* **19:** 2581–2593.

Kong J, Kim SR, Binley K, Pata I, Doi K, Mannik J, Zernant-Rajang J, Kan O, Iqball S, Naylor S, et al. 2008. Correction of the disease phenotype in the mouse model of Stargardt disease by lentiviral gene therapy. *Gene Ther* **15:** 1311–1320.

Lai CM, Yu MJ, Brankov M, Barnett NL, Zhou X, Redmond TM, Narfstrom K, Rakoczy PE. 2004. Recombinant adeno-associated virus type 2-mediated gene delivery into the Rpe65$^{-/-}$ knockout mouse eye results in limited rescue. *Genet Vaccines Ther* **2:** 3.

Lai Y, Li D, Yue Y, Duan D. 2008. Design of trans-splicing adeno-associated viral vectors for Duchenne muscular dystrophy gene therapy. *Methods Mol Biol* **433:** 259–275.

Lebherz C, Maguire A, Tang W, Bennett J, Wilson JM. 2008. Novel AAV serotypes for improved ocular gene transfer. *J Gene Med* **10:** 375–382.

Lorenz B, Gyurus P, Preising M, Bremser D, Gu S, Andrassi M, Gerth C, Gal A. 2000. Early-onset severe rod-cone dystrophy in young children with *RPE65* mutations. *Invest Ophthalmol Vis Sci* **41:** 2735–2742.

MacLaren RE, Groppe M, Barnard AR, Cottriall CL, Tolmachova T, Seymour L, Clark KR, During MJ, Cremers FP,

Black GC, et al. 2014. Retinal gene therapy in patients with choroideremia: Initial findings from a phase 1/2 clinical trial. *Lancet* **383:** 1129–1137.

Maguire AM, Simonelli F, Pierce EA, Pugh EN Jr, Mingozzi F, Bennicelli J, Banfi S, Marshall KA, Testa F, Surace EM, et al. 2008. Safety and efficacy of gene transfer for Leber's congenital amaurosis. *N Engl J Med* **358:** 2240–2248.

Maguire AM, High KA, Auricchio A, Wright JF, Pierce EA, Testa F, Mingozzi F, Bennicelli JL, Ying GS, Rossi S, et al. 2009. Age-dependent effects of RPE65 gene therapy for Leber's congenital amaurosis: A phase 1 dose-escalation trial. *Lancet* **374:** 1597–1605.

Mao H, James T Jr, Schwein A, Shabashvili AE, Hauswirth WW, Gorbatyuk MS, Lewin AS. 2011. AAV delivery of wild-type rhodopsin preserves retinal function in a mouse model of autosomal dominant retinitis pigmentosa. *Hum Gene Ther* **22:** 567–575.

Marlhens F, Bareil C, Friffoin J-M, Zrenner E, Amalric P, Eliaou C, Liu S-Y, Harris E, Redmond TM, Arnaud B, et al. 1997a. Mutations in *RPE65* cause Leber's congenital amaurosis. *Nat Genet* **17:** 139–141.

Marlhens F, Bareil C, Griffoin JM, Zrenner E, Amalric P, Eliaou C, Liu SY, Harris E, Redmond TM, Arnaud B, et al. 1997b. Mutations in *RPE65* cause Leber's congenital amaurosis. *Nat Genet* **17:** 139–140.

Michaelides M, Hardcastle AJ, Hunt DM, Moore AT. 2006. Progressive cone and cone-rod dystrophies: Phenotypes and underlying molecular genetic basis. *Surv Ophthalmol* **51:** 232–258.

Mihelec M, Pearson RA, Robbie SJ, Buch PK, Azam SA, Bainbridge JW, Smith AJ, Ali RR. 2011. Long-term preservation of cones and improvement in visual function following gene therapy in a mouse model of Leber congenital amaurosis caused by guanylate cyclase-1 deficiency. *Hum Gene Ther* **22:** 1179–1190.

Min SH, Molday LL, Seeliger MW, Dinculescu A, Timmers AM, Janssen A, Tonagel F, Tanimoto N, Weber BH, Molday RS, et al. 2005. Prolonged recovery of retinal structure/function after gene therapy in an *Rs1h*-deficient mouse model of X-linked juvenile retinoschisis. *Mol Ther* **12:** 644–651.

Moiseyev G, Takahashi Y, Chen Y, Gentleman S, Redmond TM, Crouch RK, Ma JX. 2006. RPE65 is an iron(II)-dependent isomerohydrolase in the retinoid visual cycle. *J Biol Chem* **281:** 2835–2840.

Narfstrom K, Wrigstad A, Nilsson S. 1989. The Briard dogs: A new animal model of congenital stationary night blindness. *Brit J Ophthalmol* **73:** 750–756.

Narfstrom K, Katz ML, Bragadottir R, Seeliger M, Boulanger A, Redmond TM, Caro L, Lai CM, Rakoczy PE. 2003. Functional and structural recovery of the retina after gene therapy in the *RPE65* null mutation dog. *Invest Ophthalmol Vis Sci* **44:** 1663–1672.

Nathwani AC, Tuddenham EG, Rangarajan S, Rosales C, McIntosh J, Linch DC, Chowdary P, Riddell A, Pie AJ, Harrington C, et al. 2011. Adenovirus-associated virus vector-mediated gene transfer in hemophilia B. *N Engl J Med* **365:** 2357–2365.

Neveling K, Collin RW, Gilissen C, van Huet RA, Visser L, Kwint MP, Gijsen SJ, Zonneveld MN, Wieskamp N, de Ligt J, et al. 2012. Next-generation genetic testing for retinitis pigmentosa. *Hum Mutat* **33:** 963–972.

Pang JJ, Chang B, Kumar A, Nusinowitz S, Noorwez SM, Li J, Rani A, Foster TC, Chiodo VA, Doyle T, et al. 2006. Gene therapy restores vision-dependent behavior as well as retinal structure and function in a mouse model of RPE65 Leber congenital amaurosis. *Mol Ther* **13(3):** 565–572.

Pang JJ, Boye SL, Kumar A, Dinculescu A, Deng W, Li J, Li Q, Rani A, Foster TC, Chang B, et al. 2008. AAV-mediated gene therapy for retinal degeneration in the rd10 mouse containing a recessive PDEβ mutation. *Invest Ophthalmol Vis Sci* **49:** 4278–4283.

Pang JJ, Deng WT, Dai X, Lei B, Everhart D, Umino Y, Li J, Zhang K, Mao S, Boye SL, et al. 2012. AAV-mediated cone rescue in a naturally occurring mouse model of CNGA3-achromatopsia. *PLoS ONE* **7:** e35250.

Pawlyk BS, Bulgakov OV, Liu X, Xu X, Adamian M, Sun X, Khani SC, Berson EL, Sandberg MA, Li T. 2010. Replacement gene therapy with a human *RPGRIP1* sequence slows photoreceptor degeneration in a murine model of Leber congenital amaurosis. *Hum Gene Ther* **21:** 993–1004.

Perrault I, Rozet JM, Gerber S, Ghazi I, Leowski C, Ducroq D, Souied E, DuFier JL, Munnich A, Kaplan J. 1999. Leber congenital amaurosis. *Mol Genet Metab* **68:** 200–208.

Puppo A, Cesi G, Marrocco E, Piccolo P, Jacca S, Shayakhmetov DM, Parks RJ, Davidson BL, Colloca S, Brunetti-Pierri N, et al. 2014. Retinal transduction profiles by high-capacity viral vectors. *Gene Ther* doi: 10.1038/gt.2014.57.

Redmond TM, Yu S, Lee E, Bok D, Hamasaki D, Chen N, Goletz P, Ma JX, Crouch RK, Pfeifer K. 1998. *Rpe65* is necessary for production of 11-*cis*-vitamin A in the retinal visual cycle. *Nat Genet* **20:** 344–351.

Redmond TM, Poliakov E, Yu S, Tsai JY, Lu Z, Gentleman S. 2005. Mutation of key residues of *RPE65* abolishes its enzymatic role as isomerohydrolase in the visual cycle. *Proc Natl Acad Sci* **102:** 13658–13663.

RetNet. 2014. RetNet web site. http://www.sph.uth.tmc.edu/Retnet/.

Shanks ME, Downes SM, Copley RR, Lise S, Broxholme J, Hudspith KA, Kwasniewska A, Davies WI, Hankins MW, Packham ER, et al. 2013. Next-generation sequencing (NGS) as a diagnostic tool for retinal degeneration reveals a much higher detection rate in early-onset disease. *Eur J Hum Genet* **21:** 274–280.

Simonelli F, Ziviello C, Testa F, Rossi S, Fazzi E, Bianchi PE, Fossarello M, Signorini S, Bertone C, Galantuomo S, et al. 2007. Clinical and molecular genetics of Leber's congenital amaurosis: A multicenter study of Italian patients. *Invest Ophthalmol Vis Sci* **48:** 4284–4290.

Simonelli F, Maguire AM, Testa F, Pierce EA, Mingozzi F, Bennicelli JL, Rossi S, Marshall K, Banfi S, Surace EM, et al. 2010. Gene therapy for Leber's congenital amaurosis is safe and effective through 1.5 years after vector administration. *Mol Ther* **18:** 643–650.

Simons DL, Boye SL, Hauswirth WW, Wu SM. 2011. Gene therapy prevents photoreceptor death and preserves retinal function in a Bardet-Biedl syndrome mouse model. *Proc Natl Acad Sci* **108:** 6276–6281.

Snodderly DM, Sandstrom MM, Leung IY, Zucker CL, Neuringer M. 2002. Retinal pigment epithelial cell distribution in central retina of rhesus monkeys. *Invest Ophthalmol Vis Sci* **43:** 2815–2818.

Stone EM. 2007. Genetic testing for inherited eye disease. *Arch Ophthalmol* **125:** 205–212.

Sun X, Pawlyk B, Xu X, Liu X, Bulgakov OV, Adamian M, Sandberg MA, Khani SC, Tan MH, Smith AJ, et al. 2010. Gene therapy with a promoter targeting both rods and cones rescues retinal degeneration caused by AIPL1 mutations. *Gene Ther* **17:** 117–131.

Tam LC, Kiang AS, Kennan A, Kenna PF, Chadderton N, Ader M, Palfi A, Aherne A, Ayuso C, Campbell M, et al. 2008. Therapeutic benefit derived from RNAi-mediated ablation of IMPDH1 transcripts in a murine model of autosomal dominant retinitis pigmentosa (RP10). *Hum Mol Genet* **17:** 2084–2100.

Testa F, Maguire AM, Rossi S, Pierce EA, Melillo P, Marshall K, Banfi S, Surace EM, Sun J, Acerra C, et al. 2013. Three-year follow-up after unilateral subretinal delivery of adeno-associated virus in patients with Leber congenital Amaurosis type 2. *Ophthalmology* **120:** 1283–1291.

Trapani I, Colella P, Sommella A, Iodice C, Cesi G, de Simone S, Marrocco E, Rossi S, Giunti M, Palfi A, et al. 2014. Effective delivery of large genes to the retina by dual AAV vectors. *EMBO Mol Med* **6:** 194–211.

Travis GH, Golczak M, Moise AR, Palczewski K. 2007. Diseases caused by defects in the visual cycle: Retinoids as potential therapeutic agents. *Annu Rev Pharmacol Toxicol* **47:** 469–512.

Vandenberghe L, Bell P, Maguire A, Cearley C, Xiao R, Calcedo R, Wang L, Castle M, Maguire A, Grant R, et al. 2011. Dosage thresholds for AAV2 and AAV8 photoreceptor gene therapy in monkey. *Sci Transl Med* **3:** 88ra54.

Veske A, Nilsson SE, Narfstrom K, Gal A. 1999. Retinal dystrophy of Swedish briard/briard–beagle dogs is due to a 4-bp deletion in *RPE65*. *Genomics* **57:** 57–61.

Weleber RG. 2002. Infantile and childhood retinal blindness: A molecular perspective. *Ophthalmic Genet* **23:** 71–97.

Wojno AP, Pierce EA, Bennett J. 2013. Seeing the light. *Sci Transl Med* **5:** 175fs178.

Yin L, Greenberg K, Hunter JJ, Dalkara D, Kolstad KD, Masella BD, Wolfe R, Visel M, Stone D, Libby RT, et al. 2011. Intravitreal injection of AAV2 transduces macaque inner retina. *Invest Ophthalmol Vis Sci* **52:** 2775– 2783.

Young RW, Bok D. 1969. Participation of the retinal pigment epithelium in the rod outer segment renewal process. *J Cell Biol* **42:** 392–403.

Gene Therapy for Choroideremia Using an Adeno-Associated Viral (AAV) Vector

Alun R. Barnard[1], Markus Groppe[1,2], and Robert E. MacLaren[1,2]

[1]Nuffield Laboratory of Ophthalmology, Department of Clinical Neurosciences and Oxford Biomedical Research Centre, University of Oxford, The John Radcliffe Hospital, Oxford OX3 9DU, United Kingdom

[2]Moorfields Eye Hospital and NIHR Biomedical Research Centre for Ophthalmology, London EC1V 2PD, United Kingdom

Correspondence: alun.barnard@eye.ox.ac.uk

Choroideremia is an outer retinal degeneration with a characteristic clinical appearance that was first described in the nineteenth century. The disorder begins with reduction of night vision and gradually progresses to blindness by middle age. The appearance of the fundus in sufferers is recognizable by the characteristic pale color caused by the loss of the outer retina, retinal-pigmented epithelium, and choroidal vessels, leading to exposure of the underlying sclera. Choroideremia shows X-linked recessive inheritance and the choroideremia gene (*CHM*) was one of the first to be identified by positional cloning in 1990. Subsequent identification and characterization of the *CHM* gene, which encodes Rab escort protein 1 (REP1), has led to better comprehension of the disease and enabled advances in genetic diagnosis. Despite several decades of work to understand the exact pathogenesis, no established treatments currently exist to stop or even slow the progression of retinal degeneration in choroideremia. Encouragingly, several specific molecular and clinical features make choroideremia an ideal candidate for treatment with gene therapy. This work describes the considerations and challenges in the development of a new clinical trial using adeno-associated virus (AAV) encoding the *CHM* gene.

Choroideremia (CHM; OMIM Phenotype MIM number: 303100; ICD10 code H31.2) is an X-linked, recessive, degenerative disease of the retina. In males, the condition is gradually progressive: This begins with reduced night vision in adolescence and develops with a gradual loss of peripheral vision and blindness in middle age (MacDonald et al. 2009). In contrast to Leber congenital amaurosis and many other visual cycle disorders, choroideremia is not thought to affect eye formation and early visual development. The retinal pigment epithelium (RPE), retina, and choroid do, however, begin to slowly undergo atrophy at an early age. The name of the disease refers to the clinical appearance of atrophy of the choroid, and the appearance of the fundus in sufferers is normally easily recognizable because of the characteristic pale color resulting from exposure of the underlying white sclera at later stages of the degeneration (Fig. 1). Male patients generally maintain good visual acuity until the degener-

Cite this article as *Cold Spring Harb Perspect Med* doi: 10.1101/cshperspect.a017293

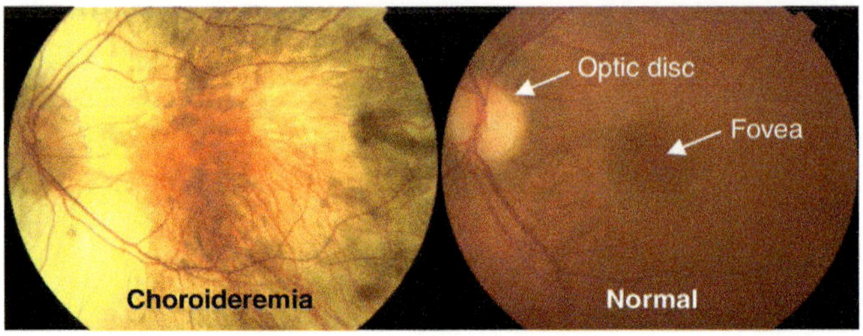

Figure 1. A fundus photograph of a patient with advanced choroideremia. Patient eye (*left*) compared with a normal eye (*right*). In the choroideremia eye, there is a residual island of healthy tissue in the central macula and fovea.

ation encroaches on the fovea, but underlying changes in the retina can be identified in childhood and are associated with significant reductions in parafoveal retinal sensitivity as measured by psychophysical testing (Jacobson et al. 2006b). Because disease progression is relatively slow and occurs after the period of visual development, patients have largely unaffected vision, particularly in early life. Hence, the majority of patients would likely benefit from successful therapeutic intervention to preserve remaining vision, even at late stages of the disease.

When examined, most carrier females show characteristic pigmentary changes of the fundus but these are generally nonprogressive if the X-inactivation occurs late during development—in other words, if there is an even and fine distribution of affected and unaffected RPE cells. These individuals remain predominantly asymptomatic in early years, but may develop reduced night vision in later years. In contrast, X-inactivation very early during development can result in large areas of retina affected by choroideremia caused by clonal expansion of cells expressing only the defective *CHM* gene (the "good" copy on the other X chromosome having been silenced). These rare, severe cases can lead to blindness in female carriers (Bonilha et al. 2008).

Choroideremia is caused by mutations in the *CHM* gene (OMIM Gene/Locus MIM number: 300390), which is located on the long arm of the X chromosome (Cremers et al. 1990). *CHM* encodes Rab escort protein 1 (REP1), which is sometimes also referred to as component A of Rab geranylgeranyl-transferase (Seabra et al. 1992, 1993). This protein is expressed ubiquitously and is found in all cell types and tissues throughout the body. Through its action on Rab GTPases, REP1 plays a role in the fundamental cellular processes of intracellular vesicle trafficking and recycling. Despite about two decades of work to understand the role of REP1 deficiency in the pathogenesis of the disease (e.g., Seabra et al. 1992, 1993, 1995; Larijani et al. 2003; Pylypenko et al. 2003; Tolmachova et al. 2006, 2010), no established treatments currently exist to stop or even slow the progression of retinal degeneration in choroideremia.

Nevertheless, in vivo gene augmentation therapy, in which a working and healthy copy of the gene is introduced into the cells within the body that need it, is an appealing strategy for this currently incurable, blinding disease. The slow rate of degeneration means that there is a long therapeutic window in which to replace the gene in ocular cells before they are lost. In addition, virtually all cases reported so far are functionally null mutations and are often predicted to result in the severe truncation or absence of endogenous REP1 protein (van den Hurk et al. 1997, 2003; McTaggart et al. 2002; Esposito et al. 2011). This is useful because the product of the therapeutic gene will not have to compete with a large pool of mutant protein. This would limit latent dominant negative effects and in theory would mean only a small amount of vector-delivered REP1 might be needed to arrest degeneration. Furthermore, recent reports showing that replacement gene therapy can be safely and successfully used to treat the retinal disease (Leber congenital am-

 Cite this article as *Cold Spring Harb Perspect Med* doi: 10.1101/cshperspect.a017293

aurosis type 2) (Bainbridge et al. 2008; Hauswirth et al. 2008; Maguire et al. 2008), provide encouragement that a similar technique could be applied to choroideremia.

THE HISTORY, PREVALENCE, AND MOLECULAR-GENETIC DIAGNOSIS OF CHOROIDEREMIA

Choroideremia was first described in the nineteenth century by the Austrian ophthalmologist Ludwig Mauthner (1872). Seemingly as a result of the barren appearance of the fundus, Mauthner named the condition "Chorioideremie," which is thought to be a combination of the ancient Greek "erēmia," meaning barren land or desert, as a suffix to the stem word "chorioid" a common alternative spelling of "choroid" (also originally from ancient Greek words for skin—"chorion," and form/type—"eidos") (Myers 2006). Thus, the disease name means "an area barren of choroid." This entered English usage as choroideremia, but an alternative spelling, choroideraemia, has been used extensively (e.g., Martin 2010). It is unclear if the addition of an "a" comes from a desire to differentiate the first and second vowel sounds in "erēmia" (which indeed are different Greek letters). Alternatively, it may have been believed that the disease name was derived by adding the prefix "er-" (possibly from the Latin "ir-" meaning not/negation) to the suffix "aemia" (derived from ancient Greek and in usage in British medicine as referring to the state or condition of the blood), thereby meaning an observation of "no blood in the choroid." Whatever the case, the preferred modern English spelling is Choroideremia, as the "ae" diphthong, seen increasingly as archaic, is being replaced by a simple "e."

Originally, the disease was thought of as a congenital absence of the majority of the choroid, probably caused by a developmental disorder (Mauthner 1872). In fact, Theodor Leber saw the same case and classified it as one of retinitis pigmentosa with extreme atrophy of the choroid (reported by Wolf 1930). Although closer to the truth, Leber's analysis seems to have been rejected at the time, and the idea of the disease being caused by a congenital (and largely stationary) absence of the choroid predominated for several decades. After more cases were studied, it became clear that the stationary nature of the disease was questionable and the idea was flatly rejected by Pameyer et al. (1960) who said that choroideremia should be considered as an "abiotrophic process of the 'tapetum nigrum' (a reference to the RPE) with a secondary progressive dystrophy of the choriocapillary layer and outer retinal layers" and were clear that "the hypothesis of a dysplasia of the choroid as a primary cause of the fundus alterations must be rejected." Even though choroideremia is now accepted as being a progressive degenerative disease, the idea that degeneration of the choroid is the primary cause still lingers in some medical definitions (e.g., Myers 2006). We now know that the name choroideremia, although an apt description of the fundus appearance of atrophy of the choroid at later stages of the disease, does not reflect the etiology of the disease very well. This is an important consideration when developing therapeutic strategies (see below).

Choroideremia has a prevalence of approximately 1:50,000 in people of European descent, with the highest prevalence in northern Finland (Sankila et al. 1992). There are thought to be more than 500 affected male patients in the United Kingdom and around 3000 throughout Europe (MacDonald et al. 2009). Thus, although relatively rare, a significant patient population exists for this blinding disease, which lacks any major treatment options.

The characteristic appearance of the fundus can be used to first identify choroideremia clinically. A family history consistent with an X-linked recessive disease can help rule out other diseases with a similar appearance (e.g., gyrate atrophy, Oliver-McFarlane syndrome, bifocal chorio-retinal atrophy). Mutations that cause choroideremia invariably lead to a complete absence of the REP1 protein. Because of this, it has been suggested that clinical diagnosis of choroideremia can be confirmed by the absence of REP1 protein in peripheral blood samples in an immunoblot analysis with anti-REP1 antibody (MacDonald et al. 1998). However, genetic testing and molecular diagnosis of a pathogenic mutation in the *CHM* gene should be used to support the clinical diagnosis. It is possible to order routine sequencing of CHM via health service approved diagnostic laboratories in many countries, including the UK, although in some cases a more thorough examination of the genomic DNA or the mRNA must be performed to detect the molecular cause of CHM (Furgoch et al. 2014).

THE EXPRESSION AND FUNCTION OF REP1 PROTEIN

In many inherited retinal dystrophies, the protein product of the causative gene directly contributes to a process that is essential for the light-sensitive function of the eye (such as phototransduction in the retina or the visual cycle in the RPE). This is not the case in choroideremia. Instead, the gene product, REP1, is involved in lipid modification of Rab GTPases, members of the Ras superfamily of monomeric G proteins (Fig. 2) (Seabra et al. 1992, 1995; Pylypenko et al. 2003). This modification, known as prenylation, involves the covalent attachment of one or more prenyl groups (geranylgeranyl or farnesyl) to carboxy-terminal cysteines of a Rab protein. REP1 binds newly synthesized, unprenylated Rabs and presents them to a catalytic Rab geranylgeranyltransferase (GGTase) subunit for the geranylgeranyl transfer reaction. REP1 also helps escort prenylated Rabs to their specific destination membrane by binding the hydrophobic, insoluble prenyl groups and carrying them through the cytoplasm (Pylypenko et al. 2003). Rabs themselves have an important function in intracellular vesicle trafficking, for which the addition of a prenyl moiety "lipid anchor" is essential (Seabra et al. 1995). Thus, in choroideremia, the affected gene plays a role in fundamental cellular processes.

Within the eye, there are a number of processes reliant on Rab protein function. In the photoreceptor, proteins destined for the outer segment, such as rhodopsin, travel from the Golgi apparatus to the connecting cilium via vesicular transport that is regulated by Rab8 and Rab6. In the RPE, intracellular trafficking controls the phagocytosis and degradation of disk

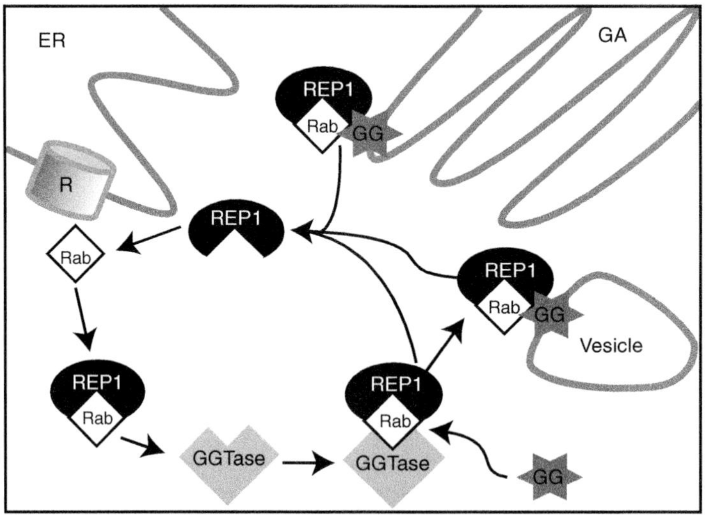

Figure 2. A schematic of the cellular function of Rab escort protein (REP1). REP1 binds Rabs (member of the Ras subfamily of small GTPases, ~70 members) as they are made by ribosomes (R) on the endoplasmic reticulum (ER). REP1 present newly synthesized, unprenylated Rabs to a catalytic Rab geranylgeranyltransferase (GGTase) subunit. Rabs undergo prenylation, which involves the covalent attachment of one or more hydrophobic prenyl groups (geranylgeranyl, GG shown here) to carboxy-terminal cysteine residues. REP1 also escorts prenylated Rabs to specific destination membranes in the Golgi apparatus (GA) and of diverse cellular vesicles (Vesicle, represents various cellular vesicles, e.g., lysosomes or transport vesicles).

membranes shed from the apical tips of photoreceptor outer segments. It is believed that Rab proteins function during phagocytosis by the RPE, possibly through an effector-mediated interaction with myosin VIIA, which is required for phagosome transport (Gibbs et al. 2003).

Although choroideremia is almost exclusively a disease affecting the eye, REP1 is expressed in all cells and tissues throughout the body. As an additional complexity, mammals (including man) also produce REP2, a protein very similar to REP1, with an (amino acid sequence 75% identical, 90% similar to REP1) (Cremers et al. 1994). REP2 is encoded by the gene *CHML* (choroideremia-like), which resides on chromosome 1 and is thought to have arisen from a retrogene insertion of the REP1 mRNA transcript sometime during vertebrate evolution (as evidenced by the lack of introns). REP2, like REP1, is expressed ubiquitously. Thus, loss of REP1 function can in theory be compensated for by the action of REP2, at least in cells outside the eye.

It is thought, therefore, that the phenotype of choroideremia is not so much dictated by the cells in which REP1 is normally expressed, but by those in which REP2 is unable to compensate for its function, for whatever reason. It has been shown that some Rabs, such as Rab27a, are preferentially prenylated by REP1 (Larijani et al. 2003). Rab27a has a key role in the retina (Tolmachova et al. 1999), and its affinity toward REP1 and REP2 proteins is similar. However, the Rab27a-REP1 and Rab27a-REP2 complexes have different affinities for the Rab GGTase enzyme, which might explain why REP2 is unable to support Rab27a prenylation in the retina of choroideremia patients over the long term (Larijani et al. 2003).

INVESTIGATING THE PATHOLOGY OF REP1 DEFICIENCY USING LABORATORY ANIMAL MODELS

To investigate the pathology of choroideremia, researchers have attempted to develop laboratory animal models of the disease. However, the global ablation of *CHM* gene function appears to be more severe in animal models than in humans. In the zebrafish, a common nonmammalian vertebrate model organism, mutation of the *chm* gene leading to a completely nonfunctional (null) allele manifests as an extremely severe systemic illness resulting in early lethality at postnatal day 6 (Starr et al. 2004; Moosajee et al. 2009). This may be explained by the fact that *chml/Rep2* is not present in the zebrafish genome (Moosajee et al. 2009). In mice, despite the presence of the *Chml* gene, the genetic deletion of *Chm* causes embryonic lethality in hemizygous male mice (Chm^{null}/Y), caused by abnormalities in extraembryonic tissues such as the placenta and yolk sac (Shi et al. 2004). Interestingly, carrier female mice ($Chm^{null/+}$) are viable and do show progressive retinal degeneration (van den Hurk et al. 1997; Tolmachova et al. 2006). Thus, the $Chm^{null/+}$ female mouse seems to best model the phenotype of affected hemizygous male patients. The reasons for this are not completely clear, but subtle species differences in RabGGT compatibility with REP2-Rab complexes and differences in X-inactivation may partially explain why the sex-linked phenotype of choroideremia differs substantially between species.

An important question in choroideremia pathology has been whether one cell type/tissue layer acts as a primary site of degeneration (which then leads to the demise of the other cell types/tissue layers) or if the disease appears in multiple cell types/tissue layers independently and/or simultaneously. The answer dictates which cell types need to be targeted by for gene replacement therapy (and which can or should be avoided). The question is complicated by the fact that the three affected eye layers (choroid, photoreceptors, and RPE) are highly interdependent. For example, genetically normal photoreceptors will degenerate secondary to loss of the RPE by any cause (for instance, in myopic and dry age-related macular degeneration), and the morphology and distribution of RPE cells will change in response to photoreceptor loss (as in many forms of retinitis pigmentosa, for example).

Therefore, more complex animal models have been used in an attempt to dissect the intricate pathologic changes that occur during the choroideremia degenerative process. Krock et al.

(2007) used the *chm* zebrafish model to create genetically mosaic mutant/wild-type eyes (by transplanting cells in blastula stage embryos) and found that REP1 appears to be critical for the pigment epithelium but not photoreceptors. In the mouse, a conditional knockout allele (*Chm*^{Flox}) has been made that allows for the selective ablation of the *Chm* gene in a particular cell/tissue type (Tolmachova et al. 2006). When *Chm* was selectively ablated in either the neurosensory retina or the RPE, it was found that different subsets of Rabs were underprenylated, implying that both layers have an intrinsic prenylation defect (Tolmachova et al. 2006). In further work, *Chm* was selectively ablated in photoreceptor cells or the RPE, resulting in independent degeneration of both layers (Tolmachova et al. 2010). Although neither condition could initiate significant degeneration of the other layer, the inherent and cell-autonomous need for REP1 function in the photoreceptors and RPE means that both layers could be considered primary sites of the disease (Tolmachova et al. 2010). Furthermore, when ablation of *Chm* in the RPE and photoreceptors was combined in the same mouse line, the phenotype was greater than the sum of the effects observed by ablating *Chm* in each cell type separately (Tolmachova et al. 2010). This highlights once again that the adjacent cell layers in the eye influence each other and that these interactions are important factors that can determine the degenerative process in choroideremia.

Overall, the animal models indicate that REP1 deficiency causes cell-autonomous problems in the eye and that both the RPE and retina/photoreceptors can be considered primary sites of the disease. It is logical therefore to propose that future gene therapy approaches for choroideremia should use viral vectors that target both photoreceptors and RPE.

FURTHER CONSIDERATIONS FOR CHOROIDEREMIA PATHOLOGY BASED ON HUMAN DATA

Caution is needed when extrapolating observations from laboratory models directly to humans, because of potential species differences as mentioned above. It is therefore crucial to use human data wherever possible to identify the retinal layers that are wholly dependent on REP1. This information can come from multiple sources, using a range of techniques.

In human female carriers, skewed X-inactivation across the retinal layers can leave affected clones of photoreceptors against normal pigment epithelial cells, and histological postmortem specimens suggest that photoreceptors degenerate independently of the RPE (Flannery et al. 1990; Syed et al. 2001; Bonilha et al. 2008). There is also evidence from optical coherence tomography scans of male choroideremia patients that the photoreceptor layer thins in advance of degeneration of the RPE (Jacobson et al. 2006b).

This data confirm the logic of designing a REP1-expressing vector that targets both the photoreceptor layer and the RPE, but further refinement might also be necessary. Because the early stages of choroideremia manifest as loss of night vision, with central, cone-mediated vision preserved until very late stages of the disease, it seems reasonable to assume that rods are affected significantly more than cones. For reasons that are not completely clear, cones are known to be dependent on surrounding rods, and any genetic condition that causes rod death will also lead to complete loss of cones in a centripetal pattern as a secondary phenomenon. In a postmortem analysis of the retina from an X-linked carrier female, apparently normal-looking, REP1-deficient cones could be identified within regions containing REP1 expressing rods (Syed et al. 2001). The differential expression of REP1 in these two photoreceptor subclasses results from differential X-inactivation (Reese et al. 1995) and provides further evidence that cones may exist without REP1 when surrounded by rods. It therefore seems reasonable to assume that cone death may occur as a phenomenon secondary to loss of rods and RPE, rather than a dependency on REP1. Hence, from a safety perspective, it might actually be better to avoid transduction of cone cells as much as possible.

It might seem ironic that despite the characteristic and defining atrophy of the choroid in choroideremia, the relative importance of REP1 deficiency in the choroidal layers has not been dealt with comprehensively in the available animal models. Fortunately, human data and observations exist that are more illuminating. Studies from postmortem carrier females show no focal loss or abnormalities of the choroid except underlying areas of severe retinal degeneration (Syed et al. 2001), which suggests that the choroidal vascular system is not dependent on REP1. Similarly, choroideremia is not known to affect blood vessels elsewhere in the body. It is therefore likely that choroidal atrophy occurs secondary to loss of the overlying RPE. In other retinal conditions, the choroid undergoes progressive atrophy many years after subretinal surgery if the pigment epithelium is damaged, leading to a gradual and focal unmasking of scleral autofluorescence, which is similar to the progression of choroideremia (MacLaren et al. 2005). Despite this, a slow primary degeneration of the choroid cannot be excluded completely.

CHOOSING A GENE THERAPY VECTOR

For gene replacement therapy to work, the genetic material (DNA/RNA) needs a delivery system (vector), and it is common in clinical trials to use a modified virus to carry the gene into cells. Adeno-associated virus (AAV) is currently a popular vector for clinical trials, particularly for ocular gene therapy, but is it applicable for use in choroideremia?

An important issue is the amount of genetic material that can be placed into each viral particle. This is known as the packaging capacity or limit, and for AAV vectors it is thought to be <5 kb of single-stranded DNA (Wu et al. 2010). Although this capacity is considered to be small, and a potential limitation of using AAV, it is more than sufficient to include the full coding sequence of REP1 (at 1.9 kb), while still allowing space for a choice of promoters and other regulatory elements.

Another consideration is whether the viral vector can effectively target and transfer DNA to (transduce) the specific cell types and tissues that need to be treated. There are many different AAV subtypes, each with slightly different DNA sequences and capsid proteins on their outer shell (serotypes). These serotypes have different cellular tropism; they preferentially target specific cell types within a given host species. Many AAV vectors target neurons effectively, but only AAV serotype 2 has been shown to transduce both photoreceptors and the RPE after subretinal injection in nonhuman primates (Bennett et al. 1999; Jacobson et al. 2006a). AAV2 therefore appears to be a good choice, as rod photoreceptors and RPE cells both need to be targeted for REP1 replacement in choroideremia.

In the photoreceptor layer, AAV2 appears to predominantly target rods rather than cones (Bennett et al. 1999). This is also beneficial because cone photoreceptors do not intrinsically suffer in the absence of REP1 in choroideremia and therefore, from a safety perspective, it might be better to avoid transduction of cone cells as much as possible. However, avoiding cone transduction completely by using AAV2 cannot be guaranteed in the degenerating retina. For instance, in the absence of rods, viral particles are likely to have greater access to cone cells. There may also be promoter-serotype interactions. AAV5, for example, does not transduce macaque primate cones effectively with the CMV promoter (Lotery et al. 2003), but it is effective in cones of the squirrel monkey when using a cone-specific promoter (Mancuso et al. 2007). It is impossible to precisely predict whether AAV2 will limit photoreceptor gene expression exclusively to rod photoreceptors in any given human retinal degeneration; however, it is probably safe to say that AAV2 will target rods more effectively than cones in humans. The tropism of AAV2 for the deeper vascular layers of the choroid is relatively unexplored in animal models and is therefore hard to predict in humans. It seems unlikely that AAV2 will be able to bypass the combined barriers of the RPE and Bruch's membrane, but any possible transduction and treatment of choroidal layers could only be beneficial. As REP1 is ubiquitously expressed, the unlikely event of a more widespread transduction pattern of the gene therapy virus might not be considered a major cause for concern, even in cells and tissue outside the eye.

AAV2 seems a suitable choice for use in choroideremia gene therapy for reasons beyond those described above. Although it is not currently known to cause disease, AAV naturally infects humans (and some other primate species). Consequently, antibodies against capsid antigens of wildtype AAVs can be detected in a significant percentage of humans (Mingozzi et al. 2007). Despite this, there are extensive safety data in primates (Jacobson et al. 2006a) and from recent *RPE65* gene therapy trials for (LCA2) (Bainbridge et al. 2008; Hauswirth et al. 2008; Maguire et al. 2008) that show subretinal administration of AAV2 does not cause significant immunogenicity, inflammation, or toxicity. In addition, data from dog models of LCA2 treated with AAV2.*RPE65* show that the treated dogs maintain vision without reduction for several years, and even over a decade in some cases (Bennicelli et al. 2008; Cideciyan et al. 2013). In humans, clinical trials have shown that visual gains following gene transfer using AAV2.RPE65 are sustained vision for at least 3 yr (Jacobson et al. 2012; Cideciyan et al. 2013; Testa et al. 2013). Clearly, the lifelong effects in humans will not be known for some time, but these data suggest that expression from the AAV2 vector is sustained, and early loss of therapeutic transgene expression through gene silencing, such as by methylation of the promoter DNA, is not a significant issue. It should be noted, however, that follow-up results from one study (Bainbridge et al. 2008) were never published and, although a maze navigation test in the one reported patient looked impressive, close inspection of the data shows that a similarly dramatic improvement in maze navigation time was seen in the control eye as well. Because *RPE65* patients dark-adapt with great difficulty, variation in pretest dark adaptation is a possible explanation for the alleged improvement in vision, as this would also benefit the control eye. In any case, the absence of any follow-up data or further analysis of visual function in this patient raises the possibility that the reported improvement in vision may have been an artifact of testing. It is also unclear why, after 5 yr, there are no reported results for the other nine patients who underwent gene therapy in this trial. The results may have been unspectacular, perhaps owing to the choice of an unsuitable promoter (MacLaren 2009).

Taken together, AAV2 displays tropism for the correct cell types needed, is capable of packaging the full REP1 coding sequence and has been shown to be safe and effective in ocular gene therapy trials for a different eye disease (LCA2) up to 3 yr after treatment. For these reasons, AAV2 was selected for use in a *CHM*-replacement gene therapy strategy for choroideremia. As AAV2 is such a compelling choice, other types of virus, such as lentiviruses and adenoviruses, were not considered.

DESIGNING AN EFFICIENT AAV2-REP1 EXPRESSION CASSETTE

Because REP1 is ubiquitously expressed, there was little point in using its 5′ upstream promoter sequence to drive regulated transgene expression. Instead, a well-characterized ubiquitous promoter, capable of driving sustained, high levels of expression, was chosen: a hybrid of the human cytomegalovirus (CMV) upstream enhancer with the chicken β-actin promoter. This promoter, variously termed CBA or CAG, has been used extensively in preclinical studies. The original CBA promoter construct was generated in Japan (Miyazaki et al. 1989; Niwa et al. 1991) and first used successfully in AAV in vivo by Mark Sands in the USA (Daly et al. 1999). A later study showed that an AAV vector with the CBA promoter administered via portal vein injection yielded 9.5-fold higher expression compared to an AAV vector with the EF1α promoter and 137-fold higher expression compared to an AAV vector with the CMV promoter/enhancer, and the CBA-mediated expression was sustained for at least a year (Xu et al. 2001). CBA promoters have provided highly effective transduction in retinal gene therapy clinical trials (Hauswirth et al. 2008; Maguire et al. 2008) and appear to sustain expression for over a decade in dogs (Bennicelli et al. 2008; Cideciyan et al. 2013) and at least 3 yr in humans (Jacobson et al. 2012; Cideciyan et al. 2013; Testa et al. 2013).

 Cite this article as *Cold Spring Harb Perspect Med* doi: 10.1101/cshperspect.a017293

Other sequences in the transgene expression cassette can be used to improve expression of the therapeutic gene. The inclusion of a woodchuck hepatitis virus posttranscriptional regulatory element (WPRE) downstream from the gene coding sequence enhanced AAV transgene expression in the rat brain (Paterna et al. 2000; Klein et al. 2002), in human embryonic kidney cells (HEK293), and human skin fibroblasts in vitro by up to 10-fold (Loeb et al. 1999). Although such an element has not been used previously in retinal gene therapy trials, the same WPRE sequence was approved by the United States Food and Drug Administration and, when used in the AAV2-GAD vector for gene therapy of Parkinson's disease, did not lead to any severe adverse events (Kaplitt et al. 2007). Importantly, this WPRE has been modified to ablate the translation initiation site of the viral X antigen, expression of which has previously been linked to increased tumor susceptibility in the liver of mice (Flajolet et al. 1998). The choice of polyadenylation signal sequence type can also be used to enhance gene expression. Bovine growth hormone polyA sequence has been shown to yield threefold higher expression levels than do other polyA sequences such as SV40 and human collagen polyA, and this increased expression is largely independent of the type of upstream promoter or transgene (Pfarr et al. 1986).

Thus, AAV transgene expression levels can be maximized by a combination of an optimized promoter and polyA signal, along with the inclusion of the WPRE sequence. This allows a lower overall dose of AAV vector to achieve the same therapeutic effect, which is likely to help minimize the immune response to viral proteins in patients. One might argue that this could also be achieved by using other AAV serotypes, such as AAV8, that appear to produce more efficient expression, especially in photoreceptors (Lebherz et al. 2008). However, as long-term data on safety and sustained expression are currently only available for AAV2, it is preferential to optimize the expression cassette rather than switch capsids.

AAV expression cassettes must be flanked by identical inverted terminal repeat sequences. These are part of the genome of wild-type AAV and are important in packaging the single-stranded DNA into virions and also in somehow protecting and maintaining the unpackaged DNA in an episomal state in transduced cells. Most inverted terminal repeat sequences used for clinical trials are derived from the genome of AAV2, regardless of which capsid serotype they are packaged into. The full annotation AAV2/2 is used to indicate that AAV2 ITRs have been used to package the expression cassette into the AAV2 serotype.

The final necessary component of the cassette is, of course, the cDNA sequence encoding human REP1. Fortunately, this has previously been fully cloned and characterized (Cremers et al. 1990; van Bokhoven et al. 1994). Overall, each AAV virion would contain a single stranded DNA sequence of ~4.2 kb in length comprising a CMV enhancer/CBA hybrid promoter, human REP1 cDNA, WPRE, and bovine growth hormone polyadenylation sequence (BGH-polyA). This would all be flanked by inverted terminal repeat sequences from the wild-type AAV2 genome. The structural organization of the AAV-REP1 vector is shown in Fig. 3.

PRECLINICAL TESTING OF THE VECTOR

To translate seamlessly and safely from the laboratory to a clinical trial, the AAV2 expression cassette was produced using protocols that had previously been scaled up to good manufacturing practice grade, approved by the United States Food and Drug Association and used safely in patients in another trial (Kaplitt et al. 2007). All preclinical work was conducted using AAV2-REP1 that had been packaged and purified to a research grade standard, but was otherwise identical to the good manufacturing practice-grade vector that could be used in a choroideremia clinical trial (Tolmachova et al. 2013).

Preclinical testing of the gene therapy expression cassette also involved creation of a green fluorescent protein (GFP) reporter vector. In the reporter vector, the coding sequence of GFP replaced the *REP1/Chm* cDNA, but otherwise, the structure and sequence were identical.

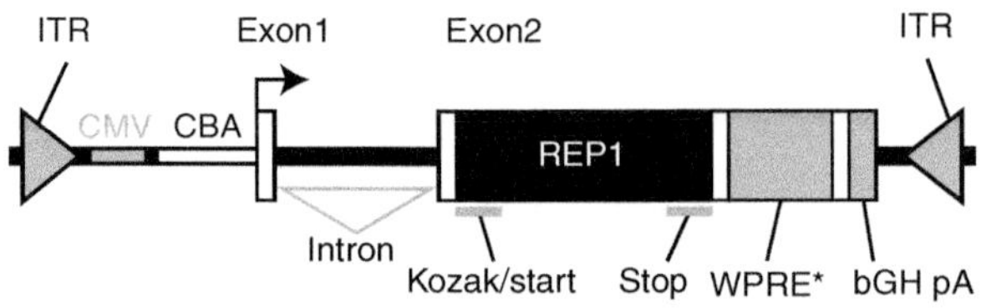

Figure 3. Design of the AAV2/2-REP1 vector used for choroideremia gene therapy. ITR, AAV2 inverted terminal repeats; CMV, cytomegalovirus enhancer element; CBA, chicken β actin promoter; Exon1, chicken β-actin exon 1; Intron, hybrid chicken β-actin and rabbit β-globin intron; Exon2, rabbit β-globin exon 3 fragment (creates an artificial splice site) and human REP1 cDNA (REP1) containing Kozak consensus sequence and start codon initiating translation (Kozak/start) and stop codon terminating translation (stop); WPRE*, modified woodchuck hepatitis virus posttranscriptional regulatory element; bGH pA, bovine growth hormone polyadenylation signal.

Subretinal injection of AAV2-GFP reporter vector in mice confirmed targeting of the transgene to RPE and a high level of expression in photoreceptors (Tolmachova et al. 2013). Furthermore, in vitro treatment of explants of human retina in culture with the AAV2-GFP vector confirmed that the gene therapy expression cassette and capsid type were capable of transducing photoreceptors and driving a high level of transgene expression (Tolmachova et al. 2013).

Importantly, the AAV2-REP1 vector was able to produce therapeutic protein in cultured fibroblasts of choroideremia patients. By examining prenylation activity in these transduced cells, correct function of the REP1 transgene product could be confirmed (Tolmachova et al. 2013). Subretinal injection of AAV2-REP1 in wild type mice did not significantly impair retinal function (as assessed by electroretinography), and thus no obvious toxic effects are evident following overexpression of REP1 (Tolmachova et al. 2013). When subretinal injection of AAV2-REP1 was used to treat *Chm*$^{null/+}$ mice, a dose dependent improvement/preservation of retinal function was observed after several months in treated eyes compared to paired, sham-injected control eyes (Tolmachova et al. 2013). Although large animal models have been used in the preclinical assessment of gene therapy for retinal disease such as LCA2 (Bennicelli et al. 2008; Cideciyan et al. 2013) and achromatopsia (Komaromy et al. 2010), no such large animal model exists for choroideremia. Thus, using a range of techniques and experiments, preclinical work confirmed the effectiveness and safety of the AAV2-REP1 gene therapy vector.

THE INITIATION OF A GENE THERAPY CLINICAL TRIAL FOR CHOROIDEREMIA

The necessary funding and regulatory and ethical approvals were obtained to embark on a gene therapy trial for choroideremia (ClinicalTrials.gov Identifier: NCT01461213). After a period of enrolment and baseline testing, the first treatment was given in October 2011. In all, the clinical trial will assess the effects of the AAV2.REP1 vector in 12 male patients with a clinical phenotype of choroideremia and a confirmed molecular diagnosis of a null mutation in the gene encoding REP1.

Choroideremia presents a number of challenges for gene therapy. Treatment must be performed when retinal structure relatively intact (i.e., before major cell loss) and when "good" foveal vision is still retained. The potential risks are significant, as delivery of the vector involves detachment of the fovea in a patient with good visual acuity, although if no form of treatment is given, vision will eventually be lost because of the ongoing degeneration. Although there is no preclinical evidence that REP1 is toxic, and it is present in virtually all nucleated cells in nonchoroideremia patients, it is possible that REP1 (over)expression might have a detrimental effect on retinal cells, in particular functional photoreceptors. In addition, this is the first gene therapy trial for retinal degeneration that specifically targets photoreceptor cells (in trials for RPE65-LCA2, the RPE cells were the primary target).

To ensure that photoreceptor cells are not compromised, the trial involves an escalation of the vector dose from a low baseline level. The starting dose of AAV2 (10^{10} genome particles) is at the lower end of the range (10^{10}–10^{12}) that has been shown to be safe in current AAV2 ocular gene therapy trials (Bainbridge et al. 2008; Hauswirth et al. 2008; Maguire et al. 2008). Because of this, reactions to AAV capsid protein are unlikely, even allowing for a large number of empty vector particles. The low initial dose also addresses the concern that, because the REP1 protein will be expressed against a null background, there is a theoretical risk of immune reaction to a new protein. The starting dose will be used in the first group of six patients and, if no serious adverse effects or reactions are seen, this will then be increased to a dose of AAV2 that is 10-fold higher (10^{11} genome particles) in the second group of six patients.

The primary objective of the study is to assess the safety and tolerability of the AAV2-REP1 vector. This will be performed by monitoring for evidence of ocular inflammation or detrimental effects to visual function in patients for 24 mo after administration. Changes in the treated eye can be compared to baseline measurements and to the fellow untreated eye. Gene transfer to the photoreceptors and RPE cells might enable the cells to survive long-term. The secondary endpoint of the study is to identify any therapeutic benefit of subretinal injection of AAV2-REP1 vector. As choroideremia is a progressive disease, this would be evidenced by a decrease in both loss of visual function and retinal degeneration in the treated eye compared to the control eye at 24 mo after gene delivery. Ophthalmological tests used to assess this will include microperimetry, optical coherence tomography scans and fundus autofluorescence imaging.

Although it is not expected that any anatomical parameter will show an improvement posttreatment compared to baseline, it is possible that there will be some recovery and restoration of vision when measured by the functional tests. These gains might be detected by microperimetry testing. Although male patients generally maintain good visual acuity until the degeneration encroaches on the fovea, significant deficits in parafoveal retinal sensitivity can be seen in more-discriminating tests (Jacobson et al. 2006b).

If the primary and secondary objectives are met, follow-up clinical trials will be initiated using the same vector at the efficacious dose. Beyond the 24 mo of formal testing, patients will continue long-term follow-up, with further assessments taking place annually as part of normal National Health Service care. This will continue for the lifetime of the patient, and the data will continue to be analyzed by members of the study group to determine if AAV2 transduction of the human retina can result in lifelong gene expression.

CONCLUDING REMARKS

More than 130 yr since the first description of choroideremia, a clinical trial involving gene therapy to treat the disease has begun. The conception and design of the clinical trial has been built on several decades of research focusing on the causes and pathology of the disease. Recent advances in the use of viral vectors for ocular gene therapy have also been invaluable. The trial is the first time photoreceptors have been specifically targeted for treatment in retinal degeneration. It is also the first time treatment of nondegenerated foveas with normal visual acuity has been attempted. Preclinical data on the testing of the AAV2-REP1 gene therapy vector have been encouraging, and the results of the human trial are awaited with great anticipation (MacLaren et al. 2014)

ACKNOWLEDGMENTS

The authors' work is supported by the National Institute for Health Research (NIHR) Biomedical Research Centres at the Oxford University Hospitals and Moorfields Eye Hospital NHS Trusts. Additional funding is provided by the Health Foundation, Fight for Sight, the Lanvern

Foundation, the Special Trustees of Moorfields Eye Hospital, the Royal College of Surgeons of Edinburgh. The CHM gene therapy clinical trial is funded by the Health Innovation Challenge Fund, a parallel funding partnership between the Wellcome Trust and the United Kingdom Department of Health.

REFERENCES

Bainbridge JW, Smith AJ, Barker SS, Robbie S, Henderson R, Balaggan K, Viswanathan A, Holder GE, Stockman A, Tyler N, et al. 2008. Effect of gene therapy on visual function in Leber's congenital amaurosis. *N Engl J Med* **358:** 2231–2239.

Bennett J, Maguire AM, Cideciyan AV, Schnell M, Glover E, Anand V, Aleman TS, Chirmule N, Gupta AR, Huang Y, et al. 1999. Stable transgene expression in rod photoreceptors after recombinant adeno-associated virus-mediated gene transfer to monkey retina. *Proc Natl Acad Sci* **96:** 9920–9925.

Bennicelli J, Wright JF, Komaromy A, Jacobs JB, Hauck B, Zelenaia O, Mingozzi F, Hui D, Chung D, Rex TS, et al. 2008. Reversal of blindness in animal models of Leber congenital amaurosis using optimized AAV2-mediated gene transfer. *Mol Ther* **16:** 458–465.

Bonilha VL, Trzupek KM, Li Y, Francis PJ, Hollyfield JG, Rayborn ME, Smaoui N, Weleber RG. 2008. Choroideremia: Analysis of the retina from a female symptomatic carrier. *Ophthalmic Genet* **29:** 99–110.

Cideciyan AV, Jacobson SG, Beltran WA, Sumaroka A, Swider M, Iwabe S, Roman AJ, Olivares MB, Schwartz SB, Komaromy AM, et al. 2013. Human retinal gene therapy for Leber congenital amaurosis shows advancing retinal degeneration despite enduring visual improvement. *Proc Natl Acad Sci* **110:** E517–E525.

Cremers FP, van de Pol DJ, van Kerkhoff LP, Wieringa B, Ropers HH. 1990. Cloning of a gene that is rearranged in patients with choroideraemia. *Nature* **347:** 674–677.

Cremers FP, Armstrong SA, Seabra MC, Brown MS, Goldstein JL. 1994. REP-2, a Rab escort protein encoded by the choroideremia-like gene. *J Biol Chem* **269:** 2111–2117.

Daly TM, Okuyama T, Vogler C, Haskins ME, Muzyczka N, Sands MS. 1999. Neonatal intramuscular injection with recombinant adeno-associated virus results in prolonged beta-glucuronidase expression in situ and correction of liver pathology in mucopolysaccharidosis type VII mice. *Hum Gene Ther* **10:** 85–94.

Esposito G, De Falco F, Tinto N, Testa F, Vitagliano L, Tandurella IC, Iannone L, Rossi S, Rinaldi E, Simonelli F, et al. 2011. Comprehensive mutation analysis (20 families) of the choroideremia gene reveals a missense variant that prevents the binding of REP1 with Rab geranylgeranyl transferase. *Hum Mutat* **32:** 1460–1469.

Flajolet M, Tiollais P, Buendia MA, Fourel G. 1998. Woodchuck hepatitis virus enhancer I and enhancer II are both involved in N-*myc2* activation in woodchuck liver tumors. *J Virol* **72:** 6175–6180.

Flannery JG, Bird AC, Farber DB, Weleber RG, Bok D. 1990. A histopathologic study of a choroideremia carrier. *Invest Ophthalmol Vis Scie* **31:** 229–236.

Furgoch MJ, Mewes-Ares J, Radziwon A, MacDonald IM. 2014. Molecular genetic diagnostic techniques in choroideremia. *Mol Vis* **20:** 535–544.

Gibbs D, Kitamoto J, Williams DS. 2003. Abnormal phagocytosis by retinal pigmented epithelium that lacks myosin VIIa, the Usher syndrome 1B protein. *Proc Natl Acad Sci* **100:** 6481–6486.

Hauswirth WW, Aleman TS, Kaushal S, Cideciyan AV, Schwartz SB, Wang L, Conlon TJ, Boye SL, Flotte TR, Byrne BJ, et al. 2008. Treatment of Leber congenital amaurosis due to *RPE65* mutations by ocular subretinal injection of adeno-associated virus gene vector: Short-term results of a phase I trial. *Hum Gene Ther* **19:** 979–990.

Jacobson SG, Boye SL, Aleman TS, Conlon TJ, Zeiss CJ, Roman AJ, Cideciyan AV, Schwartz SB, Komaromy AM, Doobrajh M, et al. 2006a. Safety in nonhuman primates of ocular AAV2-*RPE65*, a candidate treatment for blindness in Leber congenital amaurosis. *Hum Gene Ther* **17:** 845–858.

Jacobson SG, Cideciyan AV, Sumaroka A, Aleman TS, Schwartz SB, Windsor EA, Roman AJ, Stone EM, MacDonald IM. 2006b. Remodeling of the human retina in choroideremia: Rab escort protein 1 (*REP-1*) mutations. *Invest Ophthalmol Vis Sci* **47:** 4113–4120.

Jacobson SG, Cideciyan AV, Ratnakaram R, Heon E, Schwartz SB, Roman AJ, Peden MC, Aleman TS, Boye SL, Sumaroka A, et al. 2012. Gene therapy for Leber congenital amaurosis caused by *RPE65* mutations: Safety and efficacy in 15 children and adults followed up to 3 years. *Arch Ophthalmol* **130:** 9–24.

Kaplitt MG, Feigin A, Tang C, Fitzsimons HL, Mattis P, Lawlor PA, Bland RJ, Young D, Strybing K, Eidelberg D, et al. 2007. Safety and tolerability of gene therapy with an adeno-associated virus (AAV) borne *GAD* gene for Parkinson's disease: An open label, phase I trial. *Lancet* **369:** 2097–2105.

Klein RL, Hamby ME, Gong Y, Hirko AC, Wang S, Hughes JA, King MA, Meyer EM. 2002. Dose and promoter effects of adeno-associated viral vector for green fluorescent protein expression in the rat brain. *Exp Neurol* **176:** 66–74.

Komaromy AM, Alexander JJ, Rowlan JS, Garcia MM, Chiodo VA, Kaya A, Tanaka JC, Acland GM, Hauswirth WW, Aguirre GD. 2010. Gene therapy rescues cone function in congenital achromatopsia. *Hum Mol Genet* **19:** 2581–2593.

Krock BL, Bilotta J, Perkins BD. 2007. Noncell-autonomous photoreceptor degeneration in a zebrafish model of choroideremia. *Proc Natl Acad Sci* **104:** 4600–4605.

Larijani B, Hume AN, Tarafder AK, Seabra MC. 2003. Multiple factors contribute to inefficient prenylation of Rab27a in Rab prenylation diseases. *J Biol Chem* **278:** 46798–46804.

Lebherz C, Maguire A, Tang W, Bennett J, Wilson JM. 2008. Novel AAV serotypes for improved ocular gene transfer. *J Gene Med* **10:** 375–382.

Loeb JE, Cordier WS, Harris ME, Weitzman MD, Hope TJ. 1999. Enhanced expression of transgenes from adeno-associated virus vectors with the woodchuck hepatitis virus posttranscriptional regulatory element: Implications for gene therapy. *Hum Gene Ther* **10:** 2295–2305.

Lotery AJ, Yang GS, Mullins RF, Russell SR, Schmidt M, Stone EM, Lindbloom JD, Chiorini JA, Kotin RM, Davidson BL. 2003. Adeno-associated virus type 5: Transduction efficiency and cell-type specificity in the primate retina. *Hum Gene Ther* **14:** 1663–1671.

MacDonald IM, Mah DY, Ho YK, Lewis RA, Seabra MC. 1998. A practical diagnostic test for choroideremia. *Ophthalmology* **105:** 1637–1640.

MacDonald IM, Russell L, Chan CC. 2009. Choroideremia: New findings from ocular pathology and review of recent literature. *Surv Ophthalmol* **54:** 401–407.

MacLaren RE. 2009. An analysis of retinal gene therapy clinical trials. *Curr Opin Mol Ther* **11:** 540–546.

MacLaren RE, Bird AC, Sathia PJ, Aylward GW. 2005. Long-term results of submacular surgery combined with macular translocation of the retinal pigment epithelium in neovascular age-related macular degeneration. *Ophthalmology* **112:** 2081–2087.

MacLaren RE, Groppe M, Barnard AR, Cottriall CL, Tolmachova T, Seymour L, Clark KR, During MJ, Cremers FPM, Black GCM, et al. 2014. Initial observations in patients undergoing retinal gene therapy for choroideremia. *Lancet* (in press).

Maguire AM, Simonelli F, Pierce EA, Pugh EN Jr, Mingozzi F, Bennicelli J, Banfi S, Marshall KA, Testa F, Surace EM, et al. 2008. Safety and efficacy of gene transfer for Leber's congenital amaurosis. *N Engl J Med* **358:** 2240–2248.

Mancuso K, Hendrickson AE, Connor TB Jr, Mauck MC, Kinsella JJ, Hauswirth WW, Neitz J, Neitz M. 2007. Recombinant adeno-associated virus targets passenger gene expression to cones in primate retina. *J Opt Soc Am A* **24:** 1411–1416.

Martin EA. 2010. *Concise medical dictionary.* Oxford University Press, Oxford.

Mauthner L. 1872. Ophthalmologische. Mittheilungen: 2. Ein fall von chorioideremie. in *Berichte des naturwissenschaftlichen-medizinischen Verein Innsbruck*, pp. 191–197. Medical and Scientific Association Innsbruck.

McTaggart KE, Tran M, Mah DY, Lai SW, Nesslinger NJ, MacDonald IM. 2002. Mutational analysis of patients with the diagnosis of choroideremia. *Hum Mutat* **20:** 189–196.

Mingozzi F, Maus MV, Hui DJ, Sabatino DE, Murphy SL, Rasko JE, Ragni MV, Manno CS, Sommer J, Jiang H, et al. 2007. $CD8^+$ T-cell responses to adeno-associated virus capsid in humans. *Nat Med* **13:** 419–422.

Miyazaki J, Takaki S, Araki K, Tashiro F, Tominaga A, Takatsu K, Yamamura K. 1989. Expression vector system based on the chicken β-actin promoter directs efficient production of interleukin-5. *Gene* **79:** 269–277.

Moosajee M, Tulloch M, Baron RA, Gregory-Evans CY, Pereira-Leal JB, Seabra MC. 2009. Single choroideremia gene in nonmammalian vertebrates explains early embryonic lethality of the zebrafish model of choroideremia. *Invest Ophthalmol Vis Sci* **50:** 3009–3016.

Myers T. 2006. *Mosby's dictionary of medicine, nursing & health professions.* Elsevier, London.

Niwa H, Yamamura K, Miyazaki J. 1991. Efficient selection for high-expression transfectants with a novel eukaryotic vector. *Gene* **108:** 193–199.

Pameyer JK, Waardenburg PJ, Henkes HE. 1960. Choroid eremia. *Br J Ophthalmol* **44:** 724–738.

Paterna JC, Moccetti T, Mura A, Feldon J, Bueler H. 2000. Influence of promoter and WHV post-transcriptional regulatory element on AAV-mediated transgene expression in the rat brain. *Gene Ther* **7:** 1304–1311.

Pfarr DS, Rieser LA, Woychik RP, Rottman FM, Rosenberg M, Reff ME. 1986. Differential effects of polyadenylation regions on gene expression in mammalian cells. *DNA* **5:** 115–122.

Pylypenko O, Rak A, Reents R, Niculae A, Sidorovitch V, Cioaca MD, Bessolitsyna E, Thoma NH, Waldmann H, Schlichting I, et al. 2003. Structure of Rab escort protein-1 in complex with Rab geranylgeranyltransferase. *Mol Cell* **11:** 483–494.

Reese BE, Harvey AR, Tan SS. 1995. Radial and tangential dispersion patterns in the mouse retina are cell-class specific. *Proc Natl Acad Sci* **92:** 2494–2498.

Sankila EM, Tolvanen R, van den Hurk JA, Cremers FP, de la Chapelle A. 1992. Aberrant splicing of the *CHM* gene is a significant cause of choroideremia. *Nat Genet* **1:** 109–113.

Seabra MC, Brown MS, Slaughter CA, Sudhof TC, Goldstein JL. 1992. Purification of component A of Rab geranylgeranyl transferase: Possible identity with the choroideremia gene product. *Cell* **70:** 1049–1057.

Seabra MC, Brown MS, Goldstein JL. 1993. Retinal degeneration in choroideremia: Deficiency of Rab geranylgeranyl transferase. *Science* **259:** 377–381.

Seabra MC, Ho YK, Anant JS. 1995. Deficient geranylgeranylation of Ram/Rab27 in choroideremia. *J Biol Chem* **270:** 24420–24427.

Shi W, van den Hurk JA, Alamo-Bethencourt V, Mayer W, Winkens HJ, Ropers HH, Cremers FP, Fundele R. 2004. Choroideremia gene product affects trophoblast development and vascularization in mouse extra-embryonic tissues. *Dev Biol* **272:** 53–65.

Starr CJ, Kappler JA, Chan DK, Kollmar R, Hudspeth AJ. 2004. Mutation of the zebrafish choroideremia gene encoding Rab escort protein 1 devastates hair cells. *Proc Natl Acad Sci* **101:** 2572–2577.

Syed N, Smith JE, John SK, Seabra MC, Aguirre GD, Milam AH. 2001. Evaluation of retinal photoreceptors and pigment epithelium in a female carrier of choroideremia. *Ophthalmology* **108:** 711–720.

Testa F, Maguire AM, Rossi S, Pierce EA, Melillo P, Marshall K, Banfi S, Surace EM, Sun J, Acerra C, et al. 2013. Three-year follow-up after unilateral subretinal delivery of adeno-associated virus in patients with Leber congenital amaurosis type 2. *Ophthalmology* **120:** 1283–1291.

Tolmachova T, Ramalho JS, Anant JS, Schultz RA, Huxley CM, Seabra MC. 1999. Cloning, mapping and characterization of the human *RAB27A* gene. *Gene* **239:** 109–116.

Tolmachova T, Anders R, Abrink M, Bugeon L, Dallman MJ, Futter CE, Ramalho JS, Tonagel F, Tanimoto N, Seeliger MW, et al. 2006. Independent degeneration of photoreceptors and retinal pigment epithelium in conditional knockout mouse models of choroideremia. *J Clin Invest* **116:** 386–394.

Tolmachova T, Wavre-Shapton ST, Barnard AR, MacLaren RE, Futter CE, Seabra MC. 2010. Retinal pigment epithelium defects accelerate photoreceptor degeneration in cell type-specific knockout mouse models of choroideremia. *Invest Ophthalmol Vis Sci* **51:** 4913–4920.

Tolmachova T, Tolmachov OE, Barnard AR, de Silva SR, Lipinski DM, Walker NJ, Maclaren RE, Seabra MC. 2013. Functional expression of Rab escort protein 1 following AAV2-mediated gene delivery in the retina of choroideremia mice and human cells ex vivo. *J Mol Med* **91:** 825–837.

van Bokhoven H, van den Hurk JA, Bogerd L, Philippe C, Gilgenkrantz S, de Jong P, Ropers HH, Cremers FP. 1994. Cloning and characterization of the human choroideremia gene. *Hum Mol Genet* **3:** 1041–1046.

van den Hurk JA, Hendriks W, van de Pol DJ, Oerlemans F, Jaissle G, Ruther K, Kohler K, Hartmann J, Zrenner E, van Bokhoven H, et al. 1997. Mouse choroideremia gene mutation causes photoreceptor cell degeneration and is not transmitted through the female germline. *Hum Mol Genet* **6:** 851–858.

van den Hurk JA, van de Pol DJ, Wissinger B, van Driel MA, Hoefsloot LH, de Wijs IJ, van den Born LI, Heckenlively JR, Brunner HG, Zrenner E, et al. 2003. Novel types of mutation in the *choroideremia* (*CHM*) gene: A full-length L1 insertion and an intronic mutation activating a cryptic exon. *Hum Genet* **113:** 268–275.

Wolf S. 1930. Choroideremia. *Arch Ophthalmol* **3:** 80–87.

Wu Z, Yang H, Colosi P. 2010. Effect of genome size on AAV vector packaging. *Mol Ther* **18:** 80–86.

Xu L, Daly T, Gao C, Flotte TR, Song S, Byrne BJ, Sands MS, Parker Ponder K. 2001. CMV-β-actin promoter directs higher expression from an adeno-associated viral vector in the liver than the cytomegalovirus or elongation factor 1α promoter and results in therapeutic levels of human factor X in mice. *Hum Gene Ther* **12:** 563–573.

 Cite this article as *Cold Spring Harb Perspect Med* doi: 10.1101/cshperspect.a017293

Gene Therapy of *ABCA4*-Associated Diseases

Alberto Auricchio[1], Ivana Trapani[1], and Rando Allikmets[2]

[1]Telethon Institute of Genetics and Medicine, Naples, 80131 Italy

[2]Department of Ophthalmology, and Department of Pathology and Cell Biology, Columbia University, New York, New York 10032

Correspondence: rla22@cumc.columbia.edu

The ATP-binding cassette (ABC) transporter gene, *ABCA4 (ABCR)*, was characterized in 1997 as the causal gene for autosomal recessive Stargardt disease (STGD1). Shortly thereafter several other phenotypes were associated with mutations in *ABCA4*, which now have collectively emerged as the most frequent cause of retinal degeneration phenotypes of Mendelian inheritance. ABCA4 functions as an important transporter (or "flippase") of vitamin A derivatives in the visual cycle. Several ways to alleviate the effects of the defective ABCA4 protein, which cause accumulation of 11-*cis* and all-*trans*-retinal in photoreceptors and lipofuscin in the retinal pigment epithelium, have been proposed. Although *ABCA4* has proven to be a difficult research target, substantial progress through genetic, functional, and translational studies has allowed major advances in therapeutic applications for ABCA4-associated pathology, which should be available to patients in the (near) future. Here, we summarize the status of the gene therapy-based treatment options of *ABCA4*-associated diseases.

Somatic gene therapy has shown success in several animal models of (recessive) retinal degeneration (Campochiaro 2002; Allocca et al. 2006). Most well known have been reports that a recombinant adeno-associated virus (rAAV) carrying wild-type Rpe65 (rAAV-Rpe65) improved visual function in the Briard dog model of childhood blindness (Acland et al. 2001; Narfstrom et al. 2003; Le Meur et al. 2007). Similar successes have been reported for the $Rpe65^{-/-}$ and $Lrat^{-/-}$ mouse models with AAV and lentiviral vectors (Dejneka et al. 2004; Batten et al. 2005; Bemelmans et al. 2006; Yanez-Munoz et al. 2006).

Direct gene replacement represents an attractive therapeutic option also for treatment of all *ABCA4*-associated diseases, including Stargardt disease (STGD1) (Allikmets et al. 1997; Molday and Zhang 2010). Delivering a normally functioning gene to photoreceptors harboring mutant *ABCA4* via gene therapy should therefore be considered as a possible "cure" for *ABCA4*-associated diseases because: (1) All *ABCA4*-associated diseases are recessive, so that adding a functional gene could fully restore visual function and, (2) degeneration of the retinal cells in all *ABCA4*-associated diseases is relatively delayed, allowing a reasonable time window for therapeutic intervention.

Currently, two major approaches for the delivery of the genetic material to the eye are used: one based on viral vectors as delivery vehicles

Cite this article as *Cold Spring Harb Perspect Med* doi: 10.1101/cshperspect.a017301

and the other including nonviral gene delivery methods. So far, the identification of an efficient vector for the delivery of the *ABCA4* gene to the retina has been hampered by the large size of the *ABCA4* coding sequence (6.8 kb) and by the expression of the ABCA4 gene/protein exclusively in photoreceptor (PR) cells, therefore requiring vectors with large cargo capacity and able to transduce PRs efficiently. Most delivery vehicles that accept large cargo capacity, such as lentiviruses, adenoviruses, and nonviral vectors, have been suggested not to able to efficiently transduce PRs, at least in the mouse models. At the same time, vectors with efficient PR transduction capability, for example those based on adeno-associated viruses (AAVs), have a packaging capacity limited to about 4.7 kb (Colella and Auricchio 2012; Lipinski et al. 2013) and therefore would not be able to package the large *ABCA4* coding sequence of ~7 kb. Recently, significant efforts have been directed toward both the development of AAV-based systems, which are able to deliver large genes and the identification of lentiviral and nonviral vectors with higher PR tropism. Here we will review the current status of *ABCA4* gene therapy development.

NONVIRAL GENE DELIVERY IN *ABCA4*-ASSOCIATED DISEASES

Nonviral vectors offer a number of advantages over viral-based strategies including: (1) reduced toxicity from the vector, (2) lack of an immune response against the vector and possibility to readminister the vector, (3) a large transgene capacity, and (4) simple and relatively inexpensive clinical grade production (Charbel Issa and MacLaren 2012). However, although viruses have evolved to optimize the delivery of the viral gene into the nucleus of the human host cell, "naked" DNA delivered by nonviral vectors needs to overcome several barriers to be expressed, such as: (1) extracellular degradation and immune response mediated by sensor of single stranded or double stranded DNA molecules, such as toll-like receptors, (2) cytoplasmic degradation, and (3) passage through the nuclear envelope during cell division, which is not possible in postmitotic cells, such as PRs. In addition, the presence of physical barriers in the eye, such as the vitreous, inner/outer limiting membranes, the inter-PR matrix, and the high concentrations of glycosaminoglycans present throughout the eye that sequester the DNA, further limit cellular access (Lipinski et al. 2013). As a consequence, many studies have provided evidence of the higher efficiency of viral versus nonviral retinal gene delivery (Andrieu-Soler et al. 2006). In particular, injection of naked DNA via subretinal injection between the PR and retinal pigment epithelium (RPE) (Liang et al. 2000) is highly inefficient (Charbel Issa and MacLaren 2012). Therefore, chemical or physical methods have been used to enhance the efficiency of nonviral vectors gene delivery to the outer retina. Chemical methods, such as liposomes, polymers, and compacted nanoparticles, are based on the conjugation of the DNA with synthetic or natural cationic compound that both protect DNA from nuclease-mediated degradation and allow passage through/into cell membranes via endocytosis and, in some instances, receptor-mediated uptake. Physical methods, such as electroporation or iontophoresis, typically use an electrical stimulus to temporarily permeabilize the membrane and allow the DNA to cross the cellular membranes. To date, however, evidence for effective gene delivery to outer retinal cells remains scarce and the success of the majority of the nonviral delivery technology has been limited to the RPE cell layer (Kachi et al. 2005; Johnson et al. 2008; Souied et al. 2008). However, recently, the polylysine-based compacted DNA nanoparticle (NP) CK30-NP has shown significant improvement in the efficacy of ocular gene transfer in comparison to the previous nonviral methods (Farjo et al. 2006). In the compacted nanoparticles, in particular, the DNA molecule is compacted by polyethylene glycol (PEG)-substituted 30-mer lysine peptides (CK30PEG) (Liu et al. 2003). Their minimal diameter (usually 8–20 nm) is such that allows to readily enter the nucleus (Liu et al. 2003) of dividing and nondividing cells, remaining episomal. Importantly, these particles have no theoretical DNA packaging limitations and have been successfully tested with plasmids up to 20 kb in length

(Fink et al. 2006). Notably, subretinal administration of CK30-NPs results in extensive PR transduction, even though with some unexplained patterns of transgene expression (Kumar-Singh 2008) in the absence of detectable immune responses or toxicity (Farjo et al. 2006; Ding et al. 2009). In addition, in contrast with other nonviral approaches, CK30-NPs drive long-term gene expression after subretinal delivery to the mouse eye (Conley and Naash 2010). Given the success of CK30-NPs to mediate phenotypic rescue in rodent models of retinitis pigmentosa (Cai et al. 2009, 2010) and their favorable safety and efficacy profile in a human clinical trial for cystic fibrosis (Konstan et al. 2004). Han et al. (2012) have recently tested CK30-NPs for *ABCA4* delivery in the *Abca4*$^{-/-}$ mouse model of Stargardt disease. This mouse model shows some of the clinical features associated with STGD1, such as accumulation of lipofuscin (A2E) in RPE (Weng et al. 1999; Mata et al. 2001), thickening of the RPE cells (Allocca et al. 2008; Radu et al. 2008; Conley et al. 2012), delayed recovery from light desensitization (Weng et al. 1999; Maiti et al. 2006; Allocca et al. 2008; Radu et al. 2008), and thinning of the outer nuclear (PR cell) layer in albino KO mice (Radu et al. 2008; Wu et al. 2010a). In this mouse model, after subretinal injection of the CK30-NPs carrying the human *ABCA4* gene, Han et al. (2012) detected *ABCA4* transgene expression for up to 8 months after injection and found both improved recovery of dark adaptation and reduced lipofuscin accumulation. These promising data have provided the first evidence of effective nonviral vector-mediated delivery of large genes, such as *ABCA4*, to the PR cell layer.

AAV GENE DELIVERY IN *ABCA4*-ASSOCIATED DISEASES

AAV-derived vectors are currently the most favored vehicles for therapeutic gene delivery to the retina, because they have low immunogenicity, favorable safety profile and support long-term transgene expression after a single administration (Colella and Auricchio 2012; Vandenberghe and Auricchio 2012). AAV is a small (25 nm), nonenveloped virus that packages a linear single-stranded DNA genome of ~4.7 kb. One of the strengths of the AAV vector platform is the availability of more than 100 different forms called AAV serotypes, which are isolated either as infectious or as molecular clones, and which differ in their external surface capsids proteins. Capsids can be easily exchanged among various AAVs to generate hybrid vectors that contain a genome with the same AAV inverted terminal repeats (ITRs) and the capsid from a different serotype (Auricchio 2003). AAVs obtained through this transcapsidation system are named AAV2/n, where the first number refers to the ITRs and the second to the capsid (Surace and Auricchio 2008). Different capsids confer different tropism and transduction characteristics. Initial AAV vectors were based on AAV serotype 2 (AAV2/2), the most prevalent serotype in humans. However, AAV2/2, although an excellent gene transfer vector for transducing RPE or retinal ganglion cells, is relatively inefficient at transducing other retinal cell types such as PR. Because the majority of mutations causing inherited retinal degeneration, including STGD1, occurs in genes expressed in PRs (Vandenberghe and Auricchio 2012), this concern prompted the search for AAV serotypes able to overcome this limitation. AAV2/5, 2/7, 2/8, and 2/9 vectors have all efficiently transduced PRs, in addition to RPE (Auricchio et al. 2001; Lotery et al. 2003; Allocca et al. 2007), with the AAV2/8 being the most efficient serotype in mice (Auricchio et al. 2001; Lotery et al. 2003; Allocca et al. 2007), pigs (Mussolino et al. 2011), dogs (Stieger et al. 2008), and nonhuman primates (Vandenberghe et al. 2011). The major limitation to the use of AAVs for gene replacement remains their packaging capacity, which is considered to be restricted to the size of the parental genome (4.7 kb), and thus hampers the treatment of certain forms of inherited retinal diseases caused by mutations in genes where cDNA exceeds 5 kb, such as *ABCA4*. Thus, different strategies to overcome AAV cargo limitations have been investigated. One is based on packaging of oversized genomes, that is, larger than 5 kb (Table 1) (Grieger and Samulski 2005; Allocca et al.

Table 1. Schematic representation of AAV-based strategies for large gene transduction

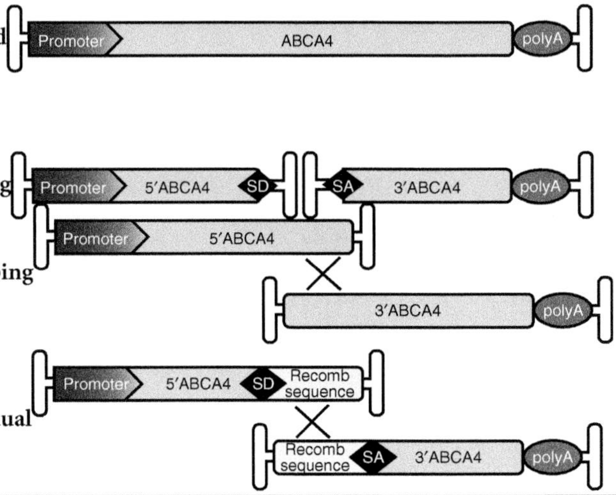

Approach	Mechanism for reconstitution
Oversized	Reassembly of truncated genomes
Trans-splicing	ITR-mediated concatemerization followed by splicing
Overlapping	Homologous recombination
Hybrid dual	Homologous recombination followed by splicing

SD, splicing donor signal; SA, splicing acceptor signal; polyA, poly-adenylation signal. Crosses show overlapping regions available for homologous recombination.

2008; Hirsch et al. 2010). Notably, oversized AAVs have been successfully used to express *ABCA4* in the PR of *Abca4*$^{-/-}$ mice resulting in significant and stable morphological and functional improvement of the *Abca4*$^{-/-}$ retina (Allocca et al. 2008). However, the mechanism underlying oversized AAV-mediated PR transduction remains elusive as the genomes contained in oversized AAV vectors appear highly heterogeneous in size and are predominantly shorter than expected (Dong et al. 2010; Hirsch et al. 2010; Lai et al. 2010; Wu et al. 2010b; Hirsch et al. 2013), which limits their use in clinical setting.

Alternatively, the ability of heterologous AAV genomes to form intermolecular concatemers in the nucleus of target cells (Duan et al. 1998) can be exploited to express large genes, which can be split into two halves, independently packaged in two different (dual) AAV vectors. Various dual AAVs strategies have been described (referred to as trans-splicing, overlapping, and hybrid dual-vector strategies, Table 1) and have been used to efficiently delivery large genes to different tissues. In the trans-splicing approach the 5′-half vector has a splice donor (SD) signal at the 3′ end, whereas the 3′-half vector carries a splice acceptor (SA) signal at the 5′end that allow trans-splicing of a single large mRNA molecule following head-to-tail concatemerization of the two AAVs (Yan et al. 2000). In the overlapping approach, the dual AAV genomes share overlapping sequences, thus the reconstitution of the large gene expression cassette relies on homologous recombination (Duan et al. 2001). The third dual AAV approach (hybrid dual) is a combination of the two previous approaches and it is based on the addition of a highly recombinogenic exogenous sequence to the trans-splicing vectors, to increase their recombination efficiency (Ghosh et al. 2008, 2011; Trapani et al. 2014). This recombinogenic sequence is placed downstream from the SD signal in the 5′-half vector and upstream of the SA signal in the 3′-half vector, so that, after recombination, it is spliced out from the mature RNA (Table 1). The recombinogenic sequences used so far to induce the recombination between dual AAV hybrid vectors derive from regions of either the alkaline phosphatase gene (AP) (Ghosh et al. 2008, 2011) or the F1 phage genome (AK) (Trapani et al. 2014). We recently compared side-by-side the efficiency of the various oversized, dual AAV overlapping, trans-splicing, and hybrid strategies for AAV-mediated large gene transduction in the mouse and pig retina (Trapani et al. 2014), and found that dual AAV trans-splicing and hybrid AK vectors efficiently reconstitute the large *ABCA4* gene in mouse PRs. Notably, subretinal administration of dual AAV trans-splicing and hybrid AK vectors improved the phenotype of a mouse model of STGD1, providing evidence for the efficacy of these strategies for *ABCA4* gene therapy. Dozens of successful proofs of concept of the efficacy of AAV mediated gene therapy for recessive and dominant inherited retinal diseases have been generated in small and large animal models (Stieger et al. 2010) and have paved the way to the first clinical trials using AAV in patients with Leber congenital amaurosis, a severe form of childhood blindness (Bainbridge et al. 2008; Maguire et al. 2008, 2009; Cideciyan et al. 2009; Simonelli et al. 2010). The results from these initial trials suggest that retinal gene therapy with AAV is safe in humans, that vision can be improved in patients that have suffered from severe impairment of visual function, in some cases for decades, and that readministration of AAV to the subretinal space is feasible, effective, and safe. This, as well as the recent evidence of the efficacy of dual AAV-mediated *ABCA4* delivery in mice (Trapani et al. 2014), strongly supports further investigation using AAV for treatment of diseases caused by *ABCA4* mutation.

LENTIVIRAL GENE DELIVERY IN *ABCA4*-ASSOCIATED DISEASES

Lentiviral vectors offer several advantages for gene therapy applications in general, as well as in the specific case of *ABCA4*-associated diseases. First and foremost, lentiviruses are capable of delivering genes stably and permanently into the genome of transduced cells in vivo (Lois et al. 2002; Gouze et al. 2003; Kostic et al. 2003). Second, they can transduce nondividing cells, a crucial requirement for terminally differentiated cells such as photoreceptors (Kingsman 2003). Third, they can carry relatively large expression cassettes, which is essential in this case because the human *ABCA4* cDNA is almost 7 kb, which exceeds the capacity of the commonly used AAV vectors. However, two major problems associated with lentiviral-based gene therapy are, as suggested, the relatively low PR tropism of lentiviral vectors in mouse models and possible tumorigenic side effects resulting from uncontrolled, random integration of lentiviruses to the host genome.

The reported low efficiency of PR transduction with lentiviruses in (adult) rodents has been considered a major limiting factor for gene therapy of eye diseases with lentiviral vectors. Although the early experiments with rats were successful (Miyoshi et al. 1997; Takahashi et al. 1999), they were not confirmed subsequently, especially in adult rodent models (Kostic et al. 2003; Gruter et al. 2005). The best efficacy of PR transduction in mice (5%–15%) was achieved after subretinal injection of mice at postnatal 4 and 5 d (Kong et al. 2008). In adult mice, the efficacy rarely exceeded 5%, even after chemical modification of the subretinal space by neuraminidase X or chondroitinase ABC (Gruter et al. 2005). It had been noted, however, that the PR transduction by lentiviruses was more efficient in other animals, such as chicken and nonhuman primates (Lotery et al. 2002; Williams et al. 2006). Subsequently, we were able to show a more efficient PR transduction of the NHP retina by EIAV lentivectors using either GFP (Binley et al. 2013) or LacZ (data not shown) as reporters under the constitutive CMV promoter. Transduction of PRs, in addition to RPE, in the injected area of adult macaques suggests that lentiviral vectors can more efficiently transduce PRs in adult NHPs than in mice, thus raising hope for gene therapy in humans, especially for delivering large genes such as *ABCA4*. Additional studies with PR-specific promoters should unequivocally address the PR transduction efficiency issue for lentiviral vectors in NHPs.

However, Abca4$^{-/-}$ mice are still the only animal model for STGD1 disease, therefore all preclinical models have used this mouse strain. An efficient amelioration of a major disease marker, A2E accumulation, was successfully achieved in studies utilizing lentiviral vectors in the Abca4$^{-/-}$ mouse model (Kong et al. 2008). After demonstrating safety and acceptable biodistribution of EIAV vectors carrying the human ABCA4 gene under the constitutive CMV promoter, phase I/II clinical trials for patients with STGD1 were started in 2012 by Oxford BioMedica (NCT01367444; see http://www.clinicaltrials.gov).

In addition to the suggested low PR transduction efficiency by lentiviruses in mice, two other concerns have slowed the development of the lentiviral platform. First, despite greatly improved biosafety, psychological concerns regarding using vectors derived from primate lentiviruses HIV-1, HIV-2, and simian immunodeficiency virus (SIV) have not been completely overcome, despite highly remote possibility of generating replication-competent lentivirus in clinical application. These concerns have been alleviated by using nonprimate lentiviral vectors, which cannot replicate in human cells (Maury 1998), such as those derived from equine infectious anemia virus (EIAV), bovine immunodeficiency virus (BIV), or feline immunodeficiency viruses (FIV) (Olsen 2001). Second, serious complications in early gene therapy clinical trials for X-linked SCID3 using retroviral vectors raised ethical and safety concerns about the use of retrovirus-based therapies in humans because of uncontrolled integration into genome (Kohn et al. 2003). These concerns are being addressed by creating either integration-deficient lentiviral vectors or vectors with targeted, clinically safe integration (Wanisch and Yanez-Munoz 2009).

CONCLUDING REMARKS

Several gene therapy applications are being used for *ABCA4*-associated diseases. Although currently only lentivirus-based therapy is in clinical trials, those based on AAV or nonviral vectors are close to follow. Another delivery vehicles not discussed above, but which are tried in preclinical studies are adenoviral (Ad) vectors. Although the Ad vectors, which are nonintegrating and transduce both dividing and nondividing cells, used to elicit immune responses that limited the duration of transgene expression, the current, helper-dependent Ad vectors, can substantially extend the duration of the expression of the transgene (Lamartina et al. 2007). Comparison of all methods will reveal which one is the most efficient and safe for patients; however, regardless of the final outcome, it is clear that efficient gene therapy will soon be available to patients affected with all *ABCA4*-associated diseases.

ACKNOWLEDGMENTS

Supported, in part, by grants from the National Eye Institute (NIH) EY021163, EY019861, and EY019007 (Core Support for Vision Research); Foundation Fighting Blindness (Owings Mills, Maryland), and unrestricted funds from Research to Prevent Blindness (New York, NY) to the Department of Ophthalmology, Columbia University.

REFERENCES

Acland GM, Aguirre GD, Ray J, Zhang Q, Aleman TS, Cideciyan AV, Pearce-Kelling SE, Anand V, Zeng Y, Maguire AM, et al. 2001. Gene therapy restores vision in a canine model of childhood blindness. *Nat Genet* **28:** 92–95.

Allikmets R, Singh N, Sun H, Shroyer NF, Hutchinson A, Chidambaram A, Gerrard B, Baird L, Stauffer D, Peiffer A, et al. 1997. A photoreceptor cell-specific ATP-binding transporter gene (*ABCR*) is mutated in recessive Stargardt macular dystrophy. *Nat Genet* **15:** 236–246.

Allocca M, Tessitore A, Cotugno G, Auricchio A. 2006. AAV-mediated gene transfer for retinal diseases. *Expert Opin Biol Ther* **6:** 1279–1294.

Allocca M, Mussolino C, Garcia-Hoyos M, Sanges D, Iodice C, Petrillo M, Vandenberghe LH, Wilson JM, Marigo V, Surace EM, et al. 2007. Novel adeno-associated virus serotypes efficiently transduce murine photoreceptors. *J Virol* **81:** 11372–11380.

Allocca M, Doria M, Petrillo M, Colella P, Garcia-Hoyos M, Gibbs D, Kim SR, Maguire A, Rex TS, Di Vicino U, et al. 2008. Serotype-dependent packaging of large genes in adeno-associated viral vectors results in effective gene delivery in mice. *J Clin Invest* **118:** 1955–1964.

Andrieu-Soler C, Bejjani RA, de Bizemont T, Normand N, BenEzra D, Behar-Cohen F. 2006. Ocular gene therapy: A review of nonviral strategies. *Mol Vis* **12:** 1334–1347.

Auricchio A. 2003. Pseudotyped AAV vectors for constitutive and regulated gene expression in the eye. *Vision Res* **43:** 913–918.

Auricchio A, Kobinger G, Anand V, Hildinger M, O'Connor E, Maguire AM, Wilson JM, Bennett J. 2001. Exchange of surface proteins impacts on viral vector cellular specificity and transduction characteristics: The retina as a model. *Hum Mol Genet* **10:** 3075–3081.

Bainbridge JW, Smith AJ, Barker SS, Robbie S, Henderson R, Balaggan K, Viswanathan A, Holder GE, Stockman A, Tyler N, et al. 2008. Effect of gene therapy on visual function in Leber's congenital amaurosis. *N Engl J Med* **358:** 2231–2239.

Batten ML, Imanishi Y, Tu DC, Doan T, Zhu L, Pang J, Glushakova L, Moise AR, Baehr W, Van Gelder RN, et al. 2005. Pharmacological and rAAV gene therapy rescue of visual functions in a blind mouse model of Leber congenital amaurosis. *PLoS Med* **2:** e333.

Bemelmans AP, Kostic C, Crippa SV, Hauswirth WW, Lem J, Munier FL, Seeliger MW, Wenzel A, Arsenijevic Y. 2006. Lentiviral gene transfer of *Rpe65* rescues survival and function of cones in a mouse model of Leber congenital amaurosis. *PLoS Med* **3:** e347.

Binley K, Widdowson P, Loader J, Kelleher M, Iqball S, Ferrige G, de Belin J, Carlucci M, Angell-Manning D, Hurst F, et al. 2013. Transduction of photoreceptors with equine infectious anemia virus lentiviral vectors: Safety and biodistribution of StarGen for Stargardt disease. *Invest Ophthalmol Vis Sci* **54:** 4061–4071.

Cai X, Nash Z, Conley SM, Fliesler SJ, Cooper MJ, Naash MI. 2009. A partial structural and functional rescue of a retinitis pigmentosa model with compacted DNA nanoparticles. *PLoS ONE* **4:** e5290.

Cai X, Conley SM, Nash Z, Fliesler SJ, Cooper MJ, Naash MI. 2010. Gene delivery to mitotic and postmitotic photoreceptors via compacted DNA nanoparticles results in improved phenotype in a mouse model of retinitis pigmentosa. *FASEB J* **24:** 1178–1191.

Campochiaro PA. 2002. Gene therapy for retinal and choroidal diseases. *Expert Opin Biol Ther* **2:** 537–544.

Charbel Issa P, MacLaren RE. 2012. Non-viral retinal gene therapy: A review. *Clin Experiment Ophthalmol* **40:** 39–47.

Cideciyan AV, Hauswirth WW, Aleman TS, Kaushal S, Schwartz SB, Boye SL, Windsor EA, Conlon TJ, Sumaroka A, Roman AJ, et al. 2009. Vision 1 year after gene therapy for Leber's congenital amaurosis. *N Engl J Med* **361:** 725–727.

Colella P, Auricchio A. 2012. Gene therapy of inherited retinopathies: A long and successful road from viral vectors to patients. *Hum Gene Ther* **23:** 796–807.

Conley SM, Naash MI. 2010. Nanoparticles for retinal gene therapy. *Prog Retin Eye Res* **29:** 376–397.

Conley SM, Cai X, Makkia R, Wu Y, Sparrow JR, Naash MI. 2012. Increased cone sensitivity to ABCA4 deficiency provides insight into macular vision loss in Stargardt's dystrophy. *Biochim Biophys Acta* **1822:** 1169–1179.

Dejneka NS, Surace EM, Aleman TS, Cideciyan AV, Lyubarsky A, Savchenko A, Redmond TM, Tang W, Wei Z, Rex TS, et al. 2004. In utero gene therapy rescues vision in a murine model of congenital blindness. *Mol Ther* **9:** 182–188.

Ding XQ, Quiambao AB, Fitzgerald JB, Cooper MJ, Conley SM, Naash MI. 2009. Ocular delivery of compacted DNA-nanoparticles does not elicit toxicity in the mouse retina. *PLoS ONE* **4:** e7410.

Dong B, Nakai H, Xiao W. 2010. Characterization of genome integrity for oversized recombinant AAV vector. *Mol Ther* **18:** 87–92.

Duan D, Sharma P, Yang J, Yue Y, Dudus L, Zhang Y, Fisher KJ, Engelhardt JF. 1998. Circular intermediates of recombinant adeno-associated virus have defined structural characteristics responsible for long-term episomal persistence in muscle tissue. *J Virol* **72:** 8568–8577.

Duan D, Yue Y, Engelhardt JF. 2001. Expanding AAV packaging capacity with trans-splicing or overlapping vectors: A quantitative comparison. *Mol Ther* **4:** 383–391.

Farjo R, Skaggs J, Quiambao AB, Cooper MJ, Naash MI. 2006. Efficient non-viral ocular gene transfer with compacted DNA nanoparticles. *PLoS ONE* **1:** e38.

Fink TL, Klepcyk PJ, Oette SM, Gedeon CR, Hyatt SL, Kowalczyk TH, Moen RC, Cooper MJ. 2006. Plasmid size up to 20 kbp does not limit effective in vivo lung gene transfer using compacted DNA nanoparticles. *Gene Ther* **13:** 1048–1051.

Ghosh A, Yue Y, Lai Y, Duan D. 2008. A hybrid vector system expands adeno-associated viral vector packaging capacity in a transgene-independent manner. *Mol Ther* **16:** 124–130.

Ghosh A, Yue Y, Duan D. 2011. Efficient transgene reconstitution with hybrid dual AAV vectors carrying the minimized bridging sequences. *Hum Gene Ther* **22:** 77–83.

Gouze E, Pawliuk R, Gouze JN, Pilapil C, Fleet C, Palmer GD, Evans CH, Leboulch P, Ghivizzani SC. 2003. Lentiviral-mediated gene delivery to synovium: Potent intraarticular expression with amplification by inflammation. *Mol Ther* **7:** 460–466.

Grieger JC, Samulski RJ. 2005. Packaging capacity of adeno-associated virus serotypes: Impact of larger genomes on infectivity and postentry steps. *J Virol* **79:** 9933–9944.

Gruter O, Kostic C, Crippa SV, Perez MT, Zografos L, Schorderet DF, Munier FL, Arsenijevic Y. 2005. Lentiviral vector-mediated gene transfer in adult mouse photoreceptors is impaired by the presence of a physical barrier. *Gene Ther* **12:** 942–947.

Han Z, Conley SM, Makkia RS, Cooper MJ, Naash MI. 2012. DNA nanoparticle-mediated *ABCA4* delivery rescues Stargardt dystrophy in mice. *J Clin Invest* **122:** 3221–3226.

Hirsch ML, Agbandje-McKenna M, Samulski RJ. 2010. Little vector, big gene transduction: Fragmented genome reassembly of adeno-associated virus. *Mol Ther* **18:** 6–8.

Hirsch ML, Li C, Bellon I, Yin C, Chavala S, Pryadkina M, Richard I, Samulski RJ. 2013. Oversized AAV transductifon is mediated via a DNA-PKcs-independent, Rad51C-dependent repair pathway. *Mol Ther* **21:** 2205–2216.

Johnson CJ, Berglin L, Chrenek MA, Redmond TM, Boatright JH, Nickerson JM. 2008. Technical brief: Subretinal injection and electroporation into adult mouse eyes. *Mol Vis* **14:** 2211–2226.

Kachi S, Oshima Y, Esumi N, Kachi M, Rogers B, Zack DJ, Campochiaro PA. 2005. Nonviral ocular gene transfer. *Gene Ther* **12:** 843–851.

Kingsman SM. 2003. Lentivirus: A vector for nervous system applications. *Ernst Schering Res Found Workshop* **43:** 179–207.

Kohn DB, Sadelain M, Glorioso JC. 2003. Occurrence of leukaemia following gene therapy of X-linked SCID. *Nat Rev Cancer* **3:** 477–488.

Kong J, Kim SR, Binley K, Pata I, Doi K, Mannik J, Zernant-Rajang J, Kan O, Iqball S, Naylor S, et al. 2008. Correction of the disease phenotype in the mouse model of Stargardt disease by lentiviral gene therapy. *Gene Ther* **15:** 1311–1320.

Konstan MW, Davis PB, Wagener JS, Hilliard KA, Stern RC, Milgram LJ, Kowalczyk TH, Hyatt SL, Fink TL, Gedeon CR, et al. 2004. Compacted DNA nanoparticles administered to the nasal mucosa of cystic fibrosis subjects are safe and demonstrate partial to complete cystic fibrosis transmembrane regulator reconstitution. *Hum Gene Ther* **15:** 1255–1269.

Kostic C, Chiodini F, Salmon P, Wiznerowicz M, Deglon N, Hornfeld D, Trono D, Aebischer P, Schorderet DF, Munier FL, et al. 2003. Activity analysis of housekeeping promoters using self-inactivating lentiviral vector delivery into the mouse retina. *Gene Ther* **10:** 818–821.

Kumar-Singh R. 2008. Barriers for retinal gene therapy: Separating fact from fiction. *Vision Res* **48:** 1671–1680.

Lai Y, Yue Y, Duan D. 2010. Evidence for the failure of adeno-associated virus serotype 5 to package a viral genome≥8.2 kb. *Mol Ther* **18:** 75–79.

Lamartina S, Cimino M, Roscilli G, Dammassa E, Lazzaro D, Rota R, Ciliberto G, Toniatti C. 2007. Helper-dependent adenovirus for the gene therapy of proliferative retinopathies: Stable gene transfer, regulated gene expression and therapeutic efficacy. *J Gene Med* **9:** 862–874.

Le Meur G, Stieger K, Smith AJ, Weber M, Deschamps JY, Nivard D, Mendes-Madeira A, Provost N, Pereon Y, Cherel Y, et al. 2007. Restoration of vision in RPE65-deficient Briard dogs using an AAV serotype 4 vector that specifically targets the retinal pigmented epithelium. *Gene Ther* **14:** 292–303.

Liang FQ, Anand V, Maguire AM, Bennett J. 2000. *Intraocular delivery of recombinant virus.* Humana, Totowa, NJ.

Lipinski DM, Thake M, MacLaren RE. 2013. Clinical applications of retinal gene therapy. *Prog Retin Eye Res* **32:** 22–47.

Liu G, Li D, Pasumarthy MK, Kowalczyk TH, Gedeon CR, Hyatt SL, Payne JM, Miller TJ, Brunovskis P, Fink TL, et al. 2003. Nanoparticles of compacted DNA transfect postmitotic cells. *J Biol Chem* **278:** 32578–32586.

Lois C, Hong EJ, Pease S, Brown EJ, Baltimore D. 2002. Germline transmission and tissue-specific expression of transgenes delivered by lentiviral vectors. *Science* **295:** 868–872.

Lotery AJ, Derksen TA, Russell SR, Mullins RF, Sauter S, Affatigato LM, Stone EM, Davidson BL. 2002. Gene transfer to the nonhuman primate retina with recombinant feline immunodeficiency virus vectors. *Hum Gene Ther* **13:** 689–696.

Lotery AJ, Yang GS, Mullins RF, Russell SR, Schmidt M, Stone EM, Lindbloom JD, Chiorini JA, Kotin RM, Davidson BL. 2003. Adeno-associated virus type 5: Transduction efficiency and cell-type specificity in the primate retina. *Hum Gene Ther* **14:** 1663–1671.

Maguire AM, Simonelli F, Pierce EA, Pugh EN Jr, Mingozzi F, Bennicelli J, Banfi S, Marshall KA, Testa F, Surace EM, et al. 2008. Safety and efficacy of gene transfer for Leber's congenital amaurosis. *N Engl J Med* **358:** 2240–2248.

Maguire AM, High KA, Auricchio A, Wright JF, Pierce EA, Testa F, Mingozzi F, Bennicelli JL, Ying GS, Rossi S, et al. 2009. Age-dependent effects of *RPE65* gene therapy for Leber's congenital amaurosis: A phase 1 dose-escalation trial. *Lancet* **374:** 1597–1605.

Maiti P, Kong J, Kim SR, Sparrow JR, Allikmets R, Rando RR. 2006. Small molecule RPE65 antagonists limit the visual cycle and prevent lipofuscin formation. *Biochemistry* **45:** 852–860.

Mata NL, Tzekov RT, Liu X, Weng J, Birch DG, Travis GH. 2001. Delayed dark-adaptation and lipofuscin accumulation in abcr+/− mice: Implications for involvement of *ABCR* in age-related macular degeneration. *Invest Ophthalmol Vis Sci* **42:** 1685–1690.

Maury W. 1998. Regulation of equine infectious anemia virus expression. *J Biomed Sci* **5:** 11–23.

Miyoshi H, Takahashi M, Gage FH, Verma IM. 1997. Stable and efficient gene transfer into the retina using an HIV-based lentiviral vector. *Proc Natl Acad Sci* **94:** 10319–10323.

Molday RS, Zhang K. 2010. Defective lipid transport and biosynthesis in recessive and dominant Stargardt macular degeneration. *Prog Lipid Res* **49:** 476–492.

Mussolino C, della Corte M, Rossi S, Viola F, Di Vicino U, Marrocco E, Neglia S, Doria M, Testa F, Giovannoni R, et al. 2011. AAV-mediated photoreceptor transduction of the pig cone-enriched retina. *Gene Ther* **18:** 637–645.

Narfstrom K, Katz ML, Bragadottir R, Seeliger M, Boulanger A, Redmond TM, Caro L, Lai CM, Rakoczy PE. 2003. Functional and structural recovery of the retina after gene therapy in the RPE65 null mutation dog. *Invest Ophthalmol Vis Sci* **44:** 1663–1672.

Olsen JC. 2001. EIAV, CAEV and other lentivirus vector systems. *Somat Cell Mol Genet* **26:** 131–145.

Radu RA, Yuan Q, Hu J, Peng JH, Lloyd M, Nusinowitz S, Bok D, Travis GH. 2008. Accelerated accumulation of lipofuscin pigments in the RPE of a mouse model for *ABCA4*-mediated retinal dystrophies following Vitamin A supplementation. *Invest Ophthalmol Vis Sci* **49:** 3821–3829.

Simonelli F, Maguire AM, Testa F, Pierce EA, Mingozzi F, Bennicelli JL, Rossi S, Marshall K, Banfi S, Surace EM, et al. 2010. Gene therapy for Leber's congenital amaurosis is safe and effective through 1.5 years after vector administration. *Mol Ther* **18:** 643–650.

Souied EH, Reid SN, Piri NI, Lerner LE, Nusinowitz S, Farber DB. 2008. Non-invasive gene transfer by iontophoresis for therapy of an inherited retinal degeneration. *Exp Eye Res* **87:** 168–175.

Stieger K, Colle MA, Dubreil L, Mendes-Madeira A, Weber M, Le Meur G, Deschamps JY, Provost N, Nivard D, Cherel Y, et al. 2008. Subretinal delivery of recombinant AAV serotype 8 vector in dogs results in gene transfer to neurons in the brain. *Mol Ther* **16:** 916–923.

Stieger K, Chauveau C, Rolling F. 2010. Preclinical studies on specific gene therapy for recessive retinal degenerative diseases. *Curr Gene Ther* **10:** 389–403.

Surace EM, Auricchio A. 2008. Versatility of AAV vectors for retinal gene transfer. *Vision Res* **48:** 353–359.

Takahashi M, Miyoshi H, Verma IM, Gage FH. 1999. Rescue from photoreceptor degeneration in the rd mouse by human immunodeficiency virus vector-mediated gene transfer. *J Virol* **73:** 7812–7816.

Trapani I, Colella P, Sommella A, Iodice C, Cesi G, De Simone S, Marrocco E, Rossi S, Giunti M, Palfi A, et al. 2014. Effective delivery of large genes to the retina by dual AAV vectors. *EMBO Mol Med* **6:** 194–211.

Vandenberghe LH, Auricchio A. 2012. Novel adeno-associated viral vectors for retinal gene therapy. *Gene Ther* **19:** 162–168.

Vandenberghe LH, Bell P, Maguire AM, Cearley CN, Xiao R, Calcedo R, Wang L, Castle MJ, Maguire AC, Grant R, et al. 2011. Dosage thresholds for AAV2 and AAV8 photoreceptor gene therapy in monkey. *Sci Transl Med* **3:** 88ra54.

Wanisch K, Yanez-Munoz RJ. 2009. Integration-deficient lentiviral vectors: A slow coming of age. *Mol Ther* **17:** 1316–1332.

Weng J, Mata NL, Azarian SM, Tzekov RT, Birch DG, Travis GH. 1999. Insights into the function of Rim protein in photoreceptors and etiology of Stargardt's disease from the phenotype in *abcr* knockout mice. *Cell* **98:** 13–23.

Williams ML, Coleman JE, Haire SE, Aleman TS, Cideciyan AV, Sokal I, Palczewski K, Jacobson SG, Semple-Rowland SL. 2006. Lentiviral expression of retinal guanylate cyclase-1 (RetGC1) restores vision in an avian model of childhood blindness. *PLoS Med* **3:** e201.

Wu L, Nagasaki T, Sparrow JR. 2010a. Photoreceptor cell degeneration in *Abcr* $^{-/-}$ mice. *Adv Exp Med Biol* **664:** 533–539.

Wu Z, Yang H, Colosi P. 2010b. Effect of genome size on AAV vector packaging. *Mol Ther* **18:** 80–86.

Yan Z, Zhang Y, Duan D, Engelhardt JF. 2000. Trans-splicing vectors expand the utility of adeno-associated virus for gene therapy. *Proc Natl Acad Sci* **97:** 6716–6721.

Yanez-Munoz RJ, Balaggan KS, MacNeil A, Howe SJ, Schmidt M, Smith AJ, Buch P, MacLaren RE, Anderson PN, Barker SE, et al. 2006. Effective gene therapy with nonintegrating lentiviral vectors. *Nat Med* **12:** 348–353.

Gene Therapy for the Retinal Degeneration of Usher Syndrome Caused by Mutations in *MYO7A*

Vanda S. Lopes and David S. Williams

Stein Eye Institute, University of California at Los Angeles, Los Angeles, California 90095-7000

Correspondence: dswilliams@ucla.edu

Usher syndrome is a deaf-blindness disorder. One of the subtypes, Usher 1B, is caused by loss of function of the gene encoding the unconventional myosin, MYO7A. A variety of different viral-based delivery approaches have been tested for retinal gene therapy to prevent the blindness of Usher 1B, and a clinical trial based on one of these approaches has begun. This review evaluates the different approaches.

Usher syndrome is mainly a recessive genetic disorder characterized by deafness and progressive retinal degeneration. It has been divided into types 1–3, according to the severity and time course of the hearing impairment. Further subdivision has been based on genetic linkage (Williams 2008). Usher 1B, the most prevalent form of Usher type 1, is caused by mutations in the gene encoding the unconventional molecular motor, MYO7A. Its recessive inheritance suggests that Usher 1B results from loss of protein function. Mutations have been found along the entire gene, some of which are predicted to be effective null mutations (Jacobson et al. 2011).

The loss of both hearing and vision makes Usher syndrome a particularly disabling disorder. Nowadays, the hearing deficiency can be addressed with the aid of cochlear implants, but the visual impairment has no treatment. In most cases, the deafness is congenital; Usher 1 patients are born profoundly deaf. Usher patients are therefore readily identified when infants, before onset of retinal degeneration, making them particularly good candidates for gene replacement therapy. The introduction of cDNA encoding functional MYO7A, before there is any retinal damage, should result in efficacious prevention. A phase 1 clinical trial has been approved by the Food and Drug Administration (FDA) and has been under way in the U.S. since 2012, and a second trial has been approved in France.

This review gives a historical account of preclinical work leading up to the clinical trials, and discusses some still unanswered questions, as well as the strengths and weaknesses of different viral-based strategies.

MUTANT *MYO7A*: MOUSE MODEL AND MUTANT PHENOTYPES

Mice carrying mutations in *Myo7a*, the Usher 1B ortholog, are known as shaker1. They were

Cite this article as *Cold Spring Harb Perspect Med* doi: 10.1101/cshperspect.a017319

identified readily by mouse geneticists, because of their head tossing, hyperactivity, and circling behavior, which result from cochlear and vestibular dysfunction (Gibson et al. 1995). Spontaneous or N-ethyl-N-nitrosourea (ENU)-induced mutations have now resulted in approximately 10 different alleles of shaker1 (Mburu et al. 1997). None of the alleles presents retinal degeneration under normal light conditions, a common feature among most of the Usher 1 mouse models (Williams 2008). However, the identification of mutant phenotypes in the retina has provided relatively robust assays by which to test the introduction of functional MYO7A protein. Hence, the shaker1 mouse represents a useful diagnostic tool for testing the efficacy of retinal gene therapy in vivo. Most of such studies have used the *Myo7a*$^{sh1\text{-}4626SB}$ allele, which possesses a premature stop codon that results in no detectable protein.

In the retina, MYO7A has been detected in the retinal pigment epithelium (RPE) and the photoreceptor cells. The majority of the protein is found in the RPE, where it localizes in the apical region (Hasson et al. 1995; Liu et al. 1997). In the photoreceptors, MYO7A is localized to the connecting cilium and periciliary region (Liu et al. 1997; Williams 2008); recently, it has also been reported to be present in the calycal processes of monkey and frog photoreceptors (Fig. 1) (Sahly et al. 2012).

MYO7A has been shown to be a functional actin-based motor (Udovichenko et al. 2002). Mutant phenotypes in shaker1 retinas are consistent with its role as a molecular motor. The most obvious defect, and one that has proved to be the most useful in studies testing the efficacy of gene therapy, is the absence of melanosomes from the apical RPE (Fig. 1) (Liu et al. 1998). MYO7A associates with melanosomes via two linker proteins, MYRIP and RAB27A. Without MYO7A (or either of the linker proteins), the melanosomes are unable to move along actin filaments, and are thus absent from the apical RPE (Futter et al. 2004; Gibbs et al. 2004; Klomp et al. 2007; Lopes et al. 2007). The consequences of mislocalized melanosomes are not clear, but it has been suggested that they move more apically at the time of light onset, and perhaps facilitate phagosome ingestion and degradation (Futter et al. 2004). Melanosomes may also serve as a sink for damaging reactive species resulting from processes like lipid peroxidation (Schraermeyer 1999). The knockdown of MYO7A in human RPE cells has the same effect on melanosome motility as that found in shaker1 RPE cells (Gibbs et al. 2010).

MYO7A also associates with RPE phagosomes and contributes to their motility, with lack of MYO7A resulting in slowed degradation of these organelles (Gibbs et al. 2003; VS Lopes and DS Williams, unpubl.). More recently, MYO7A has been implicated in the light-dependent translocation of the retinoid isomerase, RPE65. Shaker1 retinas have a lower amount of RPE65, which is likely responsible for an observed protection from acute light damage (Lopes et al. 2011).

In shaker1 photoreceptors, detailed analysis by immunoelectron microscopy has shown that the ciliary plasma membrane has an abnormal accumulation of rhodopsin (Liu et al. 1999), suggesting a role for MYO7A in facilitating opsin delivery to the disk membranes of the photoreceptor outer segment.

Electrophysiological studies of shaker1 mice indicated a slightly reduced a- and b-wave response (Libby and Steel 2001). More recently, in studying shaker1 mice on an albino background, a more significant electroretinogram (ERG) abnormality was observed, with a b-wave reduction of 20% at 6 mo, and ~27% at 12 mo of age. This change is accompanied by a progressive increase in the threshold of rod sensitivity to light, reaching 67% by 12 mo, and a delay in rod recovery after desensitization (Colella et al. 2013).

MYO7A has now been implicated in the translocation of transducin from the outer to the inner segment in response to light (Peng et al. 2011). In shaker1 mice, transducin translocation is impaired because of a shift in the activation threshold toward higher light intensities (Peng et al. 2011). Although this response is promising as read-out for MYO7A function in photoreceptors, it should be noted that, unlike the above mutant phenotypes, it has only been observed in one allele of shaker1 mice,

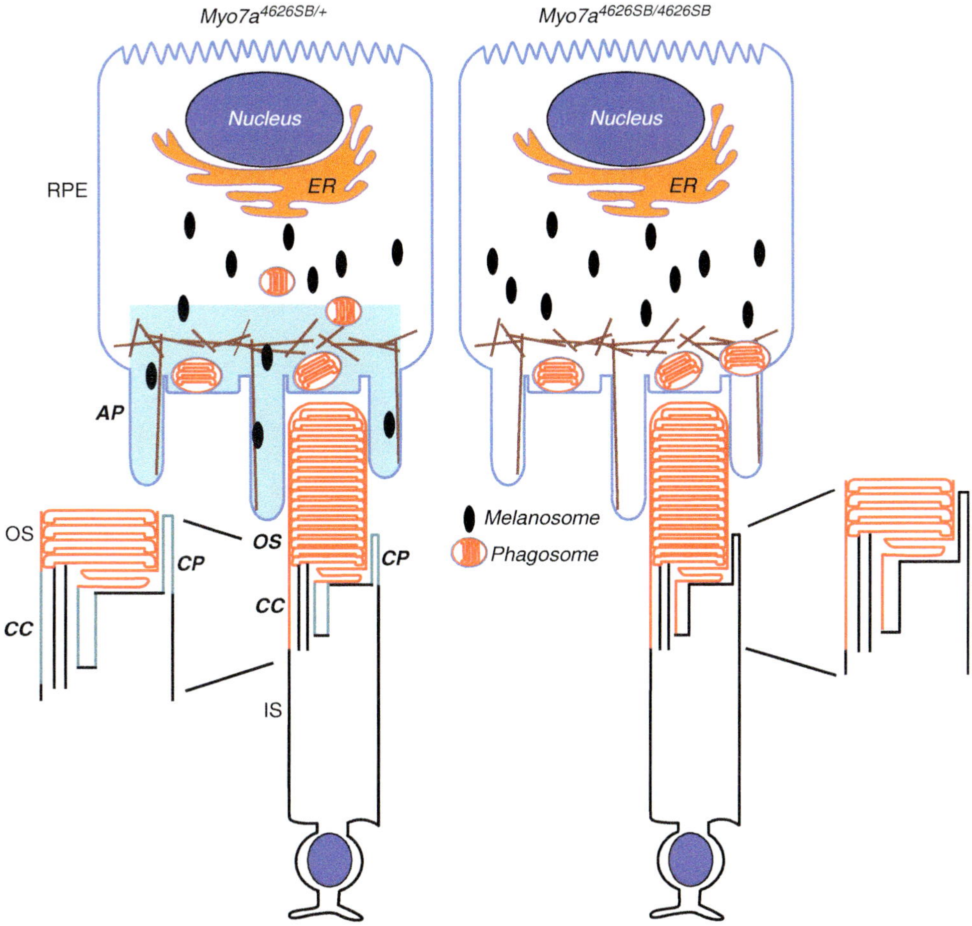

Figure 1. Diagram of MYO7A localization in the retina, and retinal mutant phenotypes identified in *Myo7a*$^{sh1\text{-}4626SB}$ mice. MYO7A (blue) has been found in the apical region of the RPE, and in the connecting cilium, periciliary membrane, and calycal processes of the photoreceptors. In the mutant RPE, phagosomes accumulate in the apical processes, whereas melanosomes are found only in the cell body. An abnormal accumulation of opsin (red) is present in the connecting cilium of mutant photoreceptors. RPE, retinal pigment epithelial cell; AP, RPE apical processes; OS, outer segment; IS, inner segment; CC, connecting cilium; CP, calycal processes.

Myo7a$^{sh1\text{-}11J}$. The specific mutation underlying this allele, and the effect that the mutation has on protein structure and levels are not known, except that mutant MYO7A protein is detectable (Zallocchi et al. 2014). The same investigators have identified an increased susceptibility to light-induced photoreceptor degeneration in *Myo7a*$^{sh1\text{-}11J}$ mice (Peng et al. 2011), which is the converse finding to that mentioned above for the null shaker1 allele, *Myo7a*$^{sh1\text{-}4626SB}$ (Lopes et al. 2011).

The above mutant phenotypes provide assays to test therapeutic efficacy in shaker1 mice. In particular, for gene therapy, mutant phenotype correction tests the presence of a fully functional MYO7A protein. The absence of retinal degeneration in this animal model is actually beneficial for such studies, because measurements can be made without concern of interference from secondary effects of cell death events. The use of a differential response to high light exposure should clearly not be used until the conflicting findings on the response are resolved.

GENE THERAPY WITH LENTIVIRUSES

As discussed later, adeno-associated viruses (AAV) have been widely used for viral delivery in gene therapy; however, the size of a gene that can be encapsulated into AAV has been reported to be limited to ~5 kb (Grieger and Samulski 2005). *MYO7A*, is a large gene of ~100 Mb and a cDNA of nearly 7 kb, so that an alternative strategy was sought for its delivery. Among the available viral gene delivery options, lentiviruses have a cargo capacity of ~10 kb and can infect postmitotic cells. Genes delivered by lentiviruses are integrated into the host genome, which typically assures long-lived gene expression, although poses a risk of insertional mutagenesis.

Human Immunodeficiency Virus (HIV)

In the late 1990s, third generation HIV-derived lentiviruses were shown to possess a number of important biosafety features (Verma and Weitzman 2005) and be effective for transduction of rodent RPE and photoreceptors (Miyoshi et al. 1997; Takahashi et al. 1999). The first gene therapy studies with *MYO7A* used the same third generation, self-inactivating, and HIV-derived lentiviral vectors (Hashimoto et al. 2007). Expression was driven by either cytomegalovirus (CMV) or a chimeric promoter, composed of CMV and 160 bp located upstream of the ATG signal in the *MYO7A* gene. Mutant phenotypes in the RPE, both in primary cell culture and in vivo, following subretinal injection, were corrected, showing the ability of HIV-derived lentiviruses to encapsulate *MYO7A* cDNA and effect expression of functional protein in infected cells. Correction of opsin distribution in the connecting cilia of shaker1 mice was also observed (Hashimoto et al. 2007).

Although this study showed successful transduction and expression of MYO7A in the targeted cells, it also highlighted the importance of the level of protein expression. With the chimeric promoter, the expression level of MYO7A in vivo was observed to vary among different RPE cells, resulting in a mosaic pattern of rescue of melanosome localization. First, the cell-to-cell variation in expression indicates a limitation with an integrating virus, because it is likely a result of variation in the number and site(s) of integration into the host genome. Second, it stresses the importance of sufficiently high expression to achieve rescue. This latter point needs to be balanced with a serious problem from overexpression. With the full CMV promoter, RPE cell death was observed in relation to high levels of expression of MYO7A, especially in primary cell culture (Hashimoto et al. 2007).

Photoreceptor cells have been reported to be transduced inefficiently by lentiviruses. It is thought that, especially in mouse retinas, where the photoreceptor cells are packed very densely, a relatively large virus has limited access to the photoreceptor cells (Gruter et al. 2005). This restriction is more of a problem for genes that are normally expressed at a higher level in photoreceptors than *MYO7A*. Indeed, it might provide some compensation for the abnormal regulation of *MYO7A* expression effected by ubiquitous promoters, because the normal expression level of *MYO7A* in photoreceptor cells is so much less than that in the RPE cells.

Equine Infectious Anemia Virus (EIAV)

Equine infectious anemia virus (EIAV) lentiviruses have been used for gene therapy of several cell types. Studies with the *ABCA4* gene, which is mutated in recessive Stargardt's macular degeneration, have shown that EIAV is able to encapsulate a large gene and transduce photoreceptors cells (Kong et al. 2008). More recent studies with EIAV delivery of *MYO7A* cDNA, under the control of a CMV promoter, have been performed with *Myo7a*$^{sh1\text{-}11J}$ mice and Rhesus monkeys (Zallocchi et al. 2014). These studies have formed preclinical support for the clinical trials underway, using the same viral delivery approach.

Delivery of the viral vector to the subretinal space led to expression of human MYO7A in the RPE and photoreceptor cells, as shown by immunofluorescence microscopy. Because *Myo7a*$^{sh1-11J}$ mice express significant levels of mutant MYO7A, and the monkeys were wild-type (WT), EIAV-*CMV-MYO7A* expression was detected by diluting MYO7A antibodies so that endogenous MYO7A could not be detected. Thus, the viral *MYO7A* expression appears to be much greater than WT levels. Moreover, MYO7A was detected in the photoreceptor outer segments, which is an abnormal localization. Given the findings of cell death resulting from overexpression of MYO7A driven by HIV-*CMV-MYO7A* (Hashimoto et al. 2007), this expression level is a concern. In photoreceptors, WT MYO7A is only present in the connecting cilium region and is usually barely detectable by epifluorescence immunomicroscopy (Liu et al. 1997).

Functional rescue was tested by studying transducin translocation profiles, which show some restoration in *Myo7a*$^{sh1-11J}$ photoreceptors. However, the majority of transducin is still retained in the outer segment, indicating incomplete rescue, even with the presumably high levels of WT MYO7A. Experiments were also performed to test for the effect of EIAV-*CMV-MYO7A* on susceptibility to light-induced degeneration. However, there was no difference between mice injected with EIAV-*CMV-MYO7A* and mice injected with saline, after maintenance under a daily cycle of 12 h 1500 lux/12 h dark for 3 mo. This result suggests that the viral vector alone may have some retinal toxicity, as the investigators themselves note. Biodistribution and toxicity studies showed that the EIAV-*CMV-MYO7A* is tolerated well in monkeys over a period of 3 mo, and that a single subretinal dose does not spread into the body, although it can raise a moderate local inflammatory response (Zallocchi et al. 2014).

In conclusion, studies show that both HIV and EIAV can be used to deliver *MYO7A* to RPE and photoreceptor cells. Both lentiviral approaches also appear to be capable of rescuing mutant phenotypes, although it is unfortunate that EIAV-*CMV-MYO7A*, which is being used in clinical trials, has not been tested for correction of phenotypes that have been identified in more than one laboratory, and with a characterized shaker1 null allele. A comparison of the two lentiviruses in vitro indicated that transgene expression was similar, but that expression derived from EIAV was more likely to be reduced over time because of instability of the RNA-transcripts (O'Rourke et al. 2002).

GENE THERAPY WITH ADENO-ASSOCIATED VIRUSES

AAV has been the most extensively studied viral tool for retinal gene therapy. These viruses can target postmitotic cells efficiently. They remain episomal, thus avoiding the insertional mutagenesis risks of lentiviruses, but still result in prolonged expression. The first retinal gene therapy approach was for treatment of Leber's congenital amaurosis (LCA2), which is caused by mutations in *RPE65*. In these studies, AAV was used to deliver normal *RPE65* cDNA to the RPE cells, and the safety and efficacy of this treatment has now been shown independently in various clinical trials (Bainbridge et al. 2008; Cideciyan et al. 2008, 2009; Hauswirth et al. 2008; Maguire et al. 2008; Jacobson et al. 2012; Testa et al. 2013). However, as noted above, its limited cargo capacity has been seen as an impediment in retinal degenerations requiring the delivery of large genes (Grieger and Samulski 2005).

AAV Single Vectors

A study by Alloca et al. (2008) indicated the potential of AAV vectors to deliver genes that are >5 kb, like *MYO7A* and *ABCA4*, to retinal cells. Although the mechanism by which such oversized AAV transduction occurs is unknown, studies on the encapsulation of large genes by AAV has shown that the vectors contain a heterogeneous population of truncated genomes that are mostly <5 kb (Dong et al. 2010; Lai et al. 2010; Wu et al. 2011). Hence, the gene is fragmented, and for functional delivery must be reconstituted by homologous recombination inside a cell (Dong et al. 2010).

Studies on the ability of oversized AAV vectors to generate MYO7A in HEK293 cells (Colella et al. 2013) and RPE primary cultures derived from *Myo7a*$^{sh1\text{-}4626SB}$ mice (Lopes et al. 2013) showed that they can indeed produce full length protein, with no major evidence of truncated products. In the RPE cultures from *Myo7a*$^{sh1\text{-}4626SB}$ mice, the expression level of MYO7A was comparable to that in cultures from heterozygous control littermates. Moreover, following injection into the subretinal space of *Myo7a*$^{sh1\text{-}4626SB}$ mice, MYO7A could be detected at WT levels in the RPE and photoreceptor cells, and at higher levels with more concentrated virus (Lopes et al. 2013). Western blot analysis of posterior eye segments, after subretinal injection, showed that expression persists for at least 15 mo (Colella et al. 2013). Two separate studies have shown that mutant retinal phenotypes of *Myo7a*$^{sh1\text{-}4626SB}$ mice could be rescued both in the RPE and photoreceptors. In a detailed study with two different serotypes, AAV2 and AAV5, melanosomes were observed in the RPE apical processes, similar to WT control mice, and the distribution of opsin in the connecting cilia of the photoreceptors was restored to normal, indicating functional protein was made in both cell types (Lopes et al. 2013). These observations were reproduced in a study, using AAV5, which showed, in addition, that the rod light desensitization threshold could be restored to normal levels (Colella et al. 2013).

AAV Dual Vectors

The major concern with oversized AAV vectors for clinical use is the apparent randomness in the resulting sizes of genomes delivered to the cells. A strategy to overcome this problem is to divide a gene or cDNA, such as *MYO7A*, into two pieces and have each piece contained within a separate AAV vector. Once inside the cells, concatemerization and homologous recombination of the two pieces will lead to the formation of full-length mRNA and protein. As described by Trapani et al. (2014), strategies include: (1) trans-splicing, where a splice donor site is introduced at the 3′ end of the first half of the gene, and an acceptor donor site is introduced at the 5′ end of the second half, resulting in full length mRNA by head to tail concatemerization of the two halves; (2) overlapping halves, where homologous overlapping sequences are introduced in similar positions as those for the trans-splice sites, and will lead to homologous recombination of the two parts in cells; and (3) hybrid alternative, where a known exogenous recombinogenic region, such as alkaline phosphatase (AP), is added to the trans-splicing vectors.

Our group has initially compared oversized single AAV2 and AAV5 vectors with an overlapping AAV2 dual vector. In primary cultures of RPE cells, we found that the oversized vector outperformed the dual system, in terms of both the average level of MYO7A protein made and the consistency of protein expression among the cells. A significant concern with the dual vector system was that, while most cells had negligible levels of MYO7A, a few cells had very high levels, and had clearly become abnormal (Lopes et al. 2013). Following subretinal injections of *Myo7a*$^{sh1\text{-}4626SB}$ mice, the overlapping dual vector was much less effective at correcting mutant phenotypes (Lopes et al. 2013). Since this study, additional reports have compared the different dual AAV vector approaches for *MYO7A* cDNA delivery.

In a study conducted by Trapani et al. (2014), the highest expression level was obtained with an AAV hybrid vector (AK), using a sequence from the F1 phage genome as the recombinogenic region. Interestingly, all AAV2 dual approaches, except the use of an AP recombinogenic hybrid, resulted in higher levels of MYO7A expression in HEK293 cells compared with the oversized single AAV2 vector, but a comparison with retinal cells was not made. Importantly, Trapani et al. (2014) found that the levels of protein expression were more variable when using the dual vectors. Consistent with the findings of Lopes et al. (2013), treatment of *Myo7a*$^{sh1\text{-}4626SB}$ mice with AAV dual vectors resulted in only a mosaic effect of RPE cells with corrected melanosome localization (Trapani et al. 2014). Still, the overlapping strategy was more efficacious in the RPE, than in photoreceptors, which may be related to the low homologous recombination that occurs in the postmitotic neurons (Fishel et al. 2007).

Western blot analysis of posterior eye segments from treated *Myo7a*$^{sh1\text{-}4626SB}$ mice showed that the trans-splicing and AK hybrid AAV dual vectors resulted in only ~20% of the MYO7A level found in heterozygous littermates, and correction of a photoreceptor phenotype could not be determined (Trapani et al. 2014).

In another study, Dyka et al. (2014) reported slightly different outcomes. In addition to the methods attempted by Trapani et al. (2014), this group tested a construct in which intronic splice sites from the native *MYO7A* gene were included. However, this additional approach resulted in very low levels of MYO7A expression. Dyka et al. found that an AP hybrid AAV vector gave the highest expression level of MYO7A, but it also generated a mix of correct and mutant sequences, which were not detected in the other approaches. When injected into WT mice, this vector resulted in abnormal levels of MYO7A in the photoreceptors, and retinal degeneration. The best performing in vivo system in this group's hands seemed to be the overlapping approach. Despite the promising results with overlapping AAV8 dual vectors, no study was conducted with shaker1 mice, so that the functionality of the protein could not be made. In addition, representative images shown by the investigators raise concerns about the distribution and levels of MYO7A produced, as strong signal is evident throughout the inner segment and outer segments (Dyka et al. 2014).

Therefore, so far, dual AAV vector approaches remain problematic. A major emphasis has been on achieving a high expression level of MYO7A. However, a fundamental problem appears to be the variation in expression level among retinal cells. To achieve sufficient expression in most cells, some cells will express at such high levels as to be toxic. A further problem is the expression of partial MYO7A protein. Published western blots indicate the additional presence of a lower mass polypeptide, and studies with fluorescent reporters (GFP and RFP) indicated that the fraction of cells cotransduced is actually less than half (Trapani et al. 2014). Ironically, the presence of partial MYO7A polypeptides has been the concern for the oversized single AAV vector approach, and a justification for testing dual AAV vectors. Yet, at least in RPE cells, transduced with single AAV2 or AAV5, carrying *MYO7A*, only full-length MYO7A was detected (Lopes et al. 2013).

WHICH ISOFORM OF *MYO7A*?

The use of a cDNA in gene therapy defines the single isoform of the gene that will be expressed. Yet, like many genes, the *MYO7A* gene is alter-

Table 1. Comparison of different strategies for viral delivery of *MYO7A* in Usher 1B retinal gene therapy

	Lentivirus		Adeno-associated virus			
	HIV-based	EIAV-based	AAV2 AAV5	AAV2 AAV8	AAV8	AAV8
Myo7a cDNA encapsulation	Single	Single	Single[a]	Dual overlapping	Dual trans-splicing	Dual hybrid
Genome integration	Yes	Yes	No	No	No	No
Retinal cell layer targeted	RPE mainly	RPE PR	RPE PR	RPE PR	RPE PR	RPE PR
Phenotype correction mouse						
RPE	Mosaic[b]	Unknown	Yes[c,d]	Mosaic[c,e]	Mosaic[e]	Mosaic[e]
PR	Yes[b]	Yes[f]	Yes[c,d]	Yes[c,e]	Unknown	Unknown

[a]Although not shown specifically for *MYO7A*, large genes are fragmented to be accommodated by AAV.
[b]Hashimoto et al. (2007), mosaic effect in RPE maybe because of variable expression levels from variable gene integration.
[c]Lopes et al. (2013).
[d]Colella et al. (2013).
[e]Trapani et al. (2014).
[f]Zallocchi et al. (2014).

natively spliced. Two closely related, long isoforms of *MYO7A*, isoforms 1 and 2, have been reported to be expressed in the retina (Weil et al. 1996). They differ by the expression of a 114-bp region in the 5′ end of exon 34. The resulting 38 amino acids in isoform 1 are located in the FERM1 domain, and may impact interaction with another Usher 1 protein, SANS (Adato et al. 2005; Wu et al. 2011). It may also affect overall protein structure and stability. Presently, no discrimination has been made in the use of isoform 1 or 2 for gene therapy trials, despite the lack of evidence toward a majority use of one or the other by retinal cells. Studies by our group and Dyka et al. (2014) have focused on isoform 2, while studies from Auricchio's group (Colella et al. 2013; Trapani et al. 2014) have used isoform 1. Thus, by accident, it appears that either isoform might do. However, it would seem that more definitive studies should be performed to determine which cDNA might be better for future clinical trials.

CONCLUDING REMARKS

A variety of viral-based delivery approaches have been tested for Usher 1B retinal gene therapy (summarized in Table 1), and most have been shown to be efficacious. Each has its advantages and disadvantages. The large size of the *MYO7A* cDNA prompted the use of lentiviruses, but integration of the gene poses a risk of insertional mutagenesis and has been shown to result in cell-to-cell variation in expression level. Clinical trials have been started with EIAV-*CMV-MYO7A*, but the preclinical studies to test efficacy have been very limited. Recent studies on the use of AAV for the delivery of *MYO7A* have been encouraging; especially because of the relatively established success of AAV in gene therapy for inherited retinal diseases such as LCA2. AAV remains episomal, thus avoiding the insertional mutagenesis risks of lentiviruses. However, the fragmentation that occurs with single AAV vectors, and the variable expression levels found with dual AAV vectors are drawbacks. One alternative that may prove to be optimal for large genes like *MYO7A* is the use of non-integrating lentiviruses; integrase-deficient vectors that can transduce retinal cells are able to persist as episomal DNA (Yáñez-Muñoz et al. 2006). However, such studies have yet to be reported.

ACKNOWLEDGMENTS

D.S.W. is supported by grants from the National Eye Institute and a Jules and Doris Stein Professorship from the Research to Prevent Blindness.

REFERENCES

Adato A, Michel V, Kikkawa Y, Reiners J, Alagramam KN, Weil D, Yonekawa H, Wolfrum U, El-Amraoui A, Petit C. 2005. Interactions in the network of Usher syndrome type 1 proteins. *Hum Mol Genet* **14:** 347–356.

Allocca M, Doria M, Petrillo M, Colella P, Garcia-Hoyos M, Gibbs D, Kim SR, Maguire A, Rex TS, Di Vicino U, et al. 2008. Serotype-dependent packaging of large genes in adeno-associated viral vectors results in effective gene delivery in mice. *J Clin Invest* **118:** 1955–1964.

Bainbridge J, Smith A, Barker S, Robbie S, Henderson R, Balaggan K, Viswanathan A, Holder GE, Stockman A, Tyler N, et al. 2008. Effect of gene therapy on visual function in Leber's congenital amaurosis. *N Engl J Med* **358:** 2231–2239.

Cideciyan A, Aleman T, Boye S, Schwartz S, Kaushal S, Roman A, Pang JJ, Sumaroka A, Windsor EA, Wilson JM, et al. 2008. Human gene therapy for RPE65 isomerase deficiency activates the retinoid cycle of vision but with slow rod kinetics. *Proc Natl Acad Sci* **105:** 15112–15117.

Cideciyan AV, Hauswirth WW, Aleman TS, Kaushal S, Schwartz SB, Boye SL, Windsor EA, Conlon TJ, Sumaroka A, Pang JJ, et al. 2009. Human RPE65 gene therapy for Leber congenital amaurosis: Persistence of early visual improvements and safety at 1 year. *Hum Gene Ther* **20:** 999–1004.

Colella P, Sommella A, Marrocco E, Di Vicino U, Polishchuk E, Garrido MG, Seeliger MW, Polishchuk R, Auricchio A. 2013. Myosin7a deficiency results in reduced retinal activity which is improved by gene therapy. *PLoS ONE* **8:** e72027.

Dong B, Nakai H, Xiao W. 2010. Characterization of genome integrity for oversized recombinant AAV vector. *Mol Ther* **18:** 87–92.

Dyka FM, Boye SL, Chiodo VA, Hauswirth WW, Boye SE. 2014. Dual adeno-associated virus vectors result in efficient in vitro and in vivo expression of an oversized gene, *MYO7A*. *Hum Gene Ther Methods* **25:** 166–177.

Fishel ML, Vasko MR, Kelley MR. 2007. DNA repair in neurons: So if they don't divide what's to repair? *Mutat Res* **614:** 24–36.

Futter CE, Ramalho JS, Jaissle GB, Seeliger MW, Seabra MC. 2004. The role of Rab27a in the regulation of melanosome distribution within retinal pigment epithelial cells. *Mol Biol Cell* **15:** 2264–2275.

Gibbs D, Kitamoto J, Williams DS. 2003. Abnormal phagocytosis by retinal pigmented epithelium that lacks myosin VIIa, the Usher syndrome 1B protein. *Proc Natl Acad Sci* **100:** 6481–6486.

Gibbs D, Azarian SM, Lillo C, Kitamoto J, Klomp AE, Steel KP, Libby RT, Williams DS. 2004. Role of myosin VIIa and Rab27a in the motility and localization of RPE melanosomes. *J Cell Sci* **117:** 6473–6483.

Gibbs D, Diemer T, Khanobdee K, Hu J, Bok D, Williams DS. 2010. Function of MYO7A in the human RPE and the validity of shaker1 mice as a model for Usher syndrome 1B. *Invest Ophthalmol Vis Sci* **51:** 1130–1135.

Gibson F, Walsh J, Mburu P, Varela A, Brown KA, Antonio M, Beisel KW, Steel KP, Brown SD. 1995. A type VII myosin encoded by the mouse deafness gene shaker-1. *Nature* **374:** 62–64.

Grieger J, Samulski R. 2005. Packaging capacity of adeno-associated virus serotypes: Impact of larger genomes on infectivity and postentry steps. *J Virol* **79:** 9933–9944.

Gruter O, Kostic C, Crippa SV, Perez MT, Zografos L, Schorderet DF, Munier FL, Arsenijevic Y. 2005. Lentiviral vector-mediated gene transfer in adult mouse photoreceptors is impaired by the presence of a physical barrier. *Gene Ther* **12:** 942–947.

Hashimoto T, Gibbs D, Lillo C, Azarian SM, Legacki E, Zhang XM, Yang XJ, Williams DS. 2007. Lentiviral gene replacement therapy of retinas in a mouse model for Usher syndrome type 1B. *Gene Ther* **14:** 584–594.

Hasson T, Heintzelman MB, Santos-Sacchi J, Corey DP, Mooseker MS. 1995. Expression in cochlea and retina of myosin VIIa, the gene product defective in Usher syndrome type 1B. *Proc Natl Acad Sci* **92:** 9815–9819.

Hauswirth WW, Aleman TS, Kaushal S, Cideciyan AV, Schwartz SB, Wang L, Conlon TJ, Boye SL, Flotte TR, Byrne BJ, et al. 2008. Treatment of Leber congenital amaurosis due to *RPE65* mutations by ocular subretinal injection of adeno-associated virus gene vector: Short-term results of a phase I trial. *Hum Gene Ther* **19:** 979–990.

Jacobson SG, Cideciyan AV, Gibbs D, Sumaroka A, Roman AJ, Aleman TS, Schwartz SB, Olivares MB, Russell RC, Steinberg JD, et al. 2011. Retinal disease course in Usher syndrome 1B due to *MYO7A* mutations. *Invest Ophthalmol Vis Sci* **52:** 7924–7936.

Jacobson SG, Cideciyan AV, Ratnakaram R, Heon E, Schwartz SB, Roman AJ, Peden MC, Aleman TS, Boye SL, Sumaroka A, et al. 2012. Gene therapy for Leber congenital amaurosis caused by *RPE65* mutations: Safety and efficacy in 15 children and adults followed up to 3 years. *Arch Ophthalmol* **130:** 9–24.

Klomp AE, Teofilo K, Legacki E, Williams DS. 2007. Analysis of the linkage of MYRIP and MYO7A to melanosomes by RAB27A in retinal pigment epithelial cells. *Cell Motil Cytoskeleton* **64:** 474–487

Kong J, Kim SR, Binley K, Pata I, Doi K, Mannik J, Zernant-Rajang J, Kan O, Iqball S, Naylor S, et al. 2008. Correction of the disease phenotype in the mouse model of Stargardt disease by lentiviral gene therapy. *Gene Ther* **15:** 1311–1320.

Lai Y, Yue Y, Duan D. 2010. Evidence for the failure of adeno-associated virus serotype 5 to package a viral genome $\geq$ 8.2 kb. *Mol Ther* **18:** 75–79.

Libby RT, Steel KP. 2001. Electroretinographic anomalies in mice with mutations in *Myo7a*, the gene involved in human Usher syndrome type 1B. *Invest Ophthalmol Vis Sci* **42:** 770–778.

Liu X, Vansant G, Udovichenko IP, Wolfrum U, Williams DS. 1997. Myosin VIIa, the product of the Usher 1B syndrome gene, is concentrated in the connecting cilia of photoreceptor cells. *Cell Motil Cytoskeleton* **37:** 240–252.

Liu X, Ondek B, Williams DS. 1998. Mutant myosin VIIa causes defective melanosome distribution in the RPE of shaker-1 mice. *Nat Genet* **19:** 117–118.

Liu X, Udovichenko IP, Brown SD, Steel KP, Williams DS. 1999. Myosin VIIa participates in opsin transport through the photoreceptor cilium. *J Neurosci* **19:** 6267–6274.

Lopes VS, Ramalho JS, Owen DM, Karl MO, Strauss O, Futter CE, Seabra MC. 2007. The ternary Rab27a-Myrip-Myosin VIIa complex regulates melanosome motility in the retinal pigment epithelium. *Traffic* **8:** 486–499.

Lopes VS, Gibbs D, Libby RT, Aleman TS, Welch DL, Lillo C, Jacobson SG, Radu RA, Steel KP, Williams DS. 2011. The Usher 1B protein, MYO7A, is required for normal localization and function of the visual retinoid cycle enzyme, RPE65. *Hum Mol Genet* **20:** 2560–2570.

Lopes VS, Boye SE, Louie CM, Boye S, Dyka F, Chiodo V, Fofo H, Hauswirth WW, Williams DS. 2013. Retinal gene therapy with a large MYO7A cDNA using adeno-associated virus. *Gene Ther* **20:** 824–833.

Maguire A, Simonelli F, Pierce E, Pugh E, Mingozzi F, Bennicelli J, Banfi S, Marshall KA, Testa F, Surace EM, et al. 2008. Safety and efficacy of gene transfer for Leber's congenital amaurosis. *N Engl J Med* **358:** 2240–2248.

Mburu P, Liu XZ, Walsh J, Saw D Jr, Cope MJ, Gibson F, Kendrick-Jones J, Steel KP, Brown SD. 1997. Mutation analysis of the mouse myosin VIIA deafness gene. *Genes Funct* **1:** 191–203.

Miyoshi H, Takahashi M, Gage FH, Verma IM. 1997. Stable and efficient gene transfer into the retina using an HIV-based lentiviral vector. *Proc Natl Acad Sci* **94:** 10319–10323.

O'Rourke JP, Newbound GC, Kohn DB, Olsen JC, Bunnell BA. 2002. Comparison of gene transfer efficiencies and gene expression levels achieved with equine infectious anemia virus- and human immunodeficiency virus type 1-derived lentivirus vectors. *J Virol* **76:** 1510–1515.

Peng YW, Zallocchi M, Wang WM, Delimont D, Cosgrove D. 2011. Moderate light-induced degeneration of rod photoreceptors with delayed transducin translocation in shaker1 mice. *Invest Ophthalmol Vis Sci* **52:** 6421–6427.

Sahly I, Dufour E, Schietroma C, Michel V, Bahloul A, Perfettini I, Pepermans E, Estivalet A, Carette D, Aghaie A, et al. 2012. Localization of Usher 1 proteins to the photoreceptor calyceal processes, which are absent from mice. *J Cell Biol* **199:** 381–399.

Schraermeyer UHK. 1999. Current understanding on the role of retinal pigment epithelium and its pigmentation. *Pigment Cell Res* **12:** 219–236.

Takahashi M, Miyoshi H, Verma IM, Gage FH. 1999. Rescue from photoreceptor degeneration in the *rd* mouse by human immunodeficiency virus vector-mediated gene transfer. *J Virol* **73:** 7812–7816.

Testa F, Maguire AM, Rossi S, Pierce EA, Melillo P, Marshall K, Banfi S, Surace EM, Sun J, Acerra C, et al. 2013. Three-year follow-up after unilateral subretinal delivery of adeno-associated virus in patients with Leber congenital amaurosis type 2. *Ophthalmology* **120:** 1283–1291.

Trapani I, Colella P, Sommella A, Iodice C, Cesi G, de Simone S, Marrocco E, Rossi S, Giunti M, Palfi A, et al. 2014. Effective delivery of large genes to the retina by dual AAV vectors. *EMBO Mol Med* **6:** 194–211.

Udovichenko IP, Gibbs D, Williams DS. 2002. Actin-based motor properties of native myosin VIIa. *J Cell Sci* **115:** 445–450.

Verma I, Weitzman M. 2005. Gene therapy: Twenty-first century medicine. *Annu Rev Biochem* **74:** 711–738.

Weil D, Levy G, Sahly I, Levi-Acobas F, Blanchard S, El-Amraoui A, Crozet F, Philippe H, Abitbol M, Petit C. 1996. Human myosin VIIA responsible for the Usher 1B syndrome: A predicted membrane-associated motor protein expressed in developing sensory epithelia. *Proc Natl Acad Sci* **93:** 3232–3237.

Williams DS. 2008. Usher syndrome: Animal models, retinal function of Usher proteins, and prospects for gene therapy. *Vision Res* **48:** 433–441.

Wu L, Pan L, Wei Z, Zhang M. 2011. Structure of MyTH4-FERM domains in myosin VIIa tail bound to cargo. *Science* **331:** 757–760.

Yáñez-Muñoz R, Balaggan K, MacNeil A, Howe S, Schmidt M, Smith A, Buch P, MacLaren R, Anderson P, Barker S, et al. 2006. Effective gene therapy with nonintegrating lentiviral vectors. *Nat Med* **12:** 348–353.

Zallocchi M, Binley K, Lad Y, Ellis S, Widdowson P, Iqball S, Scripps V, Kelleher M, Loader J, Miskin JP, et al. 2014. EIAV-based retinal gene therapy in the *shaker1* mouse model for Usher syndrome type 1B: Development of UshStat. *PLoS ONE* **9:** e94272.

Gene Therapies for Neovascular Age-Related Macular Degeneration

Peter Pechan, Samuel Wadsworth, and Abraham Scaria

Gene Therapy, Sanofi-Genzyme R&D Center, Framingham, Massachusetts 01701

Correspondence: abraham.scaria@genzyme.com

Pathological neovascularization is a key component of the neovascular form (also known as the wet form) of age-related macular degeneration (AMD) and proliferative diabetic retinopathy. Several preclinical studies have shown that antiangiogenesis strategies are effective for treating neovascular AMD in animal models. Vascular endothelial growth factor (VEGF) is one of the main inducers of ocular neovascularization, and several clinical trials have shown the benefits of neutralizing VEGF in patients with neovascular AMD or diabetic macular edema. In this review, we summarize several preclinical and early-stage clinical trials with intraocular gene therapies, which have the potential to reduce or eliminate the repeated intravitreal injections that are currently required for the treatment of neovascular AMD.

Age-related macular degeneration (AMD) is the leading cause of central vision loss in individuals 65 years of age and older. Neovascular AMD, the most severe form of AMD, is characterized by subretinal or choroidal neovascularization (CNV). It often leads to permanent vision loss and the inability to read, write, recognize faces, or drive (Klein et al. 1992). Conventional therapies approved by the United States Food and Drug Association (FDA) were laser thermal photocoagulation and photodynamic therapy with intravenous injection of verteporfin (Visudyne, Valeant Pharmaceuticals) (Miller et al. 1999). Visudyne was the first drug therapy approved for treatment of wet AMD and is efficacious in patients who have predominantly classic lesions of CNV. The first anti-VEGF drug, pegaptanib sodium (Macugen, Eyetech Inc. and Pfizer) (Gragoudas et al. 2004), was approved by the FDA in December 2004 for all angiographic subtypes of neovascular AMD. Although the previous treatments can slow the progression of vision loss, only a small percentage of treated patients experienced any improvement in visual acuity. Ranibizumab (Lucentis, Genentech), introduced earlier (Brown et al. 2006; Rosenfeld et al. 2006) and aflibercept (Eylea, also known as VEGF Trap-Eye; Regeneron) (Heier et al. 2012) were approved by the FDA in June 2006 and in November 2011, respectively, for the treatment of all subtypes of neovascular AMD. An antiplatelet-derived growth factor (anti-PDGF) aptamer agent, Fovista (Ophthotech), is currently in clinical trials and is being tested in combination with ranibizumab. The combination is showing potential to be an additional treatment alternative for wet AMD (Boyer et al. 2009).

Although these treatments maintain vision (and in some cases improve vision), they require

Cite this article as *Cold Spring Harb Perspect Med* doi: 10.1101/cshperspect.a017335

repeated treatments to remain effective. Hence, they still require years of frequent intravitreal injections, which can increase the potential risk of endophthalmitis and are inconvenient for patients, their families, and the treating physicians. An attractive alternate approach involves using a single intraocular injection of a gene therapy vector that would continuously express an antiangiogenic protein to block pathological neovascularization in AMD. Here we summarize the rationale and progress of preclinical and clinical trials using gene delivery strategies for the treatment of neovascular AMD. The gene delivery vectors used in these studies include adenoviral vectors (Ad), helper-dependent Ad vectors, adeno-associated viral vectors (AAV), and lentiviral vectors.

MOLECULES DELIVERED USING GENE THERAPY

VEGF Inhibitors

Formation of choroidal neovessels that penetrate the subretinal space, because of overproduction of growth factors such as vascular endothelial growth factor (VEGF), is the main cause of vision loss in neovascular AMD. VEGF also plays a significant role in the leakage of new intraretinal blood vessels in proliferative diabetic retinopathy (Connolly et al. 1989; Ferrara and Henzel 1989; Aiello et al. 1995; Ferrara et al. 1998). Knowing the role of VEGF in the formation of these neovessels is the determining factor in the development of anti-VEGF therapies. It has been shown that VEGF is necessary for development and maintenance of pathological neovascularization, and blockade of VEGF receptor signaling via VEGF receptor 1 (VEGFR-1, Flt) or VEGFR-2 (Flk, KDR) is sufficient to inhibit neovascularization (Aiello et al. 1995; Ozaki et al. 2000). The four main biological effects of VEGF, as determined by Ferrara and Gerber (2001), are increase in vascular permeability, growth and proliferation of vascular endothelial cells, migration of vascular endothelial cells, and survival of immature endothelial cells by preventing apoptosis. The role of VEGF in inducing retinal neovascularization and vascular leakage has been confirmed in several animal models using ocular gene delivery of VEGF (Yu et al. 1999; Rakoczy et al. 2003; Lebherz et al. 2005; Julien et al. 2008). Since the original study in rhesus monkeys (Ryan 1979), laser rupture of Bruch's membrane has become a common technique to induce CNV in different animal species. Increased expression of VEGF has been shown in laser-induced CNV in rats (Yi et al. 1997), and the blockade of VEGF receptor kinase activity (using small molecule inhibitors) has been shown to cause almost complete inhibition of laser-induced CNV in mice (Kwak et al. 2000). Blocking VEGF with antibodies or soluble VEGF receptors and inhibition of VEGF receptor tyrosine kinase activity are strategies that have shown promising preclinical and clinical results in the suppression of retinal neovascularization. Over the years, several potent VEGF inhibitor proteins have been tested in preclinical models. Intravitreal injections of VEGF-neutralizing chimeric proteins, consisting of the extracellular domain of either human Flt or mouse Flk receptors and an immunoglobulin IgG Fc region, suppressed retinal neovascularization in a murine model of ischemic retinopathy (Aiello et al. 1995). Ranibizumab (previously known as rhuFabV2), a humanized anti-VEGF monoclonal antibody fragment, has been shown to prevent laser-induced CNV in an experimental monkey model (Krzystolik et al. 2002). It has been shown that an anti-murine-VEGF antibody blocked neovascularizaton in a murine laser CNV model (Campa et al. 2008). Intravitreal injection of VEGF-Trap, a recombinant fusion protein that contains the domain 2 of Flt-1 and domain 3 of KDR fused to the Fc portion of human IgG1 (Holash et al. 2002), suppressed laser-induced CNV in a mouse model, and subcutaneous injection of VEGF-Trap also significantly inhibited subretinal neovascularization in a VEGF-overexpressing transgenic mouse model (Saishin et al. 2003). The success in preclinical models resulted in introduction of anti-VEGF protein therapy into clinical trials. Ranibizumab (Presta et al. 1997) improved vision in almost half of all treated patients with neovascular AMD (Brown et al. 2006; Rosenfeld et al. 2006), and aflibercept yielded similar benefits in patients with neovascular AMD (Heier et al. 2012). Both drugs stabilized existing vision in >90% of patients; however, they require frequent intravitreal injections (sometimes for years) by a retinal specialist.

An alternative approach, such as intraocular gene delivery of VEGF antagonists, would remove the need for frequent intravitreal injections and could provide other advantages over the current treatments. VEGF antagonists currently being investigated in this gene delivery approach are variations of the soluble VEGF receptor Flt-1 (Shibuya et al. 1990). These include the secreted form of the VEGF receptor *flt-1* (Flt-1 domains 1–6) (Kendall and Thomas 1993; Lai et al. 2002), the entire flt-1 ectodomain (Flt-1 domains 1–7) fused to the Fc portion of human IgG (Aiello et al. 1995; Honda et al. 2000), or sFLT01 (Flt-1 domain 2 fused to the Fc portion of human IgG via a 9-glycine linker) (Pechan et al. 2009).

One of the earliest studies showing inhibition of ocular neovascularization by gene delivery of a VEGF antagonist was described by Honda et al. (2000). An Ad vector expressing *flt-1* (domains 1–7) fused to IgG-Fc (flt-ExR) was shown to significantly inhibit subretinal neovascularization when the Ad vector was injected into the femoral muscle in rats (Honda et al. 2000). Several other groups used a naturally occurring soluble decoy Flt-1 receptor (sFlt1), which is an alternatively spliced form of Flt-1 consisting of the first six extracellular Ig-like domains followed by a unique carboxy-terminal extension of 31 amino acids (Kendall and Thomas 1993). Subretinal delivery of AAV-sFlt-1 under control of the cytomegalovirus (CMV) promoter was shown to suppress laser-induced CNV (Lai et al. 2002). In the mouse oxygen-induced retinopathy model, intravitreal gene delivery of the secreted form of *flt-1* using Ad and AAV vectors inhibited experimental retinal neovascularization by ~50% (Bainbridge et al. 2002). Recombinant replication-deficient adenovirus type 5 (Ad5) vectors used in these studies (Ad5.sflt) are E1a- and partially E1b- and E3- Ad5 vectors that express the secreted form of *flt-1*. The Ad5.sflt almost completely inhibited retinal neovascularization in a rat model of oxygen-induced retinopathy without affecting preexisting retinal vessels (Rota et al. 2004). In nonhuman primate studies, subretinal injection of AAV-sFlt-1 encoding the secreted form of *flt-1* resulted in long-term (8 mo) expression of sFlt-1 and prevented the development of laser photocoagulation-induced CNV in all treated monkey eyes, with regression of neovascular vessels observed in 85% of the treated eyes (Lai et al. 2005). Treatment with sFlt-1 did not change the retinal morphology, and the majority of the treated eyes (75%) retained high numbers of functional photoreceptors as measured by electroretinography (Lai et al. 2005).

In another long-term safety and efficacy study using nonhuman primates, subretinal injection of AAV2.sFlt-1, encoding the secreted form of *flt-1*, prevented the development of laser photocoagulation-induced CNV in all treated monkey eyes and yielded no evidence of damage to the eyes, no cell-mediated immunity or anterior chamber flare, and normal fundus and electroretinographic responses. Immunological analysis showed that gene therapy involving subretinal injection of AAV2.sFlt-1 did not elicit cell-mediated immunity. Biodistribution analysis showed that AAV2.sFlt-1 could be detected only in the eye and not in the other organs tested (Lai et al. 2012). A clinical trial (phase I/II) with subretinal injection of AAV2 vector expressing the secreted form of *flt-1*, sponsored by the Lions Eye Institute and Avalanche Biotechnologies, Inc., is currently ongoing in Perth, Western Australia (registration no. NCT01494805). The patients are being randomized to receive a low dose (1×10^{10} vector genomes) or high dose (1×10^{11} vector genomes) of a single subretinal injection of AAV2.sFlt-1 and will be tested to examine the baseline safety and efficacy.

Our group at Genzyme has generated a novel chimeric VEGF-binding molecule, sFLT01, containing only the second domain of Flt-1 fused to a human IgG1 Fc through a polyglycine linker, 9Gly (Pechan et al. 2009). We have shown that AAV2-mediated intravitreal gene delivery of sFLT01 efficiently inhibits angiogenesis in the mouse oxygen-induced retinopathy model (Pechan et al. 2009). Preclinical efficacy studies of intravitreally administered AAV2-sFLT01 were conducted in both C57BL/6 mouse and cynomolgus monkey models of laser-induced CNV (Lukason et al. 2011). In the mouse model, the eyes treated with AAV2-sFLT01 showed a very significant reduction in the number of burns with CNV. In cynomolgus monkeys, AAV2-sFLT01 was able to effectively inhibit laser-induced CNV in a dose-dependent manner. Two studies, with a lower dose (2×10^8 or 2×10^9 vector genomes) and a higher dose (2×10^{10} vector genomes) of AAV2-sFLT01 were conducted. With the lower dose, none of the sFLT01 treatment eyes showed a statistically significant reduction in leaking CNV lesions compared with the AAV2-Null control eyes. With the higher dose, all AAV2-sFLT01 treated eyes showed a significant reduction in the amount of CNV leakage compared with the naive contralateral control eyes with only 7% of the AAV2-sFLT01-treated burns showing leakage compared with 56% in the control eyes (Lukason et al. 2011).

Following intravitreal injection, it was also shown that AAV2-sFLT01 is well tolerated, localized in the eye, and capable of long-term expression in nonhuman primates (MacLachlan et al. 2011). Cynomolgus monkeys given an intravitreal injection of a low dose (2.4×10^9 vector genomes) or high dose (2.4×10^{10} vector genomes) of AAV2.sFLT01 showed no electroretinographic or fluorescein angiographic abnormalities for up to 12 mo, the longest time point evaluated. Mild to moderate vitreous inflammation that was transient and resolved spontaneously without any drug treatment was seen in the high-dose group, but not the low-dose group. Histopathological examinations of eyes from the low-dose group were normal and those from the high-dose group showed only occasional inflammatory cells in the trabecular meshwork, vitreous, and/or retina. Aqueous levels of sFLT01 measured in these monkey studies ranged from ~10 to 400 ng/mL at 1 mo. The expression levels were dose-dependent and decreased slightly but were still in the same general range at 12 mo. Vitreous levels of sFLT01 (when measured) were significantly higher than sFLT01 levels in the aqueous. An additional biodistribution study, performed in both Sprague-Dawley rats and cynomolgus monkeys, found only trace amounts of AAV2 vector transiently outside the injected eye (MacLachlan et al. 2011).

These encouraging preclinical efficacy and safety data have led to a Phase I dose-escalating trial testing four doses of AAV2-sFLT01 (2×10^8, 2×10^9, 6×10^9, and 2×10^{10} vector genomes) in patients with advanced neovascular AMD (registration no. NCT01024998; see http://clinicaltrials.gov/). The trial uses a single intravitreal injection with a fixed 100 μL volume of the AAV2-sFLT01 vector. Three patients were enrolled in each of the four cohorts to identify the maximal tolerated dose. Additional cohorts of patients are being treated with this maximal dose. Aqueous levels of sFLT01 are being measured in this trial and will provide useful information regarding the level and duration of transgene protein expression as well as safety and biological activity of sFLT01 as measured by optical coherence tomography of the retina. The study is being conducted at multiple medical centers in the United States.

Gene delivery of sFLT01 was studied by another group at the National Eye Institute in *Ccl2/Cx3cr1*-deficient mice, another model of AMD (Tuo et al. 2012). Previously, it was reported that *Ccl2/Cx3cr1*-deficient mice developed a broad spectrum of AMD-like pathology with early onset and high penetrance (Tuo et al. 2007). Subretinally injected AAV5.sFLT01 vector stabilized or arrested the progression of retinal lesions in *Ccl2/Cx3cr1*-deficient mice. Subretinal injection of AAV5-based vectors typically leads to significant gene expression in photoreceptors and retinal pigment epithelium. The changes in VEGF, ERK phosphorylation, and iNOS in the retinal tissues suggested the involvement of reactive nitrogen species in the retinal lesions. The findings indicate the potentially beneficial effects associated with sFLT01 gene therapy for retinal disease and possibly AMD, given the role of oxidative stress (Tuo et al. 2012).

There have been some reports that long-term systemic inhibition of VEGF in mice can be deleterious to the photoreceptors, retinal pigment epithelium, and choroid (Saint-Geniez et al. 2008, 2009). However, one report using double-transgenic mice with doxycycline-inducible expression of the soluble, secreted, full-size extracellular domain of VEGF receptor-1/sFlt-1 coupled to an IgG1 Fc fragment (sVEGFR1Fc,) indicated that constant blockade of VEGF for up to 7 mo has no identifiable deleterious effects on the retina or choroid (Ueno et al. 2008), supporting the use of VEGF antagonists in the treatment of retinal diseases. Two other studies focusing on subretinally injected AAV.sFlt-1 showed that this gene therapy approach is safe and effective for the long-term (8 mo) inhibition of pathological blood vessel growth in the eye (Lai et al. 2005, 2009).

To decrease potential long-term complications of anti-VEGF therapies, inducible, helper-dependent Ad vectors expressing sFlt-1 vectors (delivered intravitreally) have been tested for their therapeutic efficacy in a rat model of oxygen-induced retinopathy in a constitutive or doxycycline-inducible manner (Lamartina et al. 2007). The sFlt-1 cDNA used in these studies had a similar structure to the sFlt-1 form used by Rakoczy's group (Lai et al. 2005) that encodes the alternatively spliced, soluble sFlt-1 isoform. Treatment with these vectors resulted in detectable levels of sFlt-1, and retinal neovascularization was significantly inhibited. The therapeutic efficacy of the inducible, helper-dependent Ad vector was strictly doxycycline-dependent. The strategy of using an inducible vector may turn out to be a useful system for regulating protein expression in the eye.

To avoid the complications of immune responses to viral vectors, there are ongoing investigations into an alternate method involving direct injections into the ciliary muscle of a nonviral gene transfer vector expressing one of three different rat sFlt-1 variants: small-sFlt-1 (3 domains), medium-sFlt-1 (4 domains), and large sFlt-1 (6 domains). All three sflt-1 variants significantly diminished vascular leakage and neovascularization in a rat model of laser-induced CNV (El Sanharawi et al. 2013). It is not clear at this point how long expression lasts with nonviral vectors compared with AAV vectors, which have shown ocular expression for several years.

Another approach under investigation is posttranscriptional silencing of VEGF gene expression using RNA interference (RNAi). Short interfering RNA (siRNA) designed against VEGF mRNA was shown to silence VEGF gene expression and inhibit the development of laser-induced CNV in the mouse eye (Reich et al. 2003). In another experiment by the same group, it was shown that intravitreal injection of siRNA against VEGF mRNA inhibited the growth and vascular permeability of laser-induced CNV in a nonhuman primate. This effect was dose-dependent and did not cause any change in electroretinogram, hemorrhage, inflammation, or clinical signs of toxicity (Tolentino et al. 2004). Gene therapy using this approach uses short hairpin RNA (shRNA) delivered by a plasmid or viral vector. The shRNA silences the target gene through a complex process resulting in the cleavage of the target mRNA (Macrae et al. 2006). An AAV8 vector expressing an anti-VEGF shRNA, when injected subretinally, significantly reduced CNV (up to 48%) in a laser-induced murine model (Askou et al. 2012).

Pigment Epithelium-Derived Factor (PEDF)

PEDF is a 50 kDa glycoprotein belonging to the serine proteinase inhibitor (SERPIN) superfamily (Tombran-Tink et al. 1991; Becerra et al. 1995). PEDF has neuronal differentiating activities (Tombran-Tink et al. 1991) and neurotrophic activities (Steele et al. 1993) and is a potent antiangiogenic factor (Stellmach et al. 2001). The ratio between VEGF and PEDF levels is altered in the aqueous and vitreous fluids from patients with diabetic retinopathy and AMD (Ogata et al. 2001; Ohno-Matsui et al. 2001).

Three different models of ocular neovascularization have been used to investigate the efficacy of PEDF gene transfer in inhibition of neovascularization (Mori et al. 2001a). In VEGF-overexpressing transgenic mice and in the oxygen-induced retinopathy mouse model, intravitreal injection of Ad-PEDF vector resulted in significant inhibition of neovascularization as compared with null vector (Mori et al. 2001a). Both intravitreal and subretinal injection of an

Ad-PEDF vector significantly reduced CNV area in a mouse model of laser-induced CNV (Mori et al. 2001a) and even caused regression of already-established ocular neovascularization (Mori et al. 2002).

A safety study for intravitreal administration of Ad-PEDF was conducted in cynomolgus monkeys and resulted in dose-dependent, drug-induced ocular toxicity. No toxicity was detected in the eye at a low dose of 1×10^8 particle units (pu) Ad-PEDF, but dose-related inflammatory responses occurred at doses of 1×10^9 pu and higher (Rasmussen et al. 2003). Moreover, a significant decrease in electroretinographic response occurred at doses of 1×10^{10} pu or higher, correlating with more pronounced toxicity.

Periocular and intravitreal injections of E1/E4-deleted Ad vector expressing human PEDF (AdPEDF.11) was tested in a CNV model in pigs, which have eyes that are very similar to humans in size and scleral thickness. The periocular injection of 1×10^{10} or 1×10^{11} pu of Ad-PEDF gave rise to increased levels of PEDF in the periocular tissue and choroid and significantly reduced (77%) the amount of CNV at rupture sites in Bruch's membrane (Saishin et al. 2005). At a dose of 1×10^9 pu injected intravitreally the reduction in CNV area was less pronounced (38%). Periocular injections could be less invasive and potentially safer for patients.

A phase 1 clinical study (NCT00109499; GenVec) was completed in which 28 patients with advanced neovascular AMD were given a single intravitreal injection of an AdPEDF.11 in doses ranging from 10^6 to $10^{9.5}$ pu (Campochiaro et al. 2006). Six patients experienced increased intraocular pressure that was easily controlled by topical medication. Signs of mild, transient intraocular inflammation occurred in 25% of patients, but there was no severe inflammation, no serious adverse events, or dose-limiting toxicities. There were hints of anti-angiogenic activity of PEDF in the high dose patients for a few months (Campochiaro et al. 2006), and this approach may be worth investigating further with vectors that provide long-term expression of PEDF.

Endostatin and Angiostatin

Endostatin, a cleavage product of collagen XVIII, participates in physiological regression of the hyaloid vasculature and regulation of retinal vascular development and is known to inhibit tumor angiogenesis. A role for endogenous endostatin in inhibiting experimental CNV has also been shown (Marneros et al. 2007). Intravenous (tail vein) injection of Ad-endostatin under control of the CMV or Rous sarcoma virus promoter also completely prevented CNV development in a laser-induced mouse model of CNV (Mori et al. 2001b). Two different vectors for subretinal endostatin delivery were tested in the double transgenic mouse model with doxycycline-induced expression of VEGF in the retina. Both the bovine immunodeficiency lentiviral vector and the helper-dependent Ad vector with tamoxifen-inducible expression of endostatin resulted in significant suppression of leakage of intravascular [^{3}H]mannitol into the retina in this model (Takahashi et al. 2003). An equine infectious anemia virus (EIAV)-based vector encoding endostatin was evaluated in C57Bl/6J mice with experimental laser-induced CNV (Balaggan et al. 2006). The vector effectively controlled angiogenesis and hyperpermeability without long-term deleterious effects, and significantly augmented the frequency of apoptosis within the induced CNV as compared with injected controls (Balaggan et al. 2006).

Angiostatin is a fragment of plasminogen that inhibits endothelial proliferation in vitro and tumor growth in vivo. Subretinal injection of AAV-angiostatin has been shown to significantly reduce the size of CNV lesions in a rat model of laser-induced CNV (Lai et al. 2001). Intravitreal injections of HIV-based lentiviral vector encoding angiostatin have shown that gene delivery of angiostatin can inhibit retinal neovascularization in a mouse oxygen-induced retinopathy model (Igarashi et al. 2003). EIAV-based vectors encoding angiostatin or endostatin have been evaluated in an experimental laser-induced CNV mouse model (Balaggan et al. 2006). Both vectors effectively controlled angiogenesis and hyperpermeability without long-term deleterious effects; however, only the endostatin vector significantly augmented the frequency of apoptosis within the induced CNV as compared with injected controls (Balaggan et al. 2006).

The large capacity of lentiviral vectors such as EIAV enabled investigators to express both endostatin and angiostatin from a single EIAV-based vector. Subretinal injection of EIAV vectors expressing murine endostatin alone or in combination with angiostatin driven either by the CMV promoter or vitelliform macular dystrophy gene promoter caused significant suppression of CNV at laser-induced rupture sites in Bruch's membrane (Kachi et al. 2009).

Biodistribution analysis following subretinal administration of this dual vector (RetinoStat, Oxford BioMedica) into rhesus macaques and Dutch belted rabbits showed that the vector was localized within the ocular compartment, tolerated well, and capable of persistent expression (Binley et al. 2012). Following subretinal injection, endostatin and angiostatin protein levels peaked in the vitreous of rabbits at 1 mo, and the expression levels persisted for the 6-mo duration of the study. Mild to moderate ocular inflammation was seen, but it resolved by 1 mo postinjection in both species. There were no significant changes in electroretinogram or intraocular pressure in the treated eye compared with the control eye.

A phase I dose-escalation trial in patients with advanced neovascular AMD, the Gene Transfer of Endostatin/angiostatin for Macular Degeneration Trial (GEM Study, NCT01301443), has been initiated to test the safety and bioactivity of subretinal injection of EIAV.CMV-endostatin.angiostatin (RetinoStat). The study is testing safety and bioactivity of three dose levels of RetinoStat, with three subjects in each cohort and up to nine additional subjects dosed at the maximal tolerated dose. Bioactivity will be assessed by measuring changes from baseline in subretinal and intraretinal fluid by optical coherence tomography and by measuring the size of subretinal neovascular lesions by fluorescein angiography. Transgene expression will be assessed by measuring endostatin and angiostatin protein levels in aqueous samples at 3-mo intervals.

CONCLUDING REMARKS

Studies in animal models suggest that expression of antiangiogenic proteins in the eye by gene delivery could potentially benefit patients with neovascular AMD and avoid the need for repeated intraocular injections. Four different phase I/II clinical trials are in various stages of completion. Two of the trials (Ad-PEDF from GenVec and AAV2-sFLT01 from Genzyme) involve an intravitreal injection, which is currently the well-accepted method used to deliver Lucentis and Eylea in the clinic. The other two trials (EIAV-endostatin.angiostatin from Oxford BioMedica and AAV2-sflt-1 from Avalanche) involve subretinal injections in an operating room procedure. However, subretinal delivery can theoretically deliver higher levels of the therapeutic protein to the outer retina and choroid. Although these trials are not masked and are primarily safety trials, we should be able to generate some very useful data on the feasibility/safety of ocular gene delivery, protein expression levels, and biological activity of the protein as measured by retina optical coherence tomography and fluorescence angiography within the next couple of years. This could potentially set the stage for the design of larger phase III clinical trials.

REFERENCES

Aiello LP, Pierce EA, Foley ED, Takagi H, Chen H, Riddle L, Ferrara N, King GL, Smith LE. 1995. Suppression of retinal neovascularization in vivo by inhibition of vascular endothelial growth factor (VEGF) using soluble VEGF–receptor chimeric proteins. *Proc Natl Acad Sci* **92:** 10457–10461.

Askou AL, Pournaras JAC, Pihlmann M, Svalgaard JD, Arsenijevic Y, Kostic C, Bek T, Dagnaes-Hansen F, Mikkelsen JG, Jensen TG, et al. 2012. Reduction of choroidal neovascularization in mice by adeno-associated virus-delivered anti-vascular endothelial growth factor short hairpin RNA. *J Gene Med* **14:** 632–641.

Bainbridge JW, Mistry A, De Alwis M, Paleolog E, Baker A, Thrasher AJ, Ali RR. 2002. Inhibition of retinal neovascularisation by gene transfer of soluble VEGF receptor sFlt-1. *Gene Ther* **9:** 320–326.

Balaggan KS, Binley K, Esapa M, MacLaren RE, Iqball S, Duran Y, Pearson RA, Kan O, Barker SE, Smith AJ, et al. 2006. EIAV vector-mediated delivery of endostatin or angiostatin inhibits angiogenesis and vascular hyperpermeability in experimental CNV. *Gene Ther* **13:** 1153–1165.

Becerra SP, Sagasti A, Spinella P, Notario V. 1995. Pigment epithelium derived factor behaves like a noninhibitory serpin: Neurotrophic activity does not require the serpin reactive loop. *J Biol Chem* **270:** 25992–25999.

Binley K, Widdowson PS, Kelleher M, de Belin J, Loader J, Ferrige G, Carlucci M, Esapa M, Chipchase D, Angell-Manning D, et al. 2012. Safety and biodistribution of an equine infectious anemia virus-based gene therapy, RetinoStat(®), for age-related macular degeneration. *Hum Gene Ther* **23:** 980–991.

Boyer DS, Ophthotech Anti-PDGF in AMD Study Group. 2009. Combined inhibition of platelet-derived (PDGF) and vascular endothelial (VEGF) growth factors for the treatment of neovascular age-related macular degeneration (NV-AMD). Results of a phase 1 study. *Invest Ophthalmol Vis Sci* **50:** E-Abstract 1260.

Brown DM, Kaiser PK, Michels M, Soubrane G, Heier JS, Kim RY, Judy P Sy, Schneider S, ANCHOR Study Group. 2006. Ranibizumab versus verteporfin for neovascular age-related macular degeneration. *N Engl J Med* **355:** 1432–1444.

Campa C, Kasman I, Ye W, Lee WP, Fuh G, Ferrara N. 2008. Effects of an anti-VEGF-A monoclonal antibody on laser-induced choroidal neovascularization in mice: Optimizing methods to quantify vascular changes. *Invest Ophthalmol Vis Sci* **49:** 1178–1183.

Campochiaro PA, Nguyen QD, Shah SM, Klein ML, Holz E, Frank RN, Saperstein DA, Gupta A, Stout JT, Macko J, et al. 2006. Adenoviral vector-delivered pigment epithelium-derived factor for neovascular age-related macular degeneration: Results of a phase I clinical trial. *Hum Gene Ther* **17:** 167–176.

Connolly DT, Heuvelman DM, Nelson R, Olander JV, Eppley BL, Delfino JJ, Siegel NR, Leimgruber RM, Feder J. 1989. Tumor vascular permeability factor stimulates endothelial cell growth and angiogenesis. *J Clin Invest* **84:** 1470–1478.

El Sanharawi M, Touchard E, Benard R, Bigey P, Escriou V, Mehanna C, Naud MC, Berdugo M, Jeanny JC, Behar-Cohen F. 2013. Long-term efficacy of ciliary muscle gene transfer of three sFlt-1 variants in a rat model of laser-induced choroidal neovascularization. *Gene Ther* **20:** 1093–1103.

Ferrara N, Henzel WJ. 1989. Pituitary follicular cells secrete a novel heparin-binding growth factor specific for vascular endothelial cells. *Biochem Biophys Res Commun* **161:** 851–859.

Ferrara N, Gerber HP. 2001. The role of vascular endothelial growth factor in angiogenesis. *Acta Haematol* **106:** 148–156.

Ferrara N, Chen H, Davis-Smyth T, Gerber HP, Nguyen TN, Peers D, Chisholm V, Hillan KJ, Schwall RH. 1998. Vascular endothelial growth factor is essential for corpus luteum angiogenesis. *Nat Med* **4:** 336–340.

Gragoudas ES, Adamis AP, Cunningham ET, Feinsod M, Guyer DR. 2004. Pegaptanib for neovascular age-related macular degeneration. *N Engl J Med* **351:** 2805–2816.

Heier JS, Brown DM, Chong V, Korobelnik JF, Kaiser PK, Nguyen QD, Kirchhof B, Ho A, Ogura Y, Yancopoulos GD, et al. 2012. Intravitreal aflibercept (VEGF trap-eye) in wet age-related macular degeneration. *Ophthalmol* **119:** 2537–2548.

Holash J, Davis S, Papadopoulos N, Croll SD, Ho L, Russell M, Boland P, Leidich R, Hylton D, Burova E, et al. 2002. VEGF-Trap: A VEGF blocker with potent antitumor effects. *Proc Natl Acad Sci* **99:** 11393–11398.

Honda M, Sakamoto T, Ishibashi T, Inomata H, Ueno H. 2000. Experimental subretinal neovascularization is inhibited by adenovirus-mediated soluble VEGF/flt-1 receptor gene transfection: A role of VEGF and possible treatment for SRN in age-related macular degeneration. *Gene Ther* **7:** 978–985.

Igarashi T, Miyake K, Kato K, Watanabe A, Ishizaki M, Ohara K, Shimada T. 2003. Lentivirus-mediated expression of angiostatin efficiently inhibits neovascularization in a murine proliferative retinopathy model. *Gene Ther* **10:** 219–226.

Julien S, Kreppel F, Beck S, Heiduschka P, Brito V, Schnichels S, Kochanek S, Schraermeyer U. 2008. A reproducible and quantifiable model of choroidal neovascularization induced by VEGF A165 after subretinal adenoviral gene transfer in the rabbit. *Mol Vis* **14:** 1358–1372.

Kachi S, Binley K, Yokoi K, Umeda N, Akiyama H, Muramatu D, Iqball S, Kan O, Naylor S, Campochiaro PA. 2009. Equine infectious anemia viral vector-mediated codelivery of endostatin and angiostatin driven by retinal pigmented epithelium-specific VMD2 promoter inhibits choroidal neovascularization. *Hum Gene Ther* **20:** 31–39.

Kendall RL, Thomas KA. 1993. Inhibition of vascular endothelial cell growth factor activity by an endogenously encoded soluble receptor. *Proc Natl Acad Sci* **90:** 10705–10709.

Klein R, Klein BE, Linton KL. 1992. Prevalence of age-related maculopathy. The Beaver Dam Eye Study. *Ophthalmol* **99:** 933–943.

Krzystolik MG, Afshari MA, Adamis AP, Gaudreault J, Gragoudas ES, Michaud NA, Li Wenjun, Connolly E, O'Neill CA, Miller JW. 2002. Prevention of experimental choroidal neovascularization with intravitreal anti-vascular endothelial growth factor antibody fragment. *Arch Ophthalmol* **120:** 338–346.

Kwak N, Okamoto N, Wood JM, Campochiaro PA. 2000. VEGF is major stimulator in model of choroidal neovascularization. *Invest Ophthalmol Vis Sci* **41:** 3158–3164.

Lai CC , Wu WC, Chen SL, Xiao X, Tsai TC, Huan SJ, Chen TL, Tsai RJ, Tsao YP. 2001. Suppression of choroidal neovascularization by adeno-associated virus vector expressing angiostatin. *Invest Ophthalmol Vis Sci* **42:** 2401–2407.

Lai YK, Shen WY, Brankov M, Lai CM, Constable IJ, Rakoczy PE. 2002. Potential long-term inhibition of ocular neovascularisation by recombinant adeno-associated virus-mediated secretion gene therapy. *Gene Ther* **9:** 804–813.

Lai CM, Shen WY, Brankov M, Lai YK, Barnett NL, Lee SY, Yeo IYS, Mathur R, Ho JES, Pineda P, et al. 2005. Long-term evaluation of AAV-mediated sFlt-1 gene therapy for ocular neovascularization in mice and monkeys. *Mol Ther* **12:** 659–668.

Lai CM, Estcourt MJ, Wikstrom M, Himbeck RP, Barnett NL, Brankov M, Tee LBG, Dunlop SA, Degli-Esposti MA, Rakoczy EP. 2009. rAAV.sFlt-1 gene therapy achieves lasting reversal of retinal neovascularization in the absence of a strong immune response to the viral vector. *Invest Ophthalmol Vis Sci* **50:** 4279–4287.

Lai CM, Estcourt MJ, Himbeck RP, Lee SY, Yeo IYS, Luu C, Loh BK, Lee MW, Barathi A, Villano J, et al. 2012. Preclinical safety evaluation of subretinal AAV2.sFlt-1 in non-human primates. *Gene Ther* **19:** 999–1009.

Lamartina S, Cimino M, Roscilli G, Dammassa E, Lazzaro D, Rota R, Ciliberto G, Toniatti C. 2007. Helper-dependent adenovirus for the gene therapy of proliferative retinopathies: Stable gene transfer, regulated gene expression and therapeutic efficacy. *J Gene Med* **9:** 862–874.

Lebherz C, Auricchio A, Maguire AM, Rivera VM, Tang W, Grant RL, Clackson T, Bennett J, Wilson JM. 2005. Nonhuman primate models for diabetic ocular neovascularization using AAV2-mediated overexpression of vascular endothelial growth factor. *Diabetes* **54:** 1141–1149.

Lukason M, DuFresne E, Rubin H, Pechan P, Li Q, Kim I, Kiss S, Flaxel C, Collins M, Miller J, et al. 2011. Inhibition of choroidal neovascularization in a nonhuman primate model by intravitreal administration of an AAV2 vector expressing a novel anti-VEGF molecule. *Mol Ther* **19:** 260–265.

MacLachlan TK, Lukason M, Collins M, Munger R, Isenberger E, Rogers C, Malatos S, DuFresne E, Morris J, Calcedo R, et al. 2011. Preclinical safety evaluation of AAV2-sFLT01—A gene therapy for age-related macular degeneration. *Mol Ther* **19:** 326–334.

Macrae IJ, Zhou K, Li F, Repic A, Brooks AN, Cande WZ, Adams PD, Doudna JA. 2006. Structural basis for double-stranded RNA processing by Dicer. *Science* **311:** 195–198.

Marneros AG, She H, Zambarakji H, Hashizume H, Connolly EJ, Kim I, Gragoudas ES, Miller JW, Olsen BR. 2007. Endogenous endostatin inhibits choroidal neovascularization. *FASEB J* **21:** 3809–3818.

Miller JW, Schmidt-Erfurth U, Sickenberg M, Pournaras CJ, Laqua H. 1999. Photodynamic therapy with verteporfin for choroidal neovascularization caused by age-related macular degeneration: Results of a single treatment in a phase 1 and 2 study. *Arch Ophthamol* **117:** 1161–1173.

Mori K, Duh E, Gehlbach P, Ando A, Takahashi K, Pearlman J, Mori K, Yang HS, Zack DJ, Ettyreddy D, et al. 2001a. Pigment epithelium-derived factor inhibits retinal and choroidal neovascularization. *J Cell Physiol* **188:** 253–263.

Mori K, Ando A, Gehlbach P, Nesbitt D, Takahashi K, Goldsteen D, Penn M, Chen CT, Mori K, Melia M, et al. 2001b. Inhibition of choroidal neovascularization by intravenous injection of adenoviral vectors expressing secretable endostatin. *Am J Pathol* **159:** 313–320.

Mori K, Gehlbach P, Ando A, McVey D, Wei L, Campochiaro PA. 2002. Regression of ocular neovascularization in response to increased expression of pigment epithelium-derived factor. *Invest Ophthalmol Vis Sci* **43:** 2428–2434.

Ogata N, Tombran-Tink J, Nishikawa M, Nishimura T, Mitsuma Y, Sakamoto T, Matsumura M. 2001. Pigment-epithelium derived factor in the vitreous is low in diabetic retinopathy and high in rhegmatogenous detachment. *Am J Ophthalmol* **132:** 378–382.

Ohno-Matsui K, Morita I, Tombran-Tink J, Mrazek D, Onodera M, Uetama T, Hayano M, Murota SI, Mochizuki M. 2001. Novel mechanism for age-related macular degeneration: An equilibrium shift between the angiogenesis factors VEGF and PEDF. *J Cell Physiol* **189:** 323–333.

Ozaki H, Seo MS, Ozaki K, Yamada H, Yamada E, Hofmann F, Wood J, Campochiaro PA. 2000. Blockade of vascular endothelial cell growth factor receptor signaling is sufficient to completely prevent retinal neovascularization. *Am J Pathol* **156:** 679–707.

Pechan P, Rubin H, Lukason M, Ardinger J, DuFresne E, Hauswirth WW, Wadsworth SC, Scaria A. 2009. Novel anti-VEGF chimeric molecules delivered by AAV vectors for inhibition of retinal neovascularization. *Gene Ther* **16:** 10–16.

Presta LG, Chen H, O'Connor SJ, Chisholm V, Meng YG, Krummen L, Winkler M, Ferrara N. 1997. Humanization of an anti-vascular endothelial growth factor monoclonal antibody for the therapy of solid tumors and other disorders. *Cancer Res* **57:** 4593–4599.

Rakoczy PE, Brankov M, Fonceca A, Zaknich T, Rae BC, Lai CM. 2003. Enhanced recombinant adeno-associated virus-mediated vascular endothelial growth factor expression in the adult mouse retina: A potential model for diabetic retinopathy. *Diabetes* **52:** 857–863.

Rasmussen HS, Smith AC, Durham RJ, Rasmussen CS, Bee WH, Wills MC, Munger RJ, Tomlinson MJ, MacGill R, King CR. 2003. Safety of intravitreal adenoviral gene therapy containing human pigment epithelium-derived factor transgene in monkeys. *Preclinica* **1:** 77–85.

Reich SJ, Fosnot J, Kuroki A, Tang W, Yang X, Maguire AM, Bennett J, Tolentino MJ. 2003. Small interfering RNA (siRNA) targeting VEGF effectively inhibits ocular neovascularization in a mouse model. *Mol Vis* **9:** 210–216.

Rosenfeld PJ, Brown DM, Heier JS, Boyer DS, Kaiser PK, Chung CY, Kim RY, MARINA Study Group. 2006. Ranibizumab for neovascular age-related macular degeneration. *N Eng J Med* **355:** 1419–1431.

Rota R, Riccioni T, Zaccarini M, Lamartina S, Del Gallo A, Fusco A, Kovesdi I, Balestrazzi E, Abeni DC, Ali RR, et al. 2004. Marked inhibition of retinal neovascularization in rats following soluble-flt-1 gene transfer. *J Gene Med* **6:** 992–1002.

Ryan SJ. 1979. The development of an experimental model of subretinal neovascularization in disciform macular degeneration. *Trans Am Ophthalmol Soc* **77:** 707–745.

Saint-Geniez M, Maharaj ASR, Walshe TE, Tucker BA, Sekiyama E, Kurihara T, Darland DC, Young MJ, D'Amore PA. 2008. Endogenous VEGF is required for visual function: Evidence for a survival role on muller cells and photoreceptors. *PLoS ONE* **3:** e3554.

Saint-Geniez M, Kurihara T, Sekiyama E, Maldonado AE, D'Amore PA. 2009. An essential role for RPE-derived soluble VEGF in maintenance of the choriocapillaries. *Proc Natl Acad Sci* **106:** 18751–18756.

Saishin Y, Saishin Y, Takahashi K, Silva RL, Hylton D, Rudge JS, Wiegand SJ, Campochiaro PA. 2003. VEGF-TRAP(R1R2) suppresses choroidal neovascularization and VEGF-induced breakdown of the blood-retinal barrier. *J Cell Physiol* **195:** 241–248.

Saishin Y, Silva RL, Saishin Y, Kachi S, Aslam S, Gong YY, Lai H, Carrion M, Harris B, Hamilton M, et al. 2005. Periocular gene transfer of pigment epithelium-derived factor inhibits choroidal neovascularization in a human-sized eye. *Hum Gene Ther* **16:** 473–478.

Shibuya M, Yamaguchi S, Yamane A, Ikeda T, Tojo A, Matsushime H, Sato M. 1990. Nucleotide sequence and expression of a novel human receptor-type tyrosine kinase gene (*flt*) closely related to the fms family. *Oncogene* **5:** 519–524.

Steele FR, Chader GJ, Johnson LV, Tombran-Tink J. 1993. Pigment epithelium-derived factor: Neurotrophic activity and identification as a member of the serine protease inhibitor gene family. *Proc Natl Acad Sci* **90:** 1526–1530.

Stellmach V, Crawford SE, Zhou W, Bouck N. 2001. Prevention of ischemia-induced retinopathy by the natural ocular antiangiogenic agent pigment epithelium-derived factor. *Proc Natl Acad Sci* **98:** 2593–2597.

Takahashi K, Saishin Y, Saishin Y, Lima SR, Oshima Y, Oshima S, Melia M, Paszkiet B, Zerby D, Kadan MJ, et al. 2003. Intraocular expression of endostatin reduces VEGF-induced retinal vascular permeability, neovascularization, and retinal detachment. *FASEB J* **17:** 896–898.

Tolentino MJ, Brucker AJ, Fosnot J, Ying GS, Wu IH, Malik G, Wan S, Reich SJ. 2004. Intravitreal injection of vascular endothelial growth factor small interfering RNA inhibits growth and leakage in a nonhuman primate, laser-induced model of choroidal neovascularization. *Retina* **24:** 132–138.

Tombran-Tink J, Chader GC, Johnson LV. 1991. PEDF: A pigment epithelium-derived factor with potent neuronal differentiative activity. *Exp Eye Res* **53:** 411–414.

Tuo J, Bojanowski CM, Zhou M, Shen D, Ross RJ, Rosenberg KI, Cameron DJ, Yin C, Kowalak JA, Zhuang Z, et al. 2007. Murine *Ccl2/Cx3cr1* deficiency results in retinal lesions mimicking human age-related macular degeneration. *Invest Ophthalmol Vis Sci* **48:** 3827–3836.

Tuo J, Pang JJ, Cao X, Shen D, Zhang J, Scaria A, Wadsworth SC, Pechan P, Boye SL, Hauswirth WW, et al. 2012. AAV5-mediated sFLT01 gene therapy arrests retinal lesions in $Ccl2^{-/-}/Cx3cr1^{-/-}$ mice. *Neurobiol Aging* **33:** 433.e1–10.

Ueno S, Pease ME, Wersinger DMB, Masuda T, Vinores SA, Licht T, Zack DJ, Quigley H, Keshet E, Campochiaro PA. 2008. Prolonged blockade of VEGF family members does not cause identifiable damage to retinal neurons or vessels. *J Cell Physiol* **217:** 13–22.

Yi X, Ogata N, Komada M, Yamamoto C, Takahashi K, Omori K, Uyama M. 1997. Vascular endothelial growth factor expression in choroidal neovascularization in rats. *Graefes Arch Clin Exp Ophthalmol* **235:** 313–319.

Yu MJ, Shen WY, Lai MC, Constable IJ, Rakoczy PE. 1999. Generation and characterization of a recombinant adenovirus expressing vascular endothelial growth factor for studies of neovascularization in the eye. *Aust N Z J Ophthalmol* **27:** 250–253.

Leber Congenital Amaurosis Caused by Mutations in *GUCY2D*

Shannon E. Boye

Department of Ophthalmology and Department of Molecular Genetics and Microbiology, University of Florida College of Medicine, Gainesville, Florida 32610

Correspondence: shannon.boye@eye.ufl.edu

Leber congenital amaurosis (LCA) is a clinically and genetically heterogeneous group of diseases that account for the most severe form of early-onset retinal dystrophy. Mutations in retinal guanylate cyclase-1 (*GUCY2D*) are associated with LCA1, a prevalent form. *GUCY2D* encodes guanylate cyclase-1 (GC1), a protein expressed in rod and cone photoreceptors that regulates cGMP and Ca^{2+} levels within these cells. LCA1 patients present with severely impaired vision, reduced, or ablated electroretinogram and nystagmus. Despite a high degree of visual disturbance, LCA1 patients retain normal photoreceptor laminar architecture, except for foveal cone outer segment abnormalities and, in some patients, foveal cone loss. This article will summarize clinical characterization of patients and proof of concept gene replacement studies in several animal models of GC1 deficiency, both of which have laid the groundwork for clinical application of a gene therapy for treatment of LCA1.

Leber congenital amaurosis (LCA) is a clinically and genetically heterogeneous group of early-onset blinding diseases (den Hollander et al. 2008). There are currently 18 genes known to be associated with LCA, each of which encodes a retinal protein with unique function. *Guanylate cyclase-1 (GUCY2D)* was the first gene found to be associated with the disease and was thus assigned the LCA1 locus (Perrault et al. 1996). Mutations in this gene are a leading cause of LCA, accounting for 10%–20% of all cases (Perrault et al. 2000). *GUCY2D* encodes guanylate cyclase-1 (GC1), a protein expressed exclusively in the outer segments of photoreceptors (predominantly cones) in the vertebrate retina (Fig. 1) (Dizhoor et al. 1994; Liu et al. 1994).

To understand why mutations in *GUCY2D* lead to disease, one must first understand how GC1 normally contributes to the ability to see. The process of vision begins with absorption of a photon of light by a visual pigment, rhodopsin or cone opsin, in the outer segments of rod and cone photoreceptors, respectively. This interaction initiates a biochemical cascade referred to as "phototransduction." On light stimulation, cyclic guanosine monophosphate (cGMP) is hydrolyzed by cGMP phophodiesterase, leading to closure of cGMP-gated channels, reduction of intracellular Ca^{2+} and hyperpolarization of the photoreceptor. It is this reduction of intracellular calcium/hyperpolarization that signals the "recovery phase" of phototransduction

Cite this article as *Cold Spring Harb Perspect Med* doi: 10.1101/cshperspect.a017350

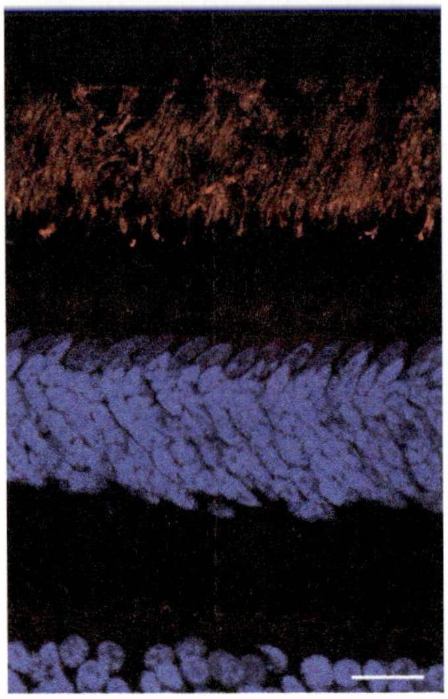

Figure 1. GC1 expression (red) in photoreceptor outer segments of a nonhuman primate retina. Frozen retinal cross sections were stained for GC1 and counterstained with DAPI. RPE, retinal pigment epithelium; OS, outer segments; IS, inner segments; ONL, outer nuclear layer; INL, inner nuclear layer. Scale bar, 7 μm.

and resets the sensitivity of photoreceptors. Photoreceptors of vertebrate species possess two guanylate cyclases (GC1 and GC2) (Lowe et al. 1995) and two guanylate cyclase activating proteins (GCAPs), GCAP1 and GCAP2 (Dizhoor et al. 1995; Gorczyca et al. 1995). GCAPs function as Ca^{2+} sensors that regulate activity of the guanylate cyclases. In the dark-adapted photoreceptor, Ca^{2+} binds GCAP1 and GCAP2, which collectively inhibit the activity of retinal GC1 and GC2. On light stimulation/hyperpolarization, Ca^{2+}-free GCAPs stimulate the activity of GCs, resulting in an increase in cGMP, reopening of the cGMP-gated channels, influx of Ca^{2+}, and return of the photoreceptor to its depolarized dark-state (Burns and Arshavsky 2005; Arshavsky and Burns 2012). In vivo, GC1 is the preferred target of GCAP1 (Olshevskaya et al. 2012). In vitro, however, GCAP1 and GCAP2 can activate both GCs, albeit with slightly different affinities and sensitivity to Ca^{2+} (Hwang et al. 2003; Peshenko and Dizhoor 2004; Peshenko et al. 2011). Mutations that reduce or abolish the ability of GC1 to replenish cGMP in photoreceptors are thought to lead to the biochemical equivalent of chronic light exposure in these cells. There are no reported cases of human disease involving mutations in *GUCY2F* (the gene encoding GC2). Deletion of GC2 from the rodent retina has little effect on retinal function (Baehr et al. 2007).

PATIENT CHARACTERIZATION

LCA1 patients present within the first year of life and are routinely described as having reduced visual acuity, reduced or nonrecordable electroretinogram (ERG) responses, nystagmus, digito-ocular signs, and apparently normal fundus (Perrault et al. 1999; Chung and Traboulsi 2009). Reports on the extent of photoreceptor degeneration associated with this disease have been conflicting. Histopathological analysis of two postmortem retinas (a 26-wk-old preterm abortus and a 12-yr-old donor) revealed signs of photoreceptor degeneration in both rods and cones (Milam et al. 2003; Porto et al. 2003). Later studies using state of the art, in-life imaging (i.e., optical coherence tomography) revealed no obvious degeneration in patients as old as 53 years of age (Simonelli et al. 2007; Pasadhika et al. 2010).

The most recent and thorough clinical characterization of LCA1 to date involved a cohort of patients ranging in age from 6 mo to 37 yr with different *GUCY2D* mutations, and has shed new light on the effects of GC1 deficiency on retinal structure and function (Jacobson et al. 2013). In agreement with previous imaging studies (Simonelli et al. 2007; Pasadhika et al. 2010), Jacobson et al. (2013) report that LCA1 patients retain normal photoreceptor laminar architecture aside from foveal cone outer segment abnormalities and, in a few patients, foveal cone loss. Outer nuclear layer and photoreceptor outer segment thickness measurements in the rod-dominant retina (i.e., outside the fovea) were normal in all patients evaluated. Contrary to previous ERG findings, Jacobson et al. report that substantial rod function can be retained in LCA1. Under dark-adapted conditions, rod sensitivity thresholds in the majority of patients were approximately 0.5 to 5 log units below that of normal. Full-field stimulus testing using blue stimuli to isolate rod responses revealed that substantial rod function remained. There was no relationship between patient age and presence of rod function. Patients with retained rod function successfully avoided obstacles in a dimly lit mobility course, revealing that rod function translates to useful vision in these cases. In contrast to the findings for the rods, ERG analysis revealed that cone function was undetectable in all LCA1 patients evaluated. Psychophysical tests revealed that the majority of patients lacked cone-mediated vision. This correlated with severely reduced visual acuity and a lack of color perception. Full-field stimulus testing, microperimetry and mobility tests revealed that a small subset of patients (four out of 11) had detectable but reduced cone function, with central fixation and some color perception.

To understand why residual, yet abnormal, cone function remained in only a subset of LCA1 patients, an elegant biochemical analysis of GC activity was performed. Human embryonic kidney (HEK293) cells were transfected with either wild-type or patient-specific GC1 mutants. Activity assays were performed by supplying cells with GCAPs under ionic conditions best suited for GC1 activity (Jacobson et al. 2013). The amount of cGMP produced by each mutant was quantified and compared relative to that produced by wild-type GC1. Not surprisingly, mutants showing biochemical evidence of catalytic activity in vitro were those expressed by patients with measurable cone function. Of these mutants, some had reduced catalytic activity (four- to fivefold lower than wild-type), whereas others demonstrated no loss-of-function in vitro. These mutations might cause defective folding, altered expression or impaired trafficking to the proper compartment of the living photoreceptor, the outer segment. However, definitive conclusions cannot be drawn until in vivo studies are performed. As expected "null" mutations that rendered GC1 biochemically inactive corresponded to patients with profound loss of cone function (Jacobson et al. 2013).

Taken together, it is now apparent that *GUCY2D*-LCA1 is unique from other forms of LCA studied in detail to date (Jacobson et al. 1998, 2003, 2005, 2007a,b, 2009, 2011; Cideciyan et al. 2007). The hallmark retinal preservation observed suggests that LCA1 is an attractive target for gene augmentation therapy and that patient retinas may better withstand the surgical manipulation of a subretinal injection. The profound visual impairment, stemming predominantly from a loss of cone function, points to the fovea as the target for treatment. In the minority of patients lacking foveal cones, the parafoveal or perifoveal retina may be targeted in the hopes that eccentric fixation will occur, as was seen in some patients in LCA2 clinical trials (Cideciyan et al. 2009). Careful consideration must be given to outcome measures when treating patients with such profound visual impairment. Tests, which control for nystagmus, such as microperimetry, can be used to assess cone-mediated central vision (Cideciyan et al. 2012), along with standard visual acuity measurements. Full-field stimulus testing, an assay for which the limits of variability have been defined in LCA patients, can be used to identify any localized improvements in rod function. Optical coherence tomography can be used both to monitor the safety of subfoveal injection and to look for any improvements in cone outer segment morphology following treatment.

PROOF OF CONCEPT STUDIES IN ANIMAL MODELS OF GC1 DEFICIENCY

Work to characterize multiple animal models of GC1 deficiency began in the 1980s. Thirty-four years later, all models have been successfully used to evaluate proof of concept for gene replacement to treat *GUCY2D*-LCA1. Below is a summary of findings for each model.

GUCY1*B Chicken

The *retinal degeneration (rd)* chicken, also referred to as the GUCY1*B chicken, was the first animal model of GC1 deficiency to be described (Cheng et al. 1980; Ulshafer et al. 1984; Ulshafer and Allen 1985a,b). This naturally occurring, cone-dominant, avian model carries a deletion/insertion mutation in the gene encoding

GC1. Exons 4–7 of the gene are replaced by an 81 bp fragment with 89% sequence identity to a portion of exon 9, in reverse orientation (Table 1). Although its reading frame is not disrupted, the mutant protein is predicted to lack a membrane spanning domain, the region essential for proper folding and enzyme activity (Polans et al. 1996). Antibodies raised against epitopes outside this deletion failed to detect any mutant protein expression in GUCY1*B chickens, suggesting that the protein is rapidly degraded. It is therefore considered to be a null allele (Semple-Rowland et al. 1998). Cyclic GMP levels in photoreceptors of posthatch day 1 GUCY1*B chickens are only ~10%–20% of those observed in age-matched, wild-type controls. Affected chickens are blind at hatch, lacking any signs of reflexive or volitional behavior, and have nonrecordable ERG responses (Ulshafer et al. 1984). The reduction in cGMP and lack of visual behavior/retinal function are evident before loss of photoreceptors, which do not begin degenerating until 1 wk posthatch (Cheng et al. 1980; Ulshafer et al. 1984). Photoreceptor loss proceeds from the central to the peripheral retina (Ulshafer and Allen 1985a). Cones, which degenerate first, are completely lost by ~3.5 mo. Rod loss follows, with all photoreceptors lost by ~8 mo (Ulshafer and Allen 1985a,b).

Table 1. Genetic bases for disease in animal models of LCA1

	Mutation	Effects on GC1 protein
GUCY1*B chicken	Naturally occurring deletion/ insertion: Exons 4–7 replaced by an 81 bp fragment with homology with sequence in exon 9, in reverse orientation	No functional enzyme produced, null
GC1KO mouse	Engineered: Disruption of exon 5 (transmembrane domain region) with neomycin resistance cassette	No functional enzyme produced, null
GC1/GC2 DKO mouse	Mouse engineered: Disruption of exon 2 (containing translation start codon and peptide leader sequence) with neomycin resistance cassette. Mice then crossed to GC1KO	No functional enzyme produced, null also no functional GC2

With the goal of providing therapy as early as possible, an in ovo treatment paradigm was developed to treat the GUCY1*B chicken. For its ability to stably transduce retinal progenitor cells (Miyoshi et al. 1997), HIV-1-based lentivirus was used to deliver a cDNA encoding bovine GC1 to the neural tube of embryonic day 2 chickens via a small, 5 mm opening in the eggshell and membrane overlying the embryo (Williams et al. 2006; Semple-Rowland and Berry 2013). The therapeutic vector was bicistronic, with GC1 expression mediated by the ubiquitous elongation factor 1α promoter and enhanced green fluorescent protein (GFP) expression coupled to a poliovirus internal ribosome entry site (Williams et al. 2006). Enhanced green fluorescent protein was included in the vector because GC1 expression cannot be reliably detected in the chicken retina. The activity of bovine GC1 in the presence of chicken GCAPs was verified in vitro before treatment (Williams et al. 2006). Posthatch chicks were subjected to behavioral analyses and ERG, and their tissues were subsequently collected for histological and molecular analyses.

Treated GUCY1*B chickens were tested for the presence of an optokinetic reflex (Wallman and Velez 1985) and volitional visual behavior beginning at 3–7 d posthatch and every few days thereafter until ~5 wk of age (Williams et al. 2006). Results were compared with those seen in untreated GUCY1*B and wild-type controls. Six of the seven treated chickens showed some degree of sight during the course of the study, and five of these six showed optokinetic reflexes and volitional visual behavior up to the end of the study; in the sixth, visual function decreased during the last week of the study. ERG analyses revealed that the five treated chickens that showed sighted behavior at the end of the study displayed modest increases in a- and b-wave amplitudes (to 6% of wild-type) under both dark- and light-adapted conditions. Quantitative genomic PCR revealed the presence of integrated transgenes in all six retinas from the treated birds that had shown sight, and that the transcript number was correlated with the degree of treatment effect. Immunohistochemical analysis of GFP expression in treated retinas revealed spotty expression of transgene throughout the photoreceptor cell bodies and possibly inner and outer segments. Histological analysis of treated, untreated, and wild-type retinas revealed that lentiviral-mediated GC1 expression slowed but did not prevent photoreceptor degeneration in affected chickens.

Results of this GUCY1*B chicken study were exciting proof of concept, albeit in a nonmammalian model, that gene replacement could be effective for treatment of LCA1. However, rescue effects noted in this and a more recent study incorporating a modified, bicistronic lentiviral vector were transient, with data only reported out to 5 wk posthatch (Williams et al. 2006; Verrier et al. 2011). Indeed, the therapeutic effect observed by Williams et al. was transient, with behavioral responses disappearing in treated GUCY1*B chickens beyond the time points discussed in that study (unpublished findings). Furthermore, results in the chicken studies were obtained following embryonic vector delivery, a currently untenable task in patients. Neural tube delivery did not allow for evaluation of an internal, untreated control because both retinas were transduced. Last, lentiviral vectors, although useful for transduction of retinal precursors, have demonstrated little to no ability to transduce the disease target in LCA1-postmitotic photoreceptors (Miyoshi et al. 1997; Bainbridge et al. 2001; Pang et al. 2006). Taken together, this highlighted the need for a more translatable animal model and gene replacement strategy with which to address a treatment for this disease.

GC1KO Mouse

In 1999, the Garbers laboratory published natural history data on the first engineered, mammalian model of GC1 deficiency, the *Gucy2e*^{tm1Gar} mouse, which is commonly referred to as the GC1 knockout (GC1KO) mouse (Yang et al. 1999). Insertion of a neomycin resistance cassette into exon 5 of *Gucy2e* (the murine homolog of *GUCY2D*) truncates GC1, rendering it null (Table 1). Western blot analysis confirmed the absence of GC1 protein and that levels of GC2 remained unchanged. Cone photoreceptors in the GC1KO mouse degenerate rapidly beginning at 4–5 wk, at a rate comparable to that seen in the GUCY1*B chicken. Loss of cone function precedes cone degeneration; cone-mediated ERG responses are barely detectable at this age. Rods do not degenerate, however, and continue to respond to light, albeit with variable and reduced amplitudes (30%–50% of wild-type). It is now known that this residual rod function is attributed to the presence of GC2 in these cells (Baehr et al. 2007). Subsequent immunohistochemical analyses of this mouse model revealed that both GCAP1 and GCAP2 are down-regulated in 4-wk-old GC1KO retinas, and GCAP1 expression is undetectable in photoreceptor outer segments of frozen retinal sections (Coleman et al. 2004). Additionally, it was found that cone arrestin translocation, a biochemical correlate of functionality, is disrupted in GC1KO cones, further supporting the notion that these cells are unable to reset their light signaling cascade (Coleman and Semple-Rowland 2005).

For its proven ability to transduce postmitotic rodent photoreceptors following subretinal injection (Yang et al. 2002), a serotype 5 adeno-associated virus (AAV5) was chosen to deliver therapeutic cDNA to the GC1KO mouse. Initial experiments, conducted by some of the same investigators working on the chicken model, also incorporated a bovine GC1 cDNA (Haire et al. 2006). Cell-specific (mouse opsin) and ubiquitous (smCBA, a truncated version of the CBA promoter, which is a fusion of the chicken β-actin promoter and the CMV immediate-early cytomegalovirus enhancer) promoters were selected to drive transgene expression

(Haire et al. 2006). Treatment by subretinal injection at postnatal day (P) 21 with either AAV5-MOP-b*Gucy2d* or AAV5-smCBA-b*Gucy2d* ($\sim 1 \times 10^9$ vg delivered) failed to restore rod or cone function to treated GC1KO mice, as assessed by full-field ERG (Haire et al. 2006). The only therapeutic effect observed in this initial experiment was a restoration of light-driven arrestin translocation in cone photoreceptors expressing AAV-mediated bGC1 (Haire et al. 2006).

In subsequent experiments, Boye et al. explored whether the lack of robust rescue noted above was owing to the species nonspecific nature of the delivered transgene. Indeed, subretinal delivery of murine *Gucy2e* with AAV5 containing either the smCBA or photoreceptor-specific, human rhodopsin kinase (hGRK1) promoter (Khani et al. 2007) led to robust rescue of the GC1KO phenotype (AAV5-smCBA-*Gucy2e*, 4×10^{10} vg delivered; AAV5-hGRK1-*Gucy2e*, 4×10^{10} vg delivered; [Boye et al. 2010]). AAV-mediated GC1 expression was found exclusively in rods and cones of treated mice, and cone photoreceptors were preserved during the course of the 3-mo study. Cone-mediated ERG was stably restored to ~45% of wild-type. Treated mice also showed cone-mediated visual behavior (optokinetic reflex) that was identical to that seen in wild-type mice. Rod-mediated behavior was not evaluated because of the residual function of this cell type in this model. This was the first demonstration of gene-based restoration of visual function/visually guided behavior and cone preservation in a mammalian model of LCA1, and thus it laid the groundwork for development of an AAV-based gene therapy for treatment of this disease.

Two follow-up studies conducted by Mihelec et al. and Boye et al. evaluated whether AAV-mediated gene replacement was therapeutic in the GC1KO mouse for >3 mo (Boye et al. 2011; Mihelec et al. 2011). Mihelec et al. demonstrated that an AAV8 vector containing the hGRK1 promoter and human *GUCY2D* cDNA effectively rescued the GC1KO mouse phenotype following subretinal injection at P10 (Mihelec et al. 2011). Two vector doses were used: a low dose of 2.1×10^8 vg delivered and a high dose of 1.2×10^{10} vg delivered. Rescue effects were assayed during the course of 6 mo. GC1 expression was found exclusively in rod/cone outer segments (Mihelec et al. 2011). Cone transducin α expression was increased, its localization to outer segments was restored, and cone photoreceptors were preserved in treated eyes for at least 6 mo (Mihelec et al. 2011). Cone function (as measured by ERG) was restored to ~20% or ~65% of wild-type following injection with low and high doses of vector, respectively. Rod function was not improved following treatment with the low dose, but was restored to 65%–100% of wild-type following injection with the high dose of vector (Mihelec et al. 2011). Incorporation of murine *Gucy2e* cDNA into AAV8-hGRK1 led to similar improvements in rod- and cone-mediated function at the high dose. Cone-mediated visual behavior (optokinetic reflex) was also significantly improved in mice treated with the high dose of vector. It is important to note, given the translational potential of this project, that these robust therapeutic effects were achieved following delivery of the human *GUCY2D* cDNA (Mihelec et al. 2011).

In the longest follow up reported to date, Boye et al. showed that subretinal delivery of AAV5-smCBA-*Gucy2e* (4×10^9 vg delivered), AAV5-hGRK1-*Gucy2e* (4×10^{10} vg delivered) and AAV8(Y733F)-hGRK1-*Gucy2e* (1×10^{10} vg delivered) in GC1KO mice (P14–P25) restored retinal function and preserved cone photoreceptors for at least 1 yr after treatment (Boye et al. 2011). The tyrosine capsid mutant AAV8(Y733F) was chosen for its improved performance relative to standard AAV8 or AAV5 in other mouse models of inherited retinal disease (Pang et al. 2011). Cones were preserved and cone-mediated ERGs were stably restored to ~45% of wild-type following treatment. AAV8(Y733F) mediated more robust ERG improvements than did either AAV5-based vector (Boye et al. 2011). Reasons for this could include the ability of AAV8-based vectors to spread beyond the injection bleb (i.e., a greater percentage of retina was transduced with this serotype) (Stieger et al. 2008), or the relative speed of transgene expression mediated by this serotype (i.e., faster onset of GC1 expression-enhanced rescue) (Petrs-Silva et al. 2009; Pang et al. 2011). Between 7 mo and 1 yr posttreatment, optic nerves and brains were analyzed for the presence of AAV5 or AAV8(Y733F) vector genomes. Whereas GC1 expression was restricted to photoreceptor outer segments, both AAV5 and AAV8(Y733F) genomes were detected in optic nerves and, in one case, the brains of treated mice. AAV8(Y733F) genomes were more abundant in the optic nerve, a result likely owed to the increased affinity of this serotype for retinal ganglion cells relative to AAV5 (Surace and Auricchio 2008; Petrs-Silva et al. 2009). Some exposure of vector to ganglion cells is expected as the syringe transverses the inner retina during subretinal injection and also because the ratio of injection volume to total eye size is high in the mouse.

One notable difference between the Boye et al. 2011 and Mihelec et al. studies was the level of functional rescue achieved. Cone-mediated ERG responses were 45% versus 65% of normal, respectively (Boye et al. 2011; Mihelec et al. 2011). In addition, only Mihelec et al. reported any significant improvements in rod function (Mihelec et al. 2011). These differences are likely attributed to the age at which therapeutic vector was delivered. Boye et al. administered vector to P14–P25 mice, after their eyes had opened naturally. Mihelec et al. administered vector at P10, before eye opening. Earlier intervention was likely more effective at combating the effects of chronic hyperpolarization that GC1KO photoreceptors endure on light stimulation. Regardless of differences in ERG improvements, treatment of GC1KO mice at all time points, with all serotypes and cDNAs tested, resulted in restoration of useful cone-mediated vision in both studies (Boye et al. 2011; Mihelec et al. 2011). Taken together, these long term studies strongly support further development of an AAV-based gene replacement therapy for LCA1.

GC1/GC2 Double Knockout (GCDKO) Mouse

The GCDKO mouse was engineered by Baehr et al. to analyze the individual contributions of GC1 and GC2 to phototransduction, and its preliminary natural history was published in 2007 (Table 1) (Baehr et al. 2007). Proof that GC2 supports 30%–50% of rod function and prevents rod degeneration in the GC1KO mouse was found via this model, as deletion of both GC1 and GC2 in the GCDKO mice renders both rod and cone photoreceptors nonfunctional (unrecordable ERG) and degenerative. Both GCAP1 and GCAP2 are down-regulated and mislocalized, and all subunits of cGMP phophodiesterase 6 are absent from GCDKO rods (Baehr et al. 2007). Cones lack cone transducin, cone cGMP phophodiesterase, and GRK1, and opsins are down-regulated and mislocalized. Down-regulation of phototransduction proteins was shown to be posttranslational, suggesting a role for GCs in the stability and/or transport of these proteins. Cone outer segments are unstable and begin to "disintegrate" (extracellular particles immunopositive for cone proteins appear adjacent to the retinal pigment epithelium) at two months of age. Overall outer segment lengths are reduced by 30%–50% in 2-mo-old mice. Appreciable thinning of the outer nuclear layer does not occur until about 3.5 to 4 mo (Boye et al. 2013). By 6 mo, only four to six nuclei remain in the outer nuclear layer (Boye et al. 2013).

The GCDKO mouse is an attractive model in which to evaluate GC1 gene replacement for two reasons. First, before its 2013 clinical characterization (Jacobson et al. 2013), multiple reports described that both cone/rod structure and cone/rod function were compromised in LCA1 (Milam et al. 2003; Porto et al. 2003), suggesting that the best model of this disease was one in which both photoreceptor subclasses were nonfunctional/degenerative. Although the GC1KO mouse is useful for evaluating therapeutic benefit to cones (Boye et al. 2010, 2011; Mihelec et al. 2011), residual rod function and preservation of rod structure in this model complicates the ability to evaluate rod therapy. The GCDKO mouse affords the opportunity to evaluate therapeutic effects on both photoreceptor subclasses. More importantly, because the GCDKO mouse lacks all retinal GC activity, it allows for testing the functional efficiency of AAV-delivered GC1. GC activity assays performed on retinal tissue cannot discriminate between cGMP produced by GC1 versus GC2. Therefore, isolating the functional efficiency of exogenous GC1 requires delivery to photoreceptors that lack endogenous GC1 and GC2. Such analysis in the GCDKO mouse would be useful as a bioassay for evaluating relative potency of clinical vectors.

Boye et al. subretinally delivered AAV (Y733F) containing the hGRK1 promoter and *Gucy2e* cDNA to GCDKO mice of various ages, ranging from P18–P108 (Boye et al. 2013). Cone-mediated ERG responses were restored to between 29%–42% of wild-type following late (P108) versus early (P18) treatment, respectively. The level of cone function achieved following early treatment is comparable to that achieved in the GC1KO mouse (Boye et al. 2010, 2011, 2013). Rod-mediated ERGs were restored to between 29%–44% of wild-type following late (P108) versus early (P18) treatment, respectively (Boye et al. 2013). This result extends the Mihelec et al. findings (Mihelec et al. 2011) by demonstrating that restoration of rod function is achievable in a model with physiologically "silent" rods. Both cone and rod responses were stable during the course of the long term study (1 yr posttreatment). Optokinetic reflex and Morris water maze tests were used to assay the presence of subcortically and cortically driven visual behavior, respectively, in GCDKO mice treated between P18 and P49. Optokinetic testing showed no significant difference in cone-mediated spatial frequency or contrast sensitivity between 1-yr-old treated GCDKO mice and age-matched wild-type controls (Boye et al. 2013). Morris water maze testing revealed no significant difference in cone- and rod- mediated behavior between 1-yr-old treated GCDKO mice and age-matched wild-type controls. Taken together, these tests show that postnatal AAV-*Gucy2e* treatment restores useful cone and rod-mediated vision in this model of LCA1. As in the GC1KO mouse, wild-type-like behavior was achieved in GCDKO mice that showed only partial ERG recovery. Optical coherence tomography was used to monitor the rate of photoreceptor degeneration in treated and untreated GCDKO and age-matched wild-type controls over time. By 7–12 mo posttreatment, significant structural preservation was seen in all treatment groups, barring the oldest (P108) cohort. Although the difference was not significant following late treatment, outer nuclear layer thickness in this group was still greater than that seen in untreated GCDKO mice. The rate of photoreceptor cell loss in GCDKO mice treated as late as P49 was comparable to the natural rate of loss in age-matched wild-type controls. As before, histological analyses confirmed that GC1 was restricted to photoreceptor outer segments and that cone photoreceptor morphology and density were preserved during the long term. Wild-type-like levels of GCAP1 and GCAP2 expression were observed in a P40-treated GCDKO mouse killed at one year of age, with expression predominantly restricted to photoreceptor outer segments. S-opsin and M-opsin were present in cones of treated mice whereas they were absent from untreated controls.

To determine the functional efficiency of the AAV-delivered GC1 enzyme, GC activity assays were performed using GCDKO retinas treated at P30–P60 with either AAV8(Y733F)-*Gucy2e* or control AAV-GFP, untreated GCDKO retinas and age-matched wild-type control retinas (Boye et al. 2013). Because GC2 is lacking from GCDKO samples, GC activity solely represents the activity of AAV-delivered GC1. Maximal GC activity in treated mice was restored to ~63% of normal (Boye et al. 2013). If the known contribution of GC2 to total GC activity in wild-type mice—20%–28% (Peshenko et al. 2011)—is subtracted from this value, levels of GC1 activity in treated GCDKO mice approach ~90% of normal. Because the area of AAV-mediated transgene expression in treated retinas is known to correspond to the area of retinal detachment (Timmers et al. 2001; Cideciyan et al. 2008), and because a "good" subretinal injection typically detaches 80%–90% of the retina, this level of GC1 activity suggests near-complete restoration for the area exposed to vector. Normalization of the maximal GC activity in wild-type and AAV-*Gucy2e*-treated GCDKO mice revealed that the calcium sensitivities for endogenous and exogenous GC were identical (Boye et al. 2013). The functional efficiency of the

AAV-delivered GC1 enzyme was therefore normal. This assay will likely be used in future experiments to evaluate the functional efficiency of GC1 encoded by human *GUCY2D* and to establish dose-response relationships in the GCDKO mouse.

CONCLUDING REMARKS

Several decisions must be made as we move beyond the aforementioned proof-of-concept studies and into the clinic. Which AAV serotype-promoter combination should be used? Which is the preferred injection route? What is the safest and most effective dose?

The answers to the first two questions are inextricably linked. Viral serotype choice is dependent on the route of administration, as transduction profiles vary greatly depending on where the vector is placed within the eye (Dalkara et al. 2009; Vandenberghe and Auricchio 2012). The route of administration is ideally dictated by the structural integrity of the retina, with subretinal injections considered "safer" under relatively less degenerated tissue that is able to withstand the impact of surgical detachment. The notable retinal preservation reported by Jacobson et al. (2013) suggests that LCA1 patients are good candidates for subretinal injection. The AAV serotypes used in proof-of-concept LCA1 studies, AAV5 and AAV8, have proven utility following subretinal injection in various mouse and dog models of photoreceptor-mediated disease (Min et al. 2005; Alexander et al. 2007; Boye et al. 2010, 2013; Gorbatyuk et al. 2010; Komaromy et al. 2010; Mao et al. 2011; Pang et al. 2011, 2012; Yao et al. 2011; Beltran et al. 2012). Because transduction can vary across species, it is essential to evaluate vectors in a species as closely related to man as possible. Toward this end, the transduction profiles of AAV5 and AAV8 have recently been described in nonhuman primates. Keeping in mind that the primary target in LCA1 is the central, cone-rich retina, focus must be placed on each serotype's ability to transduce cone photoreceptors. Only partial cone transduction was achieved following subretinal delivery of elevated doses of AAV8-CMV-GFP (10^{11} vg delivered) in nonhuman primates (Vandenberghe et al. 2011, 2013). At a lower dose (10^{10} vg delivered), this serotype failed to transduce foveal, parafoveal, or perifoveal cones (Vandenberghe et al. 2011). In contrast, foveal, parafoveal, perifoveal, and peripheral cones of nonhuman primates were all effectively transduced following subretinal delivery of AAV5-hGRK1-GFP (10^{10} vg delivered) (Boye et al. 2012). As in rodent retinas (Khani et al. 2007; Tan et al. 2009; Boye et al. 2010, 2011; Pawlyk et al. 2010; Sun et al. 2010), hGRK1 has exclusive activity in cones and rods of nonhuman primates (Boye et al. 2012). Taken together, these results support the use of a subretinally delivered AAV5 vector containing the hGRK1 promoter for delivering *GUCY2D* in a clinical setting.

Several major differences exist between *GUCY2D*-LCA1 and the form of this disease currently being treated in clinic (*RPE65*-LCA2). First, a large animal model only exists for the latter. The availability of the RPE65-deficient dog model allowed for correlations to be made between vector dose, efficacy, toxicity, and biodistribution (spread of vector genomes beyond the subretinal space) in an organism relatively similar in size (Jacobson et al. 2006a). This formed the framework for safety studies performed in normal nonhuman primates in which relationships between vector dose and toxicity/biodistribution were evaluated (Jacobson et al. 2006b). For LCA1, correlations between vector dose and efficacy are currently limited to the GC1KO and/or GCDKO mouse models. As in LCA2, relationships between vector dose and toxicity/biodistribution must be determined in nonhuman primates.

Another major difference between LCA1 and LCA2 is the disease target. LCA2 arises from defects in a protein expressed exclusively in the retinal pigment epithelium (RPE65). Of the proteins encoded by genes known to be associated with LCA—18 to date (den Hollander et al. 2008; Wang et al. 2009; Estrada-Cuzcano et al. 2011; Sergouniotis et al. 2011)—only a minority (four) are specific to the retinal pigment epithelium. The majority of LCAs (13 out of 18) are caused by defects in genes that encode photoreceptor specific proteins. More broadly, the majority of inherited retinal diseases are caused by defects in proteins expressed in photoreceptors (Wright et al. 2010), a cell type yet to be targeted in a clinical setting. Thus, developing a treatment for *GUCY2D*-LCA1 will serve as a framework for other photoreceptor-targeted gene replacement strategies.

The primary functional deficit in LCA1 (cone-mediated vision) differs from that of LCA2 (rod-mediated vision). The majority of LCA1 patients lack cone function and show severe loss of visual acuity, despite retaining foveal architecture. It is unclear how amblyopia (the inability of the retina to send visual information to the brain) in both eyes will affect patients' responses to *GUCY2D* gene replacement. It is possible that gene therapy will restore the cones' ability to reset their sensitivity (return to the dark state)/depolarize, but that this information will not be properly relayed to visual processing centers of the brain. Understanding how brains of LCA1 patients, the majority of whom have functionally silent cones, will accommodate *GUCY2D* gene replacement will only be accomplished through a clinical trial.

ACKNOWLEDGMENTS

I would like to thank Sanford L. Boye, M.S. for his thoughtful critique of this collection article and Jim Peterson, Ph.D., RN for his assistance with immunohistochemical analysis of the primate retina.

REFERENCES

Alexander JJ, Umino Y, Everhart D, Chang B, Min SH, Li Q, Timmers AM, Hawes NL, Pang JJ, Barlow RB, et al. 2007. Restoration of cone vision in a mouse model of achromatopsia. *Nat Med* **13:** 685–687.

Arshavsky VY, Burns ME. 2012. Photoreceptor signaling: Supporting vision across a wide range of light intensities. *J Biol Chem* **287:** 1620–1626.

Baehr W, Karan S, Maeda T, Luo DG, Li S, Bronson JD, Watt CB, Yau KW, Frederick JM, Palczewski K. 2007. The function of guanylate cyclase 1 and guanylate cyclase 2 in rod and cone photoreceptors. *J Biol Chem* **282:** 8837–8847.

Bainbridge JW, Stephens C, Parsley K, Demaison C, Halfyard A, Thrasher AJ, Ali RR. 2001. In vivo gene transfer to the mouse eye using an HIV-based lentiviral vector; efficient long-term transduction of corneal endothelium and retinal pigment epithelium. *Gene Ther* **8:** 1665–1668.

Beltran WA, Cideciyan AV, Lewin AS, Iwabe S, Khanna H, Sumaroka A, Chiodo VA, Fajardo DS, Roman AJ, Deng WT, et al. 2012. Gene therapy rescues photoreceptor blindness in dogs and paves the way for treating human X-linked retinitis pigmentosa. *Proc Natl Acad Sci* **109:** 2132–2137.

Boye SE, Boye SL, Pang J, Ryals R, Everhart D, Umino Y, Neeley AW, Besharse J, Barlow R, Hauswirth WW. 2010. Functional and behavioral restoration of vision by gene therapy in the guanylate cyclase-1 (GC1) knockout mouse. *PLoS ONE* **5:** e11306.

Boye SL, Conlon T, Erger K, Ryals R, Neeley A, Cossette T, Pang J, Dyka FM, Hauswirth WW, Boye SE. 2011. Long-term preservation of cone photoreceptors and restoration of cone function by gene therapy in the guanylate cyclase-1 knockout (GC1KO) mouse. *Invest Ophthalmol Vis Sci* **52:** 7098–7108.

Boye SE, Alexander JJ, Boye SL, Witherspoon CD, Sandefer KJ, Conlon TJ, Erger K, Sun J, Ryals R, Chiodo VA, et al. 2012. The human rhodopsin kinase promoter in an AAV5 vector confers rod- and cone-specific expression in the primate retina. *Hum Gene Ther* **23:** 1101–1115.

Boye SL, Peshenko IV, Huang WC, Min SH, McDoom I, Kay CN, Liu X, Dyka FM, Foster TC, Umino Y, et al. 2013. AAV-mediated gene therapy in the guanylate cyclase (RetGC1/RetGC2) double knockout mouse model of Leber congenital amaurosis. *Hum Gene Ther* **24:** 189–202.

Burns ME, Arshavsky VY. 2005. Beyond counting photons: Trials and trends in vertebrate visual transduction. *Neuron* **48:** 387–401.

Chung DC, Traboulsi EI. 2009. Leber congenital amaurosis: Clinical correlations with genotypes, gene therapy trials update, and future directions. *J AAPOS* **13:** 587–592.

Cheng KM, Shoffner RN, Gelatt KN, Gum GG, Otis JS, Bitgood JJ. 1980. An autosomal recessive blind mutant in the chicken. *Poult Sci* **59:** 2179–2181.

Cideciyan AV, Aleman TS, Jacobson SG, Khanna H, Sumaroka A, Aguirre GK, Schwartz SB, Windsor EA, He S, Chang B, et al. 2007. Centrosomal-ciliary gene *CEP290/NPHP6* mutations result in blindness with unexpected sparing of photoreceptors and visual brain: Implications for therapy of Leber congenital amaurosis. *Hum Mutat* **28:** 1074–1083.

Cideciyan AV, Aleman TS, Boye SL, Schwartz SB, Kaushal S, Roman AJ, Pang JJ, Sumaroka A, Windsor EA, Wilson JM, et al. 2008. Human gene therapy for RPE65 isomerase deficiency activates the retinoid cycle of vision but with slow rod kinetics. *Proc Natl Acad Sci* **105:** 15112–15117.

Cideciyan AV, Hauswirth WW, Aleman TS, Kaushal S, Schwartz SB, Boye SL, Windsor EA, Conlon TJ, Sumaroka A, Roman AJ, et al. 2009. Vision 1 year after gene therapy for Leber's congenital amaurosis. *N Engl J Med* **361:** 725–727.

Cideciyan AV, Swider M, Aleman TS, Feuer WJ, Schwartz SB, Russell RC, Steinberg JD, Stone EM, Jacobson SG. 2012. Macular function in macular degenerations: Repeatability of microperimetry as a potential outcome measure for *ABCA4*-associated retinopathy trials. *Invest Ophthalmol Vis Sci* **53:** 841–852.

Coleman JE, Semple-Rowland SL. 2005. GC1 deletion prevents light-dependent arrestin translocation in mouse cone photoreceptor cells. *Invest Ophthalmol Vis Sci* **46:** 12–16.

Coleman JE, Zhang Y, Brown GA, Semple-Rowland SL. 2004. Cone cell survival and downregulation of GCAP1 protein in the retinas of GC1 knockout mice. *Invest Ophthalmol Vis Sci* **45:** 3397–3403.

Dalkara D, Kolstad KD, Caporale N, Visel M, Klimczak RR, Schaffer DV, Flannery JG. 2009. Inner limiting membrane barriers to AAV-mediated retinal transduction from the vitreous. *Mol Ther* **17:** 2096–2102.

den Hollander AI, Roepman R, Koenekoop RK, Cremers FP. 2008. Leber congenital amaurosis: Genes, proteins and disease mechanisms. *Prog Retin Eye Res* **27:** 391–419.

Dizhoor AM, Lowe DG, Olshevskaya EV, Laura RP, Hurley JB. 1994. The human photoreceptor membrane guanylyl cyclase, RetGC, is present in outer segments and is regulated by calcium and a soluble activator. *Neuron* **12:** 1345–1352.

Dizhoor AM, Olshevskaya EV, Henzel WJ, Wong SC, Stults JT, Ankoudinova I, Hurley JB. 1995. Cloning, sequencing, and expression of a 24-kDa Ca^{2+}-binding protein activating photoreceptor guanylyl cyclase. *J Biol Chem* **270:** 25200–25206.

Estrada-Cuzcano A, Koenekoop RK, Coppieters F, Kohl S, Lopez I, Collin RW, De Baere EB, Roeleveld D, Marek J, Bernd A, et al. 2011. *IQCB1* mutations in patients with Leber congenital amaurosis. *Invest Ophthalmol Vis Sci* **52:** 834–839.

Gorbatyuk MS, Knox T, LaVail MM, Gorbatyuk SS, Noorwez SM, Hauswirth WW, Lin JH, Muzyczka N, Lewin AS. 2010. Restoration of visual function in P23H rhodopsin transgenic rats by gene delivery of BiP/Grp78. *Proc Natl Acad Sci* **107:** 5961–5966.

Gorczyca WA, Polans AS, Surgucheva IG, Subbaraya I, Baehr W, Palczewski K. 1995. Guanylyl cyclase activating protein. A calcium-sensitive regulator of phototransduction. *J Biol Chem* **270:** 22029–22036.

Haire SE, Pang J, Boye SE, Sokal I, Craft CM, Palczewski K, Hauswirth WW, Semple-Rowland SL. 2006. Light-driven cone arrestin translocation in cones of postnatal guanylate cyclase-1 knockout mouse retina treated with AAV-GC1. *Invest Ophthalmol Vis Sci* **47:** 3745–3753.

Hwang JY, Lange C, Helten A, Hoppner-Heitmann D, Duda T, Sharma RK, Koch KW. 2003. Regulatory modes of rod outer segment membrane guanylate cyclase differ in catalytic efficiency and Ca^{2+}-sensitivity. *Eur J Biochem* **270:** 3814–3821.

Jacobson SG, Cideciyan AV, Huang Y, Hanna DB, Freund CL, Affatigato LM, Carr RE, Zack DJ, Stone EM, McInnes RR. 1998. Retinal degenerations with truncation mutations in the cone-rod homeobox (*CRX*) gene. *Invest Ophthalmol Vis Sci* **39:** 2417–2426.

Jacobson SG, Cideciyan AV, Aleman TS, Pianta MJ, Sumaroka A, Schwartz SB, Smilko EE, Milam AH, Sheffield VC, Stone EM. 2003. *Crumbs homolog 1* (*CRB1*) mutations result in a thick human retina with abnormal lamination. *Hum Mol Genet* **12:** 1073–1078.

Jacobson SG, Aleman TS, Cideciyan AV, Sumaroka A, Schwartz SB, Windsor EA, Traboulsi EI, Heon E, Pittler SJ, Milam AH, et al. 2005. Identifying photoreceptors in blind eyes caused by *RPE65* mutations: Prerequisite for human gene therapy success. *Proc Natl Acad Sci* **102:** 6177–6182.

Jacobson SG, Acland GM, Aguirre GD, Aleman TS, Schwartz SB, Cideciyan AV, Zeiss CJ, Komaromy AM, Kaushal S, Roman AJ, et al. 2006a. Safety of recombinant adeno-associated virus type 2-*RPE65* vector delivered by ocular subretinal injection. *Mol Ther* **13:** 1074–1084.

Jacobson SG, Boye SL, Aleman TS, Conlon TJ, Zeiss CJ, Roman AJ, Cideciyan AV, Schwartz SB, Komaromy AM, Doobrajh M, et al. 2006b. Safety in nonhuman primates of ocular AAV2-*RPE65*, a candidate treatment for blindness in Leber congenital amaurosis. *Hum Gene Ther* **17:** 845–858.

Jacobson SG, Cideciyan AV, Aleman TS, Sumaroka A, Schwartz SB, Roman AJ, Stone EM. 2007a. Leber's congenital amaurosis caused by an *RPGRIP1* mutation shows treatment potential. *Ophthalmology* **114:** 895–898.

Jacobson SG, Cideciyan AV, Aleman TS, Sumaroka A, Schwartz SB, Windsor EA, Roman AJ, Heon E, Stone EM, Thompson DA. 2007b. *RDH12* and *RPE65*, visual cycle genes causing Leber congenital amaurosis, differ in disease expression. *Invest Ophthalmol Vis Sci* **48:** 332–338.

Jacobson SG, Aleman TS, Cideciyan AV, Sumaroka A, Schwartz SB, Windsor EA, Swider M, Herrera W, Stone EM. 2009. Leber congenital amaurosis caused by Lebercilin (*LCA5*) mutation: Retained photoreceptors adjacent to retinal disorganization. *Mol Vis* **15:** 1098–1106.

Jacobson SG, Cideciyan AV, Aleman TS, Sumaroka A, Roman AJ, Swider M, Schwartz SB, Banin E, Stone EM. 2011. Human retinal disease from *AIPL1* gene mutations: Foveal cone loss with minimal macular photoreceptors and rod function remaining. *Invest Ophthalmol Vis Sci* **52:** 70–79.

Jacobson SG, Cideciyan AV, Peshenko IV, Sumaroka A, Olshevskaya EV, Cao L, Schwartz SB, Roman AJ, Olivares MB, Sadigh S, et al. 2013. Determining consequences of retinal membrane guanylyl cyclase (RetGC1) deficiency in human Leber congenital amaurosis en route to therapy: Residual cone-photoreceptor vision correlates with biochemical properties of the mutants. *Hum Mol Genet* **22:** 168–183.

Khani SC, Pawlyk BS, Bulgakov OV, Kasperek E, Young JE, Adamian M, Sun X, Ali RR, Li T. 2007. AAV-mediated expression targeting of rod and cone photoreceptors with a human rhodopsin kinase promoter. *Invest Ophthalmol Vis Sci* **48:** 3954–3961.

Komaromy AM, Alexander JJ, Rowlan JS, Garcia MM, Chiodo VA, Kaya A, Tanaka JC, Acland GM, Hauswirth WW, Aguirre GD. 2010. Gene therapy rescues cone function in congenital achromatopsia. *Hum Mol Genet* **19:** 2581–2593.

Liu X, Seno K, Nishizawa Y, Hayashi F, Yamazaki A, Matsumoto H, Wakabayashi T, Usukura J. 1994. Ultrastructural localization of retinal guanylate cyclase in human and monkey retinas. *Exp Eye Res* **59:** 761–768.

Lowe DG, Dizhoor AM, Liu K, Gu Q, Spencer M, Laura R, Lu L, Hurley JB. 1995. Cloning and expression of a second photoreceptor-specific membrane retina guanylyl cyclase (RetGC), RetGC-2. *Proc Natl Acad Sci* **92:** 5535–5539.

Mao H, James T Jr, Schweln A, Shabashvili AE, Hauswirth WW, Gorbatyuk MS, Lewin AS. 2011. AAV delivery of wild-type rhodopsin preserves retinal function in a mouse model of autosomal dominant retinitis pigmentosa. *Hum Gene Ther* **22:** 567–575.

Mihelec M, Pearson RA, Robbie SJ, Buch PK, Azam SA, Bainbridge JW, Ali RR. 2011. Long-term preservation of cones and improvement in visual function following gene therapy in a mouse model of Leber congenital amaurosis caused by guanylate cyclase-1 deficiency. *Hum Gene Ther* **22:** 1179–1190.

Milam AH, Barakat MR, Gupta N, Rose L, Aleman TS, Pianta MJ, Cideciyan AV, Sheffield VC, Stone EM, Jacobson SG. 2003. Clinicopathologic effects of mutant *GUCY2D* in Leber congenital amaurosis. *Ophthalmology* **110:** 549–558.

Min SH, Molday LL, Seeliger MW, Dinculescu A, Timmers AM, Janssen A, Tonagel F, Tanimoto N, Weber BH, Molday RS, et al. 2005. Prolonged recovery of retinal structure/function after gene therapy in an *Rs1h*-deficient mouse model of X-linked juvenile retinoschisis. *Mol Ther* **12:** 644–651.

Miyoshi H, Takahashi M, Gage RH, Verma IM. 1997. Stable and efficient gene transfer into the retina using an HIV-based lentiviral vector. *Proc Natl Acad Sci* **94:** 10319–10323.

Olshevskaya EV, Peshenko IV, Savchenko AB, Dizhoor AM. 2012. Retinal guanylyl cyclase isozyme 1 is the preferential in vivo target for constitutively active GCAP1 mutants causing congenital degeneration of photoreceptors. *J Neurosci* **32:** 7208–7217.

Pang J, Cheng M, Haire SE, Barker E, Planelles V, Blanks JC. 2006. Efficiency of lentiviral transduction during development in normal and *rd* mice. *Mol Vis* **12:** 756–767.

Pang JJ, Dai X, Boye SE, Barone I, Boye SL, Mao S, Everhart D, Dinculescu A, Liu L, Umino Y, et al. 2011. Long-term retinal function and structure rescue using capsid mutant AAV8 vector in the *rd10* mouse, a model of recessive retinitis pigmentosa. *Mol Ther* **19:** 234–242.

Pang JJ, Deng WT, Dai X, Lei B, Everhart D, Umino Y, Li J, Zhang K, Mao S, Boye SL, et al. 2012. AAV-mediated cone rescue in a naturally occurring mouse model of CNGA3-achromatopsia. *PLoS ONE* **7:** e35250.

Pasadhika S, Fishman GA, Stone EM, Lindeman M, Zelkha R, Lopez I, Koenekoop RK, Shahidi M. 2010. Differential macular morphology in patients with *RPE65-*, *CEP290-*, *GUCY2D-*, and *AIPL1*-related Leber congenital amaurosis. *Invest Ophthalmol Vis Sci* **51:** 2608–2614.

Pawlyk BS, Bulgakov OV, Liu X, Xu X, Adamian M, Sun X, Khani SC, Berson EL, Sandberg MA, Li T. 2010. Replacement gene therapy with a human *RPGRIP1* sequence slows photoreceptor degeneration in a murine model of Leber congenital amaurosis. *Hum Gene Ther* **21:** 993–1004.

Perrault I, Rozet JM, Calvas P, Gerber S, Camuzat A, Dollfus H, Chatelin S, Souied E, Ghazi I, Leowski C, et al. 1996. Retinal-specific guanylate cyclase gene mutations in Leber's congenital amaurosis. *Nat Genet* **14:** 461–464.

Perrault I, Rozet JM, Gerber S, Ghazi I, Leowski C, Ducroq D, Souied E, Dufier JL, Munnich A, Kaplan J. 1999. Leber congenital amaurosis. *Mol Genet Metab* **68:** 200–208.

Perrault I, Rozet JM, Gerber S, Ghazi I, Ducroq D, Souied E, Leowski C, Bonnemaison M, Dufier JL, Munnich A, et al. 2000. Spectrum of *retGC1* mutations in Leber's congenital amaurosis. *Eur J Hum Genet* **8:** 578–582.

Peshenko IV, Dizhoor AM. 2004. Guanylyl cyclase-activating proteins (GCAPs) are Ca^{2+}/Mg^{2+} sensors: Implications for photoreceptor guanylyl cyclase (RetGC) regulation in mammalian photoreceptors. *J Biol Chem* **279:** 16903–16906.

Peshenko IV, Olshevskaya EV, Savchenko AB, Karan S, Palczewski K, Baehr W, Dizhoor AM. 2011. Enzymatic properties and regulation of the native isozymes of retinal membrane guanylyl cyclase (RetGC) from mouse photoreceptors. *Biochemistry* **50:** 5590–5600.

Petrs-Silva H, Dinculescu A, Li Q, Min SH, Chiodo V, Pang JJ, Zhong L, Zolotukhin S, Srivastava A, Lewin AS, et al. 2009. High-efficiency transduction of the mouse retina by tyrosine-mutant AAV serotype vectors. *Mol Ther* **17:** 463–471.

Polans A, Baehr W, Palczewski K. 1996. Turned on by Ca^{2+}! The physiology and pathology of Ca^{2+}-binding proteins in the retina. *Trends Neurosci* **19:** 547–554.

Porto FB, Perrault I, Hicks D, Rozet JM, Hanoteau N, Hanein S, Kaplan J, Sahel JA. 2003. Prenatal human ocular degeneration occurs in Leber's congenital amaurosis (LCA1 and 2). *Adv Exp Med Biol* **533:** 59–68.

Semple-Rowland SL, Berry J. 2013. Use of lentiviral vectors to deliver and express bicistronic transgenes in developing chicken embryos. *Methods* **66:** 466–473.

Semple-Rowland SL, Lee NR, Van Hooser JP, Palczewski K, Baehr W. 1998. A null mutation in the photoreceptor guanylate cyclase gene causes the retinal degeneration chicken phenotype. *Proc Natl Acad Sci* **95:** 1271–1276.

Sergouniotis PI, Davidson AE, Mackay DS, Li Z, Yang X, Plagnol V, Moore AT, Webster AR. 2011. Recessive mutations in *KCNJ13*, encoding an inwardly rectifying potassium channel subunit, cause Leber congenital amaurosis. *Am J Hum Genet* **89:** 183–190.

Simonelli F, Ziviello C, Testa F, Rossi S, Fazzi E, Bianchi PE, Fossarello M, Signorini S, Bertone C, Galantuomo S, et al. 2007. Clinical and molecular genetics of Leber's congenital amaurosis: A multicenter study of Italian patients. *Invest Ophthalmol Vis Sci* **48:** 4284–4290.

Stieger K, Colle MA, Dubreil L, Mendes-Madeira A, Weber M, Le MG, Deschamps JY, Provost N, Nivard D, Cherel Y, et al. 2008. Subretinal delivery of recombinant AAV serotype 8 vector in dogs results in gene transfer to neurons in the brain. *Mol Ther* **16:** 916–923.

Sun X, Pawlyk B, Xu X, Liu X, Bulgakov OV, Adamian M, Sandberg MA, Khani SC, Tan MH, Smith AJ, et al. 2010. Gene therapy with a promoter targeting both rods and cones rescues retinal degeneration caused by *AIPL1* mutations. *Gene Ther* **17:** 117–131.

Surace EM, Auricchio A. 2008. Versatility of AAV vectors for retinal gene transfer. *Vision Res* **48:** 353–359.

Tan MH, Smith AJ, Pawlyk B, Xu X, Liu X, Bainbridge JB, Basche M, McIntosh J, Tran HV, Nathwani A, et al. 2009. Gene therapy for retinitis pigmentosa and Leber congenital amaurosis caused by defects in *AIPL1*: Effective rescue of mouse models of partial and complete Aipl1 deficiency using AAV2/2 and AAV2/8 vectors. *Hum Mol Genet* **18:** 2099–2114.

Timmers AM, Zhang H, Squitieri A, Gonzalez-Pola C. 2001. Subretinal injections in rodent eyes: Effects on electrophysiology and histology of rat retina. *Mol Vis* **7:** 131–137.

Ulshafer RJ, Allen CB. 1985a. Hereditary retinal degeneration in the Rhode Island Red chicken: Ultrastructural analysis. *Exp Eye Res* **40:** 865–877.

Ulshafer RJ, Allen CB. 1985b. Ultrastructural changes in the retinal pigment epithelium of congenitally blind chickens. *Curr Eye Res* **4:** 1009–1021.

Ulshafer RJ, Allen C, Dawson WW, Wolf ED. 1984. Hereditary retinal degeneration in the Rhode Island Red chicken: I. Histology and ERG. *Exp Eye Res* **39:** 125–135.

Vandenberghe LH, Auricchio A. 2012. Novel adeno-associated viral vectors for retinal gene therapy. *Gene Ther* **19:** 162–168.

Vandenberghe LH, Bell P, Maguire AM, Cearley CN, Xiao R, Calcedo R, Wang L, Castle MJ, Maguire AC, Grant R, et al. 2011. Dosage thresholds for AAV2 and AAV8 photoreceptor gene therapy in monkey. *Sci Transl Med* **3:** 88ra54.

Vandenberghe LH, Bell P, Maguire AM, Xiao R, Hopkins TB, Grant R, Bennett J, Wilson JM. 2013. AAV9 targets cone photoreceptors in the nonhuman primate retina. *PLoS ONE* **8:** e53463.

Verrier JD, Madorsky I, Coggin WE, Geesey M, Hochman M, Walling E, Daroszewski D, Eccles KS, Ludlow R, Semple-Rowland SL. 2011. Bicistronic lentiviruses containing a viral 2A cleavage sequence reliably co-express two proteins and restore vision to an animal model of LCA1. *PLoS ONE* **6:** e20553.

Wallman J, Velez J. 1985. Directional asymmetries of optokinetic nystagmus: Developmental changes and relation to the accessory optic system and to the vestibular system. *J Neurosci* **5:** 317–329.

Wang H, den Hollander AI, Moayedi Y, Abulimiti A, Li Y, Collin RW, Hoyng CB, Lopez I, Abboud EB, Al-Rajhi AA, et al. 2009. Mutations in *SPATA7* cause Leber congenital amaurosis and juvenile retinitis pigmentosa. *Am J Hum Genet* **84:** 380–387.

Williams ML, Coleman JE, Haire SE, Aleman TS, Cideciyan AV, Sokal I, Palczewski K, Jacobson SG, Semple-Rowland SL. 2006. Lentiviral expression of retinal guanylate cyclase-1 (RetGC1) restores vision in an avian model of childhood blindness. *PLoS Med* **3:** e201.

Wright AF, Chakarova CF, Abd El-Aziz MM, Bhattacharya SS. 2010. Photoreceptor degeneration: Genetic and mechanistic dissection of a complex trait. *Nat Rev Genet* **11:** 273–284.

Yang RB, Robinson SW, Xiong WH, Yau KW, Birch DG, Garbers DL. 1999. Disruption of a retinal guanylyl cyclase gene leads to cone-specific dystrophy and paradoxical rod behavior. *J Neurosci* **19:** 5889–5897.

Yang GS, Schmidt M, Yan Z, Lindbloom JD, Harding TC, Donahue BA, Engelhardt JF, Kotin R, Davidson BL. 2002. Virus-mediated transduction of murine retina with adeno-associated virus: Effects of viral capsid and genome size. *J Virol* **76:** 7651–7660.

Yao J, Feathers KL, Khanna H, Thompson D, Tsilfidis C, Hauswirth WW, Heckenlively JR, Swaroop A, Zacks DN. 2011. XIAP therapy increases survival of transplanted rod precursors in a degenerating host retina. *Invest Ophthalmol Vis Sci* **52:** 1567–1572.

Convergence of Human Genetics and Animal Studies: Gene Therapy for X-Linked Retinoschisis

Ronald A. Bush[1], Lisa L. Wei[2], and Paul A. Sieving[2]

[1]National Institute on Deafness and Other Communication Disorders, Bethesda, Maryland 20892

[2]National Eye Institute, Bethesda, Maryland 20892

Correspondence: bushr@nidcd.nih.gov

Retinoschisis is an X-linked recessive genetic disease that leads to vision loss in males. X-linked retinoschisis (XLRS) typically affects young males; however, progressive vision loss continues throughout life. Although discovered in 1898 by Haas in two brothers, the underlying biology leading to blindness has become apparent only in the last 15 years with the advancement of human genetic analyses, generation of XLRS animal models, and the development of ocular monitoring methods such as the electroretinogram and optical coherence tomography. It is now recognized that retinoschisis results from cyst formations within the retinal layers that interrupt normal visual neurosignaling and compromise structural integrity. Mutations in the human retinoschisin gene have been correlated with disease severity of the human XLRS phenotype. Introduction of a normal human retinoschisin cDNA into retinoschisin knockout mice restores retinal structure and improves neural function, providing proof-of-concept that gene replacement therapy is a plausible treatment for XLRS.

X-linked retinoschisis (XLRS) is a developmental retinal genetic disease that impairs vision, typically beginning in young males and progressing into older age. Although the condition was first recognized in the 19th century and is readily diagnosed clinically by the characteristic intraretinal cysts arranged in a "spoke-wheel" pattern in the center of the macula, scientific progress lagged until the gene was identified about 15 years ago. This led to understanding the molecular and cellular basis of the condition, discerning the structure and function of the retinoschisin protein, generating XLRS animal models, developing suitable delivery vectors for the back of the eye, and methods to monitor structure and function of the retina in animals and humans. The culmination of these scientific discoveries poises the field for near-term clinical testing of a genetic therapy designed to restore vision and prevent further vision loss in XLRS patients.

CLINICAL DISEASE

Human retinoschisis leads to vision loss that affects boys, typically at a young age. The disease was first described in two brothers in Germany in 1898 (Haas 1898). The term retinoschisis was first used to describe the condition by Wilczek (1935) and refers to the abnormal splitting

Cite this article as *Cold Spring Harb Perspect Med* doi: 10.1101/cshperspect.a017368

through the retinal neurosensory layers. Retinoschisis is quite different from retinal detachment, in which the neurosensory tissue is elevated off and detached from the underlying retinal pigment epithelium. In 1938, the disease was recognized as an X-linked recessive trait (Mann and MacRae 1938). Today, clinical prevalence of retinoschisis is approximately 1:5000 to 1:25,000 males worldwide (George et al. 1995). Vision impairment is characteristically noticed in young males before grade school, although on occasion infants may manifest severe disease. Being an X-linked macular dystrophy, the trait is passed from mothers to affected males. Female carriers nearly never display retinal abnormalities and have normal electroretinogram (ERG) responses. On very rare occasions, female carriers will show white flecks or areas of schisis within the peripheral retina (Kaplan et al. 1991). However, because the vision of female carriers is not impacted, this indicates that haploinsufficiency does not alter apparent retinal architecture nor result in obvious visual deficiencies.

Individuals with congenital XLRS manifest a broad spectrum of clinical phenotypes, thus making initial diagnosis challenging. Schisis can involve the superficial, middle, and deep retinal layers, and is seen in both the nuclear and plexiform layers. Retinoschisis may involve the peripheral retina (Prenner et al. 2006) and lead to increased incidence of full thickness retinal detachment. In general, patients with X-linked juvenile retinoschisis show a mild reduction in central visual acuity, which gradually decreases, ranging from 20/60 to 20/120. Figure 1 shows the hallmarks of the clinical signs in the retina of a patient with a spokewheel pattern of tiny cysts that reigns in the fovea (Fig. 1A). These cavities are also readily seen by optical coherence tomography (OCT) (Fig. 1B).

The ERG is one of the most clinically informative tests for X-linked retinoschisis. The dark-adapted b-wave in XLRS patients is reduced, whereas the a-wave amplitude often remains normal (Fig. 1C) (Peachey et al. 1987). This can result in an electronegative response in which the positive-going b-wave does not increase above baseline. As the a-wave originates from photoreceptors, this indicates relatively normal photoreceptor activity. The b-wave originates from bipolar cells that lie proximal to the photoreceptors, and the electronegative response implicates defective synaptic transmission. Although an electronegative ERG response is not exclusive to XLRS individuals, only a few

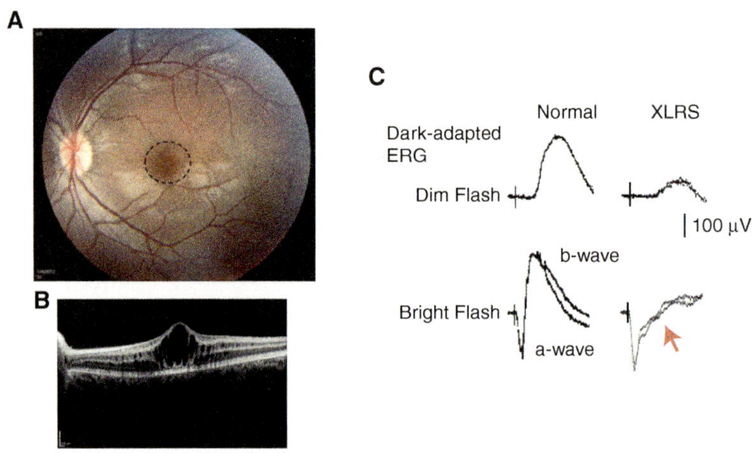

Figure 1. Fundus photo, OCT scan, and ERG typical of patients with XLRS. Color photo of macular region in X-linked retinoschisis patient (*A*) showing the characteristic intraretinal cysts arranged in a "spokewheel" pattern and corresponding OCT scan (*B*). Dark-adapted ERGs from both scotopic dim and bright stimulus flashes for an XLRS patient shows a characteristic reduction in b-wave amplitude relative to the preserved a-wave (*C*).

other retinal dystrophies result in this waveform configuration. Hence, finding this ERG type in a suspect male with a family history of retinoschisis is clinical confirmation of XLRS. However, some affected males have a more normal ERG, as was reported previously (Sieving et al. 2000; Bowles et al. 2011; Vincent et al. 2013)

MANAGEMENT OF XLRS

Currently, there are no approved treatments for the retinal degeneration or for the retinal schisis cavities. Various experimental treatment options have been considered, including the use of carbonic anhydrase inhibitors (e.g., dorzolamide and acetazolamide) with the presumed mechanism of action being the reduction of excess intraretinal fluid in cystic spaces (Apushkin and Fishman 2006; Ghajarnia and Gorin 2007). In one study, seven of eight patients showed a decrease in foveal lesions in one eye as evaluated by OCT, and six patients were reported to have a modest improvement in visual acuity (Apushkin and Fishman 2006). These findings have not been replicated and are not universally accepted. Treatment of a retinoschisin-deficient mouse model of XLRS (see below) with dorzolamide failed to produce short-term or long-term structural improvement in the retina (Zhour et al. 2012). Another proposed intervention is manipulation of the retina through surgical intraocular vitrectomy that may reduce schistic cavities (Ikeda et al. 2008). Unfortunately, these approaches do not address the fundamental pathophysiology, and no claims have been made that they alter the clinical course.

GENE AND CELL BIOLOGY OF XLRS

Genetic mutations causing XLRS are in the Retinoschisin 1 (*RS1*) gene, which maps to Xp22 and is composed of six exons (Sauer et al. 1997). Retinoschisin is a 224 amino acid secretory protein that is present throughout the neural retina (Grayson et al. 2000; Molday et al. 2001; Reid et al. 2003; Takada et al. 2004). Retinoschisin gene expression has been localized to photoreceptors in both human (Grayson et al. 2000) and mouse retina (Reid et al. 1999; Grayson et al. 2000; Molday et al. 2001; Takada et al. 2004), as well as to neurons in the inner nuclear layer (Molday et al. 2001; Takada et al. 2004), and ganglion cell layer (Takada et al. 2004) of mouse.

RS1 has a signal peptide sequence that allows for transport of the protein to the extracellular surface (Vijayasarathy et al. 2006, 2007). It also contains a single discoidin domain (Sauer et al. 1997; Grayson et al. 2000). Discoidin domains are associated with a family of extracellular cell surface proteins that are involved in cell adhesion and signaling and that interact with collagens to regulate extracellular matrix modeling (Vogel et al. 2006). Ten cysteine residues within the retinoschisin discoidin domain are important for appropriate protein folding and the formation and function of retinoschisin dimers and octamers (Wu and Molday 2003). RS1 is thought to be critical for cell adhesion during the normal development and maintenance of retinal structure. This is consistent with other discoidin domain-containing proteins and is supported by clinical observations in patients and in mouse models.

Retinoschisin expression begins during early postnatal retinal development and is maintained throughout adult life (Takada et al. 2004). As Figure 2 shows, retinoschisin is produced in the inner retina, namely, the ganglion cells, early in ocular development (top panel). However, as the eye develops, additional retinal neurons produce retinoschisin, including the outer retinal cells such as photoreceptors (bottom panel), as indicated by the presence of retinoschisin on the inner segments of rods. Interestingly, RS1 protein is also associated with bipolar cells, suggesting that it may be critical for maintaining the structural connection of postsynaptic and presynaptic elements in the outer plexiform layer that is necessary for the transmission of a visual signal from photoreceptors to bipolar cells (Molday et al. 2001; Reid et al. 2003; Takada et al. 2004). This implies that monitoring synaptic integrity by the ERG b-wave would be a suitable means for gauging this connectivity. These findings support the hypothesis that retinoschisin plays a critical role in maintaining cell–cell adhesion and in preserving retinal structure and function.

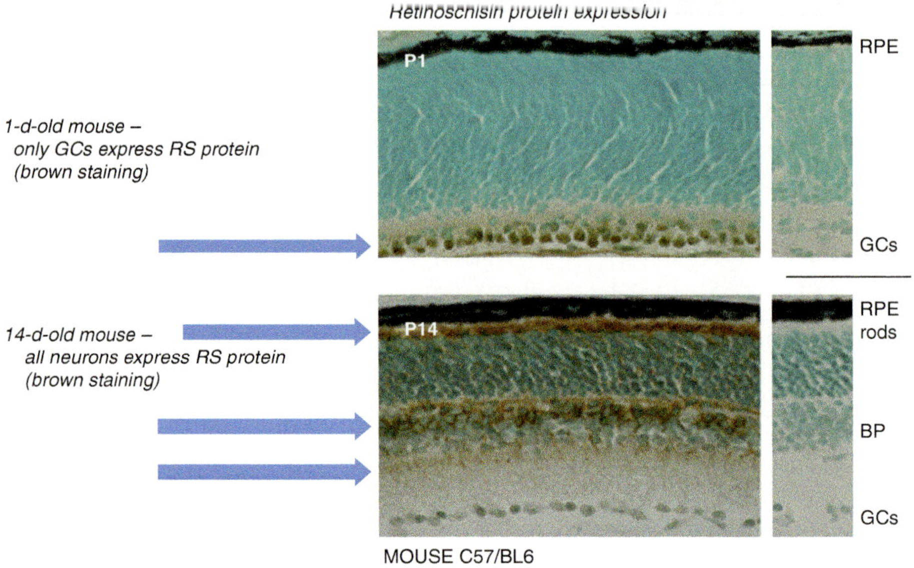

Figure 2. Retinoschisin protein expression in the mouse eye begins immediately following neuronal development and is maintained during adult life. Early in development retinoschisin is produced in the retinal ganglion cells (P1, *top* panel); later, extensive retinoschisin expression is also observed in the photoreceptors, including the rod inner segments (P14, *bottom* panel). (From Takada et al. 2004; reprinted, with express permission from the authors.)

HUMAN GENETICS FOR *RS1* MUTATIONS

In XLRS patients, numerous *RS1* mutations have been identified (The Retinal Consortium 1998; Eksandh et al. 2000; Simonelli et al. 2003). Mutations reported include missense changes, deletions, insertions, and splice site variants. Structure-function analyses reveal that the most common variants, missense mutations, interfere by three primary means: (1) interrupting normal secretion of retinoschisin; (2) disrupting proper octomerization; or (3) impacting normal function of the protein. Interestingly, a large proportion of these mutations are within the discoidin domain (exons 4–6), suggesting that the discoidin domain is a critical component for RS1 function. Examination of the nature of the *RS1* gene mutations predicts that ~40% of all the identified mutations represent null alleles and, therefore, would not produce functional retinoschisin protein (Molday et al. 2012). Such mutations represent the human equivalent of genetic knockout models in mice (see below). The majority of cases found with missense mutations had minimal structure perturbations and consequently, standard disease (Sergeev et al. 2010). However, removal or insertions of cysteine residues or changes in the hydrophobic core of retinoschisin resulted in maximum structural perturbations that caused significant changes in photopic b/a ratios (Sergeev et al. 2013). Although difficult to show, in some cases, severity of disease correlates with genotype (Sergeev et al. 2010, 2013; Bowles et al. 2011).

X-LINKED RETINOSCHISIS MOUSE MODELS

Currently, three XLRS mouse models targeting the murine ortholog of the human *RS1* gene have been developed (Table 1). All are deficient in endogenous murine retinoschisin. One model was engineered with the insertion of a LacZ/Neo^r cassette into exon 3, thus generating a null mouse model. Zeng et al. (2004) inserted a neomycin gene into intron 1 that resulted in ablation of murine retinoschisin protein expression. The last mouse model system was produced using *N*-ethyl-*N*-nitrosurea (ENU)-based ran-

Table 1. Comparison of XLRS mouse models

Source	Synonyms	Target	Category	Reported abnormal phenotypes
Bernhard H.F. Weber (Weber et al. 2002)	*Rs1h*$^{-/Y}$	Partial deletions of exon 3 and 4 and intron 3 with a Lac Z gene insertion	Targeted (reporter)	Nervous system, vision/eye
Paul A. Sieving (Zeng et al. 2004)	*Rs1*$^{-/Y}$	Deletion of all of exon 1 and partial deletion of intron 1 with a neomycin gene insertion	Targeted (knockout)	Vision/eye
Tennessee Mouse Genome Consortium (TMGC)—Monica Jablonski (distributed via TMGC, Northwestern University, and JAX Labs) (Jablonski et al. 2005)	44TNJ *Rs1*^{tmgc1}/*Rs1*^{tmgc1} and *Rs1*^{tmgc}/Y formerly called *Rs1h*^{tmgc1}	T to C transition at the second base of intron 2 of the *Rs1h* gene	Chemically induce (ENU)	Nervous system, pigmentation, vision/eye

dom mutagenesis that led to a single base-pair substitution in intron 2 (Jablonski et al. 2005). This created an alternate splice site producing two transcripts in male mice: a 10 bp insertion and a 26 bp deletion at the junction of exon 2 to intron 2. Within these two transcripts, premature stop codons are formed, preventing synthesis of full-length retinoschisin protein. All three knockout models display structural and functional retinal phenotypes very similar to that observed in humans with XLRS. ERG evaluations in the three mouse models show the characteristic reduction of the dark-adapted b-wave as observed in XLRS patients. Histologically, retina structure is disorganized, with misaligned cells and retinal splitting evident in the inner nuclear layer and structural abnormalities of synapses within the outer plexiform layer—hallmarks of the human disease. Figure 3 shows the retinal structure and dampened ERGs in the *Rs1*$^{-/Y}$ mouse (Zeng et al. 2004).

GENE THERAPY FOR XLRS

Gene Delivery Considerations

The expression of retinoschisin (*Rs1*) in mice during development and in adult tissue, along with the pathology described in the XLRS mouse retina, suggests that retinoschisin is important in normal development and maintenance of the retinal architecture, and this protein appears to be critical in sustaining functional synaptic integrity (Takada et al. 2004; Kjellstrom et al. 2007). These findings support the strategy of gene augmentation as a therapeutic approach for XLRS patients. Experimental studies introducing human *RS1* in mouse models of XLRS showed that a single administration gave sustained expression beyond a year and restored both structure and function of the retina (Zeng et al. 2004; Min et al. 2005). Based on these encouraging studies, efforts are now directed to develop a gene therapy approach for XLRS patients.

A first consideration involves selecting an appropriate means to deliver the gene. There are several methods that could be used to introduce the *RS1* gene into the eye. Viral vectors have typically shown the best efficiency with regard to delivering the gene of interest to retinal cells. Within the eye, several viral vectors have advanced or are advancing into clinical testing. Among these are vectors based on adeno-associated virus (AAV), adenovirus, retrovirus, and lentivirus (Song et al. 2003; Chevez-Barrios

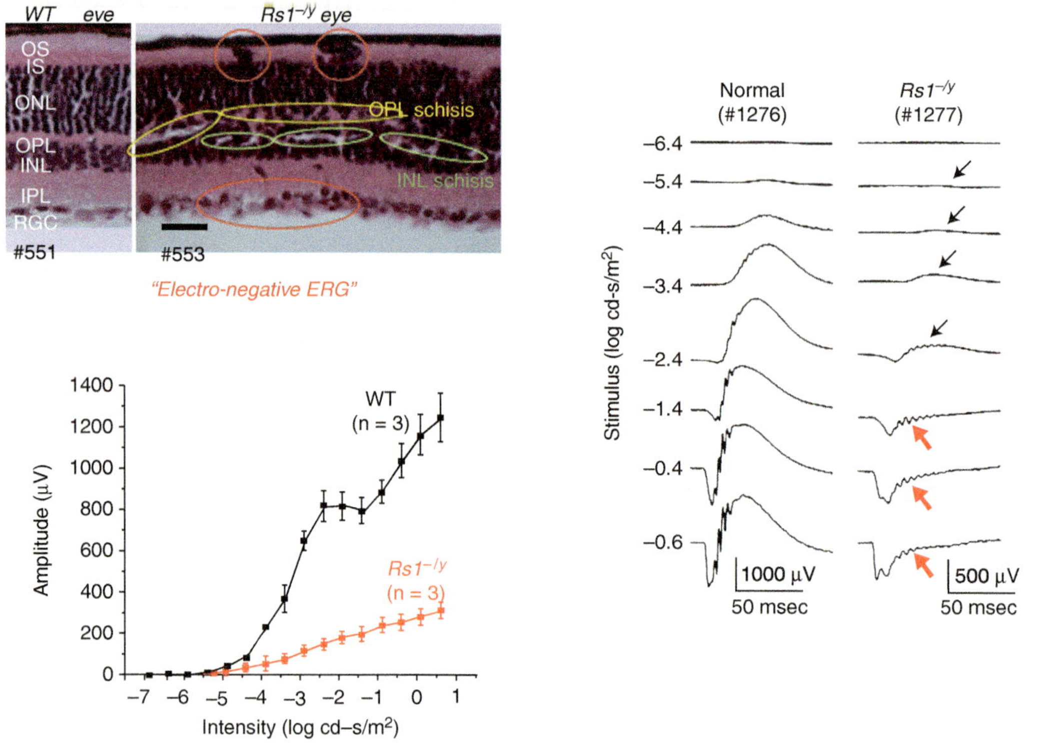

Figure 3. Retinal structure and ERG function in the *Rs1*-KO ($Rs1^{-/y}$) mouse. The retinal sections show structural changes between the normal mouse eye and the RS-KO mouse eye. The *Rs1*-KO eye shows distortions in the retinal ganglion cell layer (RGC) and random cells in the inner plexiform layer (IPL). Likewise, the synaptic connections between photoreceptors and bipolar cells are irregular in the inner nuclear layer (INL) and outer plexiform layer (OPL). Structural gaps, equivalent to "retinoschisis cavities," are evident in the INL. Photoreceptors are reduced in the retinal sections in the KO mice versus normal mice, and some photoreceptor nuclei localize to the inner and outer segment zones (IS and OS) rather than exclusively within the outer nuclear layer (ONL). As in XLRS humans, the *Rs1*-KO mouse ERG shows disproportionate b-wave reduction across the range of stimulus flash intensity, as is readily seen in the ERG wave form (arrows) and also in the graph of b-wave amplitude versus intensity. (From Zeng et al. 2004; reprinted, with express permission from the authors.)

et al. 2005; Campochiaro et al. 2006; Bainbridge et al. 2008; Hauswirth et al. 2008; Maguire et al. 2008, 2009; Simonelli et al. 2010; Balaggan and Ali 2012). Today, a large number of gene therapy constructs, in particular those for human ocular diseases, are utilizing AAV. AAV is a nonpathogenic dependovirus that replicates in the presence of another active virus infection, often adenovirus or herpes simplex virus (Berns and Giraud 1996). AAV virions are nonenveloped and typically encase single stranded DNA. There are at least 12 naturally occurring serotypes of AAV (designated AAV1–AAV12), although more than 100 nonredundant forms have been discovered (Mori et al. 2004; Daya and Berns 2008; Vandenberghe and Auricchio 2012).

AAV has two open reading frames. The first contains *rep,* which encodes four proteins necessary for viral replication. The second comprises *cap,* which encodes three structural proteins that make up the outer icosahedral capsid of the virus. The *cap* or capsid proteins have different affinities for various cell surface receptors. For instance, the primary receptors for AAV serotype 2 (AAV2) are heparin sulphate and $\alpha_V\beta_5$ integrins (Summerford and Samulski 1998; Summerford et al. 1999). AAV4 and AAV5 preferentially bind sialic acid or platelet-derived growth factor (Kaludov et al. 2002; Di Pasquale et al. 2003), whereas AAV3, AAV8, and AAV9 bind to laminin (Akache et al. 2006). Therefore, careful selection of viral serotype becomes an important consideration in choosing an appropriate vector for gene delivery for a given disease. This and the delivery route may be critical for a successful gene-based interventional approach.

Choosing the correct viral vector can help address another key component of a successful gene therapy product, namely the appropriate expression of the replacement or restorative gene. Historically, transgene expression from AAV vectors has a delayed onset, sometimes requiring up to 6 wk to achieve peak levels (Bennett et al. 1997). This would be detrimental for acute applications. However, two strategies have been devised to overcome this limitation. The first is the development of modified or mutant capsids. Mutant capsids with specific amino acid substitutions have resulted in higher transgene expression in a shorter period of time (Petrs-Silva et al. 2009). Investigators also have found that photoreceptors can be effectively transduced by intravitreal administration, a finding that has practical clinical implications for both ophthalmologists and patients (see below) (Dalkara et al. 2011; MacLachlan et al. 2011; Petrs-Silva et al. 2011).

In addition to the gene delivery vector, the second consideration is the rate-limiting requirement for synthesis of a complementary DNA strand from the original AAV single-strand DNA. Incorporating a second strand of DNA within the virus (self-complementary AAV) reduces the time required for gene expression by removing the necessity to synthesize a second DNA strand. This also eliminates the need for host DNA replication machinery. Using this approach it has been shown that transgene expression can be measured within 4 d following AAV-transgene introduction into the eye (Pang et al. 2010).

A third component that is often critical for the pharmacokinetic expression of the transgene is promoter selection. The cytomegalovirus (CMV) promoter is commonly used. This promoter can lead to high transgene expression but in many systems the expression is transient, promiscuous and in all cell types. Because XLRS involves chronic degeneration of retinal cells over years and decades in humans, an important criterion is selection of a promoter that leads to prolonged gene production in multiple cell types. Thus, for XLRS, several promoters including the rhodopsin (rho) and rhodopsin kinase (rho K) promoters have been investigated. Both of these promoters are specific to photoreceptors and give high expression, but they may also result in cell death, likely because of overexpression of retinoschisin (Y Zeng, unpubl.). Use of the retinoschisis promoter should facilitate the expression of retinoschisin in all cells in which it is normally found. By including the interphotoreceptor retinoid binding protein enhancer, gene expression levels following intravitreal injection reaches, in some animals, levels comparable to that found in wild-type animals (see Fig. 4).

Routes of Administration

In the majority of ocular gene therapy trials using AAV, the genes are delivered via subretinal injection (Bainbridge et al. 2008; Hauswirth et al. 2008; Maguire et al. 2008, 2009; Simonelli et al. 2010) with good success. This route of administration has the experimental advantage of direct dose scaling from the small mouse eye to the larger human eye. However, this procedure is complex and requires pars plana vitrectomy surgery in an operating room, which has a high risk of complications (e.g., retinal tear or retinal detachment). XLRS patients are already prone to retinal detachment, thus utilizing a method that decreases this occurrence would be preferred. Intravitreal injections into the eye have become commonplace with the advent of Macugen, Lucentis, and Eylea (three agents approved for the treatment of wet age-related macular degeneration), and can be repeated monthly. Moreover, intravitreal injections can be administered in the office and given under topical anesthesia, making this procedure less complicated and more convenient for patient, physician, and clinical staff. However, there is

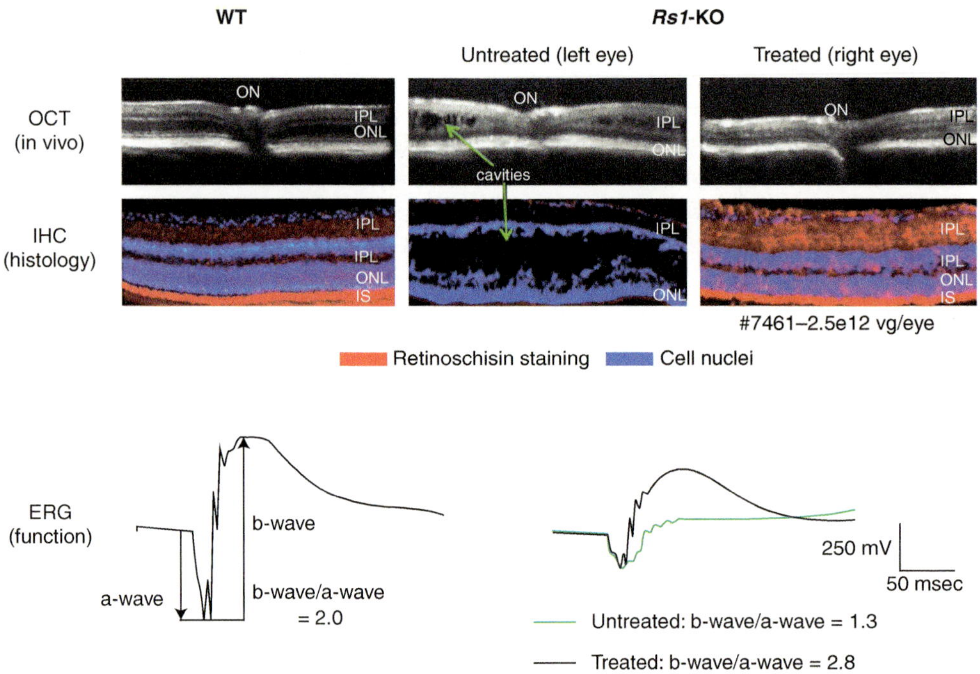

Figure 4. Retinal structure, retinoschisin expression and function in wild-type (WT), untreated- and treated-*Rs1*-KO mice. OCT in vivo images show the structure of a portion of the retinas centered on the optic nerve (ON) from a WT mouse and the right and left retinas of an *Rs1*-KO mouse treated in the right eye with 2.5×10^9 vg/eye of AAV8-retinoschisin vector. The darker bands are the nuclear layers of the retina, the thickest being the outer nuclear layer (ONL) containing the photoreceptor cells. The lighter bands *above* the ONL are the outer and inner plexiform (IPL) layers. In the untreated eye of the *Rs1*-KO mouse, these layers are much less dense and the borders between the layers less distinct. There are large cavities spanning the region between the ONL and IPL, a region that contains the second order neurons, including bipolar cells and their synapses with photoreceptors. The right eye was treated at day P21 and evaluated 16 wk later. OCT shows the cavities have closed in the treated retina, and the borders between the layers are more regular and distinct than in the untreated eyes. The layer margins are still less distinct than in the WT retina. Immunohistochemical (IHC) staining for retinoschisin protein (red) in the WT retina shows its presence in the plexiform layers, with particularly strong staining in the inner segments (IS) of the photoreceptors. Specific staining for retinoschisin is completely lacking in the untreated eye of the *Rs1*-KO mouse but is very strong in the treated eye, indicating robust expression of the therapeutic protein in the same cells as in WT. The faint staining *below* the ONL in the untreated eye is nonspecific staining of the retinal pigment epithelium. Immunohistochemistry analyses show that retinoschisin expression in photoreceptor inner segments in treated eyes are essentially comparable to WT. Image brightness intensity was adjusted against blue nuclear staining of DAPI. The ERG shows a-wave and b-wave responses to a bright flash of light, indicating phototransduction activity of photoreceptors and activity of the second order bipolar cells, respectively. Both are reduced in size in the *Rs1*-KO mouse retinas, but the ratio of the b-wave to the a-wave is pathologically reduced in the untreated eye while it is increased in the treated retina. This is consistent with the structural findings indicating severe pathology in the retina postsynaptic to photoreceptors in untreated retinas, with structure partially maintained or restored when treated by AAV8-retinoschisin. In most of our studies the vector is administered at day P21–P28, when the retina is young but fully mature. However, similar rescue of structure and function is observed when AAV8-retinoschisin is administered at 2 and 3 mo of age.

not a clear method to scale from a small animal eye to the larger human eye.

Intravitreal administration of native AAV vectors has resulted in scattered and spotty transduction of ganglion cells at the surface of the retina, but the vectors do not penetrate to reach neurons deep in the rodent or monkey eye (Dalkara et al. 2013). AAV2 variants with tyrosine mutations, or newer laboratory-created AAV vectors with capsid modifications, show the ability to penetrate deep into the retina (Petrs-Silva et al. 2009; Vandenberghe and Auricchio 2012; Dalkara et al. 2013). Consequently, intravitreal delivery of genes for retinal degenerative diseases is becoming more promising clinically. In the case of XLRS, data using an AAV8 containing the *RS1* gene (AAV8-retinoschisin) delivered into the eyes of XLRS mice by intravitreal injection show robust RS1 staining of neurons throughout the mouse retina, including photoreceptors, bipolar and amacrine cells (Park et al. 2009). This appears specific for the pathophysiology caused by XLRS, as the same vector does not penetrate the wild-type mouse retina. Additionally, a clinical trial utilizing AAV2 with soluble Flt for wet age-related macular degeneration (NCT01024998) is using intravitreal delivery, providing further support that intraocular injection is plausible for some vectors. The published preclinical studies using AAV2 to deliver an antiangiogenic molecule in primate eyes showed intraocular inflammation to the vector capsid, as the AAV2-null vector gave similar findings (MacLachlan et al. 2011). Inflammation was transitory, initially appearing in some animals at 1 mo after intravitreal injection, increasing over the next few months, and then declining.

Transition to Efficacy Studies

Preclinical safety and efficacy studies in animals can provide the foundation for human clinical trials and are helpful to establish a possible benefit to treatment that outweighs potential risks. As reviewed above, mice in which expression of the *Rs1* gene has been disrupted resulting in retinoschisin knockout (*Rs1*-KO) mice are the only animal models for XLRS. Structural and functional studies of *Rs1*-KO mice have shown a phenotype that closely mimics retinal pathology in XLRS (Zeng et al. 2004). Cavity formation reaches a maximum by 4–6 mo, in parallel with functional changes such as reduction in the ERG b-wave to a-wave ratio (b/a ratio) (Kjellstrom et al. 2007). This change is comparable to XLRS in young adults when the ERG b-wave and b/a ratio tends to reach minimum in the most severe patients (Bowles et al. 2011). AAV8-retinoschisin efficacy studies in our laboratory using *Rs1*-KO mice are described below. Retinal function was measured using ERGs, and retinal structure was evaluated in vivo with OCT imaging. Both are common clinical measures and are performed using identical or similar instruments to those used for human clinical diagnosis. In addition, retinoschisin expression was evaluated postmortem in treated animals using semiquantitative immunohistochemistry. This provides a combined assessment of therapeutic protein expression with both structural and functional benefit following vector administration.

Efficacy Study Results

Two groups of *Rs1*-KO mice received intravitreal injections in one eye between 3 and 5 wk of age of either an AAV8 vector carrying a self-complimentary copy of the human retinoschisin gene and promoter or vehicle alone. Injected doses were 2.5×10^9 vector genomes (vg)/eye down to 1×10^6 vg/eye. ERGs were recorded between 12 and 16 wk after injection, followed within 2 wk by OCT imaging and removal of the eyes for immunohistochemistry to evaluate retinoschisin expression. Figure 4 shows the results from the treated and untreated eyes of a single mouse injected with 2.5×10^9 vg/eye and evaluated 16 wk after injection compared with a wild-type mouse. The untreated eye of the *Rs1*-KO mouse has large cavities spanning the layers between the photoreceptor outer nuclear layer and the inner plexiform layer. These intermediate layers are also thicker than in wild type and have ill-defined boundaries, indicating a degree of disorganization compared with the well-defined layers in the wild-type animal.

The cavities in the untreated retina appear as empty space in the histological sections, but in vivo there are structural connections between the inner and outer margins of the cavities similar to those in human XLRS (Fig. 1). The untreated eye lacks retinoschisin expression, which is apparent in the inner nuclear layer and outer plexiform layer and is strongest in the inner segments of the photoreceptors in the wild-type retina. The structure of the treated retina in vivo and in histological sections, however, is similar to wild type in organization of the retinal layers and lack of cavities. Some disorganization is still evident in the internal structure of the layers and the indistinct or irregular margins of the layers. The treated retina shows heavy retinoschisin staining of inner segments and in the two plexiform layers between the rows of retinal cell bodies. Retinoschisin expression in this retina equals or exceeds that of wild type, although this is variable across injected eyes and sometimes within injected eyes.

The ERG of the wild-type mouse shows a dark-adapted a-wave and b-wave in response to a bright stimulus flash. The a-wave reflects phototransduction in the rods, and the b-wave originates from bipolar cells postsynaptic to the photoreceptors. Thus, a reduction of photoreceptor number or activity will produce a reduction in both the a-wave and b-wave, because postsynaptic responses depend on photoreceptor input. A reduction in the a-wave greater than in the b-wave, that is, an increase in the b/a ratio, is a hallmark of photoreceptor degenerations (Machida et al. 2000), because photoreceptors greatly outnumber the bipolar cells, and this convergence tends to reduce the effect of photoreceptor loss vis-à-vis the b-wave generation. The response from the untreated eye of the *Rs1*-KO mouse in Figure 4 shows a reduction in b/a ratio, indicating a disproportionate effect on the response of bipolar cells. This could be a result of structural and functional disruption of bipolar cells themselves and/or the synaptic signaling between photoreceptors and these second order neurons. The smaller a-wave compared with wild type indicates that there was substantial photoreceptor loss, which is also apparent as a reduction in the outer nuclear layer, as shown by OCT and histology. The increased b/a wave ratio in treated eyes is consistent with the relatively normal structural appearance of the retinal layers postsynaptic to the photoreceptors, coupled with a substantial loss of photoreceptors. Figure 5 shows dose–response results for *Rs1*-KO eyes injected with AAV8-ret-

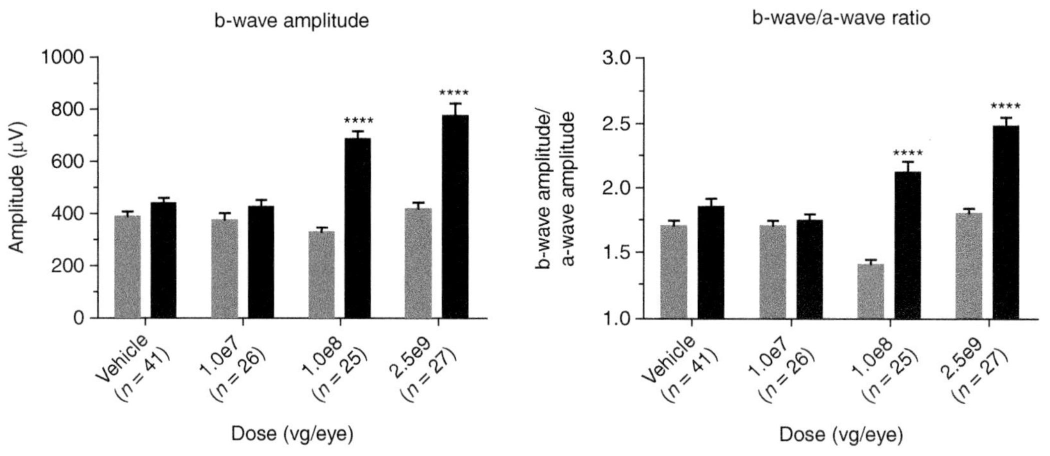

Figure 5. Dose response graphs for the ERG b-wave and b-wave to a-wave ratio in *Rs1*-KO mice treated with AAV8-retinoschisin. *Rs1*-KO mice were treated in one eye with different concentrations of vector or vehicle between 3 and 5 wk of age, and the ERG was recorded 12 to 16 wk after injection. The b-wave and the b-wave to a-wave ratio was significantly increased at doses of 1e8 and 2.5e9, relative to untreated eyes (multiple *t*-tests using Holm-Sidak correction for multiple comparisons).

inoschisin or vector controls. There was a significant improvement in the b-wave and b/a wave ratio in eyes treated with 1×10^8 and 2.5×10^9 vg/eye of AAV8-retinoschisin but not with 1×10^7 vg/eye or vehicle. The size and number of cavities were significantly reduced at 1×10^8 and 2.5×10^9 vg/eye, and these retinas showed significant retinoschisin protein expression, as assessed with immunohistochemistry, compared with untreated eyes (Fig. 4)

CONCLUDING REMARKS

Based on the very promising mouse efficacy studies, the strong transduction of the retina using AAV8 after intravitreous administration, and an acceptable safety profile in the *Rs1*-KO mouse, a next step is to advance to a phase I clinical trial in XLRS patients. The data obtained to date from animal studies suggest several issues to be considered in designing early clinical trials of *RS1* gene therapy. Each patient should be followed carefully for any clinical indication of an ocular inflammatory response to vector administration. Simultaneously, therapeutic benefit should also be measured. The first subjects for human treatment studies may have more severe disease, in which vision is already substantially compromised. Each patient should be carefully monitored to ensure that there is no detrimental effect. Then individuals with more moderate disease might be considered for treatment. In designing a human study, clinical examination methods that identify underlying cellular dysfunction should be used, if possible. In a Phase I safety study, these might include reading evaluation to monitor visual acuity, degree of ERG impairment, and OCT imaging to monitor the structure of the retina. The principles learned from genetic analyses in XLRS patients and efficacy studies in XLRS mice support clinical testing of a *RS1* gene therapy approach to reduce vision loss in retinoschisis patients.

ACKNOWLEDGMENTS

The authors are grateful to Dr. Catherine Cukras for the fundus photo and OCT scan from an XLRS patient and Cindy Best, Matthew McMahon, and Santa Tumminia for their assistance in the preparation of this review. Supported by the National Institutes of Health (NIH) Intramural Research Program through the National Institute on Deafness and Other Communication Disorders and the National Eye Institute.

REFERENCES

Akache B, Grimm D, Pandey K, Yant SR, Xu H, Kay MA. 2006. The 37/67-kilodalton laminin receptor is a receptor for adeno-associated virus serotypes 8, 2, 3, and 9. *J Virol* **80:** 9831–9836.

Apushkin MA, Fishman GA. 2006. Use of dorzolamide for patients with X-linked retinoschisis. *Retina* **26:** 741–745.

Bainbridge JW, Smith AJ, Barker SS, Robbie S, Henderson R, Balaggan K, Viswanathan A, Holder GE, Stockman A, Tyler N, et al. 2008. Effect of gene therapy on visual function in Leber's congenital amaurosis. *N Engl J Med* **358:** 2231–2239.

Balaggan KS, Ali RR. 2012. Ocular gene delivery using lentiviral vectors. *Gene Ther* **19:** 145–153.

Bennett J, Duan D, Engelhardt JF, Maguire AM. 1997. Real-time, noninvasive in vivo assessment of adeno-associated virus-mediated retinal transduction. *Invest Ophthalmol Vis Sci* **38:** 2857–2863.

Berns KI, Giraud C. 1996. Biology of adeno-associated virus. *Curr Top Microbiol Immunol* **218:** 1–23.

Bowles K, Cukras C, Turriff A, Sergeev Y, Vitale S, Bush RA, Sieving PA. 2011. X-linked retinoschisis: *RS1* mutation severity and age affect the ERG phenotype in a cohort of 68 affected male subjects. *Invest Ophthalmol Vis Sci* **52:** 9250–9256.

Campochiaro PA, Nguyen QD, Shah SM, Klein ML, Holz E, Frank RN, Saperstein DA, Gupta A, Stout JT, Macko J, et al. 2006. Adenoviral vector-delivered pigment epithelium-derived factor for neovascular age-related macular degeneration: Results of a phase I clinical trial. *Hum Gene Ther* **17:** 167–176.

Chevez-Barrios P, Chintagumpala M, Mieler W, Paysse E, Boniuk M, Kozinetz C, Hurwitz MY, Hurwitz RL. 2005. Response of retinoblastoma with vitreous tumor seeding to adenovirus-mediated delivery of thymidine kinase followed by ganciclovir. *J Clin Oncol* **23:** 7927–7935.

Dalkara D, Kolstad KD, Guerin KI, Hoffmann NV, Visel M, Klimczak RR, Schaffer DV, Flannery JG. 2011. AAV mediated GDNF secretion from retinal glia slows down retinal degeneration in a rat model of retinitis pigmentosa. *Mol Ther* **19:** 1602–1608.

Dalkara D, Byrne LC, Klimczak RR, Visel M, Yin L, Merigan WH, Flannery JG, Schaffer DV. 2013. In vivo-directed evolution of a new adeno-associated virus for therapeutic outer retinal gene delivery from the vitreous. *Sci Transl Med* **5:** 189ra176.

Daya S, Berns KI. 2008. Gene therapy using adeno-associated virus vectors. *Clin Microbiol Rev* **21:** 583–593.

Di Pasquale G, Davidson BL, Stein CS, Martins I, Scudiero D, Monks A, Chiorini JA. 2003. Identification of PDGFR as a receptor for AAV-5 transduction. *Nat Med* **9:** 1306–1312.

Eksandh LC, Ponjavic V, Ayyagari R, Bingham EL, Hiriyanna KT, Andreasson S, Ehinger B, Sieving PA. 2000. Phenotypic expression of juvenile X-linked retinoschisis in Swedish families with different mutations in the *XLRS1* gene. *Arch Ophthalmol* **118:** 1098–1104.

George ND, Yates JR, Moore AT. 1995. X linked retinoschisis. *Br J Ophthalmol* **79:** 697–702.

Ghajarnia M, Gorin MB. 2007. Acetazolamide in the treatment of X-linked retinoschisis maculopathy. *Arch Ophthalmol* **125:** 571–573.

Grayson C, Reid SN, Ellis JA, Rutherford A, Sowden JC, Yates JR, Farber DB, Trump D. 2000. Retinoschisin, the X-linked retinoschisis protein, is a secreted photoreceptor protein, and is expressed and released by Weri-Rb1 cells. *Hum Mol Genet* **9:** 1873–1879.

Haas J. 1898. Ueber das zusammenvorkommen von veraenderungen der retina und choroidea. *Arch Augenheilkd* **37:** 343–348.

Hauswirth W, Aleman TS, Kaushal S, Cideciyan AV, Schwartz SB, Wang L, Conlon T, Boye SL, Flotte TR, Byrne B, et al. 2008. Phase I trial of Leber congenital amaurosis due to *RPE65* mutations by ocular subretinal injection of adeno-associated virus gene vector: Short-term results. *Hum Gene Ther* **0:** 081015093227032.

Ikeda F, Iida T, Kishi S. 2008. Resolution of retinoschisis after vitreous surgery in X-linked retinoschisis. *Ophthalmology* **115:** 718–722 e711.

Jablonski MM, Dalke C, Wang X, Lu L, Manly KF, Pretsch W, Favor J, Pardue MT, Rinchik EM, Williams RW, et al. 2005. An ENU-induced mutation in *Rs1h* causes disruption of retinal structure and function. *Mol Vis* **11:** 569–581.

Kaludov N, Handelman B, Chiorini JA. 2002. Scalable purification of adeno-associated virus type 2, 4, or 5 using ion-exchange chromatography. *Hum Gene Ther* **13:** 1235–1243.

Kaplan J, Pelet A, Hentati H, Jeanpierre M, Briard ML, Journel H, Munnich A, Dufier JL. 1991. Contribution to carrier detection and genetic counselling in X linked retinoschisis. *J Med Genet* **28:** 83–388.

Kjellstrom S, Bush RA, Zeng Y, Takada Y, Sieving PA. 2007. Retinoschisin gene therapy and natural history in the *Rs1h*-KO mouse: Long-term rescue from retinal degeneration. *Invest Ophthalmol Vis Sci* **48:** 3837–3845.

Machida S, Kondo M, Jamison JA, Khan NW, Kononen LT, Sugawara T, Bush RA, Sieving PA. 2000. P23H rhodopsin transgenic rat: Correlation of retinal function with histopathology. *Invest Ophthalmol Vis Sci* **41:** 3200–3209.

MacLachlan TK, Lukason M, Collins M, Munger R, Isenberger E, Rogers C, Malatos S, Dufresne E, Morris J, Calcedo R, et al. 2011. Preclinical safety evaluation of AAV2-sFLT01—A gene therapy for age-related macular degeneration. *Mol Ther* **19:** 326–334.

Maguire AM, Simonelli F, Pierce EA, Pugh EN Jr, Mingozzi F, Bennicelli J, Banfi S, Marshall KA, Testa F, Surace EM, et al. 2008. Safety and efficacy of gene transfer for Leber's congenital amaurosis. *N Engl J Med* **358:** 2240–2248.

Maguire AM, High KA, Auricchio A, Wright JF, Pierce EA, Testa F, Mingozzi F, Bennicelli JL, Ying GS, Rossi S, et al. 2009. Age-dependent effects of *RPE65* gene therapy for Leber's congenital amaurosis: A phase 1 dose-escalation trial. *Lancet* **374:** 1597–1605.

Mann I, MacRae A. 1938. Congenital vascular veils in the vitreous. *Br J Ophthalmol* **22:** 1–10.

Min SH, Molday LL, Seeliger MW, Dinculescu A, Timmers AM, Janssen A, Tonagel F, Tanimoto N, Weber BH, Molday RS, et al. 2005. Prolonged recovery of retinal structure/function after gene therapy in an *Rs1h*-deficient mouse model of X-linked juvenile retinoschisis. *Mol Ther* **12:** 644–651.

Molday LL, Hicks D, Sauer CG, Weber BH, Molday RS. 2001. Expression of X-linked retinoschisis protein RS1 in photoreceptor and bipolar cells. *Invest Ophthalmol Vis Sci* **42:** 816–825.

Molday RS, Kellner U, Weber BH. 2012. X-linked juvenile retinoschisis: Clinical diagnosis, genetic analysis, and molecular mechanisms. *Prog Retin Eye Res* **31:** 195–212.

Mori S, Wang L, Takeuchi T, Kanda T. 2004. Two novel adeno-associated viruses from cynomolgus monkey: Pseudotyping characterization of capsid protein. *Virology* **330:** 375–383.

Pang J, Boye SE, Lei B, Boye SL, Everhart D, Ryals R, Umino Y, Rohrer B, Alexander J, Li J, et al. 2010. Self-complementary AAV-mediated gene therapy restores cone function and prevents cone degeneration in two models of Rpe65 deficiency. *Gene Ther* **17:** 815–826.

Park TK, Wu Z, Kjellstrom S, Zeng Y, Bush RA, Sieving PA, Colosi P. 2009. Intravitreal delivery of AAV8 retinoschisin results in cell type-specific gene expression and retinal rescue in the *Rs1*-KO mouse. *Gene Ther* **16:** 916–926.

Peachey N, Fishman G, Derlacki D, Brigell M. 1987. Psychophysical and electroretinographic findings in X-linked juvenile retinoschisis. *Arch Ophthalmol* **105:** 513–516.

Petrs-Silva H, Dinculescu A, Li Q, Min SH, Chiodo V, Pang JJ, Zhong L, Zolotukhin S, Srivastava A, Lewin AS, et al. 2009. High-efficiency transduction of the mouse retina by tyrosine-mutant AAV serotype vectors. *Mol Ther* **17:** 463–471.

Petrs-Silva H, Dinculescu A, Li Q, Deng WT, Pang JJ, Min SH, Chiodo V, Neeley AW, Govindasamy L, Bennett A, et al. 2011. Novel properties of tyrosine-mutant AAV2 vectors in the mouse retina. *Mol Ther* **19:** 293–301.

Prenner JL, Copone A Jr, Ciaccia S, Takada Y, Sieving PA, Trese MT. 2006. Congenetital X-linked retinoschisis classification system. *Retina* **26:** S61–S64.

Reid SN, Akhmedov NB, Piriev NI, Kozak CA, Danciger M, Farber DB. 1999. The mouse X-linked juvenile retinoschisis cDNA: Expression in photoreceptors. *Gene* **227:** 257–266.

Reid SN, Yamashita C, Farber DB. 2003. Retinoschisin, a photoreceptor-secreted protein, and its interaction with bipolar and muller cells. *J Neurosci* **23:** 6030–6040.

Sauer CG, Gehrig A, Warneke-Wittstock R, Marquardt A, Ewing CC, Gibson A, Lorenz B, Jurklies B, Weber BH. 1997. Positional cloning of the gene associated with X-linked juvenile retinoschisis. *Nat Genet* **17:** 164–170.

Sergeev YV, Caruso RC, Meltzer MR, Smaoui N, MacDonald IM, Sieving PA. 2010. Molecular modeling of retinoschisin with functional analysis of pathogenic mutations from human X-linked retinoschisis. *Hum Mol Genet* **19:** 1302–1313.

Sergeev YV, Vitale S, Sieving PA, Vincent A, Robson AG, Moore AT, Webster AR, Holder GE. 2013. Molecular modeling indicates distinct classes of missense variants with mild and severe XLRS phenotypes. *Hum Mol Genet* **22:** 4756–4767.

Sieving PA, Yashar BM, Ayyagari R. 2000. Juvenile retinoschisis: A model for diagnostic testing of X-linked ophthalmic disease. Trans Am ophthalmol soc 1999;v97: 451–464. *Am J Ophthalmol* **129:** 833.

Simonelli F, Cennamo G, Ziviello C, Testa F, de Crecchio G, Nesti A, Manitto MP, Ciccodicola A, Banfi S, Brancato R, et al. 2003. Clinical features of X linked juvenile retinoschisis associated with new mutations in the *XLRS1* gene in Italian families. *Br J Ophthalmol* **87:** 1130–1134.

Simonelli F, Maguire AM, Testa F, Pierce EA, Mingozzi F, Bennicelli JL, Rossi S, Marshall K, Banfi S, Surace EM, et al. 2010. Gene therapy for Leber's congenital amaurosis is safe and effective through 1.5 years after vector administration. *Mol Ther* **18:** 643–650.

Song JC, McDonnell PJ, Gordon EM, Hall FL, Anderson WF. 2003. Phase I/II evaluation of safety and efficacy of a matrix-targeted retroviral vector bearing a dominant negative cyclin G1 construct (Md-dnG1) as adjunctive intervention for superficial corneal opacity/corneal scarring. *Hum Gene Ther* **14:** 306–309.

Summerford C, Samulski RJ. 1998. Membrane-associated heparan sulfate proteoglycan is a receptor for adeno-associated virus type 2 virions. *J Virol* **72:** 1438–1445.

Summerford C, Bartlett JS, Samulski RJ. 1999. AlphaVbeta5 integrin: A co-receptor for adeno-associated virus type 2 infection. *Nat Med* **5:** 78–82.

Takada Y, Fariss RN, Tanikawa A, Zeng Y, Carper D, Bush R, Sieving PA. 2004. A retinal neuronal developmental wave of retinoschisin expression begins in ganglion cells during layer formation. *Invest Ophthalmol Vis Sci* **45:** 3302–3312.

The Retinal Consortium. 1998. Functional implications of the spectrum of mutations found in 234 cases with X-linked juvenile retinoschisis. The Retinoschisis Consortium. *Hum Mol Genet* **7:** 1185–1192.

Vandenberghe LH, Auricchio A. 2012. Novel adeno-associated viral vectors for retinal gene therapy. *Gene Ther* **19:** 162–168.

Vijayasarathy C, Gawinowicz MA, Zeng Y, Takada Y, Bush RA, Sieving PA. 2006. Identification and characterization of two mature isoforms of retinoschisin in murine retina. *Biochem Biophys Res Commun* **349:** 99–105.

Vijayasarathy C, Takada Y, Zeng Y, Bush RA, Sieving PA. 2007. Retinoschisin is a peripheral membrane protein with affinity for anionic phospholipids and affected by divalent cations. *Invest Ophthalmol Vis Sci* **48:** 991–1000.

Vincent A, Robson AG, Neveu MM, Wright GA, Moore AT, Webster AR, Holder GE. 2013. A phenotype-genotype correlation study of X-linked retinoschisis. *Ophthalmology* **120:** 1454–1464.

Vogel WF, Abdulhussein R, Ford CE. 2006. Sensing extracellular matrix: An update on discoidin domain receptor function. *Cell Signal* **18:** 1108–1116.

Weber BH, Schrewe H, Molday LL, Gehrig A, White KL, Seeliger MW, Jaissle GB, Friedburg C, Tamm E, Molday RS. 2002. Inactivation of the murine X-linked juvenile retinoschisis gene, *Rs1h*, suggests a role of retinoschisin in retinal cell layer organization and synaptic structure. *Proc Natl Acad Sci* **99:** 6222–6227.

Wilczek M. 1935. Ein der netzhautspaltung (retinoschisis) mit einer offnung. *Zeit Augenhlkd* **85:** 105–116.

Wu WW, Molday RS. 2003. Defective discoidin domain structure, subunit assembly, and endoplasmic reticulum processing of retinoschisin are primary mechanisms responsible for X-linked retinoschisis. *J Biol Chem* **278:** 28139–28146.

Zeng Y, Takada Y, Kjellstrom S, Hiriyanna K, Tanikawa A, Wawrousek E, Smaoui N, Caruso R, Bush RA, Sieving PA. 2004. *RS-1* gene delivery to an adult *Rs1h* knockout mouse model restores ERG b-wave with reversal of the electronegative waveform of X-linked retinoschisis. *Invest Ophthalmol Vis Sci* **45:** 3279–3285.

Zhour A, Bolz S, Grimm C, Willmann G, Schatz A, Weber BH, Zrenner E, Fischer MD. 2012. In vivo imaging reveals novel aspects of retinal disease progression in $Rs1h^{-/Y}$ mice but no therapeutic effect of carbonic anhydrase inhibition. *Vet Ophthalmol* **15:** 123–133.

Gene Therapy for *PRPH2*-Associated Ocular Disease: Challenges and Prospects

Shannon M. Conley and Muna I. Naash

Department of Cell Biology, University of Oklahoma Health Sciences Center, Oklahoma City, Oklahoma 73104

Correspondence: muna-naash@ouhsc.edu

The peripherin-2 (*PRPH2*) gene encodes a photoreceptor-specific tetraspanin protein called peripherin-2/retinal degeneration slow (RDS), which is critical for the formation and maintenance of rod and cone outer segments. Over 90 different disease-causing mutations in *PRPH2* have been identified, which cause a variety of forms of retinitis pigmentosa and macular degeneration. Given the disease burden associated with *PRPH2* mutations, the gene has long been a focus for preclinical gene therapy studies. Adeno-associated viruses and compacted DNA nanoparticles carrying *PRPH2* have been successfully used to mediate improvement in the $rds^{-/-}$ and $rds^{+/-}$ mouse models. However, complexities in the pathogenic mechanism for *PRPH2*-associated macular disease coupled with the need for a precise dose of peripherin-2 to combat a severe haploinsufficiency phenotype have delayed the development of clinically viable genetic treatments. Here we discuss the progress and prospects for *PRPH2*-associated gene therapy.

The peripherin-2 (*PRPH2*) gene, previously known as retinal degeneration slow (RDS), encodes a photoreceptor-specific glycoprotein, which is essential for the morphogenesis of rod and cone outer segments (OSs). Although primarily a structural protein, it is absolutely required for vision. Because of the convergence of a combination of factors, this gene has been a target for ocular gene therapy for more than two decades. First and foremost, more than 90 different mutations in *PRPH2* are known to cause varying forms of rod- and cone-dominant, blinding retinal degeneration in patients, making *PRPH2* a logical therapeutic target. In addition, there are several extremely well-characterized animal models for *PRPH2* mutations, with ocular pathologies that mimic many of the patient disease phenotypes, making preclinical testing straightforward. Finally, the *PRPH2* cDNA is relatively small ($\sim$1.1 kb coding region), making it easy to deliver using a variety of different therapeutic approaches. However, in spite of these resources and the length of time researchers have dedicated to *PRPH2* gene therapy, the complex nature of peripherin-2 protein function and regulation, combined with variability in disease mechanism, have thus far precluded development of clinically viable *PRPH2* genetic treatments. Here we discuss these complexities, consider the significant advancements that have been made, and explore barriers that will be over-

Cite this article as *Cold Spring Harb Perspect Med* doi: 10.1101/cshperspect.a017376

come as next-generation genetic therapies are developed.

THE ROLE OF PERIPHERIN-2 PROTEIN IN PHOTORECEPTOR MORPHOGENESIS AND FUNCTION

Peripherin-2 is a ~39 kDa member of the tetraspanin superfamily of proteins. In common with other family members, it has four transmembrane domains, cytoplasmic amino- and carboxy-termini, and a large extracellular loop (called EC2 or D2). Whereas most tetraspanins are located on the plasma membrane, peripherin-2 localization is restricted to the rim region of rod and cone discs/lamellae. Because the rod discs are completely separate from the plasma membrane, the peripherin-2 D2 loop is intradiscal rather than extracellular in rods. After synthesis in the photoreceptor inner segment, peripherin-2 forms noncovalently linked tetramers with itself and its nonglycosylated homolog rod outer segment membrane protein-1 (ROM1) (Goldberg and Molday 1996; Chakraborty et al. 2008a). These complexes subsequently assemble into covalently linked, larger hetero-octamers and peripherin-2 homo-oligomers that localize to the OS rim region (Goldberg et al. 1998; Loewen and Molday 2000; Chakraborty et al. 2008a).

Peripherin-2 is required for the morphogenesis and maintenance of the OS, specifically the rim region. Although the complete role of peripherin-2 in this process is not yet fully elucidated, the carboxy-terminal domain of peripherin-2 has been shown to play a role in membrane fusion (Boesze-Battagliaa and Stefano 2002, 2003), initiation of rim membrane curvature (Khattree et al. 2013), and OS targeting (Tam et al. 2004; Tian et al. 2014). The D2 loop and covalently linked peripherin-2 complexes are required for the maintenance of the flattened rim morphology (Wrigley et al. 2000; Chakraborty et al. 2009, 2010). Peripherin-2/ROM1 complexes are also thought to play a role in regulating disc size and alignment (Cheng et al. 1997; Kedzierski et al. 1997), and, in common with other tetraspanins, are hypothesized to organize a protein microdomain in the rim region (Conley et al. 2011). Interestingly, evidence from disease phenotypes and animal models (discussed below) suggests that peripherin-2 may be differentially required for rods and cones, thus adding a complicating factor for gene therapy.

RETINAL DISEASE PHENOTYPES ASSOCIATED WITH THE *PRPH2* GENE

Mutations in *PRPH2* lead to a wide variety of disease phenotypes (excellently reviewed in Boon et al. 2008). *PRPH2*-associated disease is dominantly inherited and, depending on the mutation, can manifest as autosomal-dominant retinitis pigmentosa (ADRP), digenic ADRP, pattern dystrophy (including butterfly shaped pigment dystrophy and adult vitelliform macular dystrophy), central areolar choroidal dystrophy, and other forms of late-onset macular degeneration (MD) (see http://www.retina-international.org/sci-news/*rds*mut.htm). *PRPH2*-associated monogenic and digenic forms of ADRP primarily target rod photoreceptors; patients usually present with night blindness and progressive loss of peripheral vision. They typically exhibit standard clinical signs of retinitis pigmentosa, including decline of the rod electroretinogram (ERG) response, appearance of bone spicules in the fundus and attenuation of retinal arterioles (Boon et al. 2008). Although the age of onset can be as early as the first to third decade of life in a few cases (Farrar et al. 1991; Gruning et al. 1994), disease presentation typically occurs between the third and fifth decades (Saga et al. 1993; Gruning et al. 1994).

The age of onset for macular and cone-dominant diseases is often similar to that for ADRP, but clinical signs differ dramatically. Although there is a wide spectrum of clinical phenotypes, patients with cone-dominant disease often experience central vision loss (Wickham et al. 2009) and have abnormal multifocal or pattern ERGs, even in the presence of a normal full-field ERG. When full-field ERG defects are present, consistent with the cone-dominant nature of the disease, cone function is usually affected earlier and more severely than rod function (Boon et al. 2008). Common clinical signs include abnormal fundus phenotypes characterized by central retinal pigmentation changes, regions of hyperfluorescence and hypofluorescence, and macular defects (Michaelides et al. 2005; Wickham et al. 2009). In addition, patients often exhibit atrophy of the retinal pigment epithelium (RPE) and choriocapillaris, and sometimes choroidal neovascularization (Boon et al. 2007b; Vaclavik et al. 2012), phenotypes that are thought to contribute to the severity of the vision loss (Moshfeghi et al. 2006; Vaclavik et al. 2012).

One difficulty in defining disease type is that there is often transition from one clinical classification to another; for example, patients that begin by presenting with a purely MD phenotype will later transition to a more general cone-rod or rod-cone dystrophy (Boon et al. 2008). In addition, there can be pronounced inter- and intra-familial phenotypic variability, even among patients all carrying the same mutant allele (Michaelides et al. 2005; Boon et al. 2007a; Vaclavik et al. 2012). Recently, it has been suggested that some of this variability may be a result of the presence of other genetic modifiers. Two genes have thus far been proposed as genetic modifiers: *ROM1*, mutations in which have only thus far associated with digenic RP (with *PRPH2* [Kajiwara et al. 1994]), and *ABCA4*, mutations in which are typically associated with autosomal recessive Stargardt dystrophy (Koenekoop 2003), but which have also been reported to cause some visual impairment in patients carrying only one mutant allele (Maia-Lopes et al. 2008). One study assessing potential modifiers for *PRPH2*-associated disease reported that patients carrying only the R172W *PRPH2* mutation (i.e., no alterations in *ROM1* or *ABCA4*) exhibited well-characterized MD, while those carrying only sequence alterations in *ROM1* or *ABCA4* exhibited only mild phenotypic abnormalities, such as slight lowering of multifocal ERG amplitudes in the central retina (Poloschek et al. 2010). However, clinical phenotypes were worsened and accelerated when mutations in *ROM1* and/or *ABCA4* accompanied the R172W PRPH2 mutation (Poloschek et al. 2010). However, in other families with *PRPH2*-associated disease phenotypes, changes in *ROM1* have been ruled out as a modifying factor (Leroy et al. 2007), underlining the fact that this issue remains under exploration, and the presence of modifying factors is likely to be highly variable. The multiplicity of mutant alleles and potential modifiers combined with the variability of disease phenotypes contributes to the difficulty in designing rational treatment strategies for *PRPH2*-associated diseases.

ANIMAL MODELS FOR PERIPHERIN-2-ASSOCIATED DISEASES

One of the greatest assets for the development of *PRPH2*-associated genetic therapies is the availability of a plethora of well-characterized animal models, which mimic a variety of the human disease phenotypes. In addition to serving as systems for preclinical testing, these models have also been critical for our understanding of the way peripherin-2 functions in rods and cones, both normally and in the presence of disease-causing mutations. The first, and still predominant, peripherin-2 animal model is the naturally occurring *rds* mutant mouse (also known as *rd2*). It was first described in 1978 (van Nie et al. 1978) as a model exhibiting slow retinal degeneration (Jansen and Sanyal 1984; Reuter and Sanyal 1984; Sanyal and Zeilmaker 1984; Hawkins et al. 1985), and, subsequently, the genetic and molecular defect was localized to the peripherin-2 gene (Travis et al. 1989, 1991; Arikawa et al. 1992). This mouse carries a large insertion in the first intron of the gene and no detectable peripherin-2 protein is produced (Ma et al. 1995; Ding et al. 2004), making it a functional knockout model. In addition to slow photoreceptor cell loss, mice homozygous for the mutant allele ($rds^{-/-}$) form no OSs (Jansen and Sanyal 1984). Instead, the connecting cilium terminates with a small membranous bleb, and the subretinal space is filled with abnormal membranous material. In the absence of OSs, the photopigment rhodopsin accumulates in the inner segment and in these abnormal extracellular membranes (Usukura and Bok 1987), a phenomenon thought to contribute to retinal degeneration in the $rds^{-/-}$ model. In addition to these severe structural defects, the mouse exhibits no significant rod or cone photoreceptor ERG signal (Reuter and Sanyal 1984; Chakraborty et al. 2009), emphasizing the role of peripherin-2 in OS morphogenesis and the importance of the elaborated OS structures for proper vision.

Mice heterozygous for the *rds* mutant allele exhibit a striking haploinsufficiency phenotype similar to that seen in patients with ADRP (Cheng et al. 1997). In contrast to the *rds*$^{-/-}$ mice, *rds*$^{+/-}$ mice do form OSs, but they are short and highly abnormal, characterized by whorls of disc membranes rather than properly formed and aligned discs. The *rds*$^{+/-}$ mice also exhibit gradual photoreceptor degeneration, but it is much slower than in the *rds*$^{-/-}$ animals. These structural defects are associated with severe, early onset loss of rod function, detectable as early as ERGs are recorded, with only late-onset cone dysfunction, first appearing ~4 mo of age (Cheng et al. 1997). Because of the genetic (i.e., one wild-type, WT, allele and one mutant allele) and phenotypic (early rod functional deficits followed by late cone deficits) characteristics, the *rds*$^{+/-}$ mouse has been extensively used as a model for *PRPH2*-associated ADRP.

Because *PRPH2* mutations are also associated with cone-dominant macular diseases but the WT mouse has very few cones, a cone-dominant peripherin-2 knockout was generated by crossing *rds*$^{-/-}$ mice onto the *Nrl*$^{-/-}$ background. Nrl is a transcription factor required for the development of rod cells, and in its absence developing rods adopt a cone-like fate (Mears et al. 2001). Studies in *rds*$^{-/-}$/*Nrl*$^{-/-}$ mice have highlighted the differential role of peripherin-2 in rods and cones. In contrast to rods lacking peripherin-2 (in the WT background), cones lacking peripherin-2 (in the *rds*$^{-/-}$/*Nrl*$^{-/-}$ mice) form OSs, albeit dysmorphic ones (Farjo et al. 2006b, 2007). These OSs lack the elaborate folded lamellae structure of normal cones and have no rims at all, but nonetheless retain the ability to mediate phototransduction.

In addition to knockout models, several transgenic models that express different disease-causing-mutations in peripherin-2 have been generated. These include models carrying the ADRP mutations C214S (Stricker et al. 2005; Nour et al. 2008) and P216L (Kedzierski et al. 1997, 2001), and the MD mutation R172W (Ding et al. 2004; Conley et al. 2007, 2014). By crossing these mice onto different *rds* backgrounds, researchers have been able to study the associated disease mechanisms. Expression of the C214S allele on a WT background causes no defects; however, when expressed on the *rds*$^{+/-}$ background (as would be the case in patients), the phenotype is quite similar to that of the nontransgenic *rds*$^{+/-}$ (Stricker et al. 2005). This observation suggests that the C214S mutation is a loss-of-function allele, and other biochemical studies have shown that the C214S protein is unstable, possibly misfolded, and cannot bind to ROM1, likely leading to aggregation in the inner segment and subsequent degradation (Goldberg et al. 1998; Stricker et al. 2005; Conley et al. 2010). In contrast, expression of the MD mutation R172W causes severe, dominant structural and functional degeneration of cones, on either the WT or *rds*$^{+/-}$ background. Rod function, on the other hand, is improved by the presence of the R172W transgene (i.e., R172W/*rds*$^{+/-}$ vs. *rds*$^{+/-}$) (Ding et al. 2004). On a biochemical level, the R172W protein traffics normally to the OS and assembles into complexes with ROM1, although these complexes are not quite normal, especially in cones (Ding et al. 2004; Conley et al. 2014). Combined, these data have led to an overarching hypothesis postulating that rods are more sensitive to the total amount of peripherin-2, whereas cones are more sensitive to having properly assembled peripherin-2 complexes. The corollary to this is that rod-dominant, *PRPH2*-associated disease (e.g., ADRP) is caused by haploinsufficiency, whereas cone-dominant disease is caused by toxic dominant-negative mutations.

Although this hypothesis may be generally useful, the situation is likely more complicated. In the first place, transgenic mice carrying the P216L ADRP mutation exhibit some dominant-negative rod defects such as worsening in OS ultrastructure in P216L versus WT eyes and faster degeneration in P216L/*rds*$^{+/-}$ eyes than in *rds*$^{+/-}$ eyes (Kedzierski et al. 1997). This observation suggests that while haploinsufficiency certainly causes rod-dominant disease, some ADRP mutant alleles may also have toxic gain-of-function or dominant-negative effects in rods. In addition, the mechanism by which R172W (and possibly other *PRPH2* mutations) causes MD is likely more complex than a primary defect in cones. A key phenotype of *PRPH2*-associated MD (including that associated with R172W) is maculopathy and the development of atrophic patches in the RPE, which are visible by fundus examination (Downes et al. 1999) and often appear before ERG changes or vision loss are apparent. The severe MD coupled with choroidal/RPE atrophy seen in *PRPH2*-associated MD patients is therefore likely the result of a combination of primary molecular defects in cone photoreceptors (caused by mutant peripherin-2 protein) coupled with secondary sequellae that impact the RPE as well as the choriocapillaris and choroid. These phenotypes likely present first in the macula, due to the concentration of cones in that region and the metabolic demands on the RPE there, but at a molecular level probably occur throughout the retina (Boon et al. 2008). Exploring the connection between the primary photoreceptor defect and the development of macular changes in the RPE/choroid will be critical for the development of effective genetic therapies. Unfortunately, because the mouse lacks a macula, modeling this interaction is not necessarily straightforward.

GENE THERAPY APPROACHES

There are at least four different gene therapy approaches for the treatment of *PRPH2*-associated retinal disease: (1) gene replacement therapy; (2) gene knockdown and replacement therapy; (3) delivery of neurotrophic factors; and (4) genetic treatment of disease sequellae such as neovascularization. Typical gene delivery requires packaging of the genetic material of interest (DNA or RNA) into either viral or nonviral particles, as DNA alone is not readily taken up by photoreceptors (Farjo et al. 2006a; Cai et al. 2009). Delivery is usually by subretinal injection to promote access to photoreceptors; however, the invasive nature of this approach makes development of effective alternatives a high research priority. There is great variety in the types of nucleic acid packaging approaches that can be used for ocular gene therapy, and as they have been reviewed elsewhere (e.g., Conley and Naash 2010; Han et al. 2011) we will not discuss them here.

Gene Replacement Therapy with Transgenes in Peripherin-2 Models

The earliest proof-of-principle for *PRPH2* gene replacement therapy consisted of attempts to correct the degenerative phenotypes in the $rds^{-/-}$ and $rds^{+/-}$ by transgenic expression of WT peripherin-2. These attempts were highly successful; expression of a WT peripherin-2 transgene in rods driven by the rod-opsin promoter on the $rds^{-/-}$ background preserved photoreceptors and rod OS ultrastructure (Travis et al. 1992). Similarly, subsequent studies showed that expression of a WT peripherin-2 transgene in rods and cones driven by the interphotoreceptor retinoid binding protein (IRBP) promoter rescued rod and cone OS structure and function when expressed on the $rds^{+/-}$ background (Nour et al. 2004). These studies were later extended to show that transgenic expression of WT peripherin-2 could mediate structural and functional improvement in the presence of disease-causing mutations associated with ADRP (C214S) and MD (R172W) (Conley et al. 2007; Nour et al. 2008). Several observations that arose from these studies have a direct bearing on the success of future gene therapy studies. The first was that the dose of the transgene was absolutely critical. This is not surprising given the haploinsufficiency phenotype associated with ADRP in patients, but was reemphasized in the transgenic studies. Models carrying anywhere from 10% (Travis et al. 1992) to 150% (Nour et al. 2004) of WT peripherin-2 were characterized and the amount of peripherin-2 correlated with the severity of the phenotype. Mice expressing ~80% of WT levels had significant structural and functional improvement compared with haploinsufficient $rds^{+/-}$ mice, but photoreceptors still exhibited some defects. Lower levels of expression resulted in correspondingly more severe phenotypes. Positively, overexpression of peripherin-2 elicited no toxic outcomes; so while having too little peripherin-2 results in incomplete rescue, having too much is not detrimental (Nour et al. 2004). The second interesting observation was that WT peripherin-2 expression mediated structural and functional improvements even in the presence of dominant-negative mutations such as R172W (Conley et al. 2007). Unfortunately, although some improvement was noted, it was not to the same magnitude and did not last as long as the improvement observed when WT peripherin-2 was expressed in the presence of loss-of-function mutations (e.g., C214S) associated with ADRP (Nour et al. 2008).

The partial rescue we observe with transgenesis in R172W animals suggests that the R172W mutation behaves as a dominant-negative (rather than a toxic gain-of-function mutation) and thus may be at least somewhat amenable to rescue via gene supplementation. However, it is not clear whether other dominantly inherited MD mutations in *PRPH2* are gain-of-function or dominant-negatives. Traditional gain-of-function mutations would not likely be rescued by gene supplementation, and the only partial rescue seen in the R172W model suggests that that full rescue for dominant-negative or gain-of-function mutations may require concurrent knockdown of the mutant allele.

Gene Replacement Therapy with Adeno-Associated Viruses (AAV) in Peripherin-2 Models

In the last 15 years, gene replacement therapy for peripherin-2 has been attempted using both viral and nonviral approaches. Initial studies by Dr. Robin Ali's group used recombinant AAV (rAAV) carrying a 2.2 kb fragment of the rod-opsin promoter and the murine peripherin-2 cDNA (rAAV.rho.prph2) (Ali et al. 2000). This approach has been quite promising for other ocular gene therapy studies, and AAVs are currently in clinical trials for the treatment of RPE-associated Leber congenital amaurosis (recently reviewed in Boye et al. 2013). Initially, rAAV.rho.prph2 was delivered subretinally to *rds*$^{-/-}$ animals at postnatal day (P) 10, and animals were assessed at times ranging from 3–9 wk postinjection (Ali et al. 2000). The investigators reported exciting improvements in scotopic ERG amplitudes and rod OS structure (Ali et al. 2000), although levels did not meet those seen in WT or *rds*$^{+/-}$ animals. Subsequent studies evaluated the efficacy of treatment at multiple ages (ranging from P5 to P95), with evaluation at 1 mo postinjection (Sarra et al. 2001). Although the best improvements in OS structure were observed when treatment was delivered early (P5 or P10), some minor improvements were noted at later delivery ages. Interestingly, in spite of transducing ~30%–40% of photoreceptors, there was no reduction in the rate or magnitude of photoreceptor cell loss after treatment with rAAV.rho.prph2. The investigators hypothesize that this is tied to the fact that the onset of expression of the rAAV is ~2 wk postinjection (Sarra et al. 2001), a time point at which the *rds*$^{-/-}$ retina is already undergoing significant degeneration. Although this provides another argument for early intervention and the development of treatments with rapid-onset expression, it is worth remembering that degeneration in the *rds*$^{+/-}$ retina (which more closely mimics that in patients) is much slower than in the *rds*$^{-/-}$ retina.

In a final study, researchers asked whether multiple injections could enhance the beneficial effect and how long the benefits of AAV-associated therapy would last (Schlichtenbrede et al. 2003). Repeat injection 5 d after the initial treatment (at P15) resulted in better rescue than was achieved with a single injection, but in both cases improvements in scotopic b-wave amplitude peaked at 5 wk postinjection, and by 15 wk postinjection retinal function in treated *rds*$^{-/-}$ mice was comparable to levels observed in untreated *rds*$^{-/-}$ animals (Schlichtenbrede et al. 2003). Although these results were promising, the magnitude of the improvement was fairly small; maximum b-wave amplitudes in animals treated with AAV were ~150 μV (improved from ~60 μV in uninjected *rds*$^{-/-}$ mice) compared to 400–500 μV in age-matched WT animals (Schlichtenbrede et al. 2003). Furthermore, significant improvements in scotopic a-wave amplitudes, a more direct measure of rod photoreceptor function, were not reported. Excitingly, the AAVs appeared to be well-tolerated and there was no sign of an inflammatory response in any of the eyes tested (Ali et al. 2000).

The reasons for this incomplete rescue may be tied to the partial transduction (investigators estimate ~30% transduction) or the levels of expression, but also highlight some issues related to the *rds*$^{-/-}$ model. This model has the benefit of "starting from zero"; that is, because there are no detectable OSs and no detectable function or protein, small improvements are easy to detect. On the other hand, the absence of even baseline OS structure/function and the ongoing degeneration may make it more difficult to initiate OS formation by exogenous therapeutic delivery. More importantly, this model does not accurately mimic the case in patients who have haploinsufficiency-associated disease. A more clinically relevant model would be the *rds*$^{+/-}$ mouse, which has a much slower rate of degeneration and exhibits OSs, albeit highly malformed. However, it is not clear whether improvements on the scale reported with AAV would be detectable in that model.

Gene Replacement Therapy with Nanoparticles in Peripherin-2 Models

Based on the positive initial results using AAV to deliver peripherin-2, we have more recently explored the use of compacted DNA nanoparticles (NPs) to deliver WT peripherin-2. These NPs are composed of polyethylene glycol-conjugated polylysine (CK30-PEG) and a plasmid DNA, and we have shown that they are capable of transducing a variety of retinal cell types (Farjo et al. 2006a; Han et al. 2012a). In addition to our murine studies on *PRPH2*-associated ADRP (discussed further below), we have showed that these NPs can mediate long-term ocular phenotypic improvements in mouse models of *RPE65*-associated Leber congenital amaurosis (Koirala et al. 2013a,b) and *ABCA4*-associated Stargardt macular dystrophy (Han et al. 2012b). Importantly, these NPs are well-tolerated in the retina, even after repeat injections (Ding et al. 2009; Cai et al. 2010; Han et al. 2012a,c), and have a large DNA capacity (tested up to 14 kb in the eye [Han et al. 2012b] and 20 kb in the lung [Fink et al. 2006]). To determine whether they were capable of mediating improvements in the *PRPH2*-associated retinitis pigmentosa phenotype, we generated NPs carrying the full-length mouse peripherin-2 cDNA (called NMP for normal mouse peripherin-2) under the control of the rod- and cone-specific IRBP promoter or the ubiquitously expressed chicken beta actin (CBA) promoter (Cai et al. 2009). We elected to use the *rds*$^{+/-}$ model, as it more closely mimics the patient situation, and subretinally delivered the NPs (or controls) at P5. Gene expression and disease phenotypes were tracked for up to 4 mo postinjection. We observed appreciable expression levels of the transferred gene message as early as 2 d postinjection, and by 1 wk postinjection, levels of peripherin-2 message in treated eyes had stabilized at levels two- to threefold higher than was observed in uninjected eyes, and these levels persisted throughout the study (Cai et al. 2009). As controls, we injected eyes with naked (i.e., uncompacted) plasmid; no increases in gene expression were observed in eyes treated with naked DNA compared to uninjected controls. The NP-mediated expression of peripherin-2 resulted in improved photoreceptor OS structure at both 1 and 4 mo postinjection, detected mostly in the region near the site of injection. Functionally we observed small but nonsignificant improvements in scotopic a-wave, and significant improvement in photopic (cone)-b waves, for NP-injected eyes compared to naked DNA injected eyes (Cai et al. 2009). Interestingly, there was no significant difference in efficacy for the two promoters.

To qualitatively assess the longevity of phenotypic improvement, a small subset of *rds*$^{+/-}$ animals injected at P5 with IRBP-NMP NPs were aged out to 15 mo postinjection. We observed pronounced preservation of outer nuclear layer thickness in the treated eye compared to a matched region from the uninjected contralateral eye (Fig. 1A, green bar vs. red bar in lower panels). This preservation was most pronounced in the peripheral retina and on the side

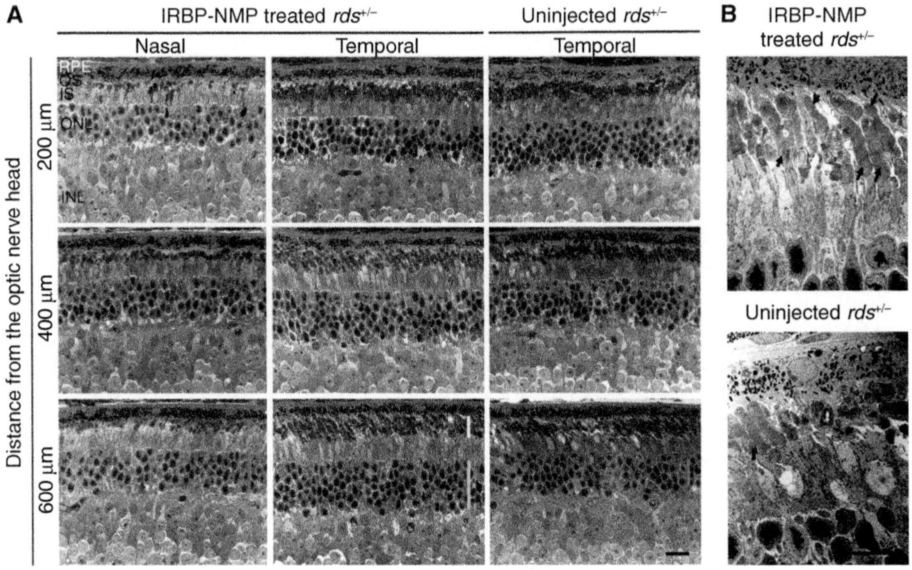

Figure 1. IRBP NPs carrying peripherin-2 mediate improvements in retinal function at 15 mo postinjection. At P5, *rds*$^{+/-}$ animals were injected in one eye with compacted DNA NPs carrying the peripherin-2 cDNA (NMP) under the control of the IRBP promoter. The contralateral eye served as an uninjected control. Fifteen months later, eyes were harvested for histological analysis. (*A*) Light micrographs showing improved outer nuclear layer (green and red bars) and OS thickness (blue and yellow bars) in the peripheral retina on the side of the eye that received the injection. NMP, peripherin-2-carrying nanoparticles; RPE, retinal pigment epithelium; OS, outer segment; IS, inner segment, ONL, outer nuclear layer; INL, inner nuclear layer. Scale bar, 25 µm. (*B*) Transmission electron micrographs of the same eyes taken from the temporal region. Black arrows identify nicely stacked OSs whereas red arrowheads show the dysmorphic swirl OS typical of *rds*$^{+/-}$ eyes. Scale bar, 10 µm.

of the eye at which injection had occurred (see the red bars in the lower left column of Fig. 1A). We also observed that the thickness of the OS layer was better preserved on the side of the eye that had been injected compared to the opposing side (Fig. 1A, yellow vs. blue bar in lower panels). This preservation was reflected on the ultrastructural level as well (Fig. 1B) in the region of injection. Whereas nicely stacked (black arrows) and highly dysmorphic (red arrowheads) OSs were observed in both the IRBP-NMP NP-treated eye and the uninjected control, overall ultrastructure was improved in the NP-treated eye (Fig. 1B). These data suggest that compacted-DNA NPs can mediate long-term improvements in retinal structure, but only in a limited region of the treated retina.

In common with those testing AAVs, we also asked whether treatment of *rds*$^{+/-}$ at a later age (P22) could mediate improvements in photoreceptor structure and function. For these studies, we elected to use NPs carrying the murine peripherin-2 cDNA (NMP) under the control of a 221 bp fragment of the mouse opsin promoter (MOP), which is expressed in rods and cones (Glushakova et al. 2006). As before, we observed only small, nonsignificant improvements in the scotopic a-wave after treatment with MOP-NMP NPs irrespective of treatment age (P5 or P22), although modest improvements in the scotopic b-wave were observed after treatment at either age. Again, we observed significant improvement in cone function (photopic b-wave) up to 4 mo posttreatment—the longest period tested—compared to controls injected with naked DNA. Although some functional improvements were detected after treatment at P22, structural improvements were quite minor compared to those seen after treatment at P5, confirming that earlier intervention yields better results. Because ERG does not always correlate with vision, we also tested visual acuity and contrast sensitivity under photopic conditions using the OptoMotry system in a subset of eyes treated at P5 with MOP-NMP NPs (Cai et al. 2010). Assessments were performed at 9–10 mo postinjection; treated animals exhibited visual acuities and contrast sensitivities similar to those observed with WT animals, whereas saline-injected eyes were not different from age-matched uninjected controls.

Combined, these studies suggest that gene augmentation with either NPs or AAV is feasible for *PRPH2*-associated RP; however, achieving full rescue has been difficult, likely because of the requirements of a precise dose of peripherin-2 to support OS structure and the difficulty in transfecting the whole retina.

Gene Knockdown Therapy in Peripherin-2 Models

Because *PRPH2*-associated disease is often caused by gain-of-function or dominant-negative alleles (such as R172W) and pure gene replacement (e.g., with transgenes) improved but did not completely correct the dominant phenotype in mice carrying that mutation (Conley et al. 2007), knockdown approaches may need to be developed to eliminate the mutant allele. From a practical standpoint, these will need to be combined with gene replacement therapy, as peripherin-2 haploinsufficiency makes knockdown of the mutant allele alone unlikely to be successful. Furthermore, the sheer number of different mutant alleles combined with the infrequency of any given allele means that developing a knockdown strategy for each mutation would be both time consuming and economically disadvantageous. As a result, development of a mutation-independent knockdown approach is desirable. This approach has been explored with relative success for rhodopsin gene therapy. Like *PRPH2*, there are a plethora of different dominant, disease-causing mutant rhodopsin alleles that cause inherited retinal degeneration, and knockdown has been attempted in vitro and in vivo with varying degrees of success using multiple methods, including ribozymes (Chakraborty et al. 2008b), siRNA (Teusner et al. 2006; Gorbatyuk et al. 2007; O'Reilly et al. 2007; Mao et al. 2012), and zinc finger nucleases (Mussolino et al. 2011). Thus far, shRNA is the most well-developed approach, and recent results suggest that a single AAV vector carrying an shRNA capable of knocking down WT- and mutant rhodopsin, coupled with a WT rhodopsin that is resistant to silencing, results in long-term (up to 9 mo of age) preservation of photoreceptor structure and function in the P23H mouse model of rhodopsin-associated ADRP (Mao et al. 2012).

Recently, the same group that has led the field in the development of rhodopsin-associated knockdown has begun to apply this approach to peripherin-2 (Petrs-Silva et al. 2012). After identifying two different siRNAs that could knockdown WT peripherin-2 in vitro, researchers packaged the shRNAs into rAAV vectors and delivered them to the subretinal space of WT mice. Peripherin-2 message was reduced by $\sim$75% in shRNA-treated eyes, and a corresponding 30%–50% decrease in the scotopic a-wave was reported. Subsequently, a version of peripherin-2 resistant to the shRNAs was placed under control of the CBA promoter in an AAV vector and codelivered with the shRNA AAV into WT mice. Codelivery of the two viruses led to rescue of the functional defect caused by the shRNA knockdown and partial recovery of total peripherin-2 protein levels (Petrs-Silva et al. 2012). A similar approach was taken by different investigators, who injected WT mice with a shRNA vector and a resistant WT peripherin-2 gene, using electroporation rather than viral compaction. They reported knockdown of the endogenous WT allele and stable expression of the resistant, exogenously delivered allele (Palfi et al. 2006). Although the efficacy of this approach in disease models has yet to be evaluated, these exciting studies show proof of principle for allele-independent knockdown combined with gene supplementation to combat *PRPH2*-associated disease.

Gene-Based Delivery of Neurotrophic Factors in the Peripherin-2 Model

Although gene augmentation therapy is the most obvious strategy for *PRPH2*-associated disease, delivery of neurotrophic factors was actually the first option to be explored. This approach does not correct the underlying genetic defect, but it has the benefit of being inherently allele- and gene-independent and therefore potentially applicable to a variety of forms of degeneration. In 1998, a French group delivered ciliary neurotrophic factor (CNTF) to the intravitreal space of *rds*$^{-/-}$ mice using an adenoviral vector (Cayouette et al. 1998). Excitingly, they reported preservation of outer nuclear layer thickness at 2 wk and 2 mo postinjection. However, they reported only very small improvements in rod function and no improvements in cone function. The retardation of retinal degeneration was enough to promote further research in that direction, however, and a separate group reported similar preservation of structure but not function after AAV-mediated delivery of CNTF in the *rds*$^{-/-}$ model (Liang et al. 2001). In later work, rAAV was also used to deliver CNTF in the P216L/*rds*$^{+/-}$ ADRP model. A rescue of retinal degeneration similar to that seen with the *rds*$^{-/-}$ mouse was reported, but the investigators also observed dose-dependent abnormalities in photoreceptor nuclei and a decrease in rod and cone function (Bok et al. 2002). Subsequent studies using this model showed that CNTF significantly altered retinal signaling pathways and down-regulated many important phototransduction genes, including cone opsins (Rhee et al. 2007). Although this toxicity precludes the further use of CNTF for *PRPH2*-associated disease, other neurotrophic factors have also been tested. Lentivirus carrying either human fibroblast growth factor-2 (FGF-2) or human pigment epithelial-derived factor (PEDF) was reported to improve scotopic a- and b-waves in *rds*$^{-/-}$ mice, but it did not improve photoreceptor survival (Miyazaki et al. 2008). Conclusions from that study are complicated, however, by significant inconsistencies between the baseline ERG values reported (Miyazaki et al. 2008) and those from other groups using the same model (Reuter and Sanyal 1984; Ali et al. 2000; Chakraborty et al. 2009). Many neurotrophic factors have been explored for the prevention of degeneration in other forms of retinal degeneration, and one may be identified which is clearly beneficial for *PRPH2*-associated disease. However, it is evident that extensive testing in the right models will be required to identify a clinically relevant choice.

Other drugs and hormones which do not fall into the category of traditional neurotrophic factors have also been used to provide some level of neuroprotection (i.e., retardation of retinal degeneration) and, in some cases, improved function, in the *rds*$^{-/-}$ and *rds*$^{+/-}$ models. These include the hormone erythropoietin (Rex et al. 2004, 2009), the calcium channel blocker nilvadipine (Takeuchi et al. 2008), and the monoamine oxidase inhibitor rasagiline (Eigeldinger-Berthou et al. 2012). It is possible that genetic interference in the pathways regulated by these compounds may prove to be a beneficial approach, or that simple delivery of pharmacologic agents in conjunction with gene supplementation therapy may be effective. Further studies will be needed to assess the safety and efficacy of this method.

Antineovascularization Therapy for Peripherin-2-Associated Disease

The final type of potential genetic therapy is targeted at the specific clinical signs of disease. Much like neurotrophic therapy, this approach does not correct the underlying genetic defect, and it is also allele- and gene-independent. As in most age-related MD, vision loss in many forms of *PRPH2*-associated macular- or pattern dystrophy is caused or exacerbated by neovascularization of the retina or choroid (Moshfeghi et al. 2006; Boon et al. 2008). In a patient carrying the *PRPH2*-pattern dystrophy mutation Y141C who exhibited choroidal neovascularization, repeat injections with the anti-VEGF drug ranibizumab ameliorated the neovascularization and improved visual acuity (Vaclavik et al. 2012). Benefits have also been reported in other studies using anti-VEGF drugs (bevacizumab or ranibizumab) to treat various forms of pattern dystrophy-associated choroidal neovascularization (Parodi et al. 2010; Gallego-Pinazo et al. 2011). Because repeated injections of this type of drug are usually required for efficacy, age-related MD research has focused on development of effective, long-lasting genetic therapies that can inhibit VEGF-associated neovascularization (e.g., Askou et al. 2012; Pihlmann et al. 2012), and has resulted in the initiation of several clinical trials (NCT01494805, NCT01367444, NCT01301443, NCT01024998). This approach has not been directly tested in *rds* models, but utilization of anti-VEGF drugs in *PRPH2* patients with neovascularization may have merit.

CONCLUDING REMARKS

Here we have discussed a variety of different options for the genetic treatment of *PRPH2*-associated ADRP and MD. Because of the differential requirements for peripherin-2 for OS structure and function in rods and cones, effective gene augmentation for loss-of-function alleles or gene knockdown plus supplementation for gain-of-function alleles will likely be a mainstay of any truly curative therapy. However, given that vision loss is sometimes associated with secondary (i.e., nonphotoreceptor) defects such as choroidal neovascularization, combinatorial therapy that includes a neuroprotective or antineovascular agent could increase treatment efficacy.

Several obstacles to the development of targeted genetic therapies for peripherin-2 remain. These include the lack of understanding of the actual disease mechanism for *PRPH2*-associated macular disease, and specifically a lack of understanding of the connection between primary photoreceptor defects that are well-tolerated for several decades and secondary RPE/choroidal defects that lead to late-onset vision loss. The lack of a mouse model with a macula and the large clinical and genetic heterogeneity in peripherin-2 patient populations further confound studies of this disease mechanism. Another complicating factor is the structural nature of the peripherin-2 protein, and the associated requirement for a very precise dose. Peripherin-2 haploinsufficiency means that effective disease treatment must generate a fairly large quantity of protein, and a result of constant OS renewal, effective treatments must result in prolonged, elevated gene expression. In addition, early treatment is clearly optimal, but the age at which treatment of mice is most effective (P5 to P10) has an in utero developmental equivalent in humans; that is, by birth the human retina has already passed the stage that has been identified as optimal for gene delivery in mice. This, combined with the fact that disease presentation often follows, rather than precedes, the onset of degeneration, means that early intervention is nearly impossible. Finally, there are obstacles that affect many forms of photoreceptor-associated gene therapy, such as the difficulty in achieving pan-retinal transfection and the difficulty of transfecting photoreceptors to any extent. Although both AAVs and compacted DNA NPs can transfect photoreceptors, they are not nearly as easy to target as other cell types (such as the adjacent RPE). This has implications for the development and targeting of delivery strategies. In addition, expression is usually limited to the region of retina detached during the subretinal injection procedure (i.e., the retinal bleb). Because retinal detachment in itself can be harmful, development of effective intravitreal gene delivery vehicles would be ideal.

Despite these limitations, advances in vector engineering to increase, prolong, and regulate gene expression, combined with advances in delivery technology, such as precisely engineered AAV capsids and targeted NPs, make the development of a clinically applicable peripherin-2 gene therapy more likely than ever before. Given that current vectors (both AAVs and NPs) are able to drive per cell gene expression at fairly high levels; key targets for immediate preclinical research in this field include increasing distribution of gene expression throughout the retina and development of therapies that are effective after intravitreal delivery.

ACKNOWLEDGMENTS

The authors thank Ms. Barb Nagel for her excellent technical assistance with the histology. This work was supported by the National Eye Institute (EY10609, EY022778, EY01865 to M.I.N.), the Foundation Fighting Blindness (M.I.N.), and the Oklahoma Center for the Advancement of Science and Technology (M.I.N. and S.M.C.).

REFERENCES

Ali RR, Sarra GM, Stephens C, Alwis MD, Bainbridge JW, Munro PM, Fauser S, Reichel MB, Kinnon C, Hunt DM, et al. 2000. Restoration of photoreceptor ultrastructure and function in retinal degeneration slow mice by gene therapy. *Nat Genet* **25**: 306–310.

Arikawa K, Molday LL, Molday RS, Williams DS. 1992. Localization of peripherin/*rds* in the disk membranes of cone and rod photoreceptors: Relationship to disk membrane morphogenesis and retinal degeneration. *J Cell Biol* **116**: 659–667.

Askou AL, Pournaras JA, Pihlmann M, Svalgaard JD, Arsenijevic Y, Kostic C, Bek T, Dagnaes-Hansen F, Mikkelsen JG, Jensen TG, et al. 2012. Reduction of choroidal neovascularization in mice by adeno-associated virus-delivered anti-vascular endothelial growth factor short hairpin RNA. *J Gene Med* **14**: 632–641.

Boesze-Battagliaa K, Stefano FP. 2002. Peripherin/rds fusogenic function correlates with subunit assembly. *Exp Eye Res* **75**: 227–231.

Boesze-Battaglia K, Goldberg AF, Dispoto J, Katragadda M, Cesarone G, Albert AD. 2003. A soluble peripherin/Rds C-terminal polypeptide promotes membrane fusion and changes conformation upon membrane association. *Exp Eye Res* **77**: 505–514.

Bok D, Yasumura D, Matthes MT, Ruiz A, Duncan JL, Chappelow AV, Zolutukhin S, Hauswirth W, LaVail MM. 2002. Effects of adeno-associated virus-vectored ciliary neurotrophic factor on retinal structure and function in mice with a P216L rds/peripherin mutation. *Exp Eye Res* **74**: 719–735.

Boon CJ, Klevering BJ, den Hollander AI, Zonneveld MN, Theelen T, Cremers FP, Hoyng CB. 2007a. Clinical and genetic heterogeneity in multifocal vitelliform dystrophy. *Arch Ophthalmol* **125**: 1100–1106.

Boon CJ, van Schooneveld MJ, den Hollander AI, van Lith-Verhoeven JJ, Zonneveld-Vrieling MN, Theelen T, Cremers FP, Hoyng CB, Klevering BJ. 2007b. Mutations in the *peripherin/RDS* gene are an important cause of multifocal pattern dystrophy simulating STGD1/fundus flavimaculatus. *Br J Ophthalmol* **91**: 1504–1511.

Boon CJ, den Hollander AI, Hoyng CB, Cremers FP, Klevering BJ, Keunen JE. 2008. The spectrum of retinal dystrophies caused by mutations in the *peripherin/RDS* gene. *Prog Retin Eye Res* **27**: 213–235.

Boye SE, Boye SL, Lewin AS, Hauswirth WW. 2013. A comprehensive review of retinal gene therapy. *Mol Ther* **21**: 509–519.

Cai X, Nash Z, Conley SM, Fliesler SJ, Cooper MJ, Naash MI. 2009. A partial structural and functional rescue of a retinitis pigmentosa model with compacted DNA nanoparticles. *PLoS ONE* **4**: e5290.

Cai X, Conley SM, Nash Z, Fliesler SJ, Cooper MJ, Naash MI. 2010. Gene delivery to mitotic and postmitotic photoreceptors via compacted DNA nanoparticles results in improved phenotype in a mouse model of retinitis pigmentosa. *FASEB J* **24**: 1178–1191.

Cayouette M, Behn D, Sendtner M, Lachapelle P, Gravel C. 1998. Intraocular gene transfer of ciliary neurotrophic factor prevents death and increases responsiveness of rod photoreceptors in the retinal degeneration slow mouse. *J Neurosci* **18**: 9282–9293.

Chakraborty D, Ding XQ, Fliesler SJ, Naash MI. 2008a. Outer segment oligomerization of Rds: Evidence from mouse models and subcellular fractionation. *Biochemistry* **47**: 1144–1156.

Chakraborty D, Whalen P, Lewin AS, Naash MI. 2008b. In vitro analysis of ribozyme-mediated knockdown of an ADRP associated rhodopsin mutation. *Adv Exp Med Biol* **613**: 97–106.

Chakraborty D, Ding XQ, Conley SM, Fliesler SJ, Naash MI. 2009. Differential requirements for retinal degeneration slow intermolecular disulfide-linked oligomerization in rods versus cones. *Hum Mol Genet* **18**: 797–808.

Chakraborty D, Conley SM, Stuck MW, Naash MI. 2010. Differences in RDS trafficking, assembly and function in cones versus rods: Insights from studies of C150S-RDS. *Hum Mol Genet* **19**: 4799–4812.

Cheng T, Peachey NS, Li S, Goto Y, Cao Y, Naash MI. 1997. The effect of peripherin/rds haploinsufficiency on rod and cone photoreceptors. *J Neurosci* **17**: 8118–8128.

Conley SM, Naash MI. 2010. Nanoparticles for retinal gene therapy. *Prog Retin Eye Res* **29**: 376–397.

Conley S, Nour M, Fliesler SJ, Naash MI. 2007. Late-onset cone photoreceptor degeneration induced by R172W mutation in Rds and partial rescue by gene supplementation. *Invest Ophthalmol Vis Sci* **48**: 5397–5407.

Conley SM, Stricker HM, Naash MI. 2010. Biochemical analysis of phenotypic diversity associated with mutations in codon 244 of the retinal degeneration slow gene. *Biochemistry* **49**: 905–911.

Conley SM, Stuck MW, Naash MI. 2011. Structural and functional relationships between photoreceptor tetraspanins and other superfamily members. *Cell Mol Life Sci.*

Conley SM, Stuck MW, Burnett JL, Chakraborty D, Azadi S, Fliesler SJ, Naash MI. 2014. Insights into the mechanisms of macular degeneration associated with the R172W mutation in RDS. *Hum Mol Genet.*

Ding XQ, Nour M, Ritter LM, Goldberg AF, Fliesler SJ, Naash MI. 2004. The R172W mutation in peripherin/*rds* causes a cone–rod dystrophy in transgenic mice. *Hum Mol Genet* **13**: 2075–2087.

Ding XQ, Quiambao AB, Fitzgerald JB, Cooper MJ, Conley SM, Naash MI. 2009. Ocular delivery of compacted DNA-nanoparticles does not elicit toxicity in the mouse retina. *PLoS ONE* **4**: e7410.

Downes SM, Fitzke FW, Holder GE, Payne AM, Bessant DA, Bhattacharya SS, Bird AC. 1999. Clinical features of codon 172 RDS macular dystrophy: Similar phenotype in 12 families. *Arch Ophthalmol* **117**: 1373–1383.

Eigeldinger-Berthou S, Meier C, Zulliger R, Lecaude S, Enzmann V, Sarra GM. 2012. Rasagiline interferes with neurodegeneration in the Prph2/rds mouse. *Retina* **32**: 617–628.

Farjo R, Skaggs J, Quiambao AB, Cooper MJ, Naash MI. 2006a. Efficient non-viral ocular gene transfer with compacted DNA nanoparticles. *PLoS ONE* **1**: e38.

Farjo R, Skaggs JS, Nagel BA, Quiambao AB, Nash ZA, Fliesler SJ, Naash MI. 2006b. Retention of function without normal disc morphogenesis occurs in cone but not rod photoreceptors. *J Cell Biol* **173**: 59–68.

Farrar GJ, Kenna P, Jordan SA, Kumar-Singh R, Humphries MM, Sharp EM, Sheils DM, Humphries P. 1991. A three-base-pair deletion in the peripherin–*RDS* gene in one form of retinitis pigmentosa. *Nature* **354**: 478–480.

Farjo R, Fliesler SJ, Naash MI. 2007. Effect of Rds abundance on cone outer segment morphogenesis, photoreceptor gene expression, and outer limiting membrane integrity. *J Comp Neurol* **504**: 619–630.

Fink TL, Klepcyk PJ, Oette SM, Gedeon CR, Hyatt SL, Kowalczyk TH, Moen RC, Cooper MJ. 2006. Plasmid size up to 20 kbp does not limit effective in vivo lung gene transfer using compacted DNA nanoparticles. *Gene Ther* **13**: 1048–1051.

Gallego-Pinazo R, Dolz-Marco R, Pardo-Lopez D, Arevalo JF, Diaz-Llopis M. 2011. Primary intravitreal ranibizumab for adult-onset foveomacular vitelliform dystrophy. *Graefes Arch Clin Exp Ophthalmol* **249**: 455–458.

Glushakova LG, Timmers AM, Issa TM, Cortez NG, Pang J, Teusner JT, Hauswirth WW. 2006. Does recombinant adeno-associated virus-vectored proximal region of mouse rhodopsin promoter support only rod-type specific expression in vivo? *Mol Vis* **12**: 298–309.

Goldberg AF, Molday RS. 1996. Subunit composition of the peripherin/rds-rom-1 disk rim complex from rod photoreceptors: Hydrodynamic evidence for a tetrameric quaternary structure. *Biochemistry* **35**: 6144–6149.

Goldberg AF, Loewen CJ, Molday RS. 1998. Cysteine residues of photoreceptor peripherin/rds: Role in subunit assembly and autosomal dominant retinitis pigmentosa. *Biochemistry* **37**: 680–685.

Gorbatyuk M, Justilien V, Liu J, Hauswirth WW, Lewin AS. 2007. Suppression of mouse rhodopsin expression in vivo by AAV mediated siRNA delivery. *Vision Res* **47**: 1202–1208.

Gruning G, Millan JM, Meins M, Beneyto M, Caballero M, Apfelstedt-Sylla E, Bosch R, Zrenner E, Prieto F, Gal A. 1994. Mutations in the human peripherin/RDS gene associated with autosomal dominant retinitis pigmentosa. *Hum Mutat* **3**: 321–323.

Han Z, Conley SM, Naash MI. 2011. AAV and compacted DNA nanoparticles for the treatment of retinal disorders: Challenges and future prospects. *Invest Ophthalmol Vis Sci* **52**: 3051–3059.

Han Z, Conley SM, Makkia R, Guo J, Cooper MJ, Naash MI. 2012a. Comparative analysis of DNA nanoparticles and AAVs for ocular gene delivery. *PLoS ONE* **7**: e52189.

Han Z, Conley SM, Makkia RS, Cooper MJ, Naash MI. 2012b. DNA nanoparticle-mediated *ABCA4* delivery rescues Stargardt dystrophy in mice. *J Clin Invest* **122**: 3221–3226.

Han Z, Koirala A, Makkia R, Cooper MJ, Naash MI. 2012c. Direct gene transfer with compacted DNA nanoparticles in retinal pigment epithelial cells: Expression, repeat delivery and lack of toxicity. *Nanomedicine (Lond)* **7**: 521–539.

Hawkins RK, Jansen HG, Sanyal S. 1985. Development and degeneration of retina in *rds* mutant mice: Photoreceptor abnormalities in the heterozygotes. *Exp Eye Res* **41**: 701–720.

Jansen HG, Sanyal S. 1984. Development and degeneration of retina in *rds* mutant mice: electron microscopy. *J Comp Neurol* **224**: 71–84.

Kajiwara K, Berson EL, Dryja TP. 1994. Digenic retinitis pigmentosa due to mutations at the unlinked peripherin/*RDS* and *ROM1* loci. *Science* **264**: 1604–1608.

Kedzierski W, Lloyd M, Birch DG, Bok D, Travis GH. 1997. Generation and analysis of transgenic mice expressing P216L-substituted rds/peripherin in rod photoreceptors. *Invest Ophthalmol Vis Sci* **38**: 498–509.

Kedzierski W, Nusinowitz S, Birch D, Clarke G, McInnes RR, Bok D, Travis GH. 2001. Deficiency of rds/peripherin causes photoreceptor death in mouse models of digenic and dominant retinitis pigmentosa. *Proc Natl Acad Sci* **98**: 7718–7723.

Khattree N, Ritter LM, Goldberg AF. 2013. Membrane curvature generation by a C-terminal amphipathic helix in peripherin-2/rds, a tetraspanin required for photoreceptor sensory cilium morphogenesis. *J Cell Sci* **126**: 4659–4670.

Koenekoop RK. 2003. The gene for Stargardt disease, *ABCA4*, is a major retinal gene: A mini-review. *Ophthalmic Genet* **24**: 75–80.

Koirala A, Conley SM, Makkia R, Liu Z, Cooper MJ, Sparrow JR, Naash MI. 2013a. Persistence of non-viral vector mediated RPE65 expression: Case for viability as a gene transfer therapy for RPE-based diseases. *J Control Release* **172**: 745–752.

Koirala A, Makkia RS, Conley SM, Cooper MJ, Naash MI. 2013b. S/MAR-containing DNA nanoparticles promote persistent RPE gene expression and improvement in RPE65-associated LCA. *Hum Mol Genet* **22**: 1632–1642.

Leroy BP, Kailasanathan A, De Laey JJ, Black GC, Manson FD. 2007. Intrafamilial phenotypic variability in families with *RDS* mutations: Exclusion of ROM1 as a genetic modifier for those with retinitis pigmentosa. *Br J Ophthalmol* **91**: 89–93.

Liang FQ, Aleman TS, Dejneka NS, Dudus L, Fisher KJ, Maguire AM, Jacobson SG, Bennett J. 2001. Long-term protection of retinal structure but not function using RAAV.CNTF in animal models of retinitis pigmentosa. *Mol Ther* **4**: 461–472.

Loewen CJ, Molday RS. 2000. Disulfide-mediated oligomerization of Peripherin/Rds and Rom-1 in photoreceptor disk membranes. Implications for photoreceptor outer segment morphogenesis and degeneration. *J Biol Chem* **275**: 5370–5378.

Ma J, Norton JC, Allen AC, Burns JB, Hasel KW, Burns JL, Sutcliffe JG, Travis GH. 1995. Retinal degeneration slow (*rds*) in mouse results from simple insertion of a *t* haplotype-specific element into protein-coding exon II. *Genomics* **28**: 212–219.

Maia-Lopes S, Silva ED, Silva MF, Reis A, Faria P, Castelo-Branco M. 2008. Evidence of widespread retinal dysfunction in patients with stargardt disease and morphologically unaffected carrier relatives. *Invest Ophthalmol Vis Sci* **49**: 1191–1199.

Mao H, Gorbatyuk MS, Rossmiller B, Hauswirth WW, Lewin AS. 2012. Long-term rescue of retinal structure and function by rhodopsin RNA replacement with a single adeno-associated viral vector in P23H *RHO* transgenic mice. *Hum Gene Ther* **23**: 356–366.

Mears AJ, Kondo M, Swain PK, Takada Y, Bush RA, Saunders TL, Sieving PA, Swaroop A. 2001. Nrl is required for rod photoreceptor development. *Nat Genet* **29**: 447–452.

Michaelides M, Holder GE, Bradshaw K, Hunt DM, Moore AT. 2005. Cone–rod dystrophy, intrafamilial variability, and incomplete penetrance associated with the R172W mutation in the peripherin/*RDS* gene. *Ophthalmology* **112**: 1592–1598.

Miyazaki M, Ikeda Y, Yonemitsu Y, Goto Y, Kohno R, Murakami Y, Inoue M, Ueda Y, Hasegawa M, Tobimatsu S, et al. 2008. Synergistic neuroprotective effect via simian lentiviral vector-mediated simultaneous gene transfer of human pigment epithelium-derived factor and human fibroblast growth factor-2 in rodent models of retinitis pigmentosa. *J Gene Med* **10**: 1273–1281.

Moshfeghi DM, Yang Z, Faulkner ND, Karan G, Thirumalaichary S, Pearson E, Zhao Y, Tsai T, Zhang K. 2006. Choroidal neovascularization in patients with adult-onset foveomacular dystrophy caused by mutations in the *RDS/peripherin* gene. *Adv Exp Med Biol* **572**: 35–40.

Mussolino C, Sanges D, Marrocco E, Bonetti C, Di Vicino U, Marigo V, Auricchio A, Meroni G, Surace EM. 2011. Zinc-finger-based transcriptional repression of rhodopsin in a model of dominant retinitis pigmentosa. *EMBO Mol Med* **3**: 118–128.

Nour M, Ding XQ, Stricker H, Fliesler SJ, Naash MI. 2004. Modulating expression of peripherin/*rds* in transgenic mice: Critical levels and the effect of overexpression. *Invest Ophthalmol Vis Sci* **45**: 2514–2521.

Nour M, Fliesler SJ, Naash MI. 2008. Genetic supplementation of RDS alleviates a loss-of-function phenotype in C214S model of retinitis pigmentosa. *Adv Exp Med Biol* **613**: 129–138.

O'Reilly M, Palfi A, Chadderton N, Millington-Ward S, Ader M, Cronin T, Tuohy T, Auricchio A, Hildinger M, Tivnan A, et al. 2007. RNA interference-mediated suppression and replacement of human rhodopsin in vivo. *Am J Hum Genet* **81**: 127–135.

Palfi A, Ader M, Kiang AS, Millington-Ward S, Clark G, O'Reilly M, McMahon HP, Kenna PF, Humphries P, Farrar GJ. 2006. RNAi-based suppression and replacement of *rds*-peripherin in retinal organotypic culture. *Hum Mutat* **27**: 260–268.

Parodi MB, Iacono P, Cascavilla M, Zucchiatti I, Kontadakis DS, Bandello F. 2010. Intravitreal bevacizumab for subfoveal choroidal neovascularization associated with pattern dystrophy. *Invest Ophthalmol Vis Sci* **51**: 4358–4361.

Petrs-Silva H, Yasumura D, Matthes MT, LaVail MM, Lewin AS, Hauswirth WW. 2012. Suppression of rds expression by siRNA and gene replacement strategies for gene therapy using rAAV vector. *Adv Exp Med Biol* **723**: 215–223.

Pihlmann M, Askou AL, Aagaard L, Bruun GH, Svalgaard JD, Holm-Nielsen MH, Dagnaes-Hansen F, Bek T, Mikkelsen JG, Jensen TG, et al. 2012. Adeno-associated virus-delivered polycistronic microRNA-clusters for knockdown of vascular endothelial growth factor in vivo. *J Gene Med* **14**: 328–338.

Poloschek CM, Bach M, Lagreze WA, Glaus E, Lemke JR, Berger W, Neidhardt J. 2010. *ABCA4* and *ROM1*: Implications for modification of the *PRPH2*-associated macular dystrophy phenotype. *Invest Ophthalmol Vis Sci* **51**: 4253–4265.

Reuter JH, Sanyal S. 1984. Development and degeneration of retina in *rds* mutant mice: The electroretinogram. *Neurosci Lett* **48**: 231–237.

Rex TS, Allocca M, Domenici L, Surace EM, Maguire AM, Lyubarsky A, Cellerino A, Bennett J, Auricchio A. 2004. Systemic but not intraocular *Epo* gene transfer protects the retina from light- and genetic-induced degeneration. *Mol Ther* **10**: 855–861.

Rex TS, Wong Y, Kodali K, Merry S. 2009. Neuroprotection of photoreceptors by direct delivery of erythropoietin to the retina of the retinal degeneration slow mouse. *Exp Eye Res* **89**: 735–740.

Rhee KD, Ruiz A, Duncan JL, Hauswirth WW, Lavail MM, Bok D, Yang XJ. 2007. Molecular and cellular alterations induced by sustained expression of ciliary neurotrophic factor in a mouse model of retinitis pigmentosa. *Invest Ophthalmol Vis Sci* **48**: 1389–1400.

Saga M, Mashima Y, Akeo K, Oguchi Y, Kudoh J, Shimizu N. 1993. A novel Cys-214-Ser mutation in the peripherin/RDS gene in a Japanese family with autosomal dominant retinitis pigmentosa. *Hum Genet* **92**: 519–521.

Sanyal S, Zeilmaker GH. 1984. Development and degeneration of retina in *rds* mutant mice: Light and electron microscopic observations in experimental chimaeras. *Exp Eye Res* **39**: 231–246.

Sarra GM, Stephens C, de Alwis M, Bainbridge JW, Smith AJ, Thrasher AJ, Ali RR. 2001. Gene replacement therapy in the retinal degeneration slow (*rds*) mouse: The effect on retinal degeneration following partial transduction of the retina. *Hum Mol Genet* **10**: 2353–2361.

Schlichtenbrede FC, da Cruz L, Stephens C, Smith AJ, Georgiadis A, Thrasher AJ, Bainbridge JW, Seeliger MW, Ali RR. 2003. Long-term evaluation of retinal function in $Prph2^{Rd2/Rd2}$ mice following AAV-mediated gene replacement therapy. *J Gene Med* **5**: 757–764.

Stricker HM, Ding XQ, Quiambao A, Fliesler SJ, Naash MI. 2005. The Cys214→Ser mutation in peripherin/*rds* causes a loss-of-function phenotype in transgenic mice. *Biochem J* **388**: 605–613.

Takeuchi K, Nakazawa M, Mizukoshi S. 2008. Systemic administration of nilvadipine delays photoreceptor degeneration of heterozygous retinal degeneration slow (rds) mouse. *Exp Eye Res* **86**: 60–69.

Tam BM, Moritz OL, Papermaster DS. 2004. The C terminus of peripherin/rds participates in rod outer segment targeting and alignment of disk incisures. *Mol Biol Cell* **15**: 2027–2037.

Teusner JT, Lewin AS, Hauswirth WW. 2006. Down-regulation of rhodopsin gene expression by AAV-vectored short interfering RNA. *Adv Exp Med Biol* **572**: 233–238.

Tian G, Ropelewski P, Nemet I, Lee R, Lodowski KH, Imanishi Y. 2014. An unconventional secretory pathway mediates the cilia targeting of peripherin/rds. *J Neurosci* **34**: 992–1006.

Travis GH, Brennan MB, Danielson PE, Kozak CA, Sutcliffe JG. 1989. Identification of a photoreceptor-specific mRNA encoded by the gene responsible for retinal degeneration slow (*rds*). *Nature* **338**: 70–73.

Travis GH, Sutcliffe JG, Bok D. 1991. The retinal degeneration slow (*rds*) gene product is a photoreceptor disc membrane-associated glycoprotein. *Neuron* **6**: 61–70.

Travis GH, Groshan KR, Lloyd M, Bok D. 1992. Complete rescue of photoreceptor dysplasia and degeneration in transgenic retinal degeneration slow (rds) mice. *Neuron* **9**: 113–119.

Usukura J, Bok D. 1987. Opsin localization and glycosylation in the developing BALB/c and *rds* mouse retina. *Prog Clin Biol Res* **247**: 195–207.

Vaclavik V, Tran HV, Gaillard MC, Schorderet DF, Munier FL. 2012. Pattern dystrophy with high intrafamilial variability associated with Y141C mutation in the peripherin/RDS gene and successful treatment of subfoveal CNV related to multifocal pattern type with anti-VEGF (ranibizumab) intravitreal injections. *Retina* **32**: 1942–1949.

van Nie R, Ivanyi D, Demant P. 1978. A new H-2-linked mutation, *rds*, causing retinal degeneration in the mouse. *Tissue Antigens* **12**: 106–108.

Wickham L, Chen FK, Lewis GP, Uppal GS, Neveu MM, Wright GA, Robson AG, Webster AR, Grierson I, Hiscott P, et al. 2009. Clinicopathological case series of four patients with inherited macular disease. *Invest Ophthalmol Vis Sci* **50**: 3553–3561.

Wrigley JD, Ahmed T, Nevett CL, Findlay JB. 2000. Peripherin/*rds* influences membrane vesicle morphology. Implications for retinopathies. *J Biol Chem* **275**: 13191–13194.

Leber Congenital Amaurosis Caused by Mutations in *RPGRIP1*

Tiansen Li

Retinal Cell Biology and Degeneration Section, Neurobiology-Neurodegeneration & Repair Laboratory, National Eye Institute, Bethesda, Maryland 20892

Correspondence: tiansen.li@nih.gov

Recessive null mutations in retinitis pigmentosa GTPase regulator interacting protein 1 (RPGRIP1) gene are the cause of LCA6 and account for 5% to 6% of the total patient population. RPGRIP1 has an essential role in the photoreceptor connecting cilia, and photoreceptors lacking RPGRIP1 are unable to maintain the light sensing outer segments. As a result, patients lose retinal functions at an early age but retain photoreceptors in the central retina well into adulthood thus holding out the prospect for gene augmentation therapies. Laboratory studies in animal models have demonstrated efficacy of gene therapy in slowing disease progression. With further refinement in the design of the replacement gene construct, clinical trials for Leber congenital amaurosis (LCA) caused by *RPGRIP1* mutations could be in the offing in the near future.

Leber congenital amaurosis (LCA) is a more severe form of retinal degeneration than retinitis pigmentosa, with visual deficit and loss of vision in early childhood (Heher et al. 1992; Fulton et al. 1996; den Hollander et al. 2008). Clinical findings indicate that both rod and cone photoreceptors are affected early on in LCA patients. Mutations in 16 different genes are currently known to cause LCA (Koenekoop 2004; den Hollander et al. 2008; Wang et al. 2009), one of which is the gene encoding retinitis pigmentosa GTPase regulator interacting protein 1 (RPGRIP1) (Dryja et al. 2001; Gerber et al. 2001; Koenekoop 2005). The rapid disease progression in LCA presents a significant challenge to gene therapy because retention of sufficient photoreceptors in the retina is a prerequisite for a satisfactory therapeutic outcome. In this regard, it is encouraging that LCA6 associated with *RPGRIP1* gene mutations have been reported to present with a more stable and somewhat nonprogressive disease course after the initial rapid decline in visual function (Hanein et al. 2004). Photoreceptors in the central retina appear to persist for long periods of time after visual function becomes immeasurable (Jacobson et al. 2007). Thus LCA6 patients with underlying *RPGRIP1* mutations have treatment potential for a gene replacement strategy if targeted to central, but not peripheral, retina. Continued improvement in retinal gene transduction vectors, validation of replacement gene design incorporating appropriate regulatory element and protein coding sequence, and better understanding of the disease pathophysiology will set the stage for clinical

Cite this article as *Cold Spring Harb Perspect Med* doi: 10.1101/cshperspect.a017384

trials of therapies targeting LCA6 in the near future.

GENETICS AND PROTEIN FUNCTION

RPGRIP1 was initially identified through protein interaction screens (Boylan and Wright 2000; Roepman et al. 2000; Hong et al. 2001) as a binding partner of retinitis pigmentosa GTPase regulator (RPGR), a protein whose defects underlie the major form of X-linked retinitis pigmentosa (RP). Recessive mutations in *RPGRIP1* cause LCA (Dryja et al. 2001; Gerber et al. 2001; Hanein et al. 2004) and have also been found to cause cone–rod dystrophy (CORD13) (Hameed et al. 2003). About 5%–6% of all cases of LCA are caused by mutations in *RPGRIP1* (Dryja et al. 2001; Gerber et al. 2001; den Hollander et al. 2008). *RPGRIP1* alleles that cause LCA mostly create premature termination codons and are therefore presumed to be "null". The less severe form of disease, cone–rod dystrophy, is linked to missense mutations that likely retain partial function and thus may be considered hypomorphic. LCA6 patients manifest loss-of-function of both rods and cones early in life and develop a severe loss of central acuity, which leads to nystagmus. Electroretinography is nonrecordable from these patients even at an early age (Dryja et al. 2001; Galvin et al. 2005; Walia et al. 2010; Khan et al. 2013). Despite the early onset nature, there is some evidence that the central retinal laminar architecture including the photoreceptor cell layer could survive until much later (Jacobson et al. 2007). The retained retinal structure corresponded to the region of visual sensitivity. Other investigators have also observed that some LCA patients with *RPGRIP1* mutations can retain a substantial number of photoreceptors even when visual function has been lost as measured by visual field and electroretinogram (ERG) (Pawlyk et al. 2010). These observations stand in contrast to LCA caused by *AIPL1* mutations, in which maculopathy or loss of photoreceptors in the center is a prominent feature (Dharmaraj et al. 2004; Jacobson et al. 2011). The residual photoreceptors could be suitable as a therapeutic target, thus raising hope for gene therapy as a means to preserve or restore some vision.

The human *RPGRIP1* gene is located on chromosome 14q11 and is expressed as multiple splice variants (Lu and Ferreira 2005). Its expression can be detected embryonically and also in tissues outside of the retina. A major retinal variant consists of 24 exons and encodes a protein of 1287 amino acid residues. This variant of RPGRIP1 contains several structurally conserved motifs. A coiled coil domain, frequently found in centrosome-associated proteins, is located within its amino-terminal half. RPGRIP1 binds to the RCC1 homology domain of RPGR via its carboxy-terminal portion, hence this region is also known as the RPGR interacting domain. A bipartite nuclear localization signal is also found in the latter domain (Arts et al. 2009). In the middle portion of the protein are two C2 domains that may bind Ca^{2+}. RPGRIP1 has no integral membrane-spanning region but C2 domains in the protein could target it to cell membranes. Its closest homolog is RPGRIP1L, a protein also implicated in certain syndromic forms of retinal degeneration, with an overall identity between the two proteins at ~34%.

RPGRIP1 expression is enriched in retinal photoreceptors where it is stably associated with the connecting cilia (structurally and functionally analogous to the transition zone of primary cilia) and is resistant to extraction with high salt and detergent (Hong et al. 2001), suggesting it is one of the core component of ciliary axoneme of photoreceptors. By immune electron microscopy, RPGRIP1 is seen between the axonemal microtubules and the plasma membrane surrounding the connecting cilia. Recombinant RPGRIP1 expressed in cultured cells spontaneously form extended filamentous structures (Zhao et al. 2003). In vivo, RPGRIP1 has been shown to be required for anchoring RPGR at the connecting cilia (Zhao et al. 2003). The connecting cilium provides the only link between the biosynthetic inner segment and the light sensing outer segment in a photoreceptor cell. As such, it is the conduit through which large amounts of nascent proteins must be trafficked in support of daily outer segment renewal. The precise function of RPGRIP1 in photoreceptors is not fully understood, but loss of RPGRIP1 leads to loss of RPGR at the connecting cilia, but not vice versa, suggesting RPGRIP1 tethers RPGR to the connecting cilia. In addition, RPGRIP1 also interacts with NPHP4, another ciliary protein, via a C2 domain (Roepman et al. 2005). Gene mutations in *NPHP4* have been shown to cause syndromic forms of retinal degeneration that also involve the kidney and other organs, known as ciliopathy. These data highlight a specific role for RPGRIP1 in ciliary structure and function. RPGRIP1 likely serves as a scaffold that anchors RPGR and additional ciliary components at the transition zone, and may play a role in ciliary trafficking in support of outer segment morphogenesis. In cells other than photoreceptors, RPGRIP1 is also localized to the ciliary/centrosomal compartment. The role of RPGRIP1 in these cells, if any, is not known. Given the fact that defects in RPGRIP1 cause only retinal degeneration, one may conclude that its function is important or nonredundant primarily in photoreceptors.

ANIMAL MODELS

A number of animal models have become available that carry recessive *RPGRIP1* mutations and recapitulate an LCA-like retinal phenotype. The first one was produced by targeted disruption of the *RPGRIP1* gene in mice (Zhao et al. 2003). Normally, the full-length mouse RPGRIP1 protein migrates on SDS-PAGE at ~200 kDa, which corresponds to the long RPGRIP1 variant mentioned earlier, and this full-length protein is ablated in the *RPGRIP1* knockout mouse. Mice lacking RPGRIP1 develop a rapid course of retinal degeneration involving both rods and cones. At the age of weaning (postnatal day 20), *RPGRIP1* knockout mice already show substantial mislocalization of photopigment in both rods and cones. Rudimentary outer segments do form but they are short and highly disorganized. ERG amplitudes are a fraction of the controls. Cell loss is relatively fast, such that by 5 mo of age, most photoreceptor cells have degenerated. In *RPGRIP1* knockout mice, RPGR is detectable by immunoblotting but is no longer found at the connecting cilium. Thus loss of RPGRIP1 leads to ectopic distribution of RPGR and therefore should abolish RPGR function as well. RPGRIP1 also likely performs additional functions at the connecting cilium, because mice lacking RPGRIP1 have a much more severe retinal phenotype than mice lacking RPGR alone. It was hypothesized that RPGRIP1 may be involved in photoreceptor disc morphogenesis. The relatively fast rate of photoreceptor degeneration in the knockout mice makes it a useful model of LCA both for studying the disease mechanism and for testing new therapies.

A second mouse model carrying a recessive *RPGRIP1* mutation, designated $Rpgrip1^{nmf247}$, was identified in an ethyl nitrosourea (ENU) chemical mutagenesis screen at the Jackson laboratory (Won et al. 2009). The mutation alters a splice site at exon 7 and results in skipping of exons 7 and 8 in the mRNA and premature termination of the open reading frame. Interestingly, this model shows a more severe retinal phenotype compared with the *RPGRIP1* knockout mice. In the homozygous $Rpgrip1^{nmf247}$ mice, disease onset is early and the rate of degeneration is faster. ERG is nonrecordable from an early age. In photoreceptors, connecting cilia emerge from the apical inner segment, but this is not followed by the elaboration of any outer segments. Most photoreceptors will degenerate by the age of postnatal day 21. These data were interpreted to indicate that the $Rpgrip1^{nmf247}$ mutation ablates an additional short variant of RPGRIP1 that escaped inactivation in the knockout model or that a truncated version of RPGRIP1 is still expressed in the knockout model giving rise to a residual RPGRIP1 function. The more severe phenotype and the accompanying protein analyses in the study indicate that the $Rpgrip1^{nmf247}$ is likely a true null and more closely recapitulates human LCA.

A canine model carrying a spontaneous mutation in *RPGRIP1* has also been reported. This mutation was originally discovered and designated as cone–rod dystrophy 1 (*cord1*) that occurs naturally in miniature longhaired dachshunds (Curtis and Barnett 1993). In the affected dogs, ERG and histological changes consistent with retinal degeneration are detectable after 10 wk of age. There is evidence that cones are affected earlier than rods. The *cord1* locus was mapped to a region of canine chromosome 15 containing the *RPGRIP1* gene. Genome sequencing identified a 44-nucleotide insertion in exon 2 of *RPGRIP1* that alters the reading frame and introduces a premature stop codon (Mellersh et al. 2006). In the initial study that identified the *RPGRIP1* mutation, affected and carrier dogs within an extended inbred pedigree were homozygous and heterozygous, respectively, for the mutation (Mellersh et al. 2006). It was therefore concluded that the *RPGRIP1* ins44 mutation was responsible for *cord1*. Subsequent studies, however, found considerable phenotypic variation and genotype–phenotype discordance (Miyadera et al. 2009), raising the possibility that the *RPGRIP1* ins44 mutation may not be the primary cause of *cord1* (Kuznetsova et al. 2012a). It was suggested that because *RPGRIP1* undergoes multiple splicing, the exon containing the insertion could be spliced out while retaining partial protein function (Kuznetsova et al. 2012b). Indeed, a genome-wide association study identified a second locus also on canine chromosome 15 that strongly influenced the manifestation of disease (Miyadera et al. 2012). Homozygosity for both *RPGRIP1* ins44 and the risk haplotype at the newly mapped locus was necessary for development of retinal degeneration. To complicate matters further, some dogs that developed retinal degeneration were neither homozygous for *RPGRIP1* ins44 nor for the second risk haplotype indicating the presence of further independent modifier loci (Miyadera et al. 2012). If this proves correct, it would make retinal degeneration in this dog breed a polygenic trait. Given the clearly showed and critical role of RPGRIP1 in human and mouse photoreceptors, it would seem certain that an *RPGRIP1* null or substantially null allele would also be causal for photoreceptor degeneration in dogs. Thus the available evidence points to *RPGRIP1* ins44 being a moderately hypomorphic allele. It is a significant contributor to disease but is not a sole determinant. Direct examination of the protein from native retinal tissues using appropriate antibodies should help resolve this puzzling question.

THERAPEUTIC STUDIES IN ANIMAL MODELS

Replacement gene therapy studies have been performed in both murine and canine models. The first study was conducted in the *RPGRIP1* knockout mice (Pawlyk et al. 2005). In that study, a mouse *RPGRIP1* cDNA was packaged into an AAV2 vector under the control of a mouse opsin promoter and delivered subretinally. Mice were followed up to 5 mo after treatment by ERG and then analyzed by immunocytochemistry and histology. Delivery of recombinant *RPGRIP1* by AAV led to the RPGRIP1 protein expression that correctly localized to the connecting cilia. The thickness of the photoreceptor layer was significantly increased in the treated retina, and the morphology of the outer segments, almost completely absent in the untreated eyes, was partly restored. Partial functional preservation was also shown by ERG. Remarkably, RPGR again localized to the photoreceptor connecting cilium in treated eyes, indicating restoration of its function. Thus the efficacy of AAV-mediated replacement gene therapy was unambiguously shown in this first study in a mouse model. Despite its apparent success, this study has left much room for further improvement. First, RPGRIP1 is known to be required in both rods and cones, and the use of an opsin promoter would limit expression primarily to rods. Second, AAV2 vector has a relatively poor tropism for photoreceptors leading to lower transduction efficacy and is slow in turning on expression of the recombinant gene. Because the mouse LCA model has a fast course of disease, by the time replacement gene is fully expressed, which could take >4–6 wk, a substantial fraction of photoreceptors would have degenerated. Lastly, the important objective of validating a human *RPGRIP1* replacement gene suitable for clinical trials was not tackled in this study.

To address some of those issues a second therapeutic study was conducted in the *RPGRIP1* knockout mice that delivered the human instead of the mouse *RPGRIP1* replacement gene (Pawlyk et al. 2010). The second study incorporated an improved version of AAV vector, AAV8. AAV8 is far more efficient at transducing photoreceptors than AAV2 and leads to a faster onset of transgene expression. This meant that in a rapidly degenerating retina, the replacement gene would be up and functional before too many photoreceptors had disappeared thus leading to a more favorable therapeutic outcome. A human rhodopsin kinase gene promoter (Khani et al. 2007) was used in place of the rhodopsin promoter to drive gene expression in both rods and cones. After subretinal delivery of the replacement gene in the mutant mice, human RPGRIP1 was expressed specifically in photoreceptors, localized correctly in the connecting cilia, and importantly restored the normal localization of RPGR. Histological examinations showed improved photoreceptor survival in the treated eyes. ERG measurements showed better preservation of rod and cone photoreceptor function: The mean rates of monthly decline without treatment were 37% for the rod a-wave, 22% for the rod b-wave, and 25% for the cone b-wave. With treatment, these rates of decline decreased to 8% for the rod a-wave and rod b-wave and to no detectable decline for the cone b-wave. This represents overall a fourfold slowing of retinal function loss (Pawlyk et al. 2010). Thus, this study showed the efficacy of a human replacement gene and validated a gene therapy design that could be adopted for future clinical trials in patients. Despite marked improvement of photoreceptor function and survival in the treated eyes compared with the control eyes, photoreceptor degeneration was slowed but not stopped. Among many possible factors that may have influenced the extent of rescue, the low degree of conservation between human and mouse genes is likely a major one. The human and mouse RPGRIP1 protein sequences are only ~60% identical, relatively low for mammalian orthologs. In fact, the conservation is so poor between the two species that an antibody raised against one species would not cross-react with the other. This means a human RPGRIP1 would not function in mouse photoreceptors as effectively as the cognate mouse RPGRIP1. If this hypothesis is correct, which seems likely, a better therapeutic outcome could reasonably be expected in future clinical studies in which a human *RPGRIP1* gene is delivered to human recipients. Other factors such as precise level of transgene expression and time of replacement gene delivery also likely play roles in determining an optical outcome.

For preclinical development of gene therapies that target a specific type of retinal degeneration, proof-of-concept studies in large animal models that share clinical features with their human counterparts would be highly desirable. A recent study evaluated gene therapy in the canine *cord1* model with homozygous *RPGRIP1* ins44 mutation (Lheriteau et al. 2014). Subretinal injection of a canine *RPGRIP1* cDNA driven by the same rhodopsin kinase promoter as that used in the mouse study and packaged into AAV vectors improved photoreceptor survival in treated retinas. The study found that photoreceptor function was significantly improved in all treated eyes for up to 24 mo postinjection. The rescue of cone function appeared to be more stable and long lasting. The treatment did not completely halt photoreceptor degeneration, similar to most gene therapy studies, as indicated by the continued thinning of the photoreceptor layer over time. It should be noted that, to achieve a measurable therapeutic benefit, the study had to use a canine RPGRIP1 cDNA in the replacement gene construct. This was again presumably because of the low degree of conservation between the human and dog RPGRIP1 primary sequences (at under 70%) such that a human RPGRIP1 would produce a weaker therapeutic effect in canine photoreceptors to the point of being difficult to show. Another issue that is relevant to assessing the outcome of the study is the findings by other investigators that the *cord1* phenotype may be inherited as a polygenic trait. Nevertheless, the demonstration of efficacy of gene therapy in this large animal model of cone–rod dystrophy is clear evidence that the *RPGRIP1* ins44 allele is a major pathogenic factor and provides promise that the model will be useful for further preclinical development of therapies for human treatment.

CONCLUDING REMARKS

Studies by many investigators in the past decade have built up a wealth of knowledge about *RPGRIP1*, from genetics, protein function, to somatic gene therapies in animal models. The remaining tasks before a clinical trial can be initiated are to finalize to choice of promoter and human RPGRIP1 coding sequence, and to carry out efficacy and toxicology validation. Although all evidence points to the long *RPGRIP1* transcript being the functionally important variant, the possibility that some shorter variants additionally contribute to photoreceptor function could bear on efforts on optimizing efficacy of therapies and should be further examined. The timing issues of gene therapy intervention also deserve some attention (Cideciyan et al. 2013). Despite potential difficulties going forward, gene therapy development for LCA caused by *RPGRIP1* mutations seems on track and the future looks promising for the emergence of a therapy that could alleviate this form of retinal degeneration.

REFERENCES

Arts HH, Cremers FP, Knoers NV, Roepman R. 2009. Focus on molecules: RPGRIP1. *Exp Eye Res* **88:** 332–333.

Boylan JP, Wright AF. 2000. Identification of a novel protein interacting with RPGR. *Hum Mol Genet* **9:** 2085–2093.

Cideciyan AV, Jacobson SG, Beltran WA, Sumaroka A, Swider M, Iwabe S, Roman AJ, Olivares MB, Schwartz SB, Komáromy AM, et al. 2013. Human retinal gene therapy for Leber congenital amaurosis shows advancing retinal degeneration despite enduring visual improvement. *Proc Natl Acad Sci* **110:** E517–E525.

Curtis R, Barnett KC. 1993. Progressive retinal atrophy in miniature longhaired dachshund dogs. *Br Vet J* **149:** 71–85.

den Hollander AI, Roepman R, Koenekoop RK, Cremers FP. 2008. Leber congenital amaurosis: Genes, proteins and disease mechanisms. *Prog Retin Eye Res* **27:** 391–419.

Dharmaraj S, Leroy BP, Sohocki MM, Koenekoop RK, Perrault I, Anwar K, Khaliq S, Devi RS, Birch DG, De Pool E, et al. 2004. The phenotype of Leber congenital amaurosis in patients with AIPL1 mutations. *Arch Ophthalmol* **122:** 1029–1037.

Dryja TP, Adams SM, Grimsby JL, McGee TL, Hong DH, Li T, Andréasson S, Berson EL. 2001. Null *RPGRIP1* alleles in patients with Leber congenital amaurosis. *Am J Hum Genet* **68:** 1295–1298.

Fulton AB, Hansen RM, Mayer DL. 1996. Vision in Leber congenital amaurosis. *Arch Ophthalmol* **114:** 698–703.

Galvin JA, Fishman GA, Stone EM, Koenekoop RK. 2005. Clinical phenotypes in carriers of Leber congenital amaurosis mutations. *Ophthalmology* **112:** 349–356.

Gerber S, Perrault I, Hanein S, Barbet F, Ducroq D, Ghazi I, Martin-Coignard D, Leowski C, Homfray T, Dufier JL, et al. 2001. Complete exon-intron structure of the RPGR-interacting protein (RPGRIP1) gene allows the identification of mutations underlying Leber congenital amaurosis. *Eur J Hum Genet* **9:** 561–571.

Hameed A, Abid A, Aziz A, Ismail M, Mehdi SQ, Khaliq S. 2003. Evidence of *RPGRIP1* gene mutations associated with recessive cone-rod dystrophy. *J Med Genet* **40:** 616–619.

Hanein S, Perrault I, Gerber S, Tanguy G, Barbet F, Ducroq D, Calvas P, Dollfus H, Hamel C, Lopponen T, et al. 2004. Leber congenital amaurosis: Comprehensive survey of the genetic heterogeneity, refinement of the clinical definition, and genotype-phenotype correlations as a strategy for molecular diagnosis. *Hum Mutat* **23:** 306–317.

Heher KL, Traboulsi EI, Maumenee IH. 1992. The natural history of Leber's congenital amaurosis. Age-related findings in 35 patients. *Ophthalmology* **99:** 241–245.

Hong DH, Yue G, Adamian M, Li T. 2001. Retinitis pigmentosa GTPase regulator (RPGR)-interacting protein is stably associated with the photoreceptor ciliary axoneme and anchors RPGR to the connecting cilium. *J Biol Chem* **276:** 12091–12099.

Jacobson SG, Cideciyan AV, Aleman TS, Sumaroka A, Schwartz SB, Roman AJ, Stone EM. 2007. Leber congenital amaurosis caused by an *RPGRIP1* mutation shows treatment potential. *Ophthalmology* **114:** 895–898.

Jacobson SG, Cideciyan AV, Aleman TS, Sumaroka A, Roman AJ, Swider M, Schwartz SB, Banin E, Stone EM. 2011. Human retinal disease from *AIPL1* gene mutations: Foveal cone loss with minimal macular photoreceptors and rod function remaining. *Invest Ophthalmol Vis Sci* **52:** 70–79.

Khan AO, Abu-Safieh L, Eisenberger T, Bolz HJ, Alkuraya FS. 2013. The *RPGRIP1*-related retinal phenotype in children. *Br J Ophthalmol* **97:** 760–764.

Khani SC, Pawlyk BS, Bulgakov OV, Kasperek E, Young JE, Adamian M, Sun X, Smith AJ, Ali RR, Li T. 2007. AAV-mediated expression targeting of rod and cone photoreceptors with a human rhodopsin kinase promoter. *Invest Ophthalmol Vis Sci* **48:** 3954–3961.

Koenekoop RK. 2004. An overview of Leber congenital amaurosis: A model to understand human retinal development. *Surv Ophthalmol* **49:** 379–398.

Koenekoop RK. 2005. *RPGRIP1* is mutated in Leber congenital amaurosis: A mini-review. *Ophthalmic Genet* **26:** 175–179.

Kuznetsova T, Iwabe S, Boesze-Battaglia K, Pearce-Kelling S, Chang-Min Y, McDaid K, Miyadera K, Kamoromy A, Aguirre GD. 2012a. Exclusion of *RPGRIP1* ins44 from primary causal association with early-onset cone–rod dystrophy in dogs. *Invest Ophthalmol Vis Sci* **53:** 5486–5501.

Kuznetsova T, Zangerl B, Aguirre GD. 2012b. *RPGRIP1* and cone–rod dystrophy in dogs. *Adv Exp Med Biol* **723:** 321–328.

Lheriteau E, Petit L, Weber M, Le Meur G, Deschamps JY, Libeau L, Mendes-Madeira A, Guihal C, François A,

Guyon R, et al. 2014. Successful gene therapy in the *RPGRIP1*-deficient dog: A large model of cone–rod dystrophy. *Mol Ther* **22:** 265–277.

Lu X, Ferreira PA. 2005. Identification of novel murine- and human-specific *RPGRIP1* splice variants with distinct expression profiles and subcellular localization. *Invest Ophthalmol Vis Sci* **46:** 1882–1890.

Mellersh CS, Boursnell ME, Pettitt L, Ryder EJ, Holmes NG, Grafham D, Forman OP, Sampson J, Barnett KC, Blanton S, et al. 2006. Canine *RPGRIP1* mutation establishes cone–rod dystrophy in miniature longhaired dachshunds as a homologue of human Leber congenital amaurosis. *Genomics* **88:** 293–301.

Miyadera K, Kato K, Aguirre-Hernandez J, Tokuriki T, Morimoto K, Busse C, Barnett K, Holmes N, Ogawa H, Sasaki N, et al. 2009. Phenotypic variation and genotype-phenotype discordance in canine cone-rod dystrophy with an *RPGRIP1* mutation. *Mol Vis* **15:** 2287–2305.

Miyadera K, Kato K, Boursnell M, Mellersh CS, Sargan DR. 2012. Genome-wide association study in *RPGRIP1*$^{-/-}$ dogs identifies a modifier locus that determines the onset of retinal degeneration. *Mamm Genome* **23:** 212–223.

Pawlyk BS, Smith AJ, Buch PK, Adamian M, Hong DH, Sandberg MA, Ali RR, Li T. 2005. Gene replacement therapy rescues photoreceptor degeneration in a murine model of Leber congenital amaurosis lacking *RPGRIP*. *Invest Ophthalmol Vis Sci* **46:** 3039–3045.

Pawlyk BS, Bulgakov OV, Liu X, Xu X, Adamian M, Sun X, Khani SC, Berson EL, Sandberg MA, Li T. 2010. Replacement gene therapy with a human *RPGRIP1* sequence slows photoreceptor degeneration in a murine model of Leber congenital amaurosis. *Hum Gene Ther* **21:** 993–1004.

Roepman R, Bernoud-Hubac N, Schick DE, Maugeri A, Berger W, Ropers H-H, Cremers FP, Ferreira PA. 2000. The retinitis pigmentosa GTPase regulator (RPGR) interacts with novel transport-like proteins in the outer segments of rod photoreceptors. *Hum Mol Genet* **9:** 2095–2105.

Roepman R, Letteboer SJ, Arts HH, van Beersum SE, Lu X, Krieger E, Ferreira PA, Cremers FP. 2005. Interaction of nephrocystin-4 and RPGRIP1 is disrupted by nephronophthisis or Leber congenital amaurosis-associated mutations. *Proc Natl Acad Sci* **102:** 18520–18525.

Walia S, Fishman GA, Jacobson SG, Aleman TS, Koenekoop RK, Traboulsi EI, Weleber RG, Pennesi ME, Heon E, Drack A, et al. 2010. Visual acuity in patients with Leber's congenital amaurosis and early childhood-onset retinitis pigmentosa. *Ophthalmology* **117:** 1190–1198.

Wang H, den Hollander AI, Moayedi Y, Abulimiti A, Li Y, Collin RW, Hoyng CB, Lopez I, Abboud EB, Al-Rajhi AA, et al. 2009. Mutations in *SPATA7* cause Leber congenital amaurosis and juvenile retinitis pigmentosa. *Am J Hum Genet* **84:** 380–387.

Won J, Gifford E, Smith RS, Yi H, Ferreira PA, Hicks WL, Li T, Naggert JK, Nishina PM. 2009. RPGRIP1 is essential for normal rod photoreceptor outer segment elaboration and morphogenesis. *Hum Mol Genet* **18:** 4329–4339.

Zhao Y, Hong DH, Pawlyk B, Yue G, Adamian M, Grynberg M, Godzik A, Li T. 2003. The retinitis pigmentosa GTPase regulator (RPGR)- interacting protein: Subserving RPGR function and participating in disk morphogenesis. *Proc Natl Acad Sci* **100:** 3965–3970.

Gene Augmentation for X-Linked Retinitis Pigmentosa Caused by Mutations in *RPGR*

William A. Beltran[1], Artur V. Cideciyan[2], Alfred S. Lewin[3], William W. Hauswirth[4], Samuel G. Jacobson[2], and Gustavo D. Aguirre[1]

[1]Section of Ophthalmology, School of Veterinary Medicine, University of Pennsylvania, Philadelphia, Pennsylvania 19104

[2]Scheie Eye Institute, Department of Ophthalmology, University of Pennsylvania Perelman School of Medicine, Philadelphia, Pennsylvania 19104

[3]Department of Molecular Genetics & Microbiology, University of Florida, Gainesville, Florida 32610

[4]Department of Ophthalmology, University of Florida, Gainesville, Florida 32610

Correspondence: wbeltran@vet.upenn.edu

X-linked retinitis pigmentosa (XLRP) caused by mutations in the *RPGR* gene is a severe and early onset form of retinal degeneration, and no treatment is currently available. Recent evidence in two clinically relevant canine models shows that adeno-associated viral (AAV)-mediated *RPGR* gene transfer to rods and cones can prevent disease onset and rescue photoreceptors at early- and mid-stages of degeneration. There is thus a strong incentive for conducting long-term, preclinical efficacy and safety studies, while concomitantly pursuing the detailed phenotypic characterization of XLRP disease in patients that may benefit from such corrective therapy.

X-linked retinitis pigmentosa (XLRP) includes some of the earliest onset and rapidly progressive forms of inherited retinal degenerations, and accounts for 6%–20% of all cases of retinitis pigmentosa (Fishman 1978; Jay 1982; Breuer et al. 2002). XLRP has been genetically mapped to six loci (RP2, RP3, RP6, RP23, RP24, and RP34); of these, RP3, which is associated with mutations in the retinitis pigmentosa GTPase regulator (*RPGR*) gene, is the predominant subtype (Meindl et al. 1996; Roepman et al. 1996). Indeed, mutations in *RPGR* are found in >70% of families affected by XLRP and ~15% of simplex retinitis pigmentosa cases (Bader et al. 2003; Sharon et al. 2003; Pelletier et al. 2007; Branham et al. 2012). Over the past decade, substantial effort has been dedicated to unveiling RPGR's function in photoreceptors, identifying novel mutations and the spectrum of disease phenotypes in humans, and characterizing small and large animal models of *RPGR*-XLRP that could be used to test novel therapeutic approaches. This review will primarily focus on the results of the preclinical studies conducted in canine models, as these provide strong evidence that a corrective gene therapy for XLRP may become a reality in the not-so-distant future.

Cite this article as *Cold Spring Harb Perspect Med* doi: 10.1101/cshperspect.a017392

RPGR AND ITS ROLES IN THE PHOTORECEPTOR CONNECTING CILIUM

The *RPGR* gene (172 kb) was initially described as containing 19 exons, and mutations in $RPGR^{ex1\text{-}19}$ accounted for only 15%–20% of XLRP patients (Meindl et al. 1996). Subsequently, an alternatively spliced carboxy-terminal exon called ORF15 was identified and found to be a hot spot for microdeletions, frameshift mutations, and premature stop mutations (Vervoort et al. 2000). Of the more than 350 *RPGR* mutations reported to date, >55% are found in exon ORF15 (see http://rpgr.hgu.mrc.ac.uk).

Among the different splice variants (Vervoort et al. 2000; Neidhardt et al. 2007; Schmid et al. 2010), $RPGR^{ex1\text{-}ORF15}$ and constitutive $RPGR^{ex1\text{-}19}$ are the most abundantly expressed RPGR isoforms in the retina. Both proteins have been immunolocalized to photoreceptor connecting cilium of both rods and cones (Hong et al. 2003; Wright et al. 2011). One group found $RPGR^{ex1\text{-}ORF15}$ in bovine and human photoreceptor outer segments (Roepman et al. 2000; Mavlyutov et al. 2002), although this was later disputed (Hong et al. 2003). The different temporal pattern of retinal expression of these two isoforms suggests that $RPGR^{ex1\text{-}19}$ may play a role in photoreceptor development whereas $RPGR^{ex1\text{-}ORF15}$ may be necessary for maintaining the integrity of mature photoreceptors (Wright et al. 2011). The constitutive human $RPGR^{ex1\text{-}19}$ isoform encodes an 815 amino acid protein (MW: 90–100 kDa) that is widely expressed, whereas the full-length human $RPGR^{ex1\text{-}ORF15}$ isoform, which encodes a 1152 amino acid, soluble protein (MW: 200–220 kDa), has been found predominantly in photoreceptors.

Both isoforms contain a common amino-terminal RCC1-like domain (Meindl et al. 1996) (encoded by exons 2 to 11), which has recently been shown to play the role of a guanine nucleotide exchange factor (GEF) by directly interacting with the GDP-bound form of the small GTPase RAB8A (Murga-Zamalloa et al. 2010a). RPGR has also been shown to interact directly or via molecular complexes with the following proteins: PDE6d (Linari et al. 1999); a number of ciliary proteins, including RPGR-interacting protein 1 (RPGRIP1) (Boylan and Wright 2000; Roepman et al. 2000; Hong et al. 2001); the nephrocystins NPHP1 (Murga-Zamalloa et al. 2010b), NPHP4 (Murga-Zamalloa et al. 2010b), NPHP5/IQCB1 (Otto et al. 2005), NPHP6/CEP290 (Chang et al. 2006), and NPHP8/RPGRIP1L (Khanna et al. 2009); the chromosome-associated proteins SMC1 and SMC3 (Khanna et al. 2005); the centrosomal protein NPM1 (Shu et al. 2005); and proteins associated with intraflagellar transport (Tg737/Polaris/IFT88) and microtubule motors (dynactin subunits, kinesin-II) (Khanna et al. 2005). Exon ORF15 encodes for a highly repetitive, glutamic acid-rich region whose function is currently unknown, yet its carboxyl terminus has been recently shown to interact with whirlin, which is a member of the Usher interactome (Wright et al. 2012). Localization of RPGR to the sensory cilia of photoreceptors (Hong et al. 2003) and its interaction with numerous complexes involved in protein transportation suggest that RPGR plays a role in regulating protein trafficking between the inner and outer segments at the level of the connecting cilium; however, its exact molecular function is still poorly understood.

Recent reports have suggested that RPGR may contribute to the biogenesis and maintenance of photoreceptor cilia and the transitional zone of motile cilia (Murga-Zamalloa et al. 2010a; Gakovic et al. 2011; Ghosh et al. 2011). This role is consistent with the occurrence of hearing dysfunction, respiratory infections, and cilia dyskinesis in some rare cases of syndromic *RPGR*-XLRP (van Dorp et al. 1992; Iannaccone et al. 2003; Koenekoop et al. 2003; Zito et al. 2003; Iannaccone et al. 2004; Moore et al. 2006; Bukowy-Bieryllo et al. 2013).

RETINAL DEGENERATION PHENOTYPE OF XLRP PATIENTS WITH *RPGR* MUTATIONS

A range of clinical diagnoses has been associated with *RPGR* mutations that cause progressive retinal degeneration of photoreceptors. *RPGR*-associated retinal degeneration most commonly presents in males of XLRP families or in simplex

 Cite this article as *Cold Spring Harb Perspect Med* doi: 10.1101/cshperspect.a017392

males as early loss of night vision and peripheral vision, abnormal electroretinograms, and relatively better retention of central vision in younger patients (Meindl et al. 1996; Roepman et al. 1996; Vervoort et al. 2000; Sandberg et al. 2007; Zahid et al. 2013). Less commonly, there is early involvement of the fovea and loss of visual acuity. Depending on the degree of abnormality in retina-wide measurements of cone versus rod function, clinical diagnoses have included X-linked cone-rod dystrophy, cone dystrophy, or macular degeneration (Mears et al. 2000; Ayyagari et al. 2002; Demirci et al. 2002; Yang et al. 2002; Ebenezer et al. 2005; Pelletier et al. 2007; Thiadens et al. 2011; Beltran et al. 2012). Retinally colocalized measures of function have often shown both rod and cone loss (Jacobson et al. 1997; Lorenz et al. 2003; Huang et al. 2012) consistent with expression of the *RPGR* gene product in rod and cone cilia (Hong et al. 2000, 2003; Roepman et al. 2000; Khanna et al. 2005; Shu et al. 2005). High allelic heterogeneity has been implied as cause for the spectrum of severity and phenotypes encountered between families carrying different *RPGR* mutations, and there is evidence that genetic modifiers may contribute to intra-familial phenotypic divergence (Keith et al. 1991; Walia et al. 2008; Ruddle et al. 2009; Fahim et al. 2011).

Carrier females with *RPGR* mutations also show a wide spectrum of retinal disease expression ranging from asymptomatic with normal electrophysiological and psychophysical test results to very severe retina-wide disease (Andreasson et al. 1997; Jacobson et al. 1997; Weleber et al. 1997; Bauer et al. 1998; Fishman et al. 1998; Flaxel et al. 1999; Ayyagari et al. 2002; Lorenz et al. 2003; Ebenezer et al. 2005; Jin et al. 2006; Ruddle et al. 2009; Thiadens et al. 2011). There tends to be significant interocular asymmetry of disease severity in most carriers (Jacobson et al. 1989; Weleber et al. 1997; Fishman et al. 1998; Lorenz et al. 2003; Ebenezer et al. 2005). A distinct golden tapetal-like reflex, hypothesized to be located at cone inner segments (Cideciyan and Jacobson 1994), or peripheral photoreceptor outer segments (Berendschot et al. 1996), has been variably described in a subset of female carriers of *RPGR* mutations (Andreasson et al. 1997; Jacobson et al. 1997; Weleber et al. 1997; Bauer et al. 1998; Fishman et al. 1998; Flaxel et al. 1999; Ayyagari et al. 2002; Lorenz et al. 2003; Ebenezer et al. 2005; Jin et al. 2006; Ruddle et al. 2009; Thiadens et al. 2011).

ANIMAL MODELS OF *RPGR*-XLRP

Murine Models

The description of the phenotypes of several mouse models of RPGR disease, including XLRP (Hong et al. 2000, 2004; Brunner et al. 2010; Wright et al. 2011; Huang et al. 2012; Thompson et al. 2012) and cone-rod dystrophy (Brunner et al. 2010), have been published. Evidence that mice sharing the same *RPGR* mutation but on a different genetic background can express a different disease phenotype further highlights the potential role of genetic modifiers (Brunner et al. 2010). Overexpression of the $RPGR^{ex1\text{-}19}$ isoform in photoreceptor cells of transgenic mice leads to early onset (2 months of age) degeneration, whereas no retinal alterations are associated with overexpression of the $RPGR^{ex1\text{-}ORF15}$ isoform (Wright et al. 2011). This finding further supports the claim that the severe phenotype described in a transgenic mouse expressing a truncated $RPGR^{ex1\text{-}ORF15}$ isoform is caused by a toxic gain-of-function and not to the overexpression of the transgene (Hong et al. 2004). With the exception of this transgenic model that shows rapid kinetics of photoreceptor loss, the other *RPGR* mutant mice, including the naturally occurring *Rd9* mouse (Thompson et al. 2012) that could be used to test a gene augmentation therapy strategy, show a slowly progressive photoreceptor degeneration resulting in retention of >50% outer nuclear layer thickness by 2 years of age (summarized in Huang et al. 2012, Supplementary Table S1, see http://www.iovs.org/lookup/suppl/doi:10.1167/iovs.12-10070/-/DCSupplemental).

Canine Models

To date, the XLPRA1 and XLPRA2 dogs are the only identified large animal models of

RPGR-XLRP. Although both diseases are caused by nearby microdeletions in the same exon ORF15, they show distinct ages of onset, rates of progression, and spatiotemporal distribution of retinal degeneration.

In XLPRA1, a five nucleotide deletion in exon ORF15 (c.1028–1032delGAGAA; GeneBank accession no. AF385621) introduces an immediate premature stop codon, and the putative protein has 230 amino acids truncated at its carboxyl-terminal end (Zhang et al. 2002). This deletion causes a rod–cone degeneration detectable by histology and electroretinogram in juvenile hemizygote male dogs (approximately one year of age) that progresses from the peripheral to the central retina (Zeiss et al. 1999; Beltran et al. 2012). Even though the research colony has been established from a single affected male, the extent of severity of the retinal changes, and their rate of progression varies from one individual to another even in animals of the same age (Zeiss et al. 1999; Guyon et al. 2007; Beltran et al. 2012), suggesting that genetic modifiers which have been implicated in humans with *RPGR*-XLRP (Fahim et al. 2011) may also be responsible for this variability in disease phenotype. As a result of random X-inactivation (also called lyonization), heterozygous female dogs undergo a patchy form of retinal degeneration (Zeiss et al. 1999; Beltran et al. 2009) that is the result of loss of photoreceptors that are clonally derived from a progenitor cell expressing the mutant XLPRA1 allele. This mosaic pattern of retinal degeneration, which is histologically detectable at 1.4 yr and is still apparent in 7.8-yr-old dogs, resembles the phenotype reported in human XLRP carriers (Szamier and Berson 1985; Jacobson et al. 1997; Aguirre et al. 2002; Vajaranant et al. 2002).

A second form of canine *RPGR*-XLRP, termed XLPRA2, is caused by a two nucleotide deletion in ORF15 (c.1084–1085delGA) (Zhang et al. 2002). This microdeletion introduces a frameshift followed by a premature stop codon. The putative protein includes 34 additional basic residues and an increased isoelectric point (4.30 vs. 4.01). XLPRA2 retinas undergo early (4 weeks of age) disorganization of photoreceptor outer segments, which is followed by increased cell death that peaks at about 7 weeks of age before returning, at 12 weeks, to a reduced yet constant rate. These photoreceptor cell death kinetics result in rapid outer nuclear layer thinning, that leads to an average thickness of three rows of nuclei by 41 weeks of age. Early cone disease has been shown to occur in the newly discovered canine fovea-like area (Beltran et al. 2014a). Mislocalization of rod opsin, short-wavelength (blue) cone opsin, and middle/long-wavelength (red/green) opsin are other early events that suggest that this canine ciliopathy affects all populations of photoreceptors. Similar evidence for altered protein trafficking through the connecting cilium has been reported in murine models (Hong et al. 2000, 2005; Brunner et al. 2010; Wright et al. 2011; Thompson et al. 2012), and in a carrier patient of XLRP (Adamian et al. 2006). Initiation of photoreceptor loss is accompanied by early retinal remodeling events such as rod neurite sprouting, retraction of rod bipolar dendrites, and Müller cell gliosis. Subsequently, other inner retinal remodeling events, including altered labeling of cell-specific markers of horizontal and amacrine cells, and loss of normal inner plexiform lamination follows (Beltran et al. 2006). Despite the severe progression of the disease, particularly in the central (visual streak) area (Beltran et al. 2012), dogs at 41 weeks of age retain sufficient rod- and cone-mediated visual function to navigate without difficulties in an obstacle avoidance course (WA Beltran, unpubl.). Similarly to XLPRA1 carriers, XLPRA2 heterozygous mutant dogs undergo random X-inactivation during embryogenesis that results in a patchy form of retinal degeneration (Fig. 1). However, unlike XLPRA1, the focal areas of cell loss do not persist. Indeed, improved outer nuclear layer lamination, loss of opsin mislocalization, and improved morphology of the outer plexiform layer and rod bipolar cell dendrites in older carriers suggests that retinal plasticity in the young XLPRA2 carriers allows tangential displacement of remaining (nonmutant) photoreceptors in the depleted foci, and rewiring with postreceptoral neurons (Beltran et al. 2009). Similar lateral dispersion of photoreceptors following focal laser damage has been

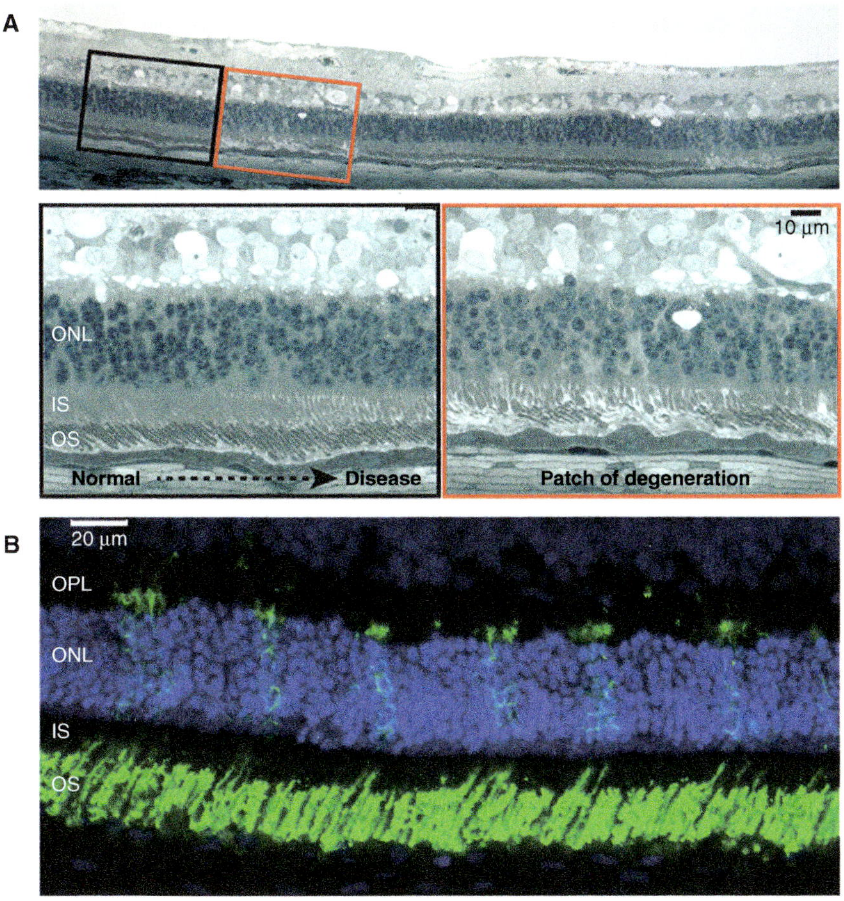

Figure 1. Mosaic pattern of retinal degeneration in XLPRA2 female carriers. (*A*) Focal patches of photoreceptor degeneration surrounded by normally laminated retina in a 24-wk-old carrier. (*B*) Numerous patches of rod opsin mislocalization to the inner segments (IS) and outer nuclear layer (ONL), and features of rod neurite sprouting in the outer plexiform layer (OPL) in a 7-wk-old carrier. (Modified from data in Figure 1 from Beltran et al. 2009).

shown in the nonhuman primate retina (Strazzeri et al. 2014).

Earlier on, we speculated that the more severe disease phenotype observed in the XLPRA2 model could be caused by a toxic gain-of-function, whereas the slower progression and delayed onset seen in XLPRA1 might be explained by a loss-of-function mechanism. These hypotheses led us to initially develop a gene augmentation strategy for the XLPRA1 disease, while preparing for the potential need to combine an allele-independent gene knockdown and a hardened (resistant) gene replacement approach to correct the XLPRA2 phenotype (see below).

OUTCOME MEASURES OF PRECLINICAL EFFICACY

Detailed analysis of the spatiotemporal features of the two canine diseases and development of staging classifications allowed establishment of outcome measures of therapeutic intervention. These are listed in Table 1.

THERAPEUTIC INTERVENTIONS: PROOF OF CONCEPT STUDIES IN CANINE MODELS OF *RPGR*-XLRP

Note: All studies reported below were carried out after approval by the University of Pennsyl-

Table 1. Outcome measures of therapeutic intervention for XLRP

Outcome measures of photoreceptor rescue	Methods	Expected positive therapeutic effect
ONL thickness	In vivo OCT, histology	Retention
IS and OS structure	In vivo OCT, histology	Preservation
Opsin mislocalization	IHC (rod, cone opsins)	Absence
Rod neurite sprouting	IHC (rod opsin, synaptophysin)	Absence
Rod function	Scotopic ERG (a wave amplitude)	Retention
Cone function	Photopic ERG (30 Hz flicker)	Retention
Bipolar cell dendrite length	Histology	Retention
IPL thickness and lamination	IHC (GABA)	Retention
Müller cell gliosis	IHC (GFAP)	Absence
Postreceptoral function	Scotopic ERG (b wave amplitude)	Retention

ERG, electroretinogram; GFAP, glial fibrillary acidic protein; IHC, immunohistochemistry; IPL, inner plexiform layer; IS, inner segment; OCT, optical coherence tomography; ONL, outer nuclear layer; OS, outer segment.

vania IACUC, and conducted in strict accordance with the recommendations in the Guide for the Care and Use of Laboratory Animals of the National Institutes of Health, the USDA's Animal Welfare Act and Animal Welfare Regulations, and in compliance with the ARVO statement for the Use of Animals in Ophthalmic and Vision Research.

Neuroprotection Fails to Rescue Photoreceptors in the XLPRA2 Dog

Following successful demonstration of neuroprotection therapy in the rcd1 dog model of autosomal recessive retinitis pigmentosa (*PDE6B* mutation) (Tao et al. 2002), we examined whether single or repeated intravitreal injections of recombinant human ciliary neurotrophic factor (CNTF) would also modify the course of retinal degeneration in the XLPRA2 dog. Our results (Beltran et al. 2007) failed to demonstrate any positive outcome even when the compound was delivered before the peak of rod loss. However, we observed an increased number of rod opsin-positive cells in the peripheral retina, suggesting the potential for CNTF-mediated photoreceptor cell proliferation in the early postnatal XLPRA2 retina.

Gene Transfer Considerations: Choice of Viral Vector, Promoters, Route of Delivery

Among the various chimeric serotypes of recombinant adeno-associated viral (AAV) vectors previously used for gene transfer to the canine retina (Beltran 2009), we selected the AAV2/5 serotype, as it had been shown in dogs to infect both rods and cones (Weber et al. 2003; Komaromy et al. 2008; Petersen-Jones et al. 2009; Beltran et al. 2010). Photoreceptor-specific promoters that would restrict transgene expression to either rods (mOP, a 476 nt segment of the proximal mouse opsin promoter), or rods and cones (hGRK1, a 292 nt segment of the human G-protein-coupled receptor kinase 1 promoter; hIRBP, a 235 nt segment of the human interphotoreceptor binding protein promoter) were used (al-Ubaidi et al. 1992; Beltran et al. 2010, 2012). Subretinal injections were performed with a subretinal cannula as previously reported (Komaromy et al. 2006; Beltran et al. 2010), and volumes injected (70–150 µL) were adjusted to the dog's age and globe size, aiming to produce a bleb that covered ~1/5–1/4 of the retinal surface.

Initial *RPGR* Gene Therapy Failures and Complications

The first viral vector constructs that were developed and tested in XLPRA1 dogs included a shortened version of the canine $RPGR^{ex1\text{-}ORF15}$ cDNA (cshort $RPGR^{ex1\text{-}ORF15}$). The decision to use this shortened RPGR transgene, which had 708 bp removed in frame from the purine-rich region of exon ORF15, was made to circumvent the DNA packaging restriction of the AAV capsid (<4.7 kb) in the event that a knockdown construct (small hairpin RNA or ribozyme) should need to be added to correct the XLPRA2 disease. This strategy was based on prior evidence that similar in-frame truncation of murine exon ORF15 did not eliminate its function (Hong et al. 2005). Five XLPRA1-affected dogs (four hemizygous males and homozygous mutant female) received, at 26–28 weeks of age (before the onset of retinal degeneration), a 150 μL subretinal injection of either an AAV2/5-mOP-cshortRPGR$^{ex1\text{-}ORF15}$ or AAV2/5-hIRBP-cshortRPGR$^{ex1\text{-}ORF15}$ vector preparation (viral titer: 1.5×10^{11} vg/mL), or balanced salt solution. At 5–7 wk postinjection retinal examination revealed multifocal hyperreflective lesions in the treated area of five out of the six eyes that received either of the two vectors. Noninvasive imaging by optical coherence tomography showed disrupted lamination, which represented photoreceptor rosettes on histologic examination (Fig. 2) (Beltran et al. 2011, 2012). The mechanism by which transduction of photoreceptors with a shortened canine RPGR$^{ex1\text{-}ORF15}$ cDNA led to these complications was not further investigated, and it was decided instead to focus only on the gene augmentation strategy by developing and testing a viral vector that would carry instead the full-length RPGR$^{ex1\text{-}ORF15}$ transgene.

Gene Augmentation with Full-Length Human RPGR$^{ex1\text{-}ORF15}$ Prevents Disease Onset in the XLPRA1 Model

With the goal of accelerating translation of gene therapy to clinical trials, we decided to include the human rather than the canine full-length RPGR$^{ex1\text{-}ORF15}$ in the new viral constructs. In addition, availability of antibodies directed against human RPGR (that do not cross-react with the canine isoform) would allow monitoring of therapeutic transgene expression. An AAV2/5 construct including the hRPGR$^{ex1\text{-}ORF15}$ transgene under the control of the hIRBP promoter was subretinally injected in two XLPRA1 dogs at 28 weeks of age (before the onset of photoreceptor loss). Dogs were monitored by noninvasive confocal scanning laser ophthalmoscopy and spectral-domain optical coherence tomography until 77 weeks of age (well after the start of retinal degeneration). Topographical mapping of the outer nuclear layer showed increased thickness in the treated region that remained within the range seen in wild-type dogs, while significant thinning was seen in the untreated region of the same eye or in the fellow, balanced salt solution-injected control eye (Fig. 3A,B). In addition, improved backscatter signal originating from the inner/outer segment layer was also detectable in the treated area (Beltran et al. 2012). Histological analysis confirmed the rescue of photoreceptors within the bleb area where *RPGR* transgene was expressed, as evidenced by an increased number of photoreceptor cells, preserved inner and outer segment structure, and absence of rod opsin and R/G opsin mislocalization (Fig. 4A–C). This positive effect on the outer retina was also associated with improved structure of the outer plexiform layer, bipolar cells, and a lack of reactivity of Müller cells (the major glial cell population in the retina) (Fig. 4D–F). These results suggest that early intervention with corrective gene augmentation can prevent the onset of photoreceptor loss and impede deleterious secondary remodeling events in the inner retina.

Gene Augmentation with Full-Length Human RPGR$^{ex1\text{-}ORF15}$ Rescues Photoreceptors in the XLPRA2 Model When Delivered at Early and Mid-Stages of Disease

The successful outcome in the XLPRA1 model led us to test whether *RPGR* gene augmentation alone could also positively alter the course of photoreceptor degeneration in the early-onset and more rapidly progressive XLPRA2 disease. An AAV2/5 construct including the hRPGR$^{ex1\text{-}ORF15}$ transgene under the control of the hIRBP promoter, and one with the hGRK1 promoter, were each subretinally injected in one XLPRA2 dog at 5 weeks of age (after disease onset, but before the peak of cell death; outer nuclear layer near normal thickness). Fellow eyes were subretinally injected with balanced salt solution. Similar longitudinal analysis (up to 36 weeks of age) of outer nuclear

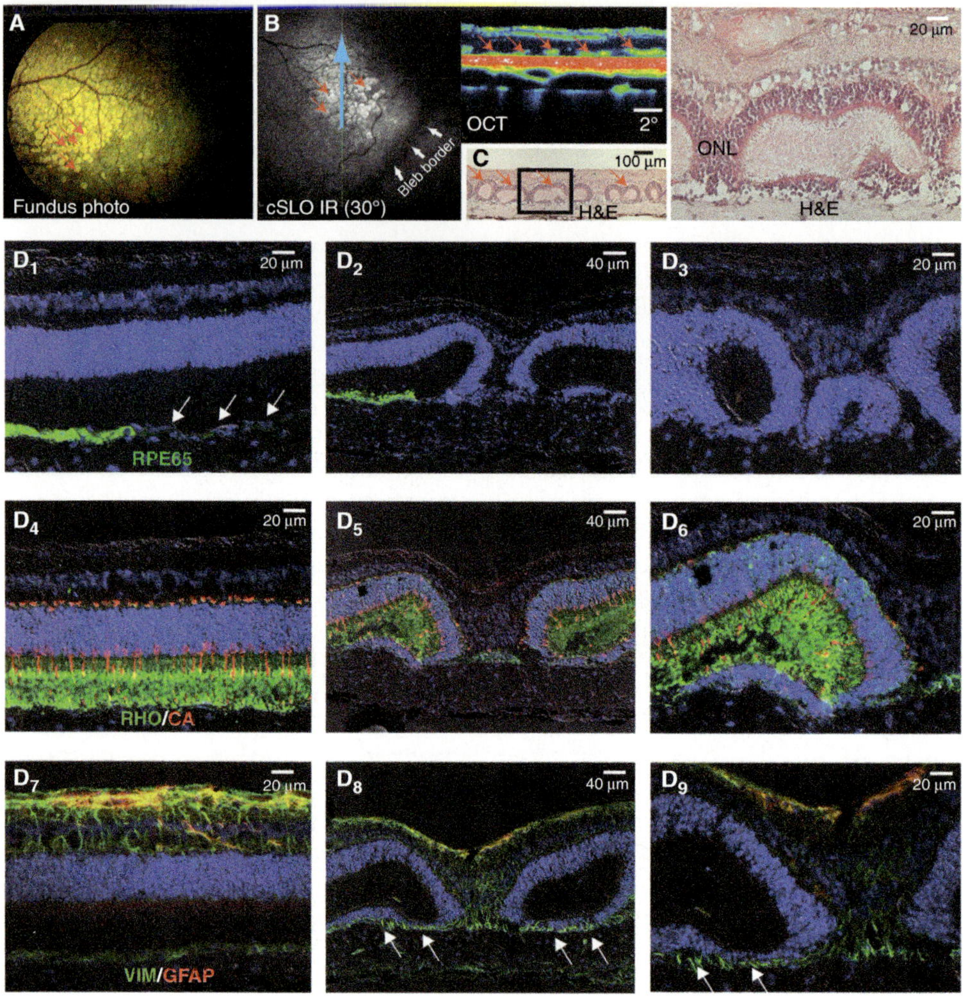

Figure 2. Retinal toxicity induced by early viral vector construct. Retinal complications in an affected XLPRA1 dog 7 wk following subretinal injection of an AAV2/5 carrying a shortened version of canine RPGR$^{ex1\text{-}ORF15}$ cDNA under the control of hIRBP promoter. (*A*) Multifocal hyperreflective lesions (red arrows) seen by ophthalmoscopy within the treated region. (*B*) Similar lesions observed by confocal scanning laser ophthalmoscopy (cSLO) and optical coherence tomography (OCT). (*C*) Histological features of photoreceptor rosettes, using hematoxylin and eosin (H&E). (*D*) Immunohistochemical characterization of the photoreceptor rosettes lesions. (D_1–D_3) Immunolabeling (green) of the retinal pigment epithelium (RPE) is lost (white arrows) at close proximity (D_1) and within (D_2–D_3) the lesions. (D_4–D_6) Normal lamination (D_4) and structure of rods (rod opsin, green) and cones (cone arrestin, red) is disrupted within the lesions (D_5–D_6). (D_7–D_9) The normal architecture of Müller cells (D_7, vimentin, green) is altered within the lesions (D_8–D_9) with prominent extension of radial processes into the vestigial subretinal space. Limited reactivity of Müller cells (GFAP, red) is seen.

layer thickness from spectral-domain optical coherence tomography-derived topographical maps illustrated a potent rescue of photoreceptors in the treated region with the AAV2/5-hIRBP-*hRPGR*$^{ex1\text{-}ORF15}$ vector (Fig. 3C,D), which was confirmed histologically (Fig. 5). Treatment corrected the mislocalization of opsins, improved expression of presynaptic markers, resulted in normal length and arborization of bipolar cell dendrites, and prevented Müller cell gliosis. Although structural preservation appeared to be more pronounced with the con-

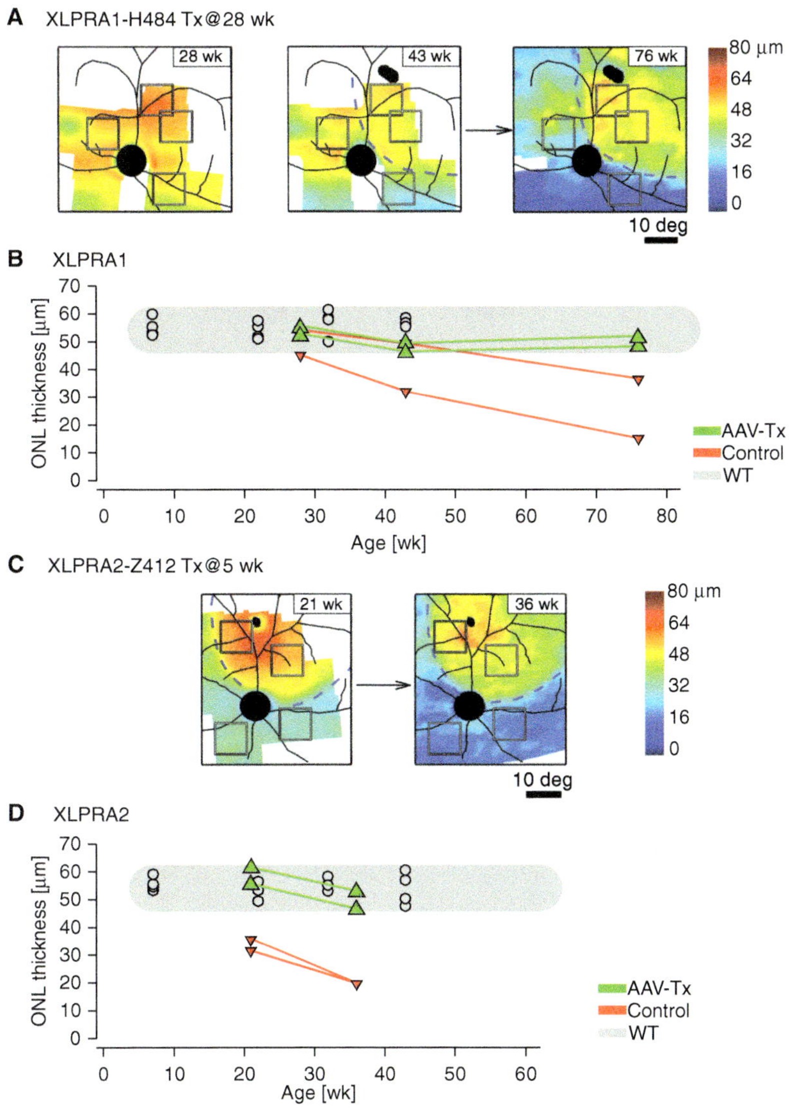

Figure 3. In vivo retinal imaging of photoreceptor rescue following gene therapy in XLPRA1 and XLPRA2 dogs. Longitudinal follow-up of outer nuclear layer (ONL) thickness changes in eyes of XLPRA1 (H484) and XLPRA2 (Z412) dogs treated with a subretinal injection of AAV2/5-hIRBP-*hRPGR*$^{ex1\text{-}ORF15}$ vector. (*A*) ONL topography of H484 measured at 28 weeks of age, immediately before the injection, and at 43 and 76 weeks of age corresponding to 15 and 48 wk after the injection, respectively. (*B*) Progression of ONL thickness at regions of interest within the injection bleb (green symbols) compared with those outside the bleb (red symbols); results from wild-type animals measured at the same retinal locations are also shown (gray symbols). (*C*) ONL topography of Z412 measured at 21 and 36 weeks of age; injection was performed at 5 weeks of age. (*B,D*) Progression of ONL thickness at regions of interest within the injection bleb (green symbols) compared with those outside the bleb (red symbols); results from wild-type animals measured at the same retinal locations are also shown (gray symbols). (*D*) Progression of ONL thickness at regions of interest within the injection bleb (green symbols) compared with those outside the bleb (red symbols); results from wild-type animals measured at the same retinal locations are also shown (gray symbols). Dashed lines in (*A*) and (*C*) demarcate the transient blebs created by the subretinal injections; retinal blood vessels and optic nerve are superimposed on the pseudocolor ONL data. Squares in (*A*) and (*C*) denote the two regions of interest chosen within the bleb boundary and two regions chosen outside the bleb boundary for the quantitative measures shown in (*B*) and (*C*). (Modified from data in Figures 2 and S1 from Beltran et al. 2012).

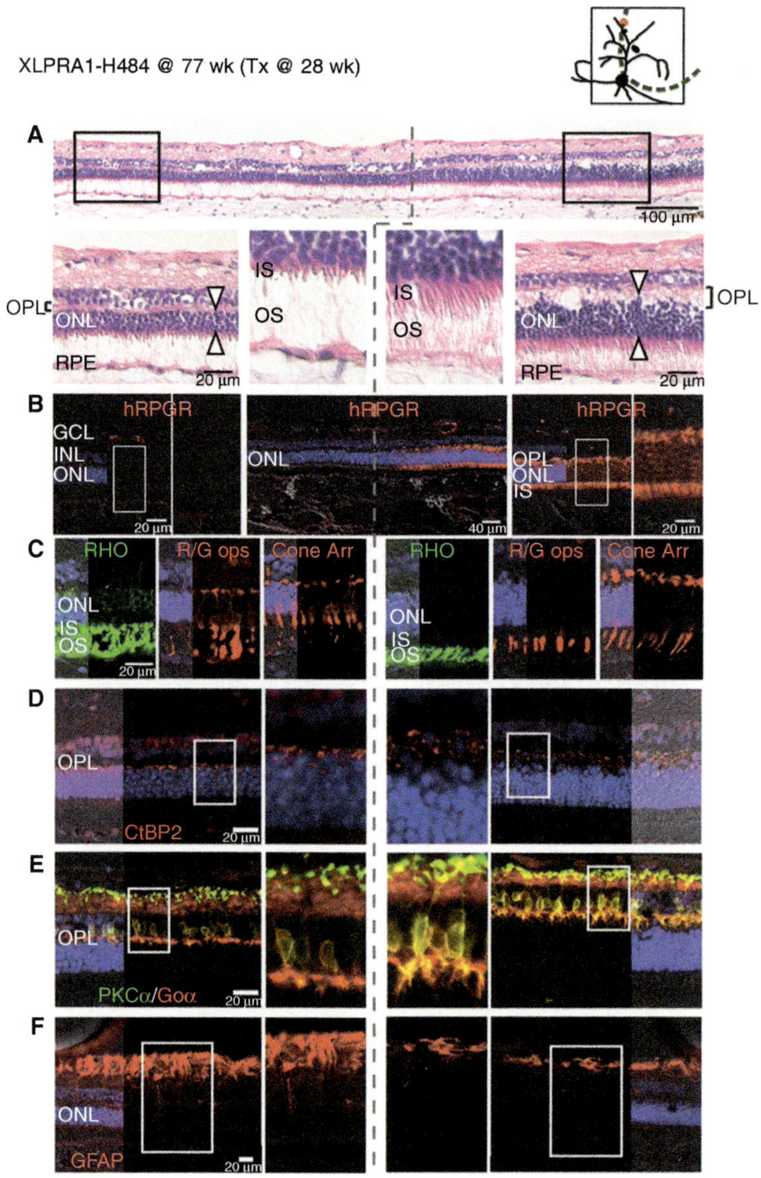

Figure 4. Gene augmentation therapy with AAV2/5-hIRBP-$hRPGR^{ex1\text{-}ORF15}$ vector prevents retinal degeneration onset in XLPRA1 disease. *Upper right* diagram shows the area of subretinal injection performed at 28 weeks of age (green dotted line), and the site of the histological sections shown below at 77 weeks of age (red line) in XLPRA1 dog H484. (*A*) H&E stained cryosection shows preserved outer nuclear layer (ONL) thickness and inner (IS) and outer segment (OS) structure in the treated region. Dotted gray line shows the abrupt demarcation between the treated and untreated regions. (*B*) RPGR immunolabeling confirms expression of the transgene exclusively in the photoreceptors of the treated area. (*C*) Mislocalization of rod opsin (RHO, green) and red/green cone opsin (R/G, red) as well as cone morphology (cone arrestin, red) is corrected in the treated area. (*D*) Preserved density of CtBP2/RIBEYE immunolabeled (red) synaptic ribbons in photoreceptor terminals and normal thickness of the outer plexiform layer (OPL) in the treated area. (*E*) Preserved dendritic arborization in rod bipolar cells immunolabeled with PKCα (green) and Goα (red) in the treated area. (*F*) Absence of Müller cell reactivity assessed by GFAP (red) immunolabeling in the treated area. (Modified from data in Figures 3 and S4 from Beltran et al. 2012).

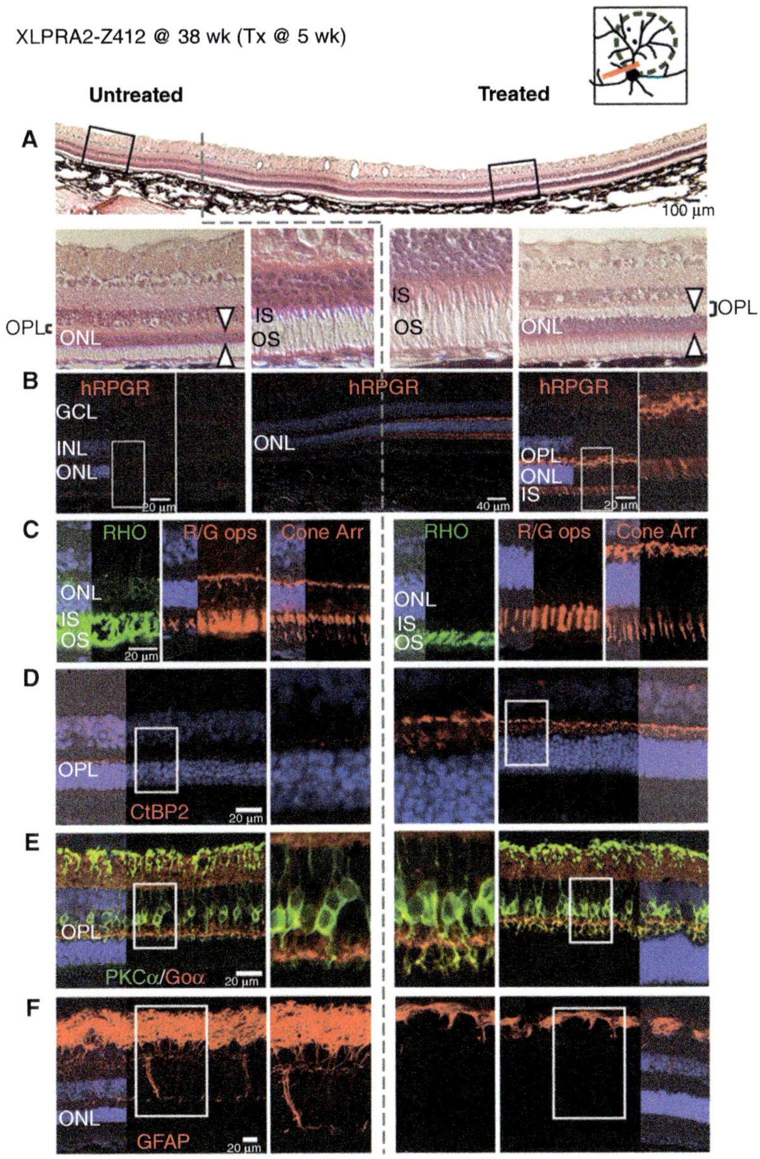

Figure 5. Gene augmentation therapy with AAV2/5-hIRBP-*hRPGR*$^{ex1\text{-}ORF15}$ vector rescues photoreceptors when delivered at early-stage of XLPRA2 disease. *Upper right* diagram shows the area of subretinal injection performed at 5 weeks of age (green dotted line), and the site of the histological sections shown below at 38 weeks of age (red line) in XLPRA2 dog Z412. (*A*) H&E stained cryosection shows increased outer nuclear layer (ONL) thickness and inner (IS) and outer segment (OS) structure in the treated region. Dotted gray line shows the abrupt demarcation between the treated and untreated regions. (*B*) RPGR immunolabeling confirms expression of the transgene exclusively in the photoreceptors of the treated area and is seen throughout the cells with the exception of the outer segments. (*C*) Mislocalization of rod opsin (RHO, green) and red/green cone opsin (R/G, red) as well as cone morphology (cone arrestin, red) is corrected in the treated area. (*D*) Increased density of CtBP2/RIBEYE immunolabeled (red) synaptic ribbons in photoreceptor terminals and increased thickness of the outer plexiform layer (OPL) in the treated area. (*E*) Preserved dendritic arborization in rod bipolar cells immunolabeled with PKCα (green) and Goα (red) in the treated area. (*F*) Absence of Müller cell reactivity assessed by GFAP (red) immunolabeling in the treated area. (Modified from data in Figures S3 and 4 from Beltran et al. 2012).

struct that included the hIRBP rather than the hGRK1 promoter, both viral vectors rescued photoreceptor- and postreceptoral electroretinogram function (Beltran et al. 2012). Comparative studies including higher numbers of animals and dose groups are warranted to adequately establish which of these two promoters is optimal.

AAV2/5-hIRBP-hRPGR$^{ex1\text{-}ORF15}$ was also delivered to three 12-wk-old XLPRA2 dogs at mid-stage disease. At this age, the outer nuclear layer thickness is ~70% of normal, retraction of rod bipolar cells has begun, and there is increased reactivity of Müller cells (Beltran et al. 2006). This is right after the peak of photoreceptor cell death and just before the beginning of the "chronic" phase of cell death, during which numerous proapoptotic and prosurvival genes are differentially expressed (Genini et al. 2013). Dogs were regularly evaluated by noninvasive retinal imaging (scanning confocal laser ophthalmoscopy and spectral-domain optical coherence tomography) and electroretinography at 39 and 42 weeks of age, respectively. Although better rescue was achieved in an age-matched XLPRA2 dog treated at five weeks of age (early disease stage), both increased outer nuclear layer thickness in the bleb area and improved electroretinogram function in the treated eye of all three dogs suggest that gene therapy intervention may be beneficial even in retinal areas that have lost >30% of their photoreceptors (Beltran et al. 2013). Ongoing studies are assessing the efficacy of therapeutic intervention at more advanced stages of disease, and whether a long-term beneficial effect can be sustained (Beltran et al. 2014b).

Positive response to gene augmentation (alone) in the early onset and rapidly progressive XLPRA2 disease challenges the original assumption that the causative frameshift mutation leads to photoreceptor cell loss through toxic gain-of-function of the mutant RPGR$^{ex1\text{-}ORF15}$ isoform. A more plausible hypothesis might be that the XLPRA2 mutation results in a loss-of-function that severely impairs photoreceptor maturation and survival, whereas the XLPRA1 disease may be caused by a hypomorphic mutation that impairs long-term rod and cone viability. While these preclinical findings in two naturally occurring large animal models of *RPGR*-XLRP provide confidence that a similar *RPGR* gene augmentation strategy may be effective and sufficient in treating patients with a wide variety of *RPGR* mutations, one must remain open to the possibility that a subset of mutations may cause photoreceptor death via a toxic gain-of-function mechanism, and would require instead a combined gene knockdown and gene replacement strategy.

CONCLUDING REMARKS

Availability of two complementary canine models that recapitulate distinct spatiotemporal features of the phenotypes reported in human *RPGR*-XLRP patients has enabled us to establish initial proof of concept that a corrective gene augmentation approach may be sufficient to both prevent and stop the degenerative process of rods and cones. These results have provided invaluable information about the viral constructs currently being considered. Indeed, there was initially concern that fine-tuning of the levels of *RPGR* transgene expression in photoreceptors may be required via supposedly less "active" promoters (e.g., the RGPR promoter [Shu et al. 2012]) than the ones currently used. Yet, the potent hRPGR immunolabeling that was observed with hIRBP and hGRK1 promoters was not limited to the connecting cilium region of transduced canine rods and cones, thus suggesting that some degree of *hRPGR*$^{ex1\text{-}ORF15}$ overexpression is tolerable and does not induce measurable cytotoxicity. A similar conclusion can be inferred on the basis of the normal retinal phenotype reported in transgenic mouse overexpressing RPGR^{ORF15} (Wright et al. 2011).

These initial proof-of-concept studies in large animals are very encouraging but will need to be monitored over a longer time period. Indeed, recent evidence in patients as well as in dogs treated by gene augmentation for the RPE65 form of Leber congenital amaurosis showed that, despite persistent functional rescue, ongoing photoreceptor loss continues (Cideciyan et al. 2013). Ongoing studies in mutant dogs should also identify the latest stage of disease that can still respond to gene therapy. Careful extrapolation of these stages from dogs to humans could provide valuable inclusion criteria for the recruitment of patients to future clinical trials. Assessing the effects of *RPGR* gene augmentation in wild-type dogs also needs to be investigated in preparation for investigational new drug-enabling preclinical safety studies. RPGR overexpression in the wild-type retina will also inform as to whether similar gene therapy intervention could be safely considered for some carrier female patients. Finally, pursuing detailed phenotypic characterization of XLRP patients (Jacobson et al. 1997; Lorenz et al. 2003; Aleman et al. 2007; Huang et al. 2012) is necessary to establish valid outcome measures of therapeutic efficacy for future human clinical trials.

ACKNOWLEDGMENTS

Supported by National Institutes of Health Grants EY-06855, EY-17549, EY-007961, EY-021721, P30 EY-001583, and 2PNEY018241, the Foundation Fighting Blindness, a Fight for Sight Nowak family grant, the Midwest Eye Banks and Transplantation Center, the Macula Vision Research Foundation, the Chatlos Foundation, Inc., the Van Sloun Fund for Canine Genetic Research, and Hope for Vision.

A patent application on AAV-mediated gene therapy for RPGR X-linked retinal degeneration has been filed (PCT/US2013/022628). W.W.H. and the University of Florida have a financial interest in the use of AAV therapies, and own equity in a company (AGTC Inc.) that might, in the future, commercialize some aspects of this work.

REFERENCES

Adamian M, Pawlyk BS, Hong DH, Berson EL. 2006. Rod and cone opsin mislocalization in an autopsy eye from a carrier of X-linked retinitis pigmentosa with a Gly436Asp mutation in the *RPGR* gene. *Am J Ophthalmol* **142:** 515–518.

Aguirre GD, Yashar BM, John SK, Smith JE, Breuer DK, Hiriyanna S, Swaroop A, Milam AH. 2002. Retinal histopathology of an XLRP carrier with a mutation in the *RPGR* exon ORF15. *Exp Eye Res* **75:** 431–443.

al-Ubaidi MR, Font RL, Quiambao AB, Keener MJ, Liou GI, Overbeek PA, Baehr W. 1992. Bilateral retinal and brain tumors in transgenic mice expressing simian virus 40 large T antigen under control of the human interphotoreceptor retinoid-binding protein promoter. *J Cell Biol* **119:** 1681–1687.

Aleman TS, Cideciyan AV, Sumaroka A, Schwartz SB, Roman AJ, Windsor EA, Steinberg JD, Branham K, Othman M, Swaroop A, et al. 2007. Inner retinal abnormalities in X-linked retinitis pigmentosa with *RPGR* mutations. *Invest Ophthalmol Vis Sci* **48:** 4759–4765.

Andreasson S, Ponjavic V, Abrahamson M, Ehinger B, Wu W, Fujita R, Buraczynska M, Swaroop A. 1997. Phenotypes in three Swedish families with X-linked retinitis pigmentosa caused by different mutations in the *RPGR* gene. *Am J Ophthalmol* **124:** 95–102.

Ayyagari R, Demirci FY, Liu J, Bingham EL, Stringham H, Kakuk LE, Boehnke M, Gorin MB, Richards JE, Sieving PA. 2002. X-linked recessive atrophic macular degeneration from *RPGR* mutation. *Genomics* **80:** 166–171.

Bader I, Brandau O, Achatz H, Apfelstedt-Sylla E, Hergersberg M, Lorenz B, Wissinger B, Wittwer B, Rudolph G, Meindl A, et al. 2003. X-linked retinitis pigmentosa: *RPGR* mutations in most families with definite X linkage and clustering of mutations in a short sequence stretch of exon ORF15. *Invest Ophthalmol Vis Sci* **44:** 1458–1463.

Bauer S, Fujita R, Buraczynska M, Abrahamson M, Ehinger B, Wu W, Falls TJ, Andreasson S, Swaroop A. 1998. Phenotype of an X-linked retinitis pigmentosa family with a novel splice defect in the *RPGR* gene. *Invest Ophthalmol Vis Sci* **39:** 2470–2474.

Beltran WA. 2009. The use of canine models of inherited retinal degeneration to test novel therapeutic approaches. *Vet Ophthalmol* **12:** 192–204.

Beltran WA, Hammond P, Acland GM, Aguirre GD. 2006. A frameshift mutation in *RPGR* exon ORF15 causes photoreceptor degeneration and inner retina remodeling in a model of X-linked retinitis pigmentosa. *Invest Ophthalmol Vis Sci* **47:** 1669–1681.

Beltran WA, Wen R, Acland GM, Aguirre GD. 2007. Intravitreal injection of ciliary neurotrophic factor (CNTF) causes peripheral remodeling and does not prevent photoreceptor loss in canine *RPGR* mutant retina. *Exp Eye Res* **84:** 753–771.

Beltran WA, Acland GM, Aguirre GD. 2009. Age-dependent disease expression determines remodeling of the retinal mosaic in carriers of *RPGR* exon ORF15 mutations. *Invest Ophthalmol Vis Sci* **50:** 3985–3995.

Beltran WA, Boye SL, Boye SE, Chiodo VA, Lewin AS, Hauswirth WW, Aguirre GD. 2010. rAAV2/5 gene-targeting to rods:dose-dependent efficiency and complications associated with different promoters. *Gene Ther* **17:** 1162–1174.

Beltran WA, Iwabe S, Fajardo D, Boye SE, Teng W-T, Hauswirth WW, Lewin AS, Aguirre GD. 2011. rAAV-mediated gene delivery of truncated canine *RPGR* causes photoreceptor dysplasia in dogs with *RPGR*-ORF15 stop mutation. *Association for Research in Vision and Ophthalmology*, 1–5 May, E-abstract 1418, Fort Lauderdale, FL.

Beltran WA, Cideciyan AV, Lewin AS, Iwabe S, Khanna H, Sumaroka A, Chiodo V, Fajardo DS, Roman AJ, Deng WT, et al. 2012. Gene therapy rescues photoreceptor blindness in dogs and paves the way for treating human X-linked retinitis pigmentosa. *Proc Natl Acad Sci* **109:** 2132–2137.

Beltran WA, Cideciyan AV, Lewin AS, Iwabe S, Boye S, Hauswirth WW, Jacobson SG, Aguirre GD. 2013. Corrective gene therapy for *RPGR*-XLRP rescues a canine model at mid-stage disease. *Association for Research in Vision & Ophthalmology*, 5–9 May, E-abstract 2707, Seattle, WA.

Beltran WA, Cideciyan AV, Guziewicz KE, Iwabe S, Swider M, Scott EM, Savina SV, Ruthel G, Stefano F, Zhang L, et al. 2014a. Canine retina has a primate fovea-like bouquet of cone photoreceptors which is affected by inherited macular degenerations. *PLoS ONE* **9:** e90390. doi:10.1371/journal.pone/0090390.

Beltran WA, Cideciyan AV, Lewin AS, Iwabe S, Swider M, Guzman JM, Boye SL, Hauswirth WW, Jacobson SG, Aguirre GD. 2014b. *RPGR* gene augmentation delivered at early, mid and late stage disease in a canine model of XLRP rescues photoreceptor function and structure. *Association for Research in Vision & Ophthalmology*, 4–8 May, E-abstract 3321, Orlando, FL.

Berendschot TT, DeLint PJ, van Norren D. 1996. Origin of tapetal-like reflexes in carriers of X-linked retinitis pigmentosa. *Invest Ophthalmol Vis Sci* **37:** 2716–2723.

Boylan JP, Wright AF. 2000. Identification of a novel protein interacting with RPGR. *Hum Mol Genet* **9:** 2085–2093.

Branham K, Othman M, Brumm M, Karoukis AJ, Atmaca-Sonmez P, Yashar BM, Schwartz SB, Stover NB, Trzupek K, Wheaton D, et al. 2012. Mutations in *RPGR* and *RP2* account for 15% of males with simplex retinal degenerative disease. *Invest Ophthalmol Vis Sci* **53:** 8232–8237.

Breuer DK, Yashar BM, Filippova E, Hiriyanna S, Lyons RH, Mears AJ, Asaye B, Acar C, Vervoort R, Wright AF, et al. 2002. A comprehensive mutation analysis of *RP2* and *RPGR* in a North American cohort of families with X-linked retinitis pigmentosa. *Am J Hum Genet* **70:** 1545–1554.

Brunner S, Skosyrski S, Kirschner-Schwabe R, Knobeloch KP, Neidhardt J, Feil S, Glaus E, Luhmann UF, Ruther K, Berger W. 2010. Cone versus rod disease in a mutant *Rpgr* mouse caused by different genetic backgrounds. *Invest Ophthalmol Vis Sci* **51:** 1106–1115.

Bukowy-Bieryllo Z, Zietkiewicz E, Loges NT, Wittmer M, Geremek M, Olbrich H, Fliegauf M, Voelkel K, Rutkiewicz E, Rutland J, et al. 2013. *RPGR* mutations might cause reduced orientation of respiratory cilia. *Pediatr Pulmonol* **48:** 352–363.

Chang B, Khanna H, Hawes N, Jimeno D, He S, Lillo C, Parapuram SK, Cheng H, Scott A, Hurd RE, et al. 2006. In-frame deletion in a novel centrosomal/ciliary protein CEP290/NPHP6 perturbs its interaction with RPGR and results in early-onset retinal degeneration in the *rd16* mouse. *Hum Mol Genet* **15:** 1847–1857.

Cideciyan AV, Jacobson SG. 1994. Image analysis of the tapetal-like reflex in carriers of X-linked retinitis pigmentosa. *Invest Ophthalmol Vis Sci* **35:** 3812–3824.

Cideciyan AV, Jacobson SG, Beltran WA, Sumaroka A, Swider M, Iwabe S, Roman AJ, Olivares MB, Schwartz SB, Komaromy AM, et al. 2013. Human retinal gene therapy for Leber congenital amaurosis shows advancing retinal degeneration despite enduring visual improvement. *Proc Natl Acad Sci* **110:** E517–E525.

Demirci FY, Rigatti BW, Wen G, Radak AL, Mah TS, Baic CL, Traboulsi EI, Alitalo T, Ramser J, Gorin MB. 2002. X-linked cone-rod dystrophy (locus *COD1*): Identification of mutations in *RPGR* exon ORF15. *Am J Hum Genet* **70:** 1049–1053.

Ebenezer ND, Michaelides M, Jenkins SA, Audo I, Webster AR, Cheetham ME, Stockman A, Maher ER, Ainsworth JR, Yates JR, et al. 2005. Identification of novel *RPGR* ORF15 mutations in X-linked progressive cone-rod dystrophy (XLCORD) families. *Invest Ophthalmol Vis Sci* **46:** 1891–1898.

Fahim AT, Bowne SJ, Sullivan LS, Webb KD, Williams JT, Wheaton DK, Birch DG, Daiger SP. 2011. Allelic heterogeneity and genetic modifier loci contribute to clinical variation in males with X-Linked retinitis pigmentosa due to *RPGR* mutations. *PLoS ONE* **6:** e23021.

Fishman GA. 1978. Retinitis pigmentosa. Genetic percentages. *Arch Ophthalmol* **96:** 822–826.

Fishman GA, Grover S, Jacobson SG, Alexander KR, Derlacki DJ, Wu W, Buraczynska M, Swaroop A. 1998. X-linked retinitis pigmentosa in two families with a missense mutation in the *RPGR* gene and putative change of glycine to valine at codon 60. *Ophthalmology* **105:** 2286–2296.

Flaxel CJ, Jay M, Thiselton DL, Nayudu M, Hardcastle AJ, Wright A, Bird AC. 1999. Difference between RP2 and RP3 phenotypes in X linked retinitis pigmentosa. *Br J Ophthalmol* **83:** 1144–1148.

Gakovic M, Shu X, Kasioulis I, Carpanini S, Moraga I, Wright AF. 2011. The role of RPGR in cilia formation and actin stability. *Hum Mol Genet* **20:** 4840–4850. doi: 10.1371/journal.pone/0085408.

Genini S, Beltran WA, Aguirre GD. 2013. Up-regulation of tumor necrosis factor superfamily genes in early phases of photoreceptor degeneration. *PLoS ONE* **8:** e85408.

Ghosh AK, Murga-Zamalloa CA, Chan L, Hitchcock PF, Swaroop A, Khanna H. 2011. Human retinopathy-associated ciliary protein retinitis pigmentosa GTPase regulator mediates cilia-dependent vertebrate development. *Hum Mol Genet* **19:** 90–98.

Guyon R, Pearce-Kelling SE, Zeiss CJ, Acland GM, Aguirre GD. 2007. Analysis of six candidate genes as potential modifiers of disease expression in canine XLPRA1, a model for human X-linked retinitis pigmentosa 3. *Mol Vis* **13:** 1094–1105.

Hong DH, Pawlyk BS, Shang J, Sandberg MA, Berson EL, Li T. 2000. A retinitis pigmentosa GTPase regulator (RPGR)-deficient mouse model for X-linked retinitis pigmentosa (RP3). *Proc Natl Acad Sci* **97:** 3649–3654.

Hong DH, Yue G, Adamian M, Li T. 2001. Retinitis pigmentosa GTPase regulator (RPGRr)-interacting protein is stably associated with the photoreceptor ciliary axoneme and anchors RPGR to the connecting cilium. *J Biol Chem* **276:** 12091–12099.

Hong DH, Pawlyk B, Sokolov M, Strissel KJ, Yang J, Tulloch B, Wright AF, Arshavsky VY, Li T. 2003. RPGR isoforms in photoreceptor connecting cilia and the transitional zone of motile cilia. *Invest Ophthalmol Vis Sci* **44:** 2413–2421.

Hong DH, Pawlyk BS, Adamian M, Li T. 2004. Dominant, gain-of-function mutant produced by truncation of RPGR. *Invest Ophthalmol Vis Sci* **45:** 36–41.

Hong DH, Pawlyk BS, Adamian M, Sandberg MA, Li T. 2005. A single, abbreviated RPGR-ORF15 variant reconstitutes RPGR function in vivo. *Invest Ophthalmol Vis Sci* **46:** 435–441.

Huang WC, Wright AF, Roman AJ, Cideciyan AV, Manson FD, Gewaily DY, Schwartz SB, Sadigh S, Limberis MP, Bell P, et al. 2012. *RPGR*-associated retinal degeneration in human X-Linked RP and a murine model. *Invest Ophthalmol Vis Sci* **53:** 5594–5608.

Iannaccone A, Breuer DK, Wang XF, Kuo SF, Normando EM, Filippova E, Baldi A, Hiriyanna S, MacDonald CB, Baldi F, et al. 2003. Clinical and immunohistochemical evidence for an X linked retinitis pigmentosa syndrome with recurrent infections and hearing loss in association with an *RPGR* mutation. *J Med Genet* **40:** e118.

Iannaccone A, Wang X, Jablonski MM, Kuo SF, Baldi A, Cosgrove D, Morton CC, Swaroop A. 2004. Increasing evidence for syndromic phenotypes associated with *RPGR* mutations. *Am J Ophthalmol* **137:** 785–786.

Jacobson SG, Yagasaki K, Feuer WJ, Roman AJ. 1989. Interocular asymmetry of visual function in heterozygotes of X-linked retinitis pigmentosa. *Exp Eye Res* **48:** 679–691.

Jacobson SG, Buraczynska M, Milam AH, Chen C, Jarvalainen M, Fujita R, Wu W, Huang Y, Cideciyan AV, Swaroop A. 1997. Disease expression in X-linked retinitis pigmentosa caused by a putative null mutation in the *RPGR* gene. *Invest Ophthalmol Vis Sci* **38:** 1983–1997.

Jay M. 1982. On the heredity of retinitis pigmentosa. *Br J Ophthalmol* **66:** 405–416.

Jin ZB, Liu XQ, Hayakawa M, Murakami A, Nao-i N. 2006. Mutational analysis of *RPGR* and *RP2* genes in Japanese patients with retinitis pigmentosa: Identification of four mutations. *Mol Vis* **12:** 1167–1174.

Keith CG, Denton MJ, Chen JD. 1991. Clinical variability in a family with X-linked retinal dystrophy and the locus at the RP3 site. *Ophthalmic Paediatr Genet* **12:** 91–98.

Khanna H, Hurd TW, Lillo C, Shu X, Parapuram SK, He S, Akimoto M, Wright AF, Margolis B, Williams DS, et al. 2005. RPGR-ORF15, which is mutated in retinitis pigmentosa, associates with SMC1, SMC3, and microtubule transport proteins. *J Biol Chem* **280:** 33580–33587.

Khanna H, Davis EE, Murga-Zamalloa CA, Estrada-Cuzcano A, Lopez I, den Hollander AI, Zonneveld MN, Othman MI, Waseem N, Chakarova CF, et al. 2009. A common allele in *RPGRIP1L* is a modifier of retinal degeneration in ciliopathies. *Nat Genet* **41:** 739–745.

Koenekoop RK, Loyer M, Hand CK, Al Mahdi H, Dembinska O, Beneish R, Racine J, Rouleau GA. 2003. Novel *RPGR* mutations with distinct retinitis pigmentosa phenotypes in French-Canadian families. *Am J Ophthalmol* **136:** 678–687.

Komaromy AM, Varner SE, de Juan E, Acland GM, Aguirre GD. 2006. Application of a new subretinal injection device in the dog. *Cell Transplantation* **15:** 511–519.

Komaromy AM, Alexander JJ, Cooper AE, Chiodo VA, Acland GM, Hauswirth WW, Aguirre GD. 2008. Targeting gene expression to cones with human cone opsin promoters in recombinant AAV. *Gene Ther* **15:** 1049–1055.

Linari M, Ueffing M, Manson F, Wright A, Meitinger T, Becker J. 1999. The retinitis pigmentosa GTPase regulator, RPGR, interacts with the delta subunit of rod cyclic GMP phosphodiesterase. *Proc Natl Acad Sci* **96:** 1315–1320.

Lorenz B, Andrassi M, Kretschmann U. 2003. Phenotype in two families with RP3 associated with *RPGR* mutations. *Ophthalmic Genet* **24:** 89–101.

Mavlyutov TA, Zhao H, Ferreira PA. 2002. Species-specific subcellular localization of RPGR and RPGRIP isoforms: Implications for the phenotypic variability of congenital retinopathies among species. *Hum Mol Genet* **11:** 1899–1907.

Mears AJ, Hiriyanna S, Vervoort R, Yashar B, Gieser L, Fahrner S, Daiger SP, Heckenlively JR, Sieving PA, Wright AF, et al. 2000. Remapping of the *RP15* locus for X-linked cone-rod degeneration to Xp11.4-p21.1, and identification of a de novo insertion in the *RPGR* exon ORF15. *Am J Hum Genet* **67:** 1000–1003.

Meindl A, Dry K, Herrmann K, Manson F, Ciccodicola A, Edgar A, Carvalho MR, Achatz H, Hellebrand H, Lennon A, et al. 1996. A gene (*RPGR*) with homology to the *RCC1* guanine nucleotide exchange factor is mutated in X-linked retinitis pigmentosa (RP3). *Nat Genet* **13:** 35–42.

Moore A, Escudier E, Roger G, Tamalet A, Pelosse B, Marlin S, Clement A, Geremek M, Delaisi B, Bridoux AM, et al. 2006. *RPGR* is mutated in patients with a complex X linked phenotype combining primary ciliary dyskinesia and retinitis pigmentosa. *J Med Genet* **43:** 326–333.

Murga-Zamalloa CA, Atkins SJ, Peranen J, Swaroop A, Khanna H. 2010a. Interaction of retinitis pigmentosa GTPase regulator (RPGR) with RAB8A GTPase: Implications for cilia dysfunction and photoreceptor degeneration. *Hum Mol Genet* **19:** 3591–3598.

Murga-Zamalloa CA, Desai NJ, Hildebrandt F, Khanna H. 2010b. Interaction of ciliary disease protein retinitis pigmentosa GTPase regulator with nephronophthisis-associated proteins in mammalian retinas. *Mol Vis* **16:** 1373–1381.

Neidhardt J, Glaus E, Barthelmes D, Zeitz C, Fleischhauer J, Berger W. 2007. Identification and characterization of a novel RPGR isoform in human retina. *Hum Mutat* **28:** 797–807.

Otto EA, Loeys B, Khanna H, Hellemans J, Sudbrak R, Fan S, Muerb U, O'Toole JF, Helou J, Attanasio M, et al. 2005. Nephrocystin-5, a ciliary IQ domain protein, is mutated in Senior-Loken syndrome and interacts with RPGR and calmodulin. *Nat Genet* **37:** 282–288.

Pelletier V, Jambou M, Delphin N, Zinovieva E, Stum M, Gigarel N, Dollfus H, Hamel C, Toutain A, Dufier JL, et al. 2007. Comprehensive survey of mutations in *RP2* and *RPGR* in patients affected with distinct retinal dystrophies: Genotype-phenotype correlations and impact on genetic counseling. *Hum Mutat* **28:** 81–91.

Petersen-Jones SM, Bartoe JT, Fischer AJ, Scott M, Boye SL, Chiodo V, Hauswirth WW. 2009. AAV retinal transduction in a large animal model species: Comparison of a self-complementary AAV2/5 with a single-stranded AAV2/5 vector. *Mol Vis* **15:** 1835–1842.

Roepman R, van Duijnhoven G, Rosenberg T, Pinckers AJ, Bleeker-Wagemakers LM, Bergen AA, Post J, Beck A,

Reinhardt R, Ropers HH, et al. 1996. Positional cloning of the gene for X-linked retinitis pigmentosa 3: Homology with the guanine-nucleotide-exchange factor RCC1. *Hum Mol Genet* **5:** 1035–1041.

Roepman R, Bernoud-Hubac N, Schick DE, Maugeri A, Berger W, Ropers HH, Cremers FP, Ferreira PA. 2000. The retinitis pigmentosa GTPase regulator (RPGR) interacts with novel transport-like proteins in the outer segments of rod photoreceptors. *Hum Mol Genet* **9:** 2095–2105.

Ruddle JB, Ebenezer ND, Kearns LS, Mulhall LE, Mackey DA, Hardcastle AJ. 2009. *RPGR ORF15* genotype and clinical variability of retinal degeneration in an Australian population. *Br J Ophthalmol* **93:** 1151–1154.

Sandberg MA, Rosner B, Weigel-DiFranco C, Dryja TP, Berson EL. 2007. Disease course of patients with X-linked retinitis pigmentosa due to *RPGR* gene mutations. *Invest Ophthalmol Vis Sci* **48:** 1298–1304.

Schmid F, Glaus E, Cremers FP, Kloeckener-Gruissem B, Berger W, Neidhardt J. 2010. Mutation- and tissue-specific alterations of *RPGR* transcripts. *Invest Ophthalmol Vis Sci* **51:** 1628–1635.

Sharon D, Sandberg MA, Rabe VW, Stillberger M, Dryja TP, Berson EL. 2003. *RP2* and *RPGR* mutations and clinical correlations in patients with X-linked retinitis pigmentosa. *Am J Hum Genet* **73:** 1131–1146.

Shu X, Fry AM, Tulloch B, Manson FD, Crabb JW, Khanna H, Faragher AJ, Lennon A, He S, Trojan P, et al. 2005. RPGR ORF15 isoform co-localizes with RPGRIP1 at centrioles and basal bodies and interacts with nucleophosmin. *Hum Mol Genet* **14:** 1183–1197.

Shu X, Simpson JR, Hart AW, Zeng Z, Patnaik SR, Gautier P, Murdoch E, Tulloch B, Wright AF. 2012. Functional characterization of the human *RPGR* proximal promoter. *Invest Ophthalmol Vis Sci* **53:** 3951–3958.

Strazzeri JM, Hunter JJ, Masella BD, Yin L, Fischer WS, Diloreto DA Jr, Libby RT, Williams DR, Merigan WH. 2014. Focal damage to macaque photoreceptors produces persistent visual loss. *Exp Eye Res* **119:** 88–96.

Szamier RB, Berson EL. 1985. Retinal histopathology of a carrier of X-chromosome-linked retinitis pigmentosa. *Ophthalmology* **92:** 271–278.

Tao W, Wen R, Goddard MB, Sherman SD, O'Rourke PJ, Stabila PF, Bell WJ, Dean BJ, Kauper KA, Budz VA, et al. 2002. Encapsulated cell based delivery of CNTF reduces photoreceptor degeneration in animal models of retinitis pigmentosa. *Invest Ophthalmol Vis Sci* **43:** 3292–3298.

Thiadens AA, Soerjoesing GG, Florijn RJ, Tjiam AG, den Hollander AI, van den Born LI, Riemslag FC, Bergen AA, Klaver CC. 2011. Clinical course of cone dystrophy caused by mutations in the *RPGR* gene. *Graefes Arch Clin Exp Ophthalmol* **249:** 1527–1535.

Thompson DA, Khan NW, Othman MI, Chang B, Jia L, Grahek G, Wu Z, Hiriyanna S, Nellissery J, Li T, et al. 2012. Rd9 is a naturally occurring mouse model of a common form of retinitis pigmentosa caused by mutations in RPGR-ORF15. *PLoS ONE* **7:** e35865. doi: 10.1371/journal.pone/0035865.

Vajaranant TS, Seiple W, Szlyk JP, Fishman GA. 2002. Detection using the multifocal electroretinogram of mosaic retinal dysfunction in carriers of X-linked retinitis pigmentosa. *Ophthalmology* **109:** 560–568.

van Dorp DB, Wright AF, Carothers AD, Bleeker-Wagemakers EM. 1992. A family with RP3 type of X-linked retinitis pigmentosa: An association with ciliary abnormalities. *Hum Genet* **88:** 331–334.

Vervoort R, Lennon A, Bird AC, Tulloch B, Axton R, Miano MG, Meindl A, Meitinger T, Ciccodicola A, Wright AF. 2000. Mutational hot spot within a new *RPGR* exon in X-linked retinitis pigmentosa. *Nat Genet* **25:** 462–466.

Walia S, Fishman GA, Swaroop A, Branham KE, Lindeman M, Othman M, Weleber RG. 2008. Discordant phenotypes in fraternal twins having an identical mutation in exon ORF15 of the *RPGR* gene. *Arch Ophthalmol* **126:** 379–384.

Weber M, Rabinowitz J, Provost N, Conrath H, Folliot S, Briot D, Cherel Y, Chenuaud P, Samulski J, Moullier P, et al. 2003. Recombinant adeno-associated virus serotype 4 mediates unique and exclusive long-term transduction of retinal pigmented epithelium in rat, dog, and nonhuman primate after subretinal delivery. *Mol Ther* **7:** 774–781.

Weleber RG, Butler NS, Murphey WH, Sheffield VC, Stone EM. 1997. X-linked retinitis pigmentosa associated with a 2-base pair insertion in codon 99 of the RP3 gene *RPGR*. *Arch Ophthalmol* **115:** 1429–1435.

Wright RN, Hong DH, Perkins B. 2011. Misexpression of the constitutive $Rpgr^{ex1-19}$ variant leads to severe photoreceptor degeneration. *Invest Ophthalmol Vis Sci* **52:** 5189–5201.

Wright RN, Hong DH, Perkins B. 2012. $Rpgr^{ORF15}$ connects to the usher protein network through direct interactions with multiple whirlin isoforms. *Invest Ophthalmol Vis Sci* **53:** 1519–1529.

Yang Z, Peachey NS, Moshfeghi DM, Thirumalaichary S, Chorich L, Shugart YY, Fan K, Zhang K. 2002. Mutations in the *RPGR* gene cause X-linked cone dystrophy. *Hum Mol Genet* **11:** 605–611.

Zahid S, Khan N, Branham K, Othman M, Karoukis AJ, Sharma N, Moncrief A, Mahmood MN, Sieving PA, Swaroop A, et al. 2013. Phenotypic conservation in patients with X-linked retinitis pigmentosa caused by *RPGR* mutations. *JAMA Ophthalmol* **131:** 1016–1025.

Zeiss CJ, Acland GM, Aguirre GD. 1999. Retinal pathology of canine X-linked progressive retinal atrophy, the locus homologue of RP3. *Invest Ophthalmol Vis Sci* **40:** 3292–3304.

Zhang Q, Acland GM, Wu WX, Johnson JL, Pearce-Kelling SE, Tulloch B, Vervoort R, Wright AF, Aguirre GD. 2002. Different *RPGR* exon ORF15 mutations in *Canids* provide insights into photoreceptor cell degeneration. *Hum Mol Genet* **11:** 993–1003.

Zito I, Downes SM, Patel RJ, Cheetham ME, Ebenezer ND, Jenkins SA, Bhattacharya SS, Webster AR, Holder GE, Bird AC, et al. 2003. *RPGR* mutation associated with retinitis pigmentosa, impaired hearing, and sinorespiratory infections. *J Med Genet* **40:** 609–615.

Gene Augmentation for adRP Mutations in *RHO*

Alfred S. Lewin, Brian Rossmiller, and Haoyu Mao

Department of Molecular Genetics and Microbiology, University of Florida College of Medicine, Gainesville, Florida 32610

Correspondence: lewin@ufl.edu

Mutations in the gene for rhodopsin, *RHO,* cause autosomal dominant retinitis pigmentosa, a disease characterized by death of rod photoreceptor cells. At the end stage, when most rods are gone, cones die too, taking central vision with them. One goal of gene therapy, therefore, is to preserve central vision by promoting rod survival in the vicinity of the macula. Dominance in *RHO* mutations is associated with two phenomena: interference with the function of normal rhodopsin and intrinsic toxicity of the mutant protein. In the case of interference, increased production of the wild-type protein may be therapeutic, but in the case of toxicity, suppression of the mutant protein may also be needed. *RHO* augmentation has made use of advances in gene delivery to the retina using adeno-associated virus (AAV). Several strategies have been developed for suppression of rhodopsin expression, but because of the heterogeneity of *RHO* mutations they are not specific for the mutant allele: They suppress both mutant and wild-type *RHO.* Experiments in autosomal dominant retinitis pigmentosa (adRP) mouse models suggest that both *RHO* augmentation and supplementation plus suppression preserve the survival of rod cells.

As many as 40% of retinitis pigmentosa cases display autosomal dominant inheritance, and approximately one quarter of these are attributable to mutations in *RHO*, the gene for rod cell opsin (Sullivan et al. 2006). A complicating feature of *RHO*-based autosomal dominant retinitis pigmentosa (adRP) is its alleleic diversity: More than 100 disease-causing mutations have been mapped to *RHO*, and the vast majority are dominant (see https://sph.uth.edu/retnet/home.htm). These mutations can be classified both by their clinical presentation and by their impact on the cellular distribution of rhodopsin. Such distinctions are critical because they determine how, or even whether, a particular patient should be considered for gene therapy.

Based on clinical observations, Cideciyan and coworkers (1998) described two classes of adRP. Class A patients lost retinal function over the entire retina and reported the onset of night blindness early in life. In contrast, class B patients exhibited a milder phenotype, normal rod activation kinetics, and preserved rod outer segment length, with anomalies in the rod visual cycle that were mutation specific. Photoreceptor degeneration in subclass B1 was not homogenous, and some patients showed an inferior to superior progression of disease. These authors conclude that the "catastrophic loss of rod func-

Cite this article as *Cold Spring Harb Perspect Med* doi: 10.1101/cshperspect.a017400

tion" in class A patients may not be correctable, so that therapy should be focused on preserving cones; whereas, in class B patients, rods have the potential to be rescued, and preserving rods is the best hope for protecting cones. The question of why cones die in retinitis pigmentosa is also crucial, because the answer will determine how many rods must be rescued to preserve central vision.

Two classes of opsin mutations were also described as a result of studies in tissue culture cells (Sung et al. 1991; Kaushal and Khorana 1994). Class I opsin mutants were expressed at high levels in cells, reconstituted rhodopsin by binding 11-*cis*-retinal and partitioned to the plasma membrane. Class II mutants were expressed at low levels, did not bind 11-*cis*-retinal and remained in the endoplasmic reticulum. The relationship between the cellular behavior of mutant opsin proteins and the clinical impact of opsin mutations is not always clear, but a few generalizations can be made. Most of the mutations that lead to opsin misfolding and instability (i.e., class II) lead to a milder disease phenotype (class B). In contrast, mutations affecting the carboxyl-terminus of opsin, such as V345L and P347S, are expressed at high levels. These mutated proteins form rhodopsin, but lead to early onset, severe retinal degeneration (class A).

Transgenic animal models of adRP have provided some clarification and some confusion. For example, rhodopsin with carboxyl-terminal chain terminating mutations (Q344X and S334X) is mislocalized to the plasma membrane of the inner segment (Sung et al. 1994; Li et al. 1996; Green et al. 2000), and this improper membrane insertion is toxic to rod photoreceptors. In contrast, class II mutations (P23H and T17M), which cause opsin to be retained in the endoplasmic reticulum, may cause cell death by continued activation of the unfolded protein response (Lin et al. 2007; Gorbatyuk et al. 2010; Kunte et al. 2012). Mendes and colleagues (2005) have refined the classification of *RHO* mutants, synthesizing results obtained in cell and transgenic models of adRP. One risk of transgenic models is related to the potential for overexpression of rhodopsin, which in itself may be toxic (Olsson et al. 1992a; Tan et al. 2001). Sakami and coworkers described a knock in mouse model of P23H *Rho* (the mouse version of *RHO*). Unlike transgenic P23H models, this line displayed the slow retinal degeneration characteristic of type B patients, and opsin did not accumulate in the endoplasmic reticulum but led to the disruption of disc membranes in rod outer segments (Sakami et al. 2011).

Two critical questions must be answered when considering rod-directed gene therapy: (1) Is the degeneration progressing too quickly for rescue by gene delivery to rod photoreceptors? If rod cells have begun their cell death program when the diagnosis is made, then therapy must be directed at macular cones (Yang et al. 2009; Punzo et al. 2009; Usui et al. 2009; Murakami et al. 2012), or alternative strategies such as stem cell therapy, retinal prosthesis or gene delivery of light sensitive channels to cells of the inner retina may be indicated. (2) How does mutant opsin kill the cell? *RHO* mutations may be dominant for either of two reasons (Wilson and Wensel 2003; Mendes et al. 2005). Rhodopsin forms dimeric complexes in the disc membrane (Fotiadis et al. 2003), and mutant proteins might interfere with the function of normal rhodopsin or its assembly in the membrane, thereby exerting dominant negative effects. Alternatively, gain-of-function mutations could cause rhodopsin to be intrinsically damaging to the rod cell. It may be possible to treat dominant negative mutations by increasing the level of the normal protein (supplementation). For mutations that cause rhodopsin to be injurious, however, suppressing the expression of the mutant proteins may also be required.

RHODOPSIN SUPPLEMENTATION

Whether or not the production of mutated opsin should be blocked, the conditions for delivery of a normal human opsin gene must be established for gene supplementation. Delivery of a wild-type copy of the defective gene is the most direct approach for gene therapy and is being tested both animal models and human clinical trials of recessive retinal degenerations, as described in many of the other reviews in this collection. Key issues that must be addressed are delivery to photoreceptors, specificity and the appropriate level of expression.

DELIVERY

For gene delivery to photoreceptors, adeno-associated virus (AAV) is currently the best-developed vehicle. Recombinant AAV leads to long-term (probably lifelong) expression of the delivered gene in nondividing cells, and because the delivered DNA is maintained as an episome (Song et al. 2004), there is little danger of insertional mutagenesis (Kaeppel et al. 2013). AAV does not cause disease and does not provoke an inflammatory response following subretinal injection, although preexisting antibodies to the virus can limit its usefulness for some applications (Mingozzi and High 2013). In three trials of gene therapy for Leber congenital amaurosis type II, AAV serotype 2 has been shown to be safe for human use (Bainbridge et al. 2008; Maguire et al. 2008; Cideciyan et al. 2009). In the eye, AAV efficiently infects both photoreceptors and the retinal pigment epithelium following subretinal injections. In rodents, a single subretinal injection of 1 or 2 µL can detach the entire retina and infect 80% of photoreceptors before the neural retina reattaches to the retinal pigment epithelium. In larger animals (such as dogs) and in humans, larger volumes on the order of 100–300 µL are delivered, and viral infection is restricted to the area of detachment. A limitation of AAV is its limited carrying capacity: 4.7 kb inserts in single stranded AAV and half of that in self-complementary AAV. Recently, genetic modifications to the viral capsid proteins have permitted transduction of photoreceptor cells from the vitreous chamber, but efficiency is currently too low, certainly in primates, to use this approach for effective replacement of rhodopsin in rods (Dalkara et al. 2013; Kay et al. 2013).

Other approaches to gene delivery to photoreceptors include the use of nanoparticles and lentivirus-based vectors (Han et al. 2012; Binley et al. 2013). Each has shown some promise, and vectors based on equine infectious anemia virus are in clinical trials for treatment of retinal disease (see http://clinicaltrials.gov, NCT01367444; NCT01301443; NCT01736592). The user communities for these systems are small, however, and for the purpose of delivering short cDNAs such as that of rhodopsin, the limited carrying capacity of AAV is not an impediment.

SPECIFICITY

AAV vectors with multiple tyrosine-to-phenylalanine modifications infect many cell types following intravitreal or subretinal injection (Petrs-Silva et al. 2011). Photoreceptor specific expression of transgenes can be achieved using several different promoters, including that of rhodopsin kinase and interphotoreceptor retinoid binding protein. The proximal rod opsin promoter of 485 bp leads to efficient transgene expression in rod photoreceptors, but delivered genes are also expressed in cone photoreceptors (Glushakova et al. 2006; Mussolino et al. 2011a). Whether production of rhodopsin in cone photoreceptors will affect cone function and vision is not known. Palfi and colleagues (2010) described a longer rod opsin promoter construct containing a 1.7 kb segment of the mouse rhodopsin promoter and two additional conserved elements from the rhodopsin promoter. In an AAV vector, this promoter led to 50% greater expression of human *RHO* mRNA than a virus using the 500-bp proximal promoter following subretinal injection in mice. Injection of this vector just after birth led to partial protection of rod cell structure and function for up to 12 wk in *Rho* knockout mice.

LEVEL OF EXPRESSION

Expression of wild-type human rhodopsin at high levels in transgenic mice leads to progressive death of photoreceptor cells (Olsson et al. 1992b; Sung et al. 1994). This phenomenon has been examined in some detail by Price et al. (2012), who expressed one or two copies of a normal human *RHO* transgene in mice with one or two copies of wild-type mouse *Rho*. Two copies of the human *RHO* gene on a $Rho^{-/-}$ background produced approximately the same level of rhodopsin protein as the two endogenous copies of mouse *Rho* in wild-type mice. Two copies of mouse *Rho* plus one copy of human *RHO* led to a 30% decrease in the thickness of the outer nuclear layer (ONL) by 6 mo of age, with most of the decline occurring in the first month of life, i.e., during photoreceptor development. A double dose of opsin genes (two *Rho* plus two *RHO*) led to a 60% decrease in ONL thickness, with a sharp decline in the first month but continued thinning over the next 5 mo. Increased expression of rhodopsin led to an increase in the volume of rod outer segments, and the authors concluded that loss of photoreceptor cell bodies (thinning of the ONL) with three copies of the gene may be caused by cellular crowding. Increased diameter of rod outer segments was also reported by Wen et al. (2009), who used transgenic mice expressing a chimeric bovine-murine opsin gene. These authors suggest that without an increase in peripherin/rds (retinal degeneration slow) that disc membranes become unstable in larger outer segments.

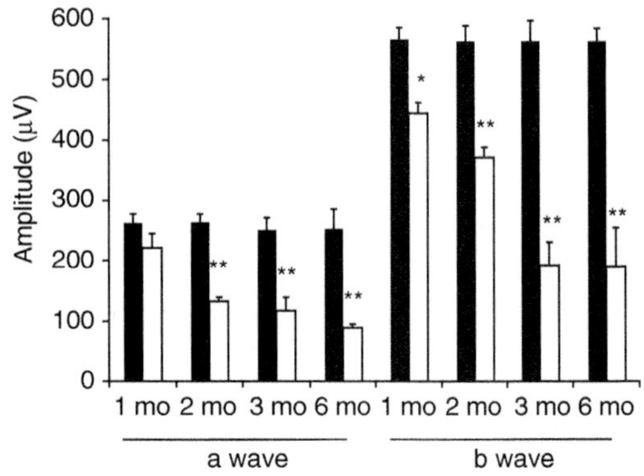

Figure 1. Virally mediated overexpression of rhodopsin leads to retinal degeneration in C57Bl/6J mice. Reduction in ERG a-wave and b-wave amplitudes in eyes injected with AAV-*Rho* (white bars) compared with the uninjected contralateral eyes (black bars) over a time course of 6 mo after injection of virus (n = 7). For the a-wave amplitudes, ** $p < 0.005$ at 2, 3, and 6 mo postinjection. For b-wave amplitudes, * $p < 0.05$ at 1 mo and ** $p < 0.005$ at 2, 3, and 6 mo postinjection. (From Mao et al. 2011; reprinted, with permission, from Mary Ann Liebert, Inc. © 2011.)

Because transgenic overexpression of rhodopsin leads to death of photoreceptors, it is logical that viral delivery of *RHO* cDNA could be harmful if too much rhodopsin is produced. Indeed, that is what we found using AAV to deliver a cDNA encoding mouse rhodopsin under the control of its own promoter (Mao et al. 2011). Subretinal delivery of this vector in wild-type mice led to a 45% increase in the level of rhodopsin monomer (similar to the presence of a single copy of a *RHO* transgene), and this level of expression caused a 70% reduction in electroretinogram (ERG) a-wave and b-wave amplitudes over the 6 mo after injection (Fig. 1). This finding suggests that rhodopsin expression from viral vectors should be carefully titrated.

Nevertheless, excess rhodopsin may not be a risk in gene therapy for adRP, because *RHO* genes will not be delivered to people with two normal copies of *RHO*. Patients harboring the P23H mutation in *RHO* have less than the normal amount of rhodopsin (Kemp et al. 1992), and this reduction is probably characteristic of many class B patients (Kemp et al. 1988). Likewise, the best-characterized transgenic mouse line expressing P23H *Rho* exhibits about one half of the normal level of rhodopsin, based on spectroscopic measurements on 1-mo-old mice (Wu et al. 1998), and the P23H *RHO* line that we developed exhibit a significant reduction in rhodopsin levels at the same age (Noorwez et al. 2009). Diminished levels of rhodopsin can be attributed to retention of the mutant protein in the endoplasmic reticulum and enhanced degradation of the wild-type protein in the presence of mutant opsin (Frederick et al. 2001; Rajan and Kopito 2005). In both people and mice, reduction in rhodopsin levels is revealed by a delayed recovery from photobleaching (Goto et al. 1995; Kemp et al. 1992). Consequently, individuals who stand to benefit from gene augmentation with rhodopsin can be identified, and those at risk of rhodopsin excess can be excluded from treatment.

PHOTORECEPTOR RESCUE BY RHODOPSIN SUPPLEMENTATION

In mice bearing a P23H *Rho* transgene, increased expression of normal rhodopsin reduces the rate of retinal degeneration. Frederick and colleagues (Frederick et al. 2001) found that in transgenic mice with no wild-type *Rho*, 80% of the photoreceptor cell bodies (ONL) were gone by postnatal day 30. In mice with one copy of the endogenous mouse gene, there was only a 50% reduction at the same time point, and in mice with a normal component of *Rho,* there was no retinal degeneration at day 30, although by postnatal day 90 photoreceptor loss was complete on all genetic backgrounds. Price and coworkers (2012) took this analysis one step further: In mice with the same P23H transgene, three wild-type rhodopsin genes (two *Rho* plus one *RHO*) retained ~70% of the ONL at 1 mo, and nearly half of the ONL at 6 mo. These results support the hypothesis of Wilson and Wensel (2003) that class II mutations such as P23H may result in a dominant negative form of opsin that is not inherently injurious to photoreceptors.

AAV-mediated delivery of a cDNA encoding wild-type rhodopsin also reduced retinal degeneration in P23H transgenic mice (Mao et al. 2011). We used a mouse line with one copy of a human P23H *RHO* gene on a wild-type background ($Rho^{+/+}$). Such mice lose 60% of the ONL and 70% of their scotopic a-wave response by 6 mo of age, but eyes injected with AAV-*Rho* retained 80% of the ONL in the superior retina and 90% in the inferior hemisphere (Fig. 2A). ERG a-wave and b-wave amplitudes also remained at ~80% of those of wild-type C57Bl/6 mice, and the decrease in ERG response seen in untreated eyes was arrested by 2 mo of age in injected eyes (Fig. 2B). These results suggest that rhodopsin supplementation by viral delivery of a wild-type *RHO* cDNA may be a viable therapeutic approach in cases of adRP associated with class II mutations in *RHO.*

That being said, models of adRP containing carboxyl-terminal mutations in rhodopsin transgenes often exhibit rapid degeneration of the outer retina even when two copies of the wild-type mouse *Rho* are present at the endogenous locus, depending on the level of expression of the transgene (Li et al. 1995, 1996; Petters et al. 1997; Pennesi et al. 2008). Millington-Ward and colleagues (2011) reported that AAV delivery of a wild-type human *RHO* cDNA driven by a 1.7 kb opsin promoter did not protect photoreceptor function (ERG b-wave) in P347S

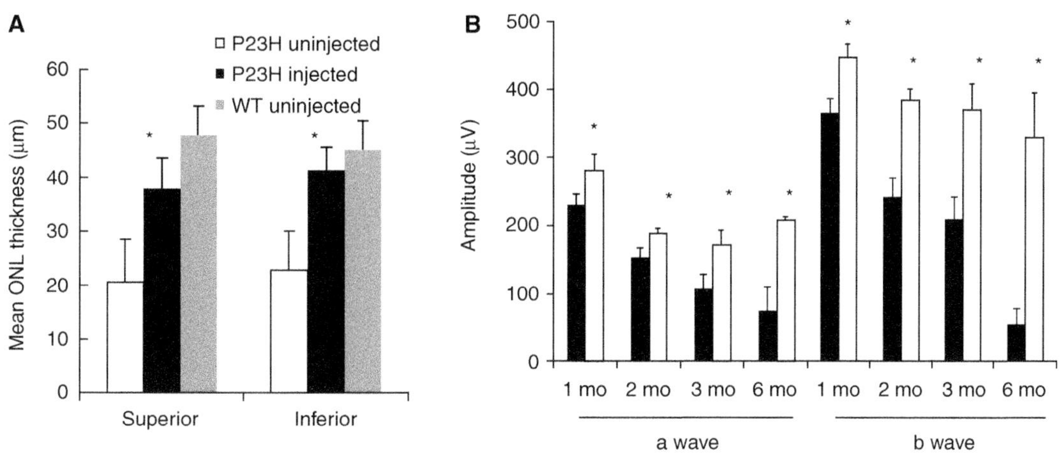

Figure 2. AAV-*Rho* protects the retinas of P23H transgenic mice for up to 6 mo. *A*. ONL from AAV-*Rho* injected eyes (black bars) were 80%–85% thicker than those of the untreated group (white bars) (* $p < 0.05$) and were slightly thinner but not significantly different from the wild-type mice at 6 mo of age (gray bars). *B*. The ERG a-wave and b-wave amplitudes of AAV-*Rho* injected eyes were elevated (white bars) in P23H transgenic mice at 1, 2, 3, and 6 mo following injection compared with uninjected eyes (black bars) (* $p < 0.05$ at 1 and 2 mo postinjection; * $p < 0.005$ at 3 and 6 mo; n = 9). (From Mao et al. 2011; reprinted, with permission, from Mary Ann Liebert, Inc. © 2011.)

RHO transgenic mice, supporting the view that gene supplementation by itself may not be sufficient for treatment of toxic gain-of-function mutations.

PHOTORECEPTOR RESCUE BY RNA REPLACEMENT

To overcome the damage caused by mutated rhodopsin in adRP, rhodopsin gene delivery can be accompanied by inhibition of synthesis of the mutant protein. Such suppression can be achieved by blockade of transcription, using zinc-finger transcriptional repressors, or can occur at the RNA level through the use of antisense techniques including antisense oligodeoxynucleotides, RNA enzymes (ribozymes) or RNA interference using short interfering RNA (siRNA). Although allele specific knockdown of P23H mRNA reduced the rate of retinal degeneration in P23H *Rho* transgenic rats over a prolonged period (LaVail et al. 2000), the large number of different adRP mutations in *RHO* make this approach challenging, because a different inhibitor would be needed for each mutation. An alternative approach is to block the expression of all endogenous rhodopsin, mutant and wild-type, and to deliver a replacement gene to support the structure and function of photoreceptors (Ader et al. 2005).

ZINC-FINGER REPRESSORS

Zinc-finger domains are features of many DNA binding proteins including transcriptional activators and repressors. The manner in which these domains interact with DNA has been studied in detail, and the rules have been established for modifying the amino acid sequence to bind a specific DNA sequence (Liu et al. 2002; Segal et al. 1999). These zinc finger domains can then be associated with transcriptional activator domains, transcriptional repressor domains or with site-specific nucleases. Mussolino and colleagues (2011b) produced a series of transcriptional repressors that silence *RHO* by combining six zinc-finger domains with the Krüppel-associated box repressor domain, screening them first in tissue culture and then in mice. Their most active repressor was specific for the human *RHO* promoter and, when delivered by subretinal injection of AAV to wild-type mice, there was no impact on ERG amplitudes or on the structure of the retinas. When injected into mice bearing one copy of the P347S *RHO* transgene and two copies of endogenous *Rho*, expression of the human transgene was reduced by 26% and ERG b-wave amplitudes were increased by nearly 30% in treated eyes 2 mo after gene transfer. In this model, normal rhodopsin was provided by the mouse gene, so that no additional supplementation was necessary.

RNA REPLACEMENT THERAPY

Combining genes for RNA inhibitors such as ribozymes or siRNAs in the same viral vector as the rhodopsin cDNA is straightforward because both genes are small (1046 nt for *RHO* cDNA, 19 bp for siRNA, 35 nt for a hammerhead ribozyme) and can be driven from short promoter sequences. For this system to operate, the *RHO* cDNA must be made resistant to the siRNA (or ribozyme) by the introduction of "silent" mutations. Although single mismatches within 4 nt of the cleavage site can inhibit cutting by hammerhead ribozymes (Fedor and Uhlenbeck 1990), three or more changes may be required to prevent the siRNA from directing digestion by the RNA-induced silencing complex, and both the position and the nature of these changes is important to prevent cleavage (Du et al. 2005). Potential problems may arise from mutations that change a commonly used codon to a less commonly used one or mutations that affect RNA secondary structure. Both phenomena can impact the rate of translation and therefore the folding of opsin (Duan et al. 2003; Cannarozzi et al. 2010).

Short interfering RNA can be produced in two ways: as short hairpin RNAs under the control of an RNA polymerase III (pol III) promoter (Paddison et al. 2002) or as artificial microRNAs (miRNA) under the control of pol II promoters (Zeng et al. 2005). Short hairpin RNA (shRNA) is processed to siRNA by the endonuclease Dicer in the cytoplasm, and has the advantage of high expression level and therefore more rhodopsin repression. However, pol III promoters are promiscuous, so that any AAV infected cell will produce the shRNA. Because of the well-known off-target effects of siRNAs, it is probably wise to restrict expression to the target cells, in this case photoreceptors. An artificial miRNA uses the processing sequences of a bona fide miRNA but replaces the sequence of the mature miRNA with that of an siRNA, in this case targeting the coding portion of *RHO*. Its synthesis can be directed by a photoreceptor-specific promoter. In fact, the gene for the artificial miRNA can be in the same transcript as the rhodopsin cDNA, either upstream in an intron sequence (Fig. 3A) or downstream in the 3′ untranslated region (Fig. 3B). Such an organization will ensure delivery of both components to the same cells, but processing of the miRNA from the *RHO* transcript is likely to reduce the level of mature mRNA either by interfering with splicing or polyadenylation. Nevertheless, delivery of artificial miRNAs with a resistant replacement gene has been successfully employed in a mouse model of liver failure associated with the PiZ allele of α-1 antitrypsin (Mueller et al. 2012).

O'Reilly and colleagues attempted the RNA replacement approach in transgenic mice bearing a P23H *RHO* gene with limited success (O'Reilly et al. 2007). Their AAV serotype 5 vector contained a pol III promoter driving the expression of an shRNA that they showed to be effective in suppressing human rhodopsin mRNA in transgenic mice. The shRNA gene was combined in the same vector with a *RHO* cDNA containing seven silent mutations to block binding of the siRNA driven by a 1.7 kb mouse *Rho* promoter. In P23H *RHO* mice injected as newborns and measured at postnatal day 10 they observed partial protection of ONL thickness (33%) compared to eyes injected with a virus expressing GFP, but only by separating their highest values from their lowest values. The transgenic mice used in these experiments exhibited rapid retinal degeneration: In untreated eyes, all photoreceptors were lost by 2 wk, so this was an extremely stringent test of therapy.

In contrast, we tested RNA replacement in a slow, progressive model of adRP based on the presence of a single human P23H transgene on the background of heterozygous disruption of the mouse *Rho* gene ($Rho^{+/-}$) (Mao et al. 2012). In these mice, maximum ERG amplitudes were decreased by 50% at 1 mo of age, and ONL thickness was half that of nontransgenic littermates by 2 mo of age. We employed an AAV5 virus expressing both an shRNA that targeted mouse *Rho* and human *RHO* and an siRNA-resistant *Rho* cDNA containing three silent mutations. Injection of this virus at postnatal day 15 led to 80% improvement in ONL thickness at 3 mo postinjection, and this difference persisted for up to 9 mo postinjection. Similarly, ERG a-wave and b-wave amplitudes remained more or less stable over the 9 mo of the experiment in injected eyes but decreased by 85% in untreated eyes (Fig. 4). Retinal degeneration was faster in this model than in the P23H *RHO*, mouse $Rho^{+/+}$ mice used for supplementation without suppression (Mao et al.

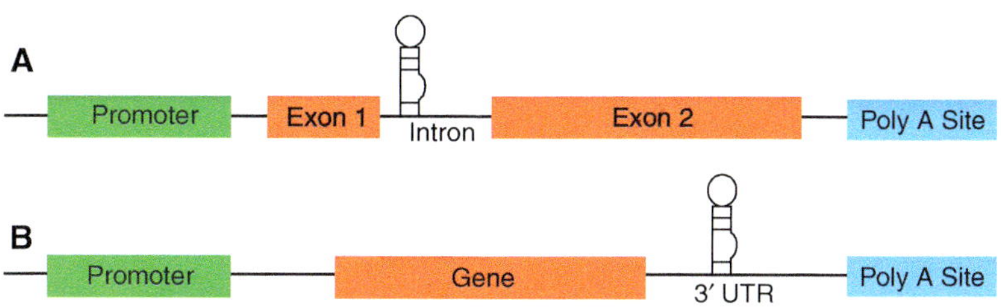

Figure 3. Constructs for mRNA suppression and replacement. Possible locations for miRNA insertion include (*A*) the intron region or (*B*) the 3′ UTR. In either case, the same promoter would be used to direct the synthesis of the artificial miRNA and the replacement gene. In the case of *RHO* adRP mutations the miRNA would be engineered to express an siRNA targeting the coding region of *RHO*, and the replacement *RHO* gene would contain synonymous changes in the third positions of codons to remove the siRNA binding site.

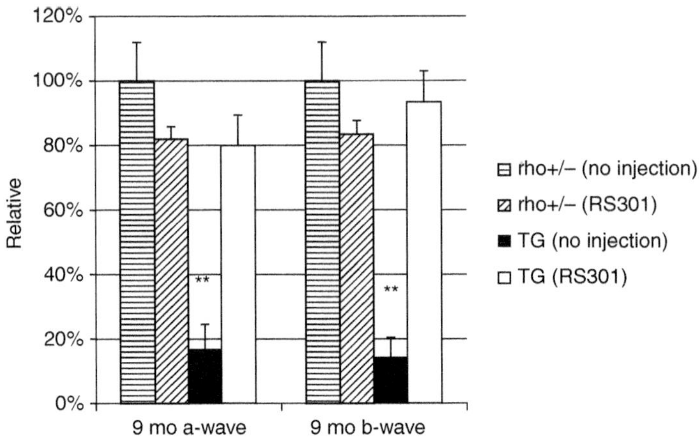

Figure 4. A single AAV RNA replacement vector preserves retinal function for 9 mo in P23H *RHO* transgenic mice. The combination vector was designated RS301. Left eyes of both strains were untreated and right eyes were injected with AAV-RS301. ERG amplitudes of the untreated, nontransgenic eyes were set at 100%. (At 9 mo, the average a-wave amplitude of these untreated eyes was 180 μV and the average b-wave amplitude was 565 μV.) By 9 mo the untreated P23H transgenic eyes showed a significantly diminished response in both a- and b-wave amplitudes, <20% of that of the untreated, nontransgenic eyes ($n = 7$; ** $p < 0.005$). P23H eyes injected with AAV-RS301 maintained 80% of the a-wave amplitude of untreated, nontransgenic eyes and 95% of the b-wave amplitude. (From Mao et al. 2012; reprinted, with permission, from Mary Ann Liebert, Inc., © 2012.)

2011), and the knockdown of endogenous rhodopsin mRNA was necessary to achieve this level of ONL preservation.

Results of Millington-Ward and colleagues (2011) suggest that RNA replacement may also work for class I mutations in rhodopsin. After using marker genes (*EGFP* and *dsRed*) to verify that photoreceptors could be infected with two AAV vectors following subretinal injection, they coinjected *RHO* P347S, $Rho^{+/-}$ mice at postnatal day 5 with AAV serotype 5 expressing an shRNA from the H1 promoter and a separate virus expressing a replacement *RHO* gene. The authors had earlier shown that delivery of the shRNA vector alone efficiently suppressed human *RHO* mRNA levels and reduced the rate of thinning of the ONL in a mouse line that carried the human P347S *RHO* gene on a mouse $Rho^{+/+}$ background (Chadderton et al. 2009). With the combined injection, they observed a 35% increase in ONL thickness compared to control injected eyes at 6 wk of age. Measurement of the ERG b-wave amplitudes suggested that the protective effect lasted up to 20 wk postinjection (Fig. 5). Although b-wave amplitudes were diminished threefold compared to the 6 wk time point, they were three times greater in the RNA-replacement eyes than in control-treated eyes.

The choice of two viruses, one for mRNA suppression and the other for mRNA replacement, is appealing in that the ratio of the two viruses can be varied depending on the level of expression of the mutant *RHO* gene in the animal model or the patient. Nevertheless, there are technical and regulatory barriers to this approach. Despite fluorescence micrographs indicating that photoreceptors can be coinfected with two viruses, it is likely that many photoreceptors will be infected with one or the other, leading to rhodopsin deficiency or excess in those cells. It is probable that a mixture of different recombinant viruses could be tested for safety and granted regulatory approval, but each variation in the ratio of viruses would be a different test compound and might require its own safety studies and regulatory review. Given the fact that a single virus expressing the shRNA and the replacement gene was effective in promoting long-term survival of photoreceptors in P23H *RHO* transgenic mice, using one vector for RNA replacement seems advisable.

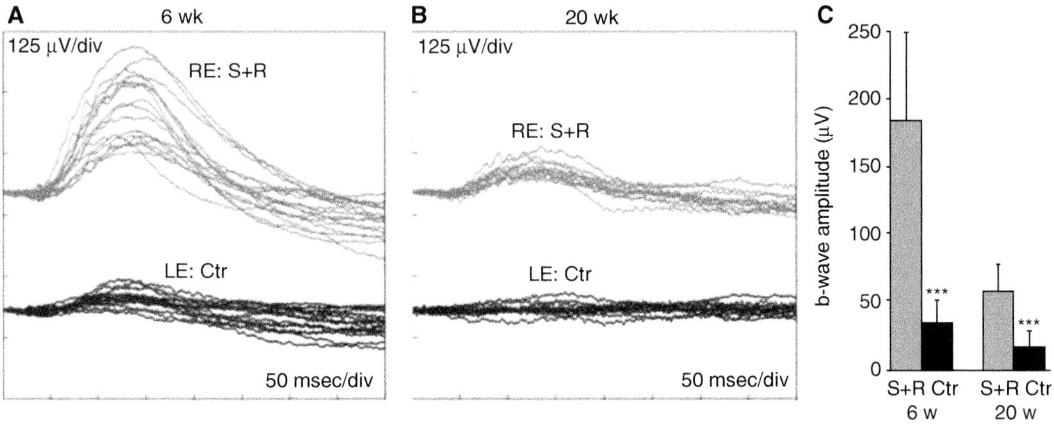

Figure 5. ERG response following suppression and replacement of P347S *RHO*. At postnatal day 5, mice were injected in one eye with a 1:30 mixture of AAV expressing the shRNA (S) and AAV expressing the siRNA-resistant replacement gene (R). Contralateral eyes were injected with a control virus expressing EGFP. Six weeks or 20 wk later, mice were dark-adapted overnight and ERG responses recorded from both eyes. (*A*,*B*) Overlays of the ERG recordings; gray and black lines represent recordings from combined suppression and replacement therapy (S+R) and control (Ctr)-injected eyes, respectively. RE, right eyes; LE, left eyes. (*C*) Mean b-wave amplitudes. Gray and black columns represent values corresponding to S+R and control-injected eyes, respectively. Error bars represent standard deviation [*** $p < 0.001$]. (From Millington-Ward et al. 2011; reprinted, with permission, from Nature Publishing Group © 2011.)

CONCLUDING REMARKS: MOVING RHODOPSIN AUGMENTATION TO THE CLINIC

Several questions must be answered before rhodopsin supplementation can be developed for clinical application. These include: How much rhodopsin is too much in a primate? Which *RHO* mutations can be treated with supplementation alone and which require supplementation plus suppression? Does this approach work in a large animal model of adRP? Where in the retina should the vector be delivered?

Although overexpression of wild-type rhodopsin, either by transgenesis or viral gene-delivery, has been demonstrated to cause photoreceptor degeneration in mice, this phenomenon has not been reported in larger animals. If the damage to photoreceptors is cell-autonomous, then there is reason to suspect that excess rhodopsin would also be harmful in people, whereas too little expression would be without benefit. Although novel capsid variants may permit infection of photoreceptor cells following intravitreal injection (Dalkara et al. 2013; Kay et al. 2013), the inner limiting membrane would prevent transduction of rod cells in the peripheral retina. Therefore, subretinal injections would be required. Because single injections of AAV will transduce photoreceptors only in the region of retinal detachment, harm or benefit should be confined to that area. To determine a therapeutic window for opsin expression, a dose escalation study should be performed in nonhuman primates using subretinal injections with AAV serotype 5 or serotype 8 expressing human *RHO* cDNA (Vandenberghe et al. 2011; Boye et al. 2012). Monitoring of retinal dimensions with spectral domain optical coherence tomography and retinal function with focal ERG should then be continued for a year or more. Some animals would have to be sacrificed after a shorter interval to assess expression levels of rhodopsin and other marker proteins.

In rodents, it is important to test AAV augmentation in as many valid models of adRP based on rhodopsin mutations as are currently available. These would include transgenic mice and rats as well as mice carrying mutations in the mouse *Rho* gene (Budzynski et al. 2010;

Sakami et al. 2011). To recapitulate adRP, the disease phenotype should be slowly progressive, so that therapy can be initiated in mature animals and after the onset of retinal degeneration. In mice and rats, it may be of value to employ self-complementary AAV for the delivery of *RHO*, because the onset of rhodopsin expression will be more rapid compared to that from single stranded AAV (McCarty et al. 2003). The goal would be to determine which, if any, of these models should be successfully treated with *RHO* augmentation and which may require supplementation plus suppression of the endogenous genes. Outcome measurements would include spectral domain optimal coherence tomography, ERG and behavioral assays such as the optokinetic response measured longitudinally in the same animals (Prusky et al. 2004).

Before moving to clinical trials, it is essential to test gene therapy by rhodopsin augmentation or replacement in large animal models of adRP. Several porcine models have been characterized, including transgenic pigs with both class I and class II mutations (Petters et al. 1997; Tso et al. 1997; Li et al. 1998; Huang et al. 2000; Ross et al. 2012). Unfortunately, all of the models, including P23H minipigs, exhibit relatively rapid retinal degeneration, so that viral delivery of *RHO* would have to be attempted soon after birth for any hope of efficacy. There is one naturally occurring canine model of *RHO* adRP that has been characterized in some detail (Kijas et al. 2002; Cideciyan et al. 2005; Gu et al. 2007). At 3 mo of age, dogs heterozygous for the T4R mutation have nearly normal ERG amplitudes, but by 13 mo, both rod and cone responses are attenuated. T4R *RHO* dogs do not recover normally from photobleaching, and are particular sensitive to light damage from clinical levels of light exposure, such as fundus imaging. The mechanism of this light damage is not known, but the mechanism appears to be different from intense light damage in albino mice, because inhibiting AP-1 activation does not block light injury (Gu et al. 2009). The extreme sensitivity to light damage is probably caused by a toxic gain-of-function by T4R rhodopsin, so that it is unlikely that *RHO* supplementation will suffice for therapy—suppression of endogenous rhodopsin may also be required. The advantage of the light damage phenotype is that success of RNA replacement can be tested simply by light exposure a few weeks after gene transfer; treated eyes should be less sensitive to intense light. A disadvantage is that retinal injections must be performed under dim red light (Komaromy et al. 2008). In contrast, it is possible that supplementation alone would prevent the slow, underlying retinal degeneration of dogs exposed only to ambient light, assuming that the mechanism for the slow retinal degeneration is distinct from the light injury response.

The large animal models of adRP will be of great use in determining the dose and distribution of gene therapy vectors. The retina of both species is cone-rich relative to rodents, particularly in the *area centralis* of the dog (Mowat et al. 2008) and the retinal streak of the pig (Hendrickson and Hicks 2002). Although the immediate objective of rhodopsin augmentation is the rescue of rod photoreceptors, the ultimate goal is preventing the loss of cones, and thus of central vision. Presumably, subretinal injections in humans would be placed in the perifoveal region to sustain rods in the vicinity of the fovea and thus promote the survival of foveal cones. Treatment near the central retina in canine and porcine models of adRP might predict whether rod-based therapies can protect central vision in this way.

ACKNOWLEDGMENTS

The authors acknowledge support from the Foundation Fighting Blindness, and from the National Eye Institute (grant 1R24EY022012, training grant T32 EY007132, vision core grant P30EY021721).

REFERENCES

Ader M, Kenna PF, Millington-Ward S, Clark G, Kennan A, O'Reilly M, Tam LC, Aherne A, McNally N, Humphries P, et al. 2005. Toward a gene therapy for dominant disease: Validation of an RNA interference-based mutation-independent approach. *Mol Ther* **12:** 555–561.

Bainbridge JW, Smith AJ, Barker SS, Robbie S, Henderson R, Balaggan K, Viswanathan A, Holder GE, Stockman A,

Tyler N, et al. 2008. Effect of gene therapy on visual function in Leber's congenital amaurosis. *N Engl J Med* **358:** 2231–2239.

Binley K, Widdowson P, Loader J, Kelleher M, Iqball S, Ferrige G, de Belin J, Carlucci M, Angell-Manning D, Hurst F, et al. 2013. Transduction of photoreceptors with equire infectious anemia virus Lentiviral Vectors: Safety and biodistribution of StarGen for Stargardt disease. *Invest Ophthal Vis Sci* **54:** 4061–4071.

Boye SE, Alexander JJ, Boye SL, Witherspoon CD, Sandefer KJ, Conlon TJ, Erger K, Sun J, Ryals R, Chiodo VA, et al. 2012. The human rhodopsin kinase promoter in an AAV5 vector confers rod- and cone-specific expression in the primate retina. *Hum Gene Ther* **23:** 1101–1115.

Budzynski E, Gross AK, McAlear SD, Peachey NS, Shukla M, He F, Edwards M, Won J, Hicks WL, Wensel TG, et al. 2010. Mutations of the Opsin gene (Y102H and I307N) lead to light-induced degeneration of photoreceptors and constitutive activation of phototransduction in mice. *J Biol Chem* **285:** 14521–14533.

Cannarozzi G, Schraudolph NN, Faty M, von RP, Friberg MT, Roth AC, Gonnet P, Gonnet G, Barral Y. 2010. A role for codon order in translation dynamics. *Cell* **141:** 355–367.

Chadderton N, Millington-Ward S, Palfi A, O'Reilly M, Tuohy G, Humphries MM, Li T, Humphries P, Kenna PF, Farrar GJ. 2009. Improved retinal function in a mouse model of dominant retinitis pigmentosa following AAV-delivered gene therapy. *Mol Ther* **17:** 593–599.

Cideciyan AV, Hood DC, Huang Y, Banin E, Li ZY, Stone EM, Milam AH, Jacobson SG. 1998. Disease sequence from mutant rhodopsin allele to rod and cone photoreceptor degeneration in man. *Proc Natl Acad Sci* **95:** 7103–7108.

Cideciyan AV, Jacobson SG, Aleman TS, Gu D, Pearce-Kelling SE, Sumaroka A, Acland GM, Aguirre GD. 2005. In vivo dynamics of retinal injury and repair in the rhodopsin mutant dog model of human retinitis pigmentosa. *Proc Natl Acad Sci* **102:** 5233–5238.

Cideciyan AV, Hauswirth WW, Aleman TS, Kaushal S, Schwartz SB, Boye SL, Windsor EA, Conlon TJ, Sumaroka A, Roman AJ, et al. 2009. Vision 1 year after gene therapy for Leber's congenital amaurosis. *N Engl J Med* **361:** 725–727.

Dalkara D, Byrne LC, Klimczak RR, Visel M, Yin L, Merigan WH, Flannery JG, Schaffer DV. 2013. In vivo-directed evolution of a new adeno-associated virus for therapeutic outer retinal gene delivery from the vitreous. *Sci Transl Med* **5:** 189ra76.

Du Q, Thonberg H, Wang J, Wahlestedt C, Liang Z. 2005. A systematic analysis of the silencing effects of an active siRNA at all single-nucleotide mismatched target sites. *Nucleic Acids Res* **33:** 1671–1677.

Duan J, Wainwright MS, Comeron JM, Saitou N, Sanders AR, Gelernter J, Gejman PV. 2003. Synonymous mutations in the human dopamine receptor *D2* (*DRD2*) affect mRNA stability and synthesis of the receptor. *Hum Mol Genet* **12:** 205–216.

Fedor MJ, Uhlenbeck OC. 1990. Substrate sequence effects on "hammerhead" RNA catalytic efficiency. *Proc Natl Acad Sci* **87:** 1668–1672.

Fotiadis D, Liang Y, Filipek S, Saperstein DA, Engel A, Palczewski K. 2003. Atomic-force microscopy: Rhodopsin dimers in native disc membranes. *Nature* **421:** 127–128.

Frederick JM, Krasnoperova NK, Hoffmann K, Church-Kopish J, Ruther K, Howes K, Lem J, Baehr W. 2001. Mutant rhodopsin transgene expression on a null background. *Invest Ophthalmol Vis Sci* **42:** 826–833.

Glushakova LG, Timmers AM, Issa TM, Cortez NG, Pang J, Teusner JT, Hauswirth WW. 2006. Does recombinant adeno-associated virus-vectored proximal region of mouse rhodopsin promoter support only rod-type specific expression in vivo? *Mol Vis* **12:** 298–309.

Gorbatyuk MS, Knox T, LaVail MM, Gorbatyuk OS, Noorwez SM, Hauswirth WW, Lin JH, Muzyczka N, Lewin AS. 2010. Restoration of visual function in P23H rhodopsin transgenic rats by gene delivery of BiP/Grp78. *Proc Natl Acad Sci* **107:** 5961–5966.

Goto Y, Peachey NS, Ripps H, Naash MI. 1995. Functional abnormalities in transgenic mice expressing a mutant rhodopsin gene. *Invest Ophthalmol Vis Sci* **36:** 62–71.

Green ES, Menz MD, LaVail MM, Flannery JG. 2000. Characterization of rhodopsin mis-sorting and constitutive activation in a transgenic rat model of retinitis pigmentosa. *Invest Ophthalmol Vis Sci* **41:** 1546–1553.

Gu D, Beltran WA, Li Z, Acland GM, Aguirre GD. 2007. Clinical light exposure, photoreceptor degeneration, and AP-1 activation: A cell death or cell survival signal in the rhodopsin mutant retina? *Invest Ophthal Vis Sci* **48:** 4907–4918.

Gu D, Beltran WA, Pearce-Kelling S, Li Z, Acland GM, Aguirre GD. 2009. Steroids do not prevent photoreceptor degeneration in the light-exposed T4R rhodopsin mutant dog retina irrespective of AP-1 inhibition. *Invest Ophthalmol Vis Sci* **50:** 3482–3494.

Han Z, Conley SM, Makkia R, Guo J, Cooper MJ, Naash MI. 2012. Comparative analysis of DNA nanoparticles and AAVs for ocular gene delivery. *PLoS ONE* **7:** e52189.

Hendrickson A, Hicks D. 2002. Distribution and density of medium- and short-wavelength selective cones in the domestic pig retina. *Exp Eye Res* **74:** 435–444.

Huang Y, Cideciyan AV, Aleman TS, Banin E, Huang J, Syed NA, Petters RM, Wong F, Milam AH, Jacobson SG. 2000. Optical coherence tomography (OCT) abnormalities in rhodopsin mutant transgenic swine with retinal degeneration [letter]. *Exp Eye Res* **70:** 247–251.

Kaeppel C, Beattie SG, Fronza R, van LR, Salmon F, Schmidt S, Wolf S, Nowrouzi A, Glimm H, von KC, et al. 2013. A largely random AAV integration profile after LPLD gene therapy. *Nat Med* **19:** 889–891.

Kaushal S, Khorana HG. 1994. Structure and function in rhodopsin. 7. Point mutations associated with autosomal dominant retinitis pigmentosa. *Biochem* **33:** 6121–6128.

Kay CN, Ryals RC, Aslanidi GV, Min SH, Ruan Q, Sun J, Dyka FM, Kasuga D, Ayala AE, Van VK, et al. 2013. Targeting photoreceptors via intravitreal delivery using novel, capsid-mutated AAV vectors. *PLoS ONE* **8:** e62097.

Kemp CM, Jacobson SG, Faulkner DJ. 1988. Two types of visual dysfunction in autosomal dominant retinitis pigmentosa. *Invest Ophthalmol Vis Sci* **29:** 1235–1241.

Kemp CM, Jacobson SG, Roman AJ, Sung CH, Nathans J. 1992. Abnormal rod dark adaptation in autosomal dominant retinitis pigmentosa with proline-23-histidine rhodopsin mutation. *Am J Ophthalmol* **113:** 165–174.

Kijas JW, Cideciyan AV, Aleman TS, Pianta MJ, Pearce-Kelling SE, Miller BJ, Jacobson SG, Aguirre GD, Acland GM. 2002. Naturally occurring rhodopsin mutation in the dog causes retinal dysfunction and degeneration mimicking human dominant retinitis pigmentosa. *Proc Natl Acad Sci* **99:** 6328–6333.

Komaromy AM, Acland GM, Aguirre GD. 2008. Operating in the dark: A night-vision system for surgery in retinas susceptible to light damage. *Arch Ophthalmol* **126:** 714–717.

Kunte MM, Choudhury S, Manheim JF, Shinde VM, Miura M, Chiodo VA, Hauswirth WW, Gorbatyuk OS, Gorbatyuk MS. 2012. ER stress is involved in T17M rhodopsin-induced retinal degeneration. *Invest Ophthalmol Vis Sci* **53:** 3792–3800.

LaVail MM, Yasumura D, Matthes MT, Drenser KA, Flannery JG, Lewin AS, Hauswirth WW. 2000. Ribozyme rescue of photoreceptor cells in P23H transgenic rats: Long-term survival and late-stage therapy. *Proc Natl Acad Sci* **97:** 11488–11493.

Li T, Franson WK, Gordon JW, Berson EL, Dryja TP. 1995. Constitutive activation of phototransduction by K296E opsin is not a cause of photoreceptor degeneration. *Proc Natl Acad Sci* **92:** 3551–3555.

Li T, Snyder WK, J Olsson JE, Dryja TP. 1996. Transgenic mice carrying the dominant rhodopsin mutation P347S: Evidence for defective vectorial transport of rhodopsin to the outer segments. *Proc Natl Acad Sci* **93:** 14176–14181.

Li ZY, Wong F, Chang JH, Possin DE, Hao Y, Petters RM, Milam AH. 1998. Rhodopsin transgenic pigs as a model for human retinitis pigmentosa. *Invest Ophthalmol Vis Sci* **39:** 808–819.

Lin JH, Li H, Yasumura D, Cohen HR, Zhang C, Panning B, Shokat KM, LaVail MM, Walter P. 2007. IRE1 signaling affects cell fate during the unfolded protein response. *Science* **318:** 944–949.

Liu Q, Xia Z, Zhong X, Case CC. 2002. Validated zinc finger protein designs for all 16 GNN DNA triplet targets. *J Biol Chem* **277:** 3850–3856.

Maguire AM, Simonelli F, Pierce EA, Pugh EN Jr, Mingozzi F, Bennicelli J, Banfi S, Marshall KA, Testa F, Surace EM, et al. 2008. Safety and efficacy of gene transfer for Leber's congenital amaurosis. *N Engl J Med* **358:** 2240–2248.

Mao H, James T, Schwein A, Shabashvili AE, Hauswirth WW, Gorbatyuk MS, Lewin AS. 2011. AAV delivery of wild-type rhodopsin preserves retinal function in a mouse model of autosomal dominant retinitis pigmentosa. *Hum Gene Ther* **22:** 567–575.

Mao H, Gorbatyuk MS, Rossmiller B, Hauswirth WW, Lewin AS. 2012. Long-term rescue of retinal structure and function by rhodopsin RNA replacement with a single adeno-associated viral vector in P23H *RHO* transgenic mice. *Hum Gene Ther* **23:** 256–266.

McCarty DM, Fu H, Monahan PE, Toulson CE, Naik P, Samulski RJ. 2003. Adeno-associated virus terminal repeat (TR) mutant generates self-complementary vectors to overcome the rate-limiting step to transduction in vivo. *Gene Ther* **10:** 2112–2118.

Mendes HF, van der SJ, Chapple JP, Cheetham ME. 2005. Mechanisms of cell death in rhodopsin retinitis pigmentosa: Implications for therapy. *Trends Mol Med* **11:** 177–185.

Millington-Ward S, Chadderton N, O'Reilly M, Palfi A, Goldmann T, Kilty C, Humphries M, Wolfrum U, Bennett J, Humphries P, et al. 2011. Suppression and replacement gene therapy for autosomal dominant disease in a murine model of dominant retinitis pigmentosa. *Mol Ther* **19:** 642–649.

Mingozzi F, High KA. 2013. Immune responses to AAV vectors: Overcoming barriers to successful gene therapy. *Blood* **122:** 23–36.

Mowat FM, Petersen-Jones SM, Williamson H, Williams DL, Luthert PJ, Ali RR, Bainbridge JW. 2008. Topographical characterization of cone photoreceptors and the area centralis of the canine retina. *Mol Vis* **14:** 2518–2527.

Mueller C, Tang Q, Gruntman A, Blomenkamp K, Teckman J, Song L, Zamore PD, Flotte TR. 2012. Sustained miRNA-mediated knockdown of mutant AAT with simultaneous augmentation of wild-type AAT has minimal effect on global liver miRNA profiles. *Mol Ther* **20:** 590–600.

Murakami Y, Matsumoto H, Roh M, Suzuki J, Hisatomi T, Ikeda Y, Miller JW, Vavvas DG. 2012. Receptor interacting protein kinase mediates necrotic cone but not rod cell death in a mouse model of inherited degeneration. *Proc Natl Acad Sci* **109:** 14598–14603.

Mussolino C, Della CM, Rossi S, Viola F, Di VU, Marrocco E, Neglia S, Doria M, Testa R, Giovannoni R, et al. 2011a. AAV-mediated photoreceptor transduction of the pig cone-enriched retina. *Gene Ther* **18:** 637–645.

Mussolino C, Sanges D, Marrocco E, Bonetti C, Di VU, Marigo V, Auricchio A, Meroni G, Surace EM. 2011b. Zinc-finger-based transcriptional repression of rhodopsin in a model of dominant retinitis pigmentosa. *EMBO Mol Med* **3:** 118–128.

Noorwez SM, Sama RR, Kaushal S. 2009. Calnexin improves the folding efficiency of mutant rhodopsin in the presence of pharmacological chaperone 11-*cis*-retinal. *J Biol Chem* **284:** 33333–33342.

O'Reilly M, Palfi A, Chadderton N, Millington-Ward S, Ader M, Cronin T, Tuohy T, Auricchio A, Hildinger M, Tivnan A, et al. 2007. RNA interference-mediated suppression and replacement of human rhodopsin in vivo. *Am J Hum Genet* **81:** 127–135.

Olsson JE, Gordon JW, Pawlyk BS, Roof D, Hayes A, Molday RS, Mukai S, Cowley GS, Berson EL, Dryja TP. 1992a. Transgenic mice with a rhodopsin mutation (Pro23His): A mouse model of autosomal dominant retinitis pigmentosa. *Neuron* **9:** 815–830.

Olsson JE, Gordon JW, Pawlyk BS, Roof D, Hayes A, Molday RS, Mukai S, Cowley GS, Berson EL, Dryja TP. 1992b. Transgenic mice with a rhodopsin mutation (Pro23His): A mouse model of autosomal dominant retinitis pigmentosa. *Neuron* **9:** 815–830.

Paddison PJ, Caudy AA, Bernstein E, Hannon GJ, Conklin DS. 2002. Short hairpin RNAs (shRNAs) induce sequence-specific silencing in mammalian cells. *Genes Dev* **16:** 948–958.

Palfi A, Millington-Ward S, Chadderton N, O'Reilly M, Goldmann T, Humphries MM, Li T, Wolfrum U, Humphries P, Kenna PF, et al. 2010. Adeno-associated virus-mediated rhodopsin replacement provides therapeutic benefit in mice with a targeted disruption of the rhodopsin gene. *Hum Gene Ther* **21:** 311–323.

Pennesi ME, Nishikawa S, Matthes MT, Yasumura D, LaVail MM. 2008. The relationship of photoreceptor degeneration to retinal vascular development and loss in mutant rhodopsin transgenic and RCS rats. *Exp Eye Res* **87:** 561–570.

Petrs-Silva H, Dinculescu A, Li Q, Deng WT, Pang JJ, Min SH, Chiodo V, Neeley AW, Govindasamy L, Bennett A, et al. 2011. Novel properties of tyrosine-mutant AAV2 vectors in the mouse retina. *Mol Ther* **19:** 293–301.

Petters RM, Alexander CA, Wells KD, Collins EB, Sommer JR, Blanton MR, Rojas G, Hao Y, Flowers WL, Banin E, et al. 1997. Genetically engineered large animal model for studying cone photoreceptor survival and degeneration in retinitis pigmentosa [see comments]. *Nat Biotechnol* **15:** 965–970.

Price BA, Sandoval IM, Chan F, Nichols R, Roman-Sanchez R, Wensel TG, Wilson JH. 2012. Rhodopsin gene expression determines rod outer segment size and rod cell resistance to a dominant-negative neurodegeneration mutant. *PLoS ONE* **7:** e49889.

Prusky GT, Alam NM, Beekman S, Douglas RM. 2004. Rapid quantification of adult and developing mouse spatial vision using a virtual optomotor system. *Invest Ophthalmol Vis Sci* **45:** 4611–4616.

Punzo C, Kornacker K, Cepko CL. 2009. Stimulation of the insulin/mTOR pathway delays cone death in a mouse model of retinitis pigmentosa. *Nat Neurosci* **12:** 44–52.

Rajan RS, Kopito RR. 2005. Suppression of wild-type rhodopsin maturation by mutants linked to autosomal dominant retinitis pigmentosa. *J Biol Chem* **280:** 1284–1291.

Ross JW, Fernandez de Castro JP, Zhao J, Samuel M, Walters E, Rios C, Bray-Ward P, Jones BW, Marc RE, Wang W, et al. 2012. Generation of an inbred miniature pig model of retinitis pigmentosa. *Invest Ophthalmol Vis Sci* **53:** 501–507.

Sakami S, Maeda T, Bereta G, Okano K, Golczak M, Sumaroka A, Roman AJ, Cideciyan AV, Jacobson SG, Palczewski K. 2011. Probing mechanisms of photoreceptor degeneration in a new mouse model of the common form of autosomal dominant retinitis pigmentosa due to P23H opsin mutations. *J Biol Chem* **286:** 10551–10567.

Segal DJ, Dreier B, Beerli RR, Barbas CF III. 1999. Toward controlling gene expression at will: Selection and design of zinc finger domains recognizing each of the 5′-GNN-3′ DNA target sequences. *Proc Natl Acad Sci* **96:** 2758–2763.

Song S, Lu Y, Choi YK, Han Y, Tang Q, Zhao G, Berns KI, Flotte TR. 2004. DNA-dependent PK inhibits adeno-associated virus DNA integration. *Proc Natl Acad Sci* **101:** 2112–2116.

Sullivan LS, Bowne SJ, Birch DG, Hughbanks-Wheaton D, Heckenlively JR, Lewis RA, Garcia CA, Ruiz RS, Blanton SH, Northrup H, et al. 2006. Prevalence of disease-causing mutations in families with autosomal dominant retinitis pigmentosa: A screen of known genes in 200 families. *Invest Ophthalmol Vis Sci* **47:** 3052–3064.

Sung CH, Schneider B, Agarwal N, Papermaster DS, Nathans J. 1991. Functional heterogeneity of mutant rhodopsins responsible for autosomal dominant retinitis pigmentosa. *Proc Natl Acad Sci* **88:** 8840–8844.

Sung CH, Makino C, Baylor D, Nathans J. 1994. A rhodopsin gene mutation responsible for autosomal dominant retinitis pigmentosa results in a protein that is defective in localization to the photoreceptor outer segment. *J Neurosci* **14:** 5818–5833.

Tan E, Wang Q, Quiambao AB, Xu X, Qtaishat NM, Peachey NS, Lem J, Fliesler SJ, Pepperberg DR, Naash MI, et al. 2001. The relationship between opsin overexpression and photoreceptor degeneration. *Invest Ophthalmol Vis Sci* **42:** 589–600.

Tso MO, Li WW, Zhang C, Lam TT, Hao Y, Petters RM, Wong F. 1997. A pathologic study of degeneration of the rod and cone populations of the rhodopsin Pro347-Leu transgenic pigs. *Trans Am Ophthalmol Soc* **95:** 467–479.

Usui S, Komeima K, Lee SY, Jo YJ, Ueno S, Rogers BS, Wu Z, Shen J, Lu L, Oveson BC, et al. 2009. Increased expression of catalase and superoxide dismutase 2 reduces cone cell death in retinitis pigmentosa. *Mol Ther* **17:** 778–786.

Vandenberghe LH, Bell P, Maguire AM, Cearley CN, Xiao R, Calcedo R, Wang L, Castle MJ, Maguire AC, Grant R, et al. 2011. Dosage thresholds for AAV2 and AAV8 photoreceptor gene therapy in monkey. *Sci Transl Med* **3:** p88ra54.

Wen XH, Shen L, Brush RS, Michaud N, Al-Ubaidi MR, Gurevich VV, Hamm HE, Lem J, DiBenedetto E, Anderson RE, et al. 2009. Overexpression of rhodopsin alters the structure and photoresponse of rod photoreceptors. *Biophys J* **96:** 939–950.

Wilson JH, Wensel TG. 2003. The nature of dominant mutations of rhodopsin and implications for gene therapy. *Mol Neurobiol* **28:** 149–158.

Wu TH, Ting TD, Okajima TI, Pepperberg DR, Ho YK, Ripps H, Naash MI. 1998. Opsin localization and rhodopsin photochemistry in a transgenic mouse model of retinitis pigmentosa. *Neuroscience* **87:** 709–717.

Yang Y, Mohand-Said S, Danan A, Simonutti M, Fontaine V, Clerin E, Picaud S, Leveillard T, Sahel JA. 2009. Functional cone rescue by RdCVF protein in a dominant model of retinitis pigmentosa. *Mol Ther* **17:** 787–795.

Zeng Y, Cai X, Cullen BR. 2005. Use of RNA polymerase II to transcribe artificial microRNAs. *Methods Enzymol* **392:** 371–380.

Curing Color Blindness—Mice and Nonhuman Primates

Maureen Neitz and Jay Neitz

Department of Ophthalmology, University of Washington, Seattle, Washington 98109

Correspondence: mneitz@uw.edu

It has been possible to use viral-mediated gene therapy to transform dichromatic (red-green color-blind) primates to trichromatic. Even though the third cone type was added after the end of developmental critical periods, treated animals acquired red-green color vision. What happened in the treated animals may represent a recapitulation of the evolution of trichromacy, which seems to have evolved with the acquisition of a third cone type without the need for subsequent modification to the circuitry. Some transgenic mice in which a third cone type was added also acquired trichromacy. However, compared with treated primates, red-green color vision in mice is poor, indicating large differences between mice and monkeys in their ability to take advantage of the new input. These results have implications for understanding the limits and opportunities for using gene therapy to treat vision disorders caused by defects in cone function.

Visual experience-dependent neural plasticity is a recognized property of the developing cortex, but what purpose is served by the ability of sensory processes to remodel their function in response to changes in experience (Hubel 1988)? An engaging hypothesis is that plasticity relieves the necessity to hard-wire all connections during development according to genetic instructions. In the adult cortex, this could allow adaptive adjustments depending on the environment and could provide a mechanism for recovering from damage (Albright et al. 2000). Classic visual deprivation experiments led to the expectation that neural connections established during development would not appropriately process an input that was not present from birth, and therefore, that treatment of congenital vision disorders would be ineffective unless administered to the very young. However, in recent experiments using adult red-green color-deficient primates, addition of a third opsin was sufficient to produce trichromatic color vision behavior (Mancuso et al. 2009), demonstrating that trichromacy does not require an early developmental process and that there are exceptions to the idea that neural inputs to the visual system cannot be appropriately processed unless they are established before a critical period in development. For example, in a recent study of surgical outcome for removal in congenital cataracts in pediatric patients, poor outcomes were associated with surgical intervention after compared with before one year of age (Khanna et al. 2013). The successes so far provide reason

Cite this article as *Cold Spring Harb Perspect Med* doi: 10.1101/cshperspect.a017418

for optimism that gene therapy can be developed as a viable treatment strategy for adult patients with disorders affecting cone photoreceptor function, and they open the way for new research to explore the possibilities and limits for gaining function by adding new inputs in adults. A better understanding of the ways in which the adult nervous system changes and does not change will be key for future development of therapies to restore visual function.

CURING COLOR BLINDNESS IN NONHUMAN PRIMATES

Experiments using gene therapy in an attempt to cure congenital red-green color blindness in nonhuman primates were performed on adult squirrel monkeys (*Saimiri sciureus*). In this species, as in many other New World primates, there is a single opsin gene on the X chromosome, but there is allelic diversity at the locus (Jacobs 1984; Mollon et al. 1984; Jacobs and Neitz 1985; Soares et al. 2010; Bunce et al. 2011). One allele encodes the equivalent to a human long-wavelength (L) opsin; another encodes the equivalent to a human middle-wavelength (M) opsin; and at least one allele encodes an opsin that gives rise to a photopigment that is spectrally intermediate between human L and M photopigments (Neitz et al. 1991; Jacobs et al. 1993). Because all male squirrel monkeys have only one X chromosome, they are dichromatic, with one cone photopigment encoded by the X chromosome plus a short wavelength (S)-sensitive cone photopigment encoded by an autosome. Females who are homozygous for the cone opsin allele encoded by the X chromosome are also dichromatic; however, females who are heterozygous have trichromatic color vision (Jacobs and Neitz 1987). The process of X inactivation segregates the expression of the two opsin alleles into separate populations of cone photoreceptors, giving rise to a mosaic containing L, M, and S cones.

Gene Therapy with L Opsin in Dichromatic Squirrel Monkeys

The gene therapy trials targeted adult squirrel monkeys that were missing the gene encoding L opsin. Adeno-associated virus serotype 2/5 (rAAV2/5) containing a recombinant human L-opsin (RHLOPS) gene under the control of the recombinant human L/M-opsin enhancer and promoter pR2.1 (Wang et al. 1992) was delivered to the photoreceptor layer by subretinal injection (Mancuso et al. 2009). Transcriptional regulatory elements contained in pR2.1 direct gene expression in M cones, but not S cones, rods, or any other retinal cell type (Li et al. 2007). These control elements include the locus control region, which is an enhancer that is required for transcription of the opsin genes on the X chromosome (Nathans et al. 1989; Wang et al. 1992; Wang et al. 1999), and the proximal promoter for the L-opsin gene. To provide the receptor basis for trichromacy, animals received three 100-μL injections in each eye. This transduced roughly one-third of the M cones such that they coexpressed the transgenic L opsin along with the endogenous M opsin, whereas the untransduced M cones expressed only the endogenous M opsin. The transduced- and wild-type cones were randomly intermixed in a relatively smooth mosaic. Before treatment, monkeys were trained to perform a computer-based color vision test, the Cambridge Colour Test (Reffin et al. 1991; Regan et al. 1994), which had been modified for use with animals (Fig. 2) (Mancuso et al. 2006). All dichromats, including humans and monkeys who are missing either the L- or the M photopigment, fail to distinguish from gray any colors near the "spectral neutral point" located in the blue-green region of color space. They also fail to distinguish complementary colors near the "extra-spectral neutral point" in the red-violet region (Jacobs 1984). Trichromats experience six basic color percepts that exist as opponent pairs: blue and yellow, red, and green, and black and white. In contrast, dichromats experience only four basic color percepts, nominally blue and yellow, and black and white, but they do not experience the normal sensations of red or green (Schmidt et al. 2014). For all dichromats there are two colors that are indistinguishable from gray, one of which appears greenish and the other reddish to normal trichromats.

Before treatment, two dichromatic monkeys completed three complete color vision tests (Mancuso et al. 2009). Each test examined the animal's ability to discriminate 16 different hues from gray. For each hue, thresholds were determined for how much color had to be added to a gray stimulus for it to be distinguishable from a gray background. Because 4–6 mo were required to test all 16 hues, baseline results represented testing conducted for >1 yr. As predicted, before treatment, the monkeys had low thresholds for colors that represent blues and yellows to their dichromatic eyes. They always failed to discriminate specific blue-green and red-violet hues from gray, as is characteristic of animals and humans with only S and M cones (protanopes). Their pretreatment thresholds, extrapolated from psychometric functions, were orders of magnitude higher for colors that activate the normal red-green system and fall along a "protan line" in color space than for colors that maximally activate the blue-yellow color opponent system and that fall along a "tritan line" (a color confusion line for people with defects in S cones). Results were highly repeatable, with no improvement between the first and third tests, demonstrating that the animals do not spontaneously improve in the absence of treatment.

Coexpressing the L-opsin transgene within a subset of endogenous M cones shifted their spectral sensitivity, allowing the transduced M cones to respond to long-wavelength light (Mancuso et al. 2009). This produced two distinct cone types absorbing in the middle-to-long wavelengths: "M+L" and M. Thus, together with S cones, the treated animals had three cone types, as required for trichromacy. The spectral sensitivity shift was readily detected using a custom-built, wide-field, color multifocal electroretinogram (mf-ERG) system (Kuchenbecker et al. 2008). In experiments performed on separate animals that were not involved in behavioral testing, the color mf-ERG was validated by treating an animal with a mixture of two viral vectors that were identical except that one carried the human L-opsin gene whereas the other carried the gene for humanized green fluorescent protein (GFP). Faint GFP fluorescence was first detected at 9 wk postinjection, and it continued to increase in area and intensity for >24 wk (Mancuso et al. 2009). Although faint signs of GFP were first detectable at 9 wk, L-opsin levels sufficient to produce suprathreshold mf-ERG signals were still not present at 16 wk postinjection. After GFP fluorescence became robust, the mf-ERG response to red light, which indicates responses from the introduced L opsin, showed highly increased response amplitudes in the area of treated retina. The two dichromatic monkeys who participated in behavioral tests of color vision were treated only with the virus carrying the L opsin gene. The treatment goal of producing a large homogeneous region was accomplished by placing injections at three well-spaced locations with centers corresponding to ~10° eccentricity from the fovea. This produced an mf-ERG response to red light that covered an area of central retina of roughly 100° in diameter. The wide-field color mf-ERG results showed that gene therapy changed the spectral sensitivity of a subset of the cones.

A priori, there were two possibilities for how a change in spectral sensitivity might change color vision behavior. First, animals may have had an increase in sensitivity to long-wavelength light, but if the neural circuitry for extracting color information from the nascent "M+L cone" submosaic was absent, they would remain dichromatic—the hallmark of which is having two hues that are indistinguishable from gray (i.e., the spectral neutral point, and extraspectral neutral point). The spectral neutral point for individuals that have only S and M cones, as the monkeys had before therapy, occurs near the dominant wavelength of 495 nm. At the limit, an increase in spectral sensitivity would shift the monkeys' neutral point toward that of individuals with only S and L cones, near the dominant wavelength of 505 nm. Thus, there would be a shift in blue-yellow color vision caused by the increased sensitivity to red light produced by the added human L cone photopigment; however, the animal could still have dichromacy.

The second, more engaging possibility is that treatment would be sufficient to expand sensory capacity in monkeys, providing them with trichromatic vision. The change in spectral sensitivity measured with the wide-field color mf-ERG is necessary but not sufficient to produce a new capacity for color vision. To give another example, individuals with L cones but no M cones (termed deuteranopes) have a relatively enhanced sensitivity to red light, but they are still as dichromatic as individuals with M cones but no L cones (protanopes) in that they are unable to distinguish particular colors (i.e., their spectral and extraspectral neutral points) from gray. In addition to neural pathways carrying blue-yellow color information about the relative spectral distribution of short versus long wavelength light, dichromats have visual channels carrying achromatic information about the relative "brightness" or luminance of objects compared with their surroundings. To determine if the animals had acquired a third neural channel carrying red-green information, it was necessary to prove that the changes in the animals' behavior were not just manifestations of changes in the achromatic and blue-yellow systems induced by the change in spectral sensitivity following addition of the L pigment. In the Cambridge Colour Test (Fig. 1) used to measure color discrimination in the monkeys, both the stimulus and the background are made up of dots that incorporate random luminance variation, which makes brightness a nonrelevant cue for detection. Luminance adjustments were made in the stimulus to ensure that brightness could not be a cue for detection, and under all conditions the treated monkeys made discriminations that were impossible for untreated animals. To confirm that the behavioral change observed in animals expressing the transgenic L pigment was not purely a shift in spectral sensitivity, monkeys were also tested using the dominant wavelengths that could represent all possible dichromacies based on S versus (L+M) pigments in which L and M might exist in different proportions. Together, these dominant wavelengths span the possible confusion points for deuteranopes and protanopes and for any

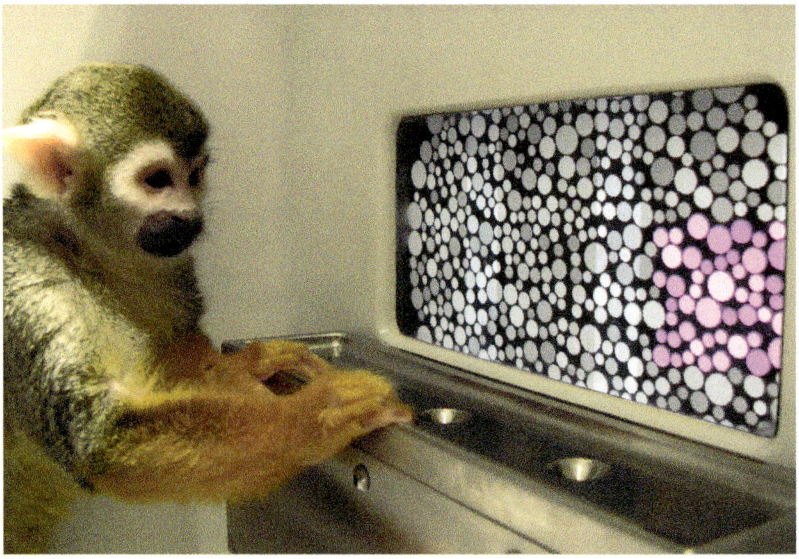

Figure 1. Color vision assayed using the Cambridge Colour Test. In this test, adapted for use with animals, the animal's task is to locate the blob of color against a background of gray dots using the touch-sensitive screen. Over trials, the positive stimulus randomly appears in one of three positions. The amount of color in the positive stimulus is reduced over trials to determine the amount needed to produce a threshold. Both stimulus and background dots vary in intensity making it impossible for the animal to locate the "blob" based on brightness cues. The animal has to use color vision to detect differences in the spectral distribution of light in the stimulus compared with the background.

intermediate dichromatic forms that could arise from expressing combinations of L pigments or combinations of M pigments (Neitz and Neitz 2011). The measured thresholds for the treated monkeys were low for all the dominant wavelengths tested, demonstrating that the monkeys lacked a spectral neutral point and had acquired a neural channel carrying red-green color vision, and as such were truly trichromatic. The treated animals discriminated colors in the red range from those in the green range and distinguished both from gray; they also discriminated between other color combinations that dichromats find impossible to tell apart. The finding that the treated monkeys were able to discriminate blue-green when it was tested against a red-violet background instead of the gray background indicated that the monkeys' newly acquired "green" and "red" percepts were distinct from one another.

A Possible Evolutionary Mechanism for a Shift from Dichromacy to Trichromacy

Classic experiments in which visual deprivation of one eye during development caused permanent vision loss led to the idea that visual inputs must be present during development for the formation of circuits to process the visual information (Hubel and Wiesel 1970). From the clear change in behavior associated with treatment, compared both between and within subjects (Mancuso et al. 2009), we conclude that the adult monkeys gained new color vision capacities because of gene therapy. These startling empirical results provide insight into the evolutionary changes in the visual system that are required for adding a new dimension of color vision. Previously, it seemed possible that a transformation from dichromacy to trichromacy would require evolutionary and developmental changes, for instance, the development of new neural circuitry in later structures along the pathway to vision—in addition to acquiring a third cone type. However, results from squirrel monkeys show that a transformation from dichromatic to trichromatic color vision behavior can occur with the addition of a third cone type after the visual system has developed.

The acquisition of new color vision was also shown in genetically engineered mice (Jacobs et al. 2007); however, the point has been made that such plasticity need not indicate that any rewiring of the neural circuitry has occurred (Makous 2007). Indeed, given that new color vision behavior in adult squirrel monkeys was observed just as levels of transgene expression became robust, we conclude that rewiring of the visual system was not associated with the change from dichromatic to trichromatic vision. We suggest that gene therapy with a new opsin recapitulates what occurred during evolution of trichromacy in primates. These experiments show that a new capacity for color vision, as defined by new discrimination abilities, can use preexisting neural circuitry. Moreover, results from squirrel monkeys suggest that full trichromatic color vision could have evolved solely by adding a gene for a third cone pigment, in the absence of any other genetic change in the visual system specific to red-green color vision. These experiments to cure color blindness are the first to use gene therapy in primates to treat a vision disorder in which all photoreceptors are intact and healthy, making it possible to assess the full potential of gene therapy to manipulate visual capacities.

Neural Plasticity: Implications for Treatment of Retinal Disorders

Treatment allowing monkeys to see new colors in adulthood provides a striking counter-example to what occurs under conditions of monocular deprivation. For instance, it is impossible to restore vision in an adult who has grown up with a unilateral congenital cataract (Birch and Stager 1996). Future technologies may allow opportunities for functions to be added or restored in the eye. Although some changes may produce irreversible outcomes analogous to monocular deprivation, others, like gene therapy for red-green color blindness, may provide new vision capabilities.

Even before the advent of gene therapy, the neural mechanisms underlying color vision were thought to represent an interesting model system for understanding neural plasticity.

Color vision may be an example of experience guiding neural function in the visual system. For example, there is amazing variation in the ratio of L to M cones in the retina (Hagstrom et al. 1998; Roorda and Williams 1999; Carroll et al. 2000; Hofer et al. 2005), yet individuals with very different ratios are not correspondingly different in their color vision—they are all categorized as having normal trichromacy by standard color vision tests (Pokorny et al. 1991; Jordan and Mollon 1997; Miyahara et al. 1998; Brainard et al. 2000). This indicates that the red/green chromatic system is able to adjust to produce the same vision in individuals with large differences in their cone mosaics.

New World primates are an exact genetic model of inherited red-green color blindness in humans and provide an interesting insight into visual plasticity. Most mammals have two types of cone photoreceptors: S and M/L. These two cone types are the basis for dichromatic color vision. In contrast, Old World primates are usually trichromatic, having the S cones and two spectrally distinct M/L cones. For example, humans have M and L cones separated in peak sensitivity by 20–30 nm. Genetic evidence suggests that uniform trichromacy arose from allelic trichromacy via a gene translocation that placed M and L pigment genes in tandem on the X chromosome (Nathans et al. 1986a,b; Vollrath et al. 1988). Most New World primates, including squirrel monkeys, show allelic trichromacy (a single gene for cone opsin with multiple alleles forming spectrally distinct pigments), which appears to be an evolutionary intermediate between Old World primates and other mammals. The majority of all squirrel monkeys are dichromatic, but about 2/3 (the heterozygous females) are trichromatic, and the visual system is plastic enough support both types of vision as normal variants.

Possible Neural Networks Used by Newly Trichromatic Primates

In the retina, there are spectrally opponent cells that are believed to serve color vision via two distinct, spectrally opponent pathways: red-green and blue-yellow. Gene therapy for color blindness in adult primates provides insight into the role of early visual experience in the development of color vision circuitry. Because of the capricious nature of viral transduction, one virtue of gene therapy for color blindness is that it produces a random mosaic of cones that closely mimics that of naturally occurring trichromats. How, then, do treated animals extract a new dimension of color vision from their new cone complement?

The squirrel monkeys might form the circuitry underlying red-green color vision by adapting components that were not previously involved in color vision in dichromats. An alternative could be called the "blue-yellow" hypothesis, in which the addition of the third cone class split formerly S versus M receptive fields into two types with differing spectral sensitivities. Adapting a portion of one color system to provide a new visual dimension could obviate the need for neural rewiring as part of the process of adopting new color vision (Shapley 2009; Neitz and Neitz 2011).

RECENT EVIDENCE POINTS TO A NEW HYPOTHESIS FOR THE BIOLOGICAL BASIS OF TRICHROMACY IN PRIMATES

The textbook version of the standard model for the physiological basis for trichromatic color vision is that blue-yellow color vision is based on retinal small bistratified S-(L+M) cells and red-green color vision is based on (L-M) and (M-L) midget ganglion cells (DeValois and DeValois 1993; Dacey 2000). If correct, then human perceptions should be predictable from the responses of those cells; however, there are conspicuous differences between human color vision and what is predicted from the responses of S-(L+M) and L versus M cells (DeValois and DeValois 1993). The contradiction between human perception and L versus M midget ganglion cell responses arises because S cones have an input to perceptual redness and greenness but they do not have an input to the putative canonical (L-M) "red-ON" and (M-L) "green-ON" midget ganglion cells of the standard model (Drum 1989; DeValois and DeValois 1993; Dacey 2000). Excitatory S-cone input contributes to the perception of both blue and red and inhibitory S-cone input contributes to the perceptions of both yellow and green. DeValois and DeValois (1993) proposed the addition of a third stage of processing at a higher level of the visual pathway that "rotates" the color axes of the cells in the lateral geniculate nucleus to give rise to the red-green and yellow-blue axes of perceptual color space.

Several recent findings have led us to propose an alternative neurobiological explanation for color appearance and hue perception (Schmidt et al. 2014), and this alternative also provides a simple explanation for why gene therapy "cures" color blindness in adult squirrel monkeys. S-cone inputs to small bistratified cells are mediated by S-cone bipolar cells and these are specifically ON-type bipolar cells. Humans with mutations in the *GRM6* gene encoding the metabotropic glutamate receptor (mGluR6) specific to ON bipolar cells have no means to transmit any ON responses to the inner retina, and thus lack S-cone input to the small bistratified ganglion cell, yet these individuals have normal color perception (Terasaki et al. 1999; Dryja et al. 2005; Neitz and Neitz 2011). This flatly contradicts the prediction of the standard model. These findings thus suggest that the small bistratified cell is not responsible for conscious color perception.

A possible alternative is as follows: There are two recent reports demonstrating that synaptic elements for GABAergic feed-forward signaling between HII horizontal cells and midget bipolar cells, which is enhanced in primates' S cones, compared with mice or ground squirrels (Puller et al. 2014a,b). These findings suggest that the feed-forward mechanism may have evolved in primates for the purpose of color vision. The GABA-mediated feed-forward mechanism would specifically inject S-cone input into the midget bipolar cells of adjacent L/M cones. To explain hue appearance, S-cone signals have to be combined with M versus L opponent signals in two different ways to produce red-green and blue-yellow axes that match human perceptions, but only a small subset of midget ganglion cells need to carry S-cone signals to account for hue perception. Recordings from large samples of cells in the lateral geniculate nucleus (Tailby et al. 2008) have identified a group of cells that have input from M cones with the same sign as S cones, for instance, they are (S+M)-L cells that we propose are the retinal locus responsible for blue perception (Schmidt et al. 2014). Moreover, one population of cells in the lateral geniculate nucleus had L-(S+M) inputs as required for the yellow side of blue-yellow hue opponency and as predicted by the hypothesis that S-OFF signals may be injected directly into midget bipolar cells by the proposed GABA feed-forward mechanism. Because the only cells in the retina known to carry opponent signals from M versus L cones are midget ganglion cells, these results could reflect the existence of a small subclass of midget ganglion cells that are the substrate for hue perception. Thus, we argue that there are two populations of midget ganglion cells, one of which makes up the majority, which are the standard L/M cells. We propose that a second, much smaller population is made up of individual midget bipolar cells that receive input from L- or M cones that are next to an S cone and that also receive a significant feed-forward input from the neighboring S cone via an HII horizontal cell. This subgroup may represent between 5% and 15% of the total midget ganglion cell population, and we propose that these cells are responsible for conscious color perception in primates. In our model (illustrated in Fig. 2), S cone signals are combined with L and M opponent signals in the outer retina to produce a small population of bipolar cells that provide the origins of what become four labeled lines for the four unique hues (Schmidt et al. 2014).

This new theory of the neural circuitry for primate color vision makes it easy to explain how gene therapy cures red-green color blindness: The addition of an opsin gene recapitulates the circuitry of normal trichromacy by converting the formerly blue-yellow system with two circuits, one for blue and one for yellow, into four circuits. The former blue circuit is split into red and blue circuits, and the former yellow circuit is split into yellow- and green circuits. According to this hypothesis, blue-yellow color vision in the untreated, dichromatic

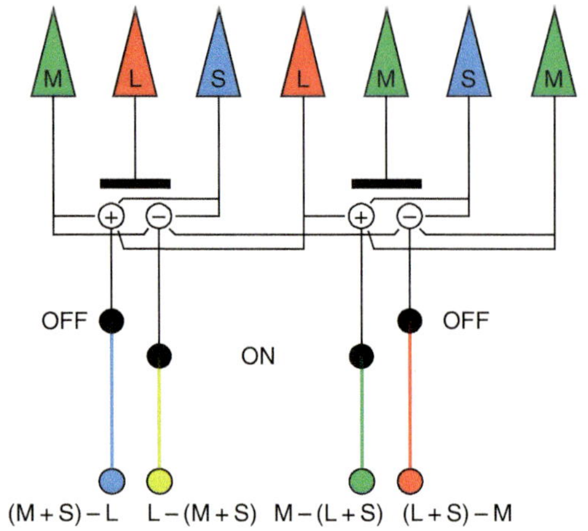

Figure 2. Schematic representation of the blue-yellow midget ganglion cell theory. A blue-yellow system that is separate from the S-(M+L) small bistratified cell system is proposed to have evolved in primates for the purpose of conscious color vision (Schmidt et al. 2014). In a dichromatic monkey, midget bipolar cells that contact M cones that are adjacent to S cones differentiate S and M signals via the inverse sign between a GABA-mediated feed-forward from S cones via HII horizontal cells and the direct feed-forward from M cones to the bipolar cell. S-ON and S-OFF signals responsible for the sensations of blue and yellow, respectively, are produced by signaling through ON and OFF bipolar cells. The introduction of L cones splits the system in two. M cone centers are responsible for red and green sensation via OFF and ON midget bipolar cells, and L cone centers mediate blue and yellow sensations via OFF and ON midget bipolar cells, respectively.

animals is served by a subset of midget ganglion cells that have S-cone input via GABA-mediated feed forward. Receptive fields for midget ganglion cells with direct input from M cones to bipolar cells and sign-inverted S-cone input from GABA-mediated feed forward via HII horizontal cells mediate the perception of blue by transmitting S-ON signals through the OFF midget bipolar cell. The same receptive fields mediate the perception of yellow via the ON midget bipolar cell. In the treated animals (Fig. 2), receptive fields that combine inputs from virally transduced "L" cones and sign-inverted inputs from S and M cones are responsible for the perception of blue via (S+M)-ON signals transmitted to the OFF midget bipolar cells, and the same receptive fields are responsible for the perception of yellow via L-ON signals transmitted through the ON midget bipolar cells of the central "L" cone. Red-green color vision in the treated animals is conferred by receptive fields, with an untransduced M cone providing direct input to the midget bipolar cell and S plus-transduced "L" cones providing sign-inverted input via GABA-mediated feed forward. In this case, the percept of red is mediated by the OFF midget bipolar neuron that receives (S+L)-ON input via the GABA-mediated HII horizontal cell feed-forward mechanism. The same receptive field mediates the perception of green via the ON midget bipolar cell receiving input directly from the M cone.

CURING COLOR BLINDNESS IN MICE COMPARED WITH PRIMATES

Trichromacy exists as a normal trait among some members of the squirrel monkey species. Thus, dichromacy exists as a variant in the monkey population much like it does in humans. The difference between squirrel monkeys and humans, however, is that although ~7%–8% of human males have some form of color vision deficiency, all male squirrel monkeys have a dichromatic form of color blindness and only a subset of females are trichromats. Is there something about the visual system in animals like squirrel monkeys, which already have trichromatic members that makes it especially permissive to the addition of trichromacy by gene therapy? What would happen if the same experiments were performed in a species that was uniformly dichromatic?

The latter question has been addressed in a series of experiments in which genetic manipulations were used to generate trichromatic mice (Smallwood et al. 2003). "Knock-in" mice were made by replacing the endogenous M-cone opsin gene (spectral peak ~511 nm) with one encoding human L opsin (spectral peak ~555 nm) (Jacobs et al. 1991). The knock-in mice were mated to wild-type mice to produce heterozygous females in which X inactivation produced two middle-to-long wavelength cone submosaics, as occurs naturally in female squirrel monkeys, and some of the heterozygous mice gained red-green color vision capacities (Jacobs et al. 2007). Interestingly, red-green color vision in the mice was very weak compared with that shown by humans with normal trichromacy or by the monkeys treated with gene therapy; it was so weak, in fact, that it was not detected in two of the five mice tested. This shows that in a species entirely lacking red-green color vision it is possible to get some trichromatic behavior simply by adding a new cone subpopulation; however, the capacity is extremely poor compared with primates with the new M-plus-L cone.

Presumably, allelic trichromacy in New World monkeys evolved from a mutation that changed the spectral sensitivity of the pigment produced by the opsin gene on the X chromosome, allowing a heterozygous female to have two spectrally distinct populations of cones and providing the basis for red-green color vision. In squirrel monkeys, the three different X chromosome opsin alleles are present at equal frequency in the population. This is consistent with the idea that the selective advantages associated with red-green color vision maximized the number of trichromats in the population. Primates are the only mammals that have red-green color vision. If trichromacy could arise in other mammals by a single point mutation in the opsin gene on the X chromosome, it seems likely that there would be many more mammals with at least allelic trichromacy. Thus, we conclude that changes in a primate ancestor's visual system for purposes other than red-green color vision occurred before the mutation that added the extra L/M photopigment could be opportunistically used to produce the dramatically better color vision of primate trichromacy (Wassle and Boycott 1991). These changes presumably include the evolution of the midget bipolar/ganglion cell system in primates, in which every cone in the central retina is associated with a private line from the retina to the central nervous system. In addition, as discussed above, our primate ancestors may have evolved a blue-yellow color vision system separate from the ancient small bistratified ganglion cell/koniocellular blue-yellow pathway in the lateral geniculate nucleus. Although the primitive koniocellular blue-yellow system may serve in the guidance of navigational movements, we might not have direct conscious awareness of the signals. The putative primate-specific blue-yellow system includes a GABA-mediated feed-forward pathway from S cones to midget bipolar cells, and we speculate that it provides the basis for conscious color vision in the ventral stream.

We suggest that once the midget ganglion cell-based blue-yellow system for color vision in the ventral stream was established in our primate ancestor, the addition of the third cone type split the system into two pathways, one for red-green color vision and the other for blue-yellow color vision (Neitz and Neitz 2011; Schmidt et al. 2014). Moreover, we suggest that the evolution of red-green color vision has been recapitulated in the acquisition of red-green color vision by gene therapy. Normally, the signals in the ventral stream are attached to specific meanings through a process of learning. Thus, the acquisition of red-green color vision would not require any rewiring, but presumably treated animals would have to learn that the subset of blue-yellow signaling neurons that are transformed to red-green signaling neurons carry a new meaning.

MEANS OF DELIVERY FOR GENE THERAPY: SUBRETINAL VERSUS INTRAVITREAL INJECTION

Previously, in treating red-green color blindness in primates, virus was injected into the subretinal space (the region between the retinal pigment epithelium and the photoreceptors) because it was the only way to ensure that the virus would have access to photoreceptors; however, subretinal injections carry risk of retinal damage (Maguire et al. 2008; Nork et al. 2012), which would be eliminated if the virus could effectively transduce cones when injected into the vitreous. If gene therapy is to be a viable option to cure color blindness in humans, the benefits must outweigh the risks. A major step toward reducing risk from the procedure will come from developing viruses that will transduce cones following a simple injection into the vitreous chamber of the eye; however, naturally occurring adeno-associated virus serotypes do not penetrate to the outer retina effectively when injected into the vitreous (Dalkara et al. 2009).

Recent efforts to develop viruses that can penetrate to the outer retina when injected into the vitreous have shown promising results (Petrs-Silva et al. 2009; Dalkara et al. 2013). AAV viruses with tyrosine mutations exposed at the surface allow the virus to escape degradation by cellular pathways, and in rodents these viruses penetrated and transduced photoreceptors when injected into the vitreous (Petrs-Silva et al. 2009; Petrs-Silva et al. 2011). However, in our preliminary experiments there was limited improvement in the extent or pattern of cells in the primate retina (macaque and baboon) transduced by tyrosine-mutated AAV2 as opposed to wild-type AAV2, or for tyrosine-mutated AAV5 compared with wild-type AAV5 (ARVO abstract) (Di et al. 1987).

Several labs have shown success using in vitro and in vivo selection to develop gene therapy vectors that target specific cell types (Muller et al. 2003; Perabo et al. 2003). In recent work, directed in vivo evolution of AAV2 libraries in the mouse retina was used to identify mutant viruses that could transduce outer retinal cells, notably photoreceptors, with greater efficiency when injected into the vitreous (Dalkara et al. 2013). Three AAV libraries were combined and injected into the vitreous of mice. One library was a collection of capsids with random oligonucleotides encoding 7mer peptides inserted in the heparin-binding domain of the capsid; a second library carried a tyrosine mutant version of the viral genome that was subjected to random mutagenesis; and the third was a chimeric capsid-encoding library generated by shuffling AAV1, -2, -4, -5, -6, -8, and -9. The combined libraries were injected into transgenic mice with GFP-labeled rods. The GFP-expressing cells were sorted using flow cytometry. The viral DNA was then recovered from the photoreceptors, packaged into virus and again injected into mice. This process was repeated to complete several rounds of viral evolution in which virus was recovered from photoreceptors, subjected to error-prone polymerase chain reactions to introduce further genetic diversity, and reinjected into mice. Of the AAV variants obtained using this approach, the majority were from the 7mer library and shared the same 7-amino-acid motif (LGETTRP), designated 7m8. When injected into the vitreous of mouse eyes, the 7m8 variant transduced photoreceptors with much higher efficiency than did a tyrosine-mutated AAV2. When the 7m8 variant of AAV2 carrying GFP was injected into the vitreous of macaque eyes, there were patchy spots of transduced photoreceptors in the peripheral retina (Dalkara et al. 2013). This approach shows great promise for recovering virus with capsid mutations that allow efficient penetration to the outer retina and transduction of photoreceptors when injected into the vitreous.

Gene therapy promises great benefits in the treatment of both rod- and cone- photoreceptor-based vision disorders. These include blue cone monochromacy, which is often caused by mutations in opsin genes or by the deletion of the locus control region, an enhancer critically important for transcription of the adjacent cone opsin genes (Nathans et al. 1989; Nathans et al. 1993). Blue cone monochromats have no functioning L- or M cones, and must rely entirely on S cones for photopic vision; as a consequence, they have low vision and no color vision. Deletions of the locus control region impairs function of cone photoreceptors, but adaptive optics imaging suggests that at least some fraction of L/M cones remain viable and amenable to gene therapy (Carroll et al. 2012; Cideciyan et al. 2013). Likewise, for the cone opsin mutation designated LIAVA (for the combination of amino acids specified by five polymorphic codons in exon 3), the cones are rendered nonfunctional but they do not appear to degenerate (Carroll et al. 2004). For these and a host of other retinal degenerations affecting photoreceptors, a virus that effectively transduces photoreceptors and cells of the retinal pigment epithelium when injected into the vitreous would have great benefit.

CONCLUDING REMARKS

The most-common inherited defects for red-green color vision in humans arise from gene rearrangements in which all genes encoding the

L- or M-cone opsin have been either deleted or displaced to a nonexpressed position in the array (Nathans et al. 1986a; Hayashi et al. 1999). The cause of red-green color blindness in squirrel monkeys—the presence of a single opsin gene on the X chromosome—is thus genetically identical to that in a subset of humans. The number of humans with red-green color vision defects is large—one in twelve males and one in ~230 females. One day, gene therapy methods may be sufficiently safe and practical that it will be possible to treat people for whom color blindness is a detriment to their quality of life. However, red-green color blindness can also be caused by point mutations in the cone opsin genes (Winderickx et al. 1992; Neitz et al. 2004; Carroll et al. 2009, 2012; Wagner-Schuman et al. 2010), which in some cases are associated with cone dystrophy (Gardner et al. 2010; McClements et al. 2013), leading to debilitating vision loss in addition to color vision deficits. It remains to be seen whether the gene therapy approach used in squirrel monkeys could rescue cone dystrophy caused by mutations in cone photopigment genes. Also, more debilitating than red-green color blindness is blue cone monochromacy. There is evidence with some mutations that at least some cones may remain viable into adulthood (Carroll et al. 2012; Cideciyan et al. 2013), making this disorder amenable to gene therapy, at least in a subset of cases.

In the broader scope, results from experiments to cure color blindness in mice and nonhuman primates provide important lessons about how preexisting circuitry may be exploited in response to new inputs added in adulthood. The unique capacity of the primate brain to adapt to new inputs by learning new associations may provide a mechanism for new capacities to be added in humans via gene therapy.

ACKNOWLEDGMENTS

Work described in this paper was funded by the National Eye Institute (NEI) grants R01EY016861, R01EY009303, R01EY009620, and P30EY001730; by the Washington National Primate Research Center (WaNPRC) through National Institutes of Health (NIH) grant P51OD010425; and Research to Prevent Blindness. J.N. is the Bishop Professor of Ophthalmology, and M.N. is the Ray H. Hill Professor of Ophthalmology.

REFERENCES

Albright TD, Jessell TM, Kandel ER, Posner MI. 2000. Neural science: A century of progress and the mysteries that remain. *Cell* **100:** S1–S55.

Birch EE, Stager DR. 1996. The critical period for surgical treatment of dense congenital unilateral cataract. *Invest Ophthalmol Vis Sci* **37:** 1532–1538.

Brainard DH, Roorda A, Yamauchi Y, Calderone JB, Metha A, Neitz M, Neitz J, Williams DR, Jacobs GH. 2000. Functional consequences of the relative numbers of L and M cones. *J Opt Soc Am A Opt Image Sci Vis* **17:** 607–614.

Bunce J, Isbell L, Neitz M, Bonci D, Surridge A, Jacobs G, Smith D. 2011. Characterization of opsin gene alleles affecting color vision in a wild population of titi monkeys (*Callicebus brunneus*). *Am J Primatol* **73:** 189–196.

Carroll J, McMahon C, Neitz M, Neitz J. 2000. Flicker-photometric electroretinogram estimates of L: M cone photoreceptor ratio in men with photopigment spectra derived from genetics. *J Opt Soc Am A Opt Image Sci Vis* **17:** 499–509.

Carroll J, Neitz M, Wolfing J, Gray D, Neitz J, Williams DR. 2004. Different genetic causes of red-green color blindness give rise to different retinal phenotypes as assessed with adaptive optics. *Invest Ophthalmol Vis Sci* **45:** U426–U426.

Carroll J, Baraas RC, Wagner-Schuman M, Rha J, Siebe CA, Sloan C, Tait DM, Thompson S, Morgan JIW, Neitz J, et al. 2009. Cone photoreceptor mosaic disruption associated with Cys203Arg mutation in the M-cone opsin. *Proc Natl Acad Sci* **106:** 20948–20953.

Carroll J, Dubra A, Gardner JC, Mizrahi-Meissonnier L, Cooper RF, Dubis AM, Nordgren R, Genead M, Connor TB Jr, Stepien KE, et al. 2012. The effect of cone opsin mutations on retinal structure and the integrity of the photoreceptor mosaic. *Invest Ophthalmol Vis Sci* **53:** 8006–8015.

Cideciyan AV, Hufnagel RB, Carroll J, Sumaroka A, Luo X, Schwartz SB, Dubra A, Land M, Michaelides M, Gardner JC, et al. 2013. Human cone visual pigment deletions spare sufficient photoreceptors to warrant gene therapy. *Hum Gene Ther* **24:** 993–1006.

Dacey DM. 2000. Parallel pathways for spectral coding in primate retina. *Ann Rev Neurosci* **23:** 743–775.

Dalkara D, Kolstad K, Caporale N, Visel M, Klimczak R, Schaffer D, Flannery J. 2009. Inner limiting membrane barriers to AAV-mediated retinal transduction from the vitreous. *Mol Ther* **17:** 2096–2102.

Dalkara D, Byrne LC, Klimczak RR, Visel M, Yin L, Merigan WH, Flannery JG, Schaffer DV. 2013. In vivo directed evolution of a new adeno-associated virus for therapeutic outer retinal gene delivery from the vitreous. *Sci Trans Med* **5:** 189ra76.

DeValois RL, DeValois KK. 1993. A multi-stage color model. *Vision Res* **33:** 1053–1065.

Dl S, Neitz J, Jacobs GH. 1987. Early color deprivation and subsequent color vision in a dichromatic monkey. *Vision Res* **27:** 2009–2013.

Drum B. 1989. Hue signals from short- and medium-wavelength sensitive cones. *J Opt Soc Am A Opt Image Sci Vis* **6:** 153–156.

Dryja TP, McGee TL, Berson EL, Fishman GA, Sandberg MA, Alexander KR, Derlacki DJ, Rajagopalan AS. 2005. Night blindness and abnormal cone electroretinogram ON responses in patients with mutations in the *GRM6* gene encoding mGluR6. *Proc Natl Acad Sci* **102:** 4884–4889.

Gardner J, Webb T, Kanuga N, Robson A, Holder G, Stockman A, Ripamonti C, Ebenezer N, Ogun O, Devery S, et al. 2010. X-linked cone dystrophy caused by mutation of the red and green cone opsins. *Am J Hum Genet* **87:** 26–39.

Hagstrom SA, Neitz J, Neitz M. 1998. Variations in cone populations for red-green color vision examined by analysis of mRNA. *NeuroReport* **9:** 1963–1967.

Hayashi T, Motulsky AG, Deeb SS. 1999. Position of a 'green-red' hybrid gene in the visual pigment array determines colour-vision phenotype. *Nat Genet* **22:** 90–93.

Hofer H, Carroll J, Neitz J, Neitz M, Williams DR. 2005. Organization of the human trichromatic cone mosaic. *J Neurosci* **25:** 9669–9679.

Hubel DH. 1988. *Eye, Brain, and Vision*. W.H. Freeman and Company, New York.

Hubel DH, Wiesel TN. 1970. The period of susceptibility to the physiological effects of unilateral eye closure in kittens. *J Physiol* **206:** 419–436.

Jacobs GH. 1984. Within-species variations in visual capacity among squirrel monkeys (*Saimiri sciureus*): Color vision. *Vision Res* **24:** 1267–1277.

Jacobs GH, Neitz J. 1985. Color vision in squirrel monkeys: Sex-related differences suggest the mode of inheritance. *Vision Res* **25:** 141–143.

Jacobs GH, Neitz J. 1987. Inheritance of color vision in a New World monkey (*Saimiri sciureus*). *Proc Natl Acad Sci* **84:** 2545–2549.

Jacobs GH, Neitz J, Deegan JF II. 1991. Retinal receptors in rodents maximally sensitive to ultraviolet light. *Nature* **353:** 655–656.

Jacobs GH, Neitz J, Neitz M. 1993. Genetic basis of polymorphism in the color vision of platyrrhine monkeys. *Vision Res* **33:** 269–274.

Jacobs GH, Williams GA, Cahill H, Nathans J. 2007. Emergence of novel color vision in mice engineered to express a human cone photopigment. *Science* **315:** 1723–1725.

Jordan G, Mollon JD. 1997. Unique hues in heterozygotes for protan and deutan deficiencies. In *Colour Vision Deficiencies XIII* (ed. Cavonius CR), pp. 67–76. Kluwer Academic Publishers, Dordrecht, Netherlands.

Khanna RC, Foster A, Krishnaiah S, Mehta MK, Gogate PM. 2013. Visual outcomes of bilateral congenital and developmental cataracts in young children in south India and causes of poor outcome. *Indian J Ophthalmol* **61:** 65–70.

Kuchenbecker J, Sahay M, Tait DM, Neitz M, Neitz J. 2008. Topography of the long- to middle-wavelength sensitive cone ratio in the human retina assessed with a wide-field color multifocal electroretinogram. *Vis Neurosci* **25:** 301–306.

Li Q, Timmers AM, Guy J, Pang J, Hauswirth WW. 2007. Cone-specific expression using a human red opsin promoter in recombinant AAV. *Vision Res* **48:** 332–338.

Maguire AM, Simonelli F, Pierce EA, Pugh ENJ, Mingozzi F, Bennicelli J, Banfi S, Marshall KA, Testa F, Surace EM, et al. 2008. Safety and efficacy of gene transfer for Leber's congenital amaurosis. *N Engl J Med* **358:** 2240–2248.

Makous W. 2007. Comment on "Emergence of novel color vision in mice engineered to express a human cone photopigment." *Science* **318:** 196.

Mancuso K, Neitz M, Neitz J. 2006. An adaptation of the Cambridge Colour Test for use with animals. *Vis Neurosci* **23:** 695–701.

Mancuso K, Hauswirth WW, Li Q, Connor TB, Kuchenbecker JA, Mauck MC, Neitz J, Neitz M. 2009. Gene therapy for red-green colour blindness in adult primates. *Nature* **461:** 784–787.

McClements M, Davies WI, Michaelides M, Carroll J, Rha J, Mollon JD, Neitz M, MacLaren RE, Moore AT, Hunt DM. 2013. X-linked cone dystrophy and colour vision deficiency arising from a missense mutation in a hybrid L/M cone opsin gene. *Vision Res* **80:** 41–50.

Miyahara E, Pokorny J, Smith VC, Baron R, Baron E. 1998. Color vision in two observers with highly biased LWS/MWS cone ratios. *Vision Res* **38:** 601–612.

Mollon JD, Bowmaker JK, Jacobs GH. 1984. Variations of colour vision in a New World primate can be explained by polymorphism of retinal photopigments. *Proc R Soc Lond B Biol Sci* **222:** 373–399.

Muller OJ, Kaul F, Weitzman MD, Pasqualini R, Arap W, Kleinschmidt JA, Trepel M. 2003. Random peptide libraries displayed on adeno-associated virus to select for targeted gene therapy vectors. *Nat Biotechnol* **21:** 1040–1046.

Nathans J, Piantanida TP, Eddy RL, Shows TB, Hogness DS. 1986a. Molecular genetics of inherited variation in human color vision. *Science* **232:** 203–210.

Nathans J, Thomas D, Hogness DS. 1986b. Molecular genetics of human color vision: The genes encoding blue, green, and red pigments. *Science* **232:** 193–202.

Nathans J, Davenport CM, Maumenee IH, Lewis RA, Hejtmancik JF, Litt M, Lovrien E, Weleber R, Bachynski B, Zwas F, et al. 1989. Molecular genetics of human blue cone monochromacy. *Science* **245:** 831–838.

Nathans J, Maumenee IA, Zrenner E, Sadowski B, Sharpe LT, Lewis RA, Hansen E, Rosenberg P, Schwartz M, Heckenlively JR, et al. 1993. Genetic heterogeneity among blue-cone monochromats. *Am J Hum Genet* **53:** 987–1000.

Neitz J, Neitz M. 2011. The genetics of normal and defective color vision. *Vision Res* **51:** 633–651.

Neitz M, Neitz J, Jacobs GH. 1991. Spectral tuning of pigments underlying red-green color vision. *Science* **252:** 971–974.

Neitz M, Carroll J, Renner A, Knau H, Werner JS, Neitz J. 2004. Variety of genotypes in males diagnosed as dichromatic on a conventional clinical anomaloscope. *Vis Neurosci* **21:** 205–216.

Nork TM, Murphy CJ, Kim CB, Ver Hoeve JN, Rasmussen CA, Miller PE, Wabers HD, Neider MW, Dubielzig RR,

McCulloh RJ, et al. 2012. Functional and anatomic consequences of subretinal dosing in the cynomolgus macaque. *Arch Ophthalmol* **130:** 65–75.

Perabo L, Buning H, Kofler DM, Ried MU, Girod A, Wendtner CM, Enssle J, Hallek M. 2003. In vitro selection of viral vectors with modified tropism: The adeno-associated virus display. *Mol Ther* **8:** 151–157.

Petrs-Silva H, Dinculescu A, Li Q, Min S, Chiodo V, JJ P, Zhong L, Zolotukhin S, Srivastava A, Lewin A, et al. 2009. High-efficiency transduction of the mouse retina by tyrosine-mutant AAV serotype vectors. *Mol Ther* **17:** 463–471.

Petrs-Silva H, Dinculescu A, Li Q, Deng W, Pang J, Min S, Chiodo V, Neeley A, Govindasamy L, Debbett A, et al. 2011. Novel properties of tyrosine-mutant AAV2 vectors in the mouse retina. *Mol Ther* **19:** 293–301.

Pokorny J, Smith VC, Wesner MF. 1991. Variability in cone populations and implications. In *From Pigments to Perception: Advances in Understanding Visual Processes* (ed. Valberg A, Lee BB), pp. 23–33. Plenum Press, New York.

Puller C, Haverkamp S, Neitz M, Neitz J. 2014a. Synaptic elements for GABAergic feed-forward signaling between HII horizontal cells and blue cone bipolar cells are enriched beneath primate S-cones. *PloS ONE* **9:** e288963.

Puller C, Manookin MB, Neitz M, Neitz J. 2014b. Specialized synaptic pathway for chromatic signals beneath S-cone photoreceptors is common to human, Old and New World primates. *J Opt Soc Am A Opt Image Sci Vis* **31:** A189–A194.

Reffin JP, Astell S, Mollon JD. 1991. Trials of a computer-controlled colour vision test that preserves the advantages of pseudo-isochromatic plates. In *Colour Vision Deficiencies X* (ed. Drum B, Moreland JD, Serra A), pp. 69–76. Kluwer Academic Publishers, Dordrecht, Netherlands.

Regan BC, Reffin JP, Mollon JD. 1994. Luminance noise and the rapid determination of discrimination ellipses in colour deficiency. *Vision Res* **34:** 1279–1299.

Roorda A, Williams DR. 1999. The arrangement of the three cone classes in the living human eye. *Nature* **397:** 520–522.

Schmidt BP, Neitz M, Neitz J. 2014. Neurobiological hypothesis of color appearance and hue perception. *J Opt Soc Am* **31:** A195–A207.

Shapley R. 2009. Vision: Gene therapy in colour. *Nature* **461:** 737–739.

Smallwood PM, Olveczky BP, Williams GL, Jacobs GH, Reese BE, Meister M, Nathans J. 2003. Genetically engineered mice with an additional class of cone photoreceptors: Implications for the evolution of color vision. *Proc Natl Acad Sci* **100:** 11706–11711.

Soares J, Fiorani M, Araujo E, Zana Y, Bonci D, Neitz M, Ventura D, Gattass R. 2010. Cone photopigment variations in *Cebus apella* monkeys evidenced by electroretinogram measurements and genetic analysis. *Vision Res* **50:** 99–106.

Tailby C, Solomon SG, Lennie P. 2008. Functional asymmetries in visual pathways carrying S-cone signals in macaque. *J Neurosci* **28:** 4078–4087.

Terasaki H, Miyake Y, Nomura R, Horiguchi M, Suzuki S, Kondo M. 1999. Blue-on-yellow perimetry in the complete type of congenital stationary night blindness. *Invest Ophthalmol Vis Sci* **40:** 2761–2764.

Vollrath D, Nathans J, Davis RW. 1988. Tandem array of human visual pigment genes at Xq28. *Science* **240:** 1669–1672.

Wagner-Schuman M, Neitz J, Rha J, Williams DR, Neitz M, Carroll J. 2010. Color-deficient cone mosaics associated with Xq28 opsin mutations: A stop codon versus gene deletions. *Vision Res* **50:** 2396–2402.

Wang Y, Macke JP, Merbs SL, Zack DJ, Klaunberg B, Bennett J, Gearhart J, Nathans J. 1992. A locus control region adjacent to the human red and green visual pigment genes. *Neuron* **9:** 429–440.

Wang Y, Smallwood PM, Cowan M, Blesh D, Lawler A, Nathans J. 1999. Mutually exclusive expression of human red and green visual pigment-reporter transgenes occurs at high frequency in murine cone photoreceptors. *Proc Natl Acad Sci* **96:** 5251–5256.

Wassle H, Boycott BB. 1991. Functional architecture of the mammalian retina. *Physiol Rev* **71:** 447–480.

Winderickx J, Sanocki E, Lindsey DT, Teller DY, Motulsky AG, Deeb SS. 1992. Defective colour vision associated with a missense mutation in the human green visual pigment gene. *Nat Genet* **1:** 251–256.

Gene Therapy Using Stem Cells

Erin R. Burnight[1], Luke A. Wiley[1], Robert F. Mullins[1], Edwin M. Stone[1,2], and Budd A. Tucker[1]

[1]The Stephen A. Wynn Institute for Vision Research, Department of Ophthalmology and Visual Sciences, University of Iowa, Iowa City, Iowa 52242

[2]Howard Hughes Medical Institute, University of Iowa, Iowa City, Iowa 52242

Correspondence: budd-tucker@uiowa.edu

Viral-mediated gene augmentation therapy has recently shown success in restoring vision to patients with retinal degenerative disorders. Key to this success was the availability of animal models that accurately presented the human phenotype to test preclinical efficacy and safety. These exciting studies support the use of gene therapy in the treatment of devastating retinal degenerative diseases. In some cases, however, in vivo gene therapy for retinal degeneration would not be effective because the cell types targeted are no longer present. The development of somatic cell reprogramming methods provides an attractive source of autologous cells for transplantation and treatment of retinal degenerative disease. This article explores the development of gene therapy and patient-derived stem cells for the purpose of restoring vision to individuals suffering from inherited retinal degenerations.

Gene therapy for the treatment of inherited disorders such as adrenoleukodystrophy (Cartier et al. 2009), adenosine deaminase-related severe combined immunodeficiency (Gaspar et al. 2011), and the childhood blindness Leber congenital amaurosis (LCA) (Bainbridge et al. 2008; Hauswirth et al. 2008; Maguire et al. 2009) have recently shown great promise. Inherent to the success of these clinical trials was the availability of animal models to test therapeutic strategies. For instance, gene replacement with an adeno-associated virus (AAV) vector to treat *RPE65*-associated LCA (LCA2) was largely successful in both the *Rpe65*$^{-/-}$ mouse and the large Briard dog model of the disease (Bennicelli et al. 2008). In comparison to contralateral sham-injected eyes, electroretinogram (ERG) responses and visual acuity increased significantly in *Rpe65*$^{-/-}$ mouse eyes treated subretinally with an AAV-*RPE65* vector. Similarly, subretinal AAV-*RPE65* delivery resulted in significant reversal of nystagmus and visual deficits in *RPE65* mutant dogs (Acland et al. 2001, 2005; Narfström et al. 2003). Notably, ERG a-waves, indicative of photoreceptor responses, also increased dramatically (by 26%–60%) and persisted for the duration of the study following injection of the therapeutic gene transfer vector. The kinetics of the a-waves were not significantly different between treated and phenotypically normal animals (Bennicelli et al. 2008). These promising findings paved the way for the development of AAV-mediated *RPE65* gene replacement therapy for patients with LCA2.

Cite this article as *Cold Spring Harb Perspect Med* doi: 10.1101/cshperspect.a017434

ANIMAL MODELS AND THERAPEUTIC GENE TRANSFER

Although animal models are invaluable for investigation of disease pathophysiology and evaluation of gene transfer strategies, not all models faithfully recapitulate the human phenotype. This is especially true when developing therapeutic strategies for the treatment of inherited macular degenerations. For example, the study of gene transfer for the treatment of age-related macular degeneration (AMD), Stargardt disease, and Best disease are hampered by the fact that the rod-dominant mouse retina lacks a macula, the central zone of the primate retina that has evolved to subserve very fine visual acuity. Similarly, many disease models have a drastically different age of onset and disease progression than is observed in the human condition. For instance, dominant Pro23His rhodopsin-associated retinitis pigmentosa typically causes relatively late-onset disease in humans, with significant vision remaining until late in life. The pig model of Pro23His rhodopsin-associated retinitis pigmentosa has a retinal disease that is significantly more aggressive than that seen in humans; as early as 3 mo of age, these animals have extensive photoreceptor cell loss (Fig. 1) (Ross et al. 2012). Similarly, in the rd16 CEP290 mouse model of LCA, mice are born with a full complement of photoreceptor cells, but the very aggressive disease results in almost complete loss of photoreceptor cells by 3 wk of age (Chang et al. 2006). The fact that a large proportion of the photoreceptor cells are lost before the eyes open makes gene transfer approaches for the treatment of this disease very difficult.

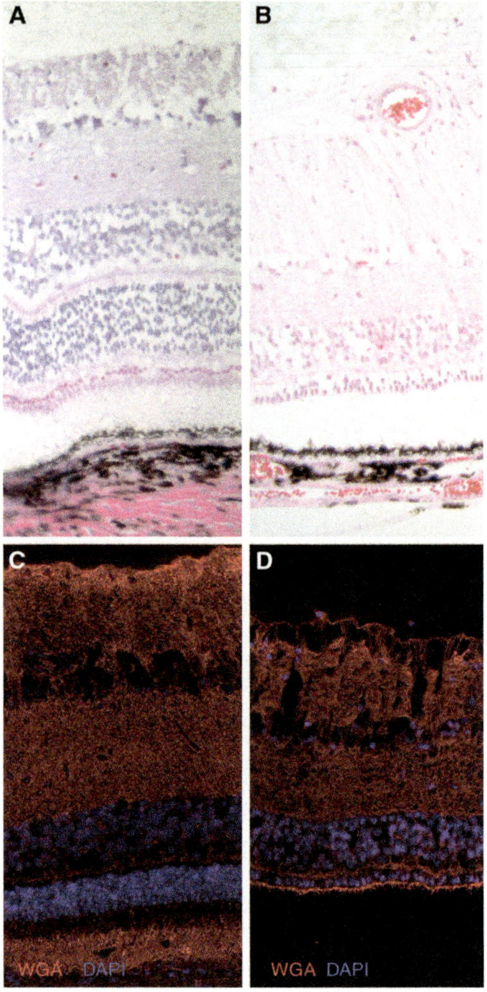

Figure 1. The transgenic pig carrying a human Pro23His rhodopsin transgene displays drastically accelerated retinal degeneration. *A–B*: Histological analysis of both wild-type (*A*) and Pro23His (*B*) pig retinal tissue at 6 mo of age. *C–D*: Cytochemical analysis of both wild-type (*C*) and Pro23His (*D*) pig retinal tissue at 6 mo of age, using wheat germ agglutinin (WGA, red) and DAPI (blue).

Advances in pluripotent stem cell technologies provide an exciting avenue for the treatment of retinal degenerative disease. For instance, human embryonic stem cell (ESC)-derived photoreceptor precursor cells transplanted into a mouse model of retinal degeneration have been shown to migrate into and integrate within the degenerative retina, express rod and cone photoreceptor markers and restore electroretinal activity (Lamba et al. 2009). However, ESC-derived photoreceptor transplants are by definition allogeneic and would likely require life-long immune modulation if used clinically (Preynat-Seauve et al. 2009; West et al. 2010). Like ESCs, patient-specific induced pluripotent stem cells (iPSCs) possess the ability to differentiate into photoreceptor precursors which can integrate into a diseased retina and give rise to new functional photoreceptor cells (Lamba et al. 2010;

Homma et al. 2013; Tucker et al. 2013b). However, unlike ESCs, iPSCs can be autologous and thus have a greatly reduced risk of being rejected by the host immune system.

Patient-derived iPSCs can be generated in 4–6 wk via forced factor expression in a variety of cell types. Takahashi and Yamanaka first showed this concept through retroviral-mediated expression of the transcription factors *OCT4*, *SOX2*, *KLF4*, and *cMYC* in mouse embryonic fibroblasts (Takahashi and Yamanaka 2006) and human primary dermal fibroblasts (Takahashi et al. 2007). In addition to the "Yamanaka factors," Yu and colleagues in the Thomson laboratory established that the factors *OCT4*, *SOX2*, *LIN28*, and *NANOG* were capable of generating induced pluripotent stem cells from mesenchymal cells (Yu et al. 2007). Many cell types have since been reprogrammed using forced factor expression including dermal keratinocytes (Carey et al. 2009), neural progenitor cells (Kim et al. 2011), hepatocytes (Liu et al. 2010), and peripheral blood cells (Loh et al. 2009). Since Yamanaka's seminal report, several groups showed reprogramming using many delivery methods—both integrating and nonintegrating. Integrating lentiviral vectors are widely used for delivery of reprogramming transgenes (Brambrink et al. 2008; Maherali et al. 2008). However, to avoid the insertional mutagenic risk associated with integrating vector systems, investigators use adenovirus (Stadtfeld et al. 2008), Sendai virus (Jin et al. 2012; Tucker et al. 2013a), and transient plasmid delivery (González et al. 2009; Si-Tayeb et al. 2010). For a more detailed description of these and other delivery methods please refer to reviews (Malik and Rao 2013; Hu 2014).

Beyond being an attractive cell source for retinal transplantation, the patient-specific nature of the iPSC makes this technology very attractive for disease modeling and investigation of disease pathophysiology. That is, the molecular causes of clinical variations in disease can be studied by comparing cells derived from mildly and severely affected individuals. For example, fibroblast cultures from *CEP290*-associated LCA patients with different genotypes show cellular phenotypes of varying degrees of severity (Burnight et al. 2014). iPSC-derived photoreceptors from each of these patients can be used to study the molecular causes of the phenotypic variation observed. The efficacy of novel therapies can also be tested on cells of the actual patients who might be treated.

INDUCED PLURIPOTENT STEM CELLS AS PATIENT-SPECIFIC MODELS TO TEST EXOGENOUS GENE DELIVERY

There are many vector systems from which to choose when developing a strategy for the treatment of an inherited retinal degenerative disease. For in vivo gene transfer, there are several obstacles to the effective delivery and expression of therapeutic transgenes. In many cases, gene delivery methods must overcome host immunity (Reichel et al. 1998; Ikeda et al. 2002; Li et al. 2008). Moreover, certain cell and tissue types are difficult to transduce in vivo, which is likely because of a combination of incompatible vector tropism and limited diffusion away from the injection site. Gene delivery to cells ex vivo (i.e., "in a dish"), circumvents many of these limitations and shifts the scientific focus from the delivery vehicle to the genetic cargo. This is of particular value when one wishes to choose among several possible promoters, evaluate gene function, and determine the optimal level of transgene expression without killing dozens, if not hundreds, of animals in the process.

One of the major considerations when determining which vector system to use is gene size. Small, nonstructural enzymes (i.e., MAK, RPE65, etc.) are often well-suited for expression via the AAV vector system (Bennicelli et al. 2008; Conlon et al. 2013; Molday et al. 2013; Dai et al. 2014). Indeed, the recent success of clinical trials involving patients with LCA2 highlights the utility of the AAV vector for in vivo gene transfer to the retina (Bainbridge et al. 2008; Hauswirth et al. 2008; Maguire et al. 2008). However, the natural serotypes of AAV do not transduce human pluripotent stem cells very efficiently. The commonly used AAV2 serotype transduces human stem cells only marginally (10% at a multiplicity of infection of 10,000 [Asuri et al. 2012]). Asuri and colleagues (2012) addressed this limitation via directed evolution of the capsid, which yielded threefold higher transduction efficiency when transduced at an equal multiplicity of infection. Another consideration when using AAV vectors in gene transfer studies is the packaging limit. Large genes such as *CEP290* (~8 kb coding sequence) or *ABCA4* (~6.5 kb coding sequence) require vectors that can accommodate more than the 4.5 kb packaging limit of AAV (Wu et al. 2010). To this end, the lentivirus is an attractive choice. The packaging limit of lentivirus is ~8 − 10 kb (Balaggan and Ali 2012) and can thus accommodate larger transgene expression cassettes. Moreover, lentiviruses can be pseudotyped with a variety of pantropic envelope glycoproteins (Calame et al. 2011)—the most common of which is the G glycoprotein of the vesicular stomatitis virus (VSVG)—and can transduce pluripotent stem cells well (Endo et al. 2007; Tucker et al. 2011).

We have employed lentiviral-mediated gene transfer to transduce pluripotent stem cell-derived photoreceptor precursor cultures from patients with LCA and retinitis pigmentosa. For example, the most common cause of retinitis pigmentosa in the Jewish population is a splice-altering insertion of an Alu element in the male germ cell-associated kinase (*MAK*) gene. Cilia formation assays showed that patient's cells generated elongated cilia when compared with phenotypically normal cells (Tucker et al. 2011). On transduction with VSVG-pseudotyped lentiviral vectors expressing *MAK*, cells formed significantly shorter cilia compared with untransduced cultures. Thus, we achieved functional gene correction in patient-specific, stem cell-derived photoreceptor precursors. For treatment of patients with LCA, we successfully packaged cDNA encoding the large structural gene *CEP290* into lentiviral vectors with the heterologous cytomegalovirus (CMV) promoter driving transgene expression (Burnight et al. 2014).

Another important consideration in developing gene transfer strategies to treat inherited disorders in vitro is the timing of the genetic correction. Is it more effective to perform gene transfer to the somatic cells (i.e., fibroblasts or keratinocytes) before reprogramming them into iPSC cultures, or to differentiate the cultures first and then transduce them? Long-term gene expression in immature cell types transduced with γ-retroviral and lentiviral vectors can be silenced because of epigenetic mechanisms such as DNA methylation or histone modification of the heterologous promoter (Ellis 2005; Herbst et al. 2012). For example, transgene silencing was observed in iPSCs derived from a murine model of tyrosinemia type 1 ($FAH^{-/-}$) after transduction with a lentivirus expressing *FAH* (Wu et al. 2011). Only 20% of cells expressed the transgene. Nonetheless, a small percentage of these genetically corrected iPSCs showed full pluripotent potential, and viable mice were generated via tetracomplementation (Wu et al. 2011).

Because phenotypic correction is not as efficient when transducing iPSCs (because of transgene silencing), it may be more advantageous to correct somatic cells before reprogramming. For example, Raya and colleagues transduced fibroblasts from Fanconi anemia patients with lentiviral vectors expressing *FANCA* or *FANCD2*. These cells, on reprogramming, expressed the pluripotency markers OCT4, SOX2, NANOG, SSEA3, SSEA4, and TRA1-60, and were indistinguishable from human embryonic stem cells and iPSCs from healthy individuals. Moreover, the genetically corrected iPSCs differentiated into phenotypically normal myeloid and erythroid progenitors (Raya et al. 2009).

Introducing therapeutic transgenes after differentiation is also a viable option in some cases. We recently showed successful lentiviral gene transfer to differentiated photoreceptor precursor cultures from patients with *CEP290*-associated LCA. Transduced photoreceptor precursor cells (identified by expression of retinal markers *OTX2*, *OPSN1SW*, and *ROM1*) expressed *CEP290* transcript and full-length protein after 90 d of differentiation (Burnight et al. 2014). Furthermore, a cilia formation defect that was identified in serum-starved fibroblasts isolated from a CEP290 patient carrying two hypomorphic alleles was rescued following transduction with the *CEP290*-expressing lentiviral vector described above (Burnight et al. 2014).

Effective gene therapy strategies must result in therapeutic transgene expression in the appropriate cell type and at the appropriate level. Transgene expression is commonly driven by strong, ubiquitously expressing promoter elements, such as CMV. However, overexpression of large structural proteins such as CEP290 or members of the BBSome, a complex of proteins associated with Bardet-Biedl syndrome, may lead to cytotoxicity and cell death (Seo et al. 2013; Burnight et al. 2014). For an inherited retinal disease, it is important to direct the appropriate level of expression in the cell type specific to the pathophysiology of the disease. Thus, developing a "molecular toolbox" of gene transfer reagents is of great interest. This array of reagents would include promoters specific to heterologous cell or tissue types with varying degrees of expressivity and a series of viral vectors with a range of carrying capacities (Fig. 2). Indeed, work from our laboratory and others indicates promoter elements from retina-specific genes such as *GRK1, IRBP, RHO, PDE, NRL,* and *RCVRN* achieve photoreceptor-specific expression both in vitro and in vivo (Nicoud et al. 2007). However, it has yet to be shown whether issues relating to the level of transgene expression and cellular toxicity will remain. For some genes, precise stoichiometry may require identification and use of the endogenous promoter of the therapeutic gene. Conversely, a series of cell type-specific promoters, such as those indicated above, with tunable expression elements may be useful. The ability to efficiently generate and test these reagents will almost certainly benefit from the ability to create disease-specific cell types from affected individuals.

GENOME EDITING

As indicated above, successful genetic correction in iPSCs was achieved through gene augmentation using exogenous vector systems. Therapeutic transgene expression in the retina persists for long periods of time, reducing the need for vector readministration (Bemelmans et al. 2008; Ikeda et al. 2009; Koirala et al. 2013; Testa et al. 2013). However, integrating vectors such as those derived from γ retrovirus carry the inherent risk of inducing insertional

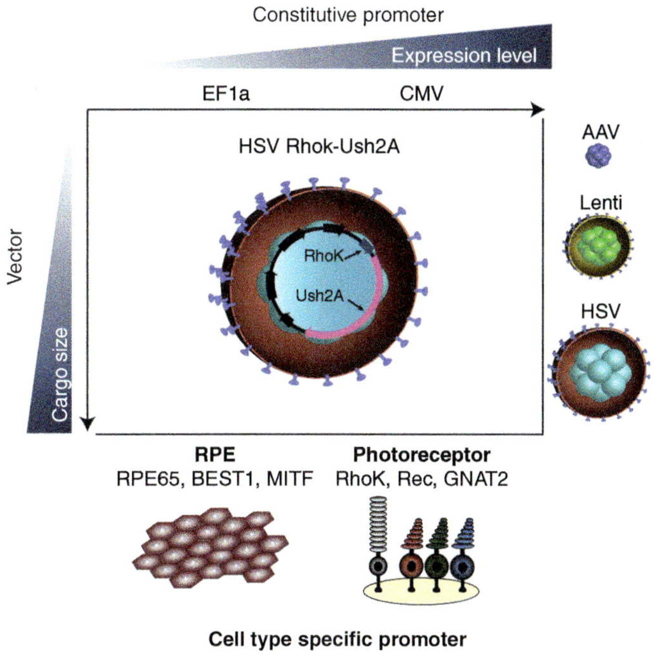

Figure 2. Schematic diagram depicting a molecular toolbox for exogenous replacement of genes. Genes of various sizes requiring various levels of expression and cell type selectivity.

mutagenesis (Hacein-Bey-Abina et al. 2003). As was shown by Hacein-Bey-Abina et al., some patients who received ex vivo gene augmentation via a γ-retroviral vector developed a T cell-like leukemia as a result of vector insertion and proto-oncogene activation in treated cells. This adverse event highlights the mutagenic risk involved with employing integrating vectors. Furthermore, given the fact that precise regulation of gene expression may be required, the ability to genetically modify defective genes in vitro provides an attractive strategy for both the creation and the repair of disease-causing mutations. Development of patient-specific autologous cells for transplantation would greatly benefit from such a strategy.

The use of genome editing tools such as zinc finger nucleases (ZFNs), transcription activator-like effector nucleases (TALENs), and the recently reported clustered regularly interspersed short tandem repeat (CRISPR)/Cas system is increasing. By editing the mutation directly through double-strand break induction by a genome editing reagent and subsequent homology-directed repair, one can take advantage of the endogenous expression control elements (i.e., promoters, enhancers, and repressors). This approach addresses some of the more serious limitations of gene replacement such as inappropriate spatial expression or incorrect levels of expression from heterologous promoters as well as the possibility of activation or inactivation of deleterious genes from vector integration.

In nature, transcription activator-like (TAL) effector proteins are transcription factors used by the plant pathogen *Xanthamonas* to evade host immune mechanisms (Gu et al. 2005; Kay et al. 2007; Sugio et al. 2007). The DNA targeting domain in the TAL effector protein consists of tandem repeats of ~34 amino acids, at the center of which is a highly variable pair of amino acids that confer nucleotide specificity (Schornack et al. 2006). The DNA recognition "code" was recently deciphered (Boch et al. 2009; Moscou and Bogdanove 2009), allowing TAL effectors to be engineered to recognize specific sites in the genome. Complexing the engineered TAL effectors with the nuclease domain of the type-II restriction endonuclease FokI can induce double-strand breaks at specific sites at or near mutations in patient-specific iPSCs. When co-delivered with a donor cassette containing a corrected sequence, homology-directed repair can result in genetic correction of these cells.

Recently Hockemeyer and colleagues (2011) targeted three endogenous loci, *PPP1RP12C*, *OCT4*, and *PITX3*, with engineered TALENs. TALEN expression constructs and donor cassettes were electroporated into both human ESCs and iPSCs. The researchers reported targeting efficiencies of 50%–100% depending on the locus. To assess binding specificity of the *PPP1RP12C* TALEN pair, Hockmeyer et al. interrogated the 19 top-ranked, maximal-likelihood potential off-target sites, as determined using systematic evolution of ligands by exponential enrichment (SELEX)-derived base-frequency matrices (Perez et al. 2008). NextGen Illumina sequencing revealed insertions or deletions at off-target sites at a very low rate (0.01%), indicating the TALENs were quite specific. Southern analysis at all three sites indicated modification at the intended site only, confirming these results (Hockemeyer et al. 2011). This valuable series of experiments provides support for the feasibility of successful genome modification in pluripotent stem cells, and suggests a powerful method for employing genetic repair in patient-specific, iPSC-derived photoreceptor precursor cells for treatment of inherited retinal degenerations. That said, before clinical use, it will be important to assess off-targeting in cells treated with genome editing reagents to prevent unwanted outcomes. Double-strand breaks are induced via heterodimerization of the FokI nuclease domains from two engineered TALENs targeted to half-recognition sequences at the intended locus. An unintended outcome of TALEN expression is the formation of homodimers, from which off-target cleavage can result. Thus, reengineering the FokI catalytic domain such that TALEN pairs form obligate heterodimers reduces the frequency of off-target cleavage (Doyon et al. 2011; Hockemeyer et al. 2011; Ramalingam et al. 2011).

Recently, the CRISPR/Cas system has been introduced (Cong et al. 2013; Jinek et al. 2013;

Mali et al. 2013) and offers several advantages for genome editing in iPSCs. First, CRISPR reagents are easier to design and work more predictably because their DNA targeting is based on RNA hybridization instead of the zinc-finger protein binding of TALENs. The guide RNA of the CRISPR system consists of an NGG sequence (protospacer adjacent motif, or PAM) downstream from the 20-nucleotide target (Cho et al. 2013; Cong et al. 2013; Mali et al. 2013). One can generate a CRISPR targeting reagent by simply synthesizing these guide sequences as complementary oligonucleotides and ligating them into a bicistronic vector that also contains a Cas9 nuclease optimized for expression in human cells (Cong et al. 2013; Ran et al. 2013b).

Recently, Mali and colleagues (2013) showed successful genome editing in human iPSCs using the CRISPR/Cas system. These researchers developed humanized CRISPR/Cas reagents targeting the endogenous AAVS1 locus. They showed homology-directed repair using a double-stranded DNA donor cassette in 2%–4% of fibroblast-derived iPSCs generated from participants in the Personal Genome Project (PGP).

As with TALEN and ZFN technology, the possibility of toxicity from off-target double-stranded breaks must also be addressed when employing the CRISPR/Cas system (Fu et al. 2013). Targeting via CRISPR/Cas can tolerate mispairing of the 20-nucleotide guide RNA (Cong et al. 2013; Jinek et al. 2013), which creates the potential for double-stranded breaks at unintended genomic loci. To address this issue, Cong et al. (2013) mutated a single amino acid in the catalytic domain of the Cas9 nuclease, thereby limiting the enzyme's activity to single-strand "nicks." These "nicks" can be repaired by the endogenous base excision repair pathway (Lindahl 1993). By using guide RNAs with a mutant Cas9 "nickase," targeted to sequences on opposite strands, one can increase editing specificity and significantly reduce off-target toxicity. For example, Ran and colleagues (2013a) recently showed efficient modification (>40%) at three loci in human cells using paired nickases targeting sequences separated by four to 20 bases on opposite strands of genomic DNA. Moreover, using deep sequencing analysis of off targets, these investigators showed a 200- to 1500-fold increase in specificity when compared with wild-type Cas9. Ran and colleagues extended these studies in vivo by coinjecting guide RNAs targeting the *Mecp2* locus and either mutant or wild-type Cas9 mRNA into single-cell mouse zygotes. These experiments yielded >80% modification at the intended locus. A previous study also supported in vivo genome editing with the CRISPR/Cas system. Wang et al. injected wild-type Cas9 and guide RNAs targeting the *Tet1* and *Tet2* loci as well as oligo repair templates into zygotes and generated mice with modification of both genes at a rate of 80% (Wang et al. 2013). This elegant set of experiments show the utility of employing nickases to increase specificity and safety of the valuable genome editing CRISPR/Cas technology for both in vitro and in vivo studies (Ran et al. 2013a; Wang et al. 2013). To treat patients who have molecularly confirmed retinal degenerative disorders, CRISPR/Cas reagents can be delivered to patient-derived iPSCs to correct disease-causing mutations before differentiating into photoreceptor precursor cells for transplantation. For in vivo therapeutic use, the addition of inducible promoters to allow transient expression of the guide RNAs may be desirable to further reduce off-target effects. Should CRISPR/Cas technology prove safe and effective for in vivo studies, many of the challenges associated with delivering large transgenes and regulating their level of expression may be overcome.

CONCLUDING REMARKS

In the not-too-distant past, the prognosis for patients affected with an inherited retinal disorder was grim. Patients were often told that there was nothing that could be performed and that their fate was irreversible blindness. Fortunately, with developments in stem cell and gene transfer technologies there is now realistic hope for treating many of these individuals. The ability to accurately identify a patient's disease-causing mutations is a prerequisite to the development of both gene-based and autologous cell-based therapies. As depicted in Figure 3, one can envision a strategy in which high-quality genetic testing, coupled with in vitro patient-specific, stem cell-based model systems, will allow for the rapid development of gene- and cell-based treatments. This process would begin by collecting blood and skin samples from the affected patient. DNA isolated from blood would be subjected to genetic screening to identify potential disease-causing mutations, and skin-derived fibroblasts or keratinocytes would be harvested for generation of iPSCs. To confirm pathogenic mutations and elucidate pathophysiologic mechanisms, iPSC-derived photoreceptor precursor cells, generated via directed differentiation, could be subjected to a variety of pathway-specific analyses. Disease-specific phenotypes identified in these studies would be used to test and confirm the efficacy of gene transfer and genome editing approaches. Gene transfer vectors shown to be effective at correcting the disease phenotype would then be used to treat patients' remaining photoreceptor cells. For patients with extensive photoreceptor cell loss, an autologous cell replacement strategy using patient-specific photoreceptor precursor cells genetically corrected via CRISPR- or TALEN-based genome editing would also be employed. This approach could be used to treat inherited retinal disorders, regardless of the clinical stage and prevalence of the disease, and regardless of the size of the causative gene.

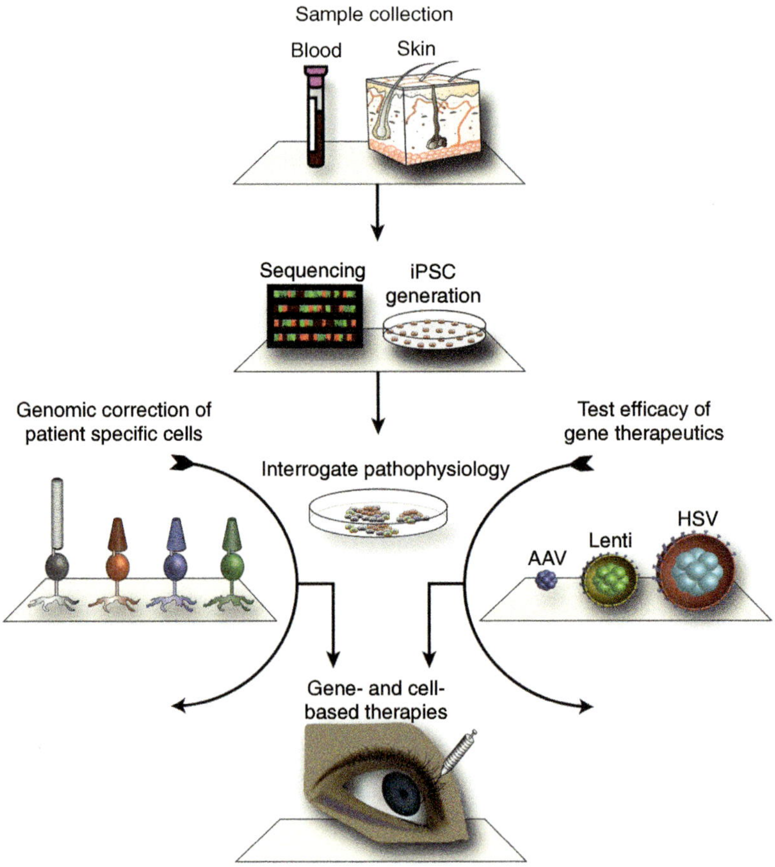

Figure 3. Schematic diagram depicting the proposed pipeline from gene discovery to treatment of inherited retinal degenerative disease.

ACKNOWLEDGMENTS

This work was supported by National Institutes of Health (NIH) Directors New Innovator Award 1-DP2-OD007483-01, NEI EY017451, F32 EY022834, Howard Hughes Medical Institute (HHMI), Foundation Fighting Blindness, Stephen A. Wynn Foundation, Grousbeck Family Foundation, and Leo, Jacques & Marion Hauser Family Vision Restoration Fund.

REFERENCES

Acland GM, Aguirre GD, Ray J, Zhang Q, Aleman TS, Cideciyan AV, Pearce-Kelling SE, Anand V, Zeng Y, Maguire AM, et al. 2001. Gene therapy restores vision in a canine model of childhood blindness. *Nat Genet* **28:** 92–95.

Acland GM, Aguirre GD, Bennett J, Aleman TS, Cideciyan AV, Bennicelli J, Dejneka NS, Pearce-Kelling SE, Maguire AM, Palczewski K, et al. 2005. Long-term restoration of rod and cone vision by single dose rAAV-mediated gene transfer to the retina in a canine model of childhood blindness. *Mol Ther* **12:** 1072–1082.

Asuri P, Bartel MA, Vazin T, Jang J-H, Wong TB, Schaffer DV. 2012. Directed evolution of adeno-associated virus for enhanced gene delivery and gene targeting in human pluripotent stem cells. *Mol Ther* **20:** 329–338.

Bainbridge JWB, Smith AJ, Barker SS, Robbie S, Henderson R, Balaggan K, Viswanathan A, Holder GE, Stockman A, Tyler N, et al. 2008. Effect of gene therapy on visual function in Leber's congenital amaurosis. *N Engl J Med* **358:** 2231–2239.

Balaggan KS, Ali RR. 2012. Ocular gene delivery using lentiviral vectors. *Gene Ther* **19:** 145–153.

Bemelmans A-P, Kostic C, Cachafeiro M, Crippa SV, Wanner D, Tekaya M, Wenzel A, Arsenijevic Y. 2008. Lentiviral gene transfer-mediated cone vision restoration in *RPE65* knockout mice. *Adv Exp Med Biol* **613:** 89–95.

Bennicelli J, Wright JF, Komaromy A, Jacobs JB, Hauck B, Zelenaia O, Mingozzi F, Hui D, Chung D, Rex TS, et al. 2008. Reversal of blindness in animal models of Leber congenital amaurosis using optimized AAV2-mediated gene transfer. *Mol Ther* **16:** 458–465.

Boch J, Scholze H, Schornack S, Landgraf A, Hahn S, Kay S, Lahaye T, Nickstadt A, Bonas U. 2009. Breaking the code of DNA binding specificity of TAL-type III effectors. *Science* **326:** 1509–1512.

Brambrink T, Foreman R, Welstead GG, Lengner CJ, Wernig M, Suh H, Jaenisch R. 2008. Sequential expression of pluripotency markers during direct reprogramming of mouse somatic cells. *Cell Stem Cell* **2:** 151–159.

Burnight ER, Wiley LA, Drack AV, Braun TA, Anfinson KR, Kaalberg EE, Halder JA, Affatigato LM, Mullins RF, Stone EM, et al. 2014. *CEP290* gene transfer rescues Leber congenital amaurosis cellular phenotype. *Gene Ther* **21:** 662–672.

Calame M, Cachafeiro M, Philippe S, Schouwey K, Tekaya M, Wanner D, Sarkis C, Kostic C, Arsenijevic Y. 2011. Retinal degeneration progression changes lentiviral vector cell targeting in the retina. *PLoS ONE* **6:** e23782.

Carey BW, Markoulaki S, Hanna J, Saha K, Gao Q, Mitalipova M, Jaenisch R. 2009. Reprogramming of murine and human somatic cells using a single polycistronic vector. *Proc Natl Acad Sci* **106:** 157–162.

Cartier N, Hacein-Bey-Abina S, Bartholomae CC, Veres G, Schmidt M, Kutschera I, Vidaud M, Abel U, Dal-Cortivo L, Caccavelli L, et al. 2009. Hematopoietic stem cell gene therapy with a lentiviral vector in X-linked adrenoleukodystrophy. *Science* **326:** 818–823.

Chang B, Khanna H, Hawes N, Jimeno D, He S, Lillo C, Parapuram SK, Cheng H, Scott A, Hurd RE, et al. 2006. In-frame deletion in a novel centrosomal/ciliary protein CEP290/NPHP6 perturbs its interaction with RPGR and results in early-onset retinal degeneration in the *rd16* mouse. *Hum Mol Genet* **15:** 1847–1857.

Cho SW, Kim S, Kim JM, Kim J-S. 2013. Targeted genome engineering in human cells with the Cas9 RNA-guided endonuclease. *Nat Biotechnol* **31:** 230–232.

Cong L, Ran FA, Cox D, Lin S, Barretto R, Habib N, Hsu PD, Wu X, Jiang W, Marraffini LA, et al. 2013. Multiplex genome engineering using CRISPR/Cas systems. *Science* **339:** 819–823.

Conlon TJ, Deng W-T, Erger K, Cossette T, Pang J-J, Ryals R, Clément N, Cleaver B, McDoom I, Boye SE, et al. 2013. Preclinical potency and safety studies of an AAV2-mediated gene therapy vector for the treatment of *MERTK* associated retinitis pigmentosa. *Hum Gene Ther Clin Dev* **24:** 23–28.

Dai X, Han J, Qi Y, Zhang H, Xiang L, Lv J, Li J, Deng W-T, Chang B, Hauswirth WW, et al. 2014. AAV-mediated lysophosphatidylcholine acyltransferase 1 (*Lpcat1*) gene replacement therapy rescues retinal degeneration in *rd11* mice. *Invest Ophthalmol Vis Sci* **55:** 1724–1734.

Doyon Y, Vo TD, Mendel MC, Greenberg SG, Wang J, Xia DF, Miller JC, Urnov FD, Gregory PD, Holmes MC. 2011. Enhancing zinc-finger-nuclease activity with improved obligate heterodimeric architectures. *Nat Methods* **8:** 74–79.

Ellis J. 2005. Silencing and variegation of γ retrovirus and lentivirus vectors. *Hum Gene Ther* **16:** 1241–1246.

Endo M, Zoltick PW, Chung DC, Bennett J, Radu A, Muvarak N, Flake AW. 2007. Gene transfer to ocular stem cells by early gestational intraamniotic injection of lentiviral vector. *Mol Ther* **15:** 579–587.

Fu Y, Foden JA, Khayter C, Maeder ML, Reyon D, Joung JK, Sander JD. 2013. High-frequency off-target mutagenesis induced by CRISPR-Cas nucleases in human cells. *Nat Biotechnol* **31:** 822–826.

Gaspar HB, Cooray S, Gilmour KC, Parsley KL, Zhang F, Adams S, Bjorkegren E, Bayford J, Brown L, Davies EG, et al. 2011. Hematopoietic stem cell gene therapy for adenosine deaminase-deficient severe combined immunodeficiency leads to long-term immunological recovery and metabolic correction. *Sci Transl Med* **3:** p97ra80.

González F, Barragan Monasterio M, Tiscornia G, Montserrat Pulido N, Vassena R, Batlle Morera L, Rodríguez-Pizà I, Izpisúa Belmonte JC. 2009. Generation of mouse-induced pluripotent stem cells by transient expression of a single nonviral polycistronic vector. *Proc Natl Acad Sci* **106:** 8918–8922.

Gu K, Yang B, Tian D, Wu L, Wang D, Sreekala C, Yang F, Chu Z, Wang G-L, White FF, et al. 2005. *R* gene expression induced by a type-III effector triggers disease resistance in rice. *Nature* **435:** 1122–1125.

Hacein-Bey-Abina S, Kalle Von C, Schmidt M, McCormack MP, Wulffraat N, Leboulch P, Lim A, Osborne CS, Pawliuk R, Morillon E, et al. 2003. *LMO2*-associated clonal T cell proliferation in two patients after gene therapy for SCID-X1. *Science* **302:** 415–419.

Hauswirth WW, Aleman TS, Kaushal S, Cideciyan AV, Schwartz SB, Wang L, Conlon TJ, Boye SL, Flotte TR, Byrne BJ, et al. 2008. Treatment of Leber congenital amaurosis due to *RPE65* mutations by ocular subretinal injection of adeno-associated virus gene vector: Short-term results of a phase I trial. *Hum Gene Ther* **19:** 979–990.

Herbst F, Ball CR, Tuorto F, Nowrouzi A, Wang W, Zavidij O, Dieter SM, Fessler S, van der Hoeven F, Kloz U, et al. 2012. Extensive methylation of promoter sequences silences lentiviral transgene expression during stem cell differentiation in vivo. *Mol Ther* **20:** 1014–1021.

Hockemeyer D, Wang H, Kiani S, Lai CS, Gao Q, Cassady JP, Cost GJ, Zhang L, Santiago Y, Miller JC, et al. 2011. Genetic engineering of human pluripotent cells using TALE nucleases. *Nat Biotechnol* **29:** 731–734.

Homma K, Okamoto S, Mandai M, Gotoh N, Rajasimha HK, Chang Y-S, Chen S, Li W, Cogliati T, Swaroop A, et al. 2013. Developing rods transplanted into the degenerating retina of Crx-knockout mice exhibit neural activity similar to native photoreceptors. *Stem Cells* **31:** 1149–1159.

Hu K. 2014. All roads lead to induced pluripotent stem cells: The technologies of iPSC generation. *Stem Cells Dev* **23:** 1285–1300.

Ikeda Y, Yonemitsu Y, Sakamoto T, Ishibashi T, Ueno H, Kato A, Nagai Y, Fukumura M, Inomata H, Hasegawa M, et al. 2002. Recombinant Sendai virus-mediated gene transfer into adult rat retinal tissue: Efficient gene transfer by brief exposure. *Exp Eye Res* **75:** 39–48.

Ikeda Y, Yonemitsu Y, Miyazaki M, Kohno R-I, Murakami Y, Murata T, Tabata T, Ueda Y, Ono F, Suzuki T, et al. 2009. Stable retinal gene expression in nonhuman primates via subretinal injection of SIVagm-based lentiviral vectors. *Hum Gene Ther* **20:** 573–579.

Jin Z-B, Okamoto S, Xiang P, Takahashi M. 2012. Integration-free induced pluripotent stem cells derived from retinitis pigmentosa patient for disease modeling. *Stem Cells Transl Med* **1:** 503–509.

Jinek M, East A, Cheng A, Lin S, Ma E, Doudna J. 2013. RNA-programmed genome editing in human cells. *eLife* **2:** e00471.

Kay S, Hahn S, Marois E, Hause G, Bonas U. 2007. A bacterial effector acts as a plant transcription factor and induces a cell size regulator. *Science* **318:** 648–651.

Kim KS, Lee HJ, Jeong HS, Li J, Teng YD, Sidman RL, Snyder EY, Kim SU. 2011. Self-renewal induced efficiently, safely, and effective therapeutically with one regulatable gene in a human somatic progenitor cell. *Proc Natl Acad Sci* **108:** 4876–4881.

Koirala A, Conley SM, Makkia R, Liu Z, Cooper MJ, Sparrow JR, Naash MI. 2013. Persistence of non-viral vector mediated *RPE65* expression: Case for viability as a gene transfer therapy for RPE-based diseases. *J Control Release* **172:** 745–752.

Lamba DA, Gust J, Reh TA. 2009. Transplantation of human embryonic stem cell-derived photoreceptors restores some visual function in *Crx*-deficient mice. *Cell Stem Cell* **4:** 73–79.

Lamba DA, McUsic A, Hirata RK, Wang P-R, Russell D, Reh TA. 2010. Generation, purification and transplantation of photoreceptors derived from human induced pluripotent stem cells. *PLoS ONE* **5:** e8763.

Li Q, Miller R, Han P-Y, Pang J, Dinculescu A, Chiodo V, Hauswirth WW. 2008. Intraocular route of AAV2 vector administration defines humoral immune response and therapeutic potential. *Mol Vis* **14:** 1760–1769.

Lindahl T. 1993. Instability and decay of the primary structure of DNA. *Nature* **362:** 709–715.

Liu H, Ye Z, Kim Y, Sharkis S, Jang Y-Y. 2010. Generation of endoderm-derived human induced pluripotent stem cells from primary hepatocytes. *Hepatology* **51:** 1810–1819.

Loh Y-H, Agarwal S, Park I-H, Urbach A, Huo H, Heffner GC, Kim K, Miller JD, Ng K, Daley GQ. 2009. Generation of induced pluripotent stem cells from human blood. *Blood* **113:** 5476–5479.

Maguire AM, Simonelli F, Pierce EA, Pugh EN, Mingozzi F, Bennicelli J, Banfi S, Marshall KA, Testa F, Surace EM, et al. 2008. Safety and efficacy of gene transfer for Leber's congenital amaurosis. *N Engl J Med* **358:** 2240–2248.

Maguire AM, High KA, Auricchio A, Wright JF, Pierce EA, Testa F, Mingozzi F, Bennicelli JL, Ying G-S, Rossi S, et al. 2009. Age-dependent effects of *RPE65* gene therapy for Leber's congenital amaurosis: A phase 1 dose-escalation trial. *Lancet* **374:** 1597–1605.

Maherali N, Ahfeldt T, Rigamonti A, Utikal J, Cowan C, Hochedlinger K. 2008. A high-efficiency system for the generation and study of human induced pluripotent stem cells. *Cell Stem Cell* **3:** 340–345.

Mali P, Yang L, Esvelt KM, Aach J, Guell M, DiCarlo JE, Norville JE, Church GM. 2013. RNA-guided human genome engineering via Cas9. *Science* **339:** 823–826.

Malik N, Rao MS. 2013. A review of the methods for human iPSC derivation. *Methods Mol Biol* **997:** 23–33.

Molday LL, Djajadi H, Yan P, Szczygiel L, Boye SL, Chiodo VA, Gregory-Evans K, Sarunic MV, Hauswirth WW, Molday RS. 2013. RD3 gene delivery restores guanylate cyclase localization and rescues photoreceptors in the *Rd3* mouse model of Leber congenital amaurosis 12. *Hum Mol Genet* **22:** 3894–3905.

Moscou MJ, Bogdanove AJ. 2009. A simple cipher governs DNA recognition by TAL effectors. *Science* **326:** 1501.

Narfström K, Katz ML, Bragadottir R, Seeliger M, Boulanger A, Redmond TM, Caro L, Lai C-M, Rakoczy PE. 2003. Functional and structural recovery of the retina after gene therapy in the *RPE65* null mutation dog. *Invest Ophthalmol Vis Sci* **44:** 1663–1672.

Nicoud M, Kong J, Iqball S, Kan O, Naylor S, Gouras P, Allikmets R, Binley K. 2007. Development of photoreceptor-specific promoters and their utility to investigate EIAV lentiviral vector mediated gene transfer to photoreceptors. *J Gene Med* **9:** 1015–1023.

Perez EE, Wang J, Miller JC, Jouvenot Y, Kim KA, Liu O, Wang N, Lee G, Bartsevich VV, Lee Y-L, et al. 2008. Establishment of HIV-1 resistance in $CD4^+$ T cells by genome editing using zinc-finger nucleases. *Nat Biotechnol* **26:** 808–816.

Preynat-Seauve O, de Rham C, Tirefort D, Ferrari-Lacraz S, Krause K-H, Villard J. 2009. Neural progenitors derived from human embryonic stem cells are targeted by allogeneic T and natural killer cells. *J Cell Mol Med* **13:** 3556–3569.

Ramalingam S, Kandavelou K, Rajenderan R, Chandrasegaran S. 2011. Creating designed zinc-finger nucleases with minimal cytotoxicity. *J Mol Biol* **405:** 630–641.

Ran FA, Hsu PD, Lin C-Y, Gootenberg JS, Konermann S, Trevino AE, Scott DA, Inoue A, Matoba S, Zhang Y, et al. 2013a. Double nicking by RNA-guided CRISPR Cas9 for enhanced genome editing specificity. *Cell* **154:** 1380–1389.

Ran FA, Hsu PD, Wright J, Agarwala V, Scott DA, Zhang F. 2013b. Genome engineering using the CRISPR-Cas9 system. *Nat Protoc* **8:** 2281–2308.

Raya A, Rodríguez-Pizà I, Guenechea G, Vassena R, Navarro S, Barrero MJ, Consiglio A, Castellà M, Río P, Sleep E, et al. 2009. Disease-corrected haematopoietic progenitors from Fanconi anaemia induced pluripotent stem cells. *Nature* **460:** 53–59.

Reichel MB, Ali RR, Thrasher AJ, Hunt DM, Bhattacharya SS, Baker D. 1998. Immune responses limit adenovirally mediated gene expression in the adult mouse eye. *Gene Ther* **5:** 1038–1046.

Ross JW, Fernandez de Castro JP, Zhao J, Samuel M, Walters E, Rios C, Bray-Ward P, Jones BW, Marc RE, Wang W, et al. 2012. Generation of an inbred miniature pig model of retinitis pigmentosa. *Invest Ophthalmol Vis Sci* **53:** 501–507.

Schornack S, Meyer A, Römer P, Jordan T, Lahaye T. 2006. Gene-for-gene-mediated recognition of nuclear-targeted AvrBs3-like bacterial effector proteins. *J Plant Physiol* **163:** 256–272.

Seo S, Mulins RF, Dumitrescu AV, Bhattarai S, Gratie D, Wang K, Stone E, Sheffield VC, Drack AV. 2013. Subretinal gene therapy of mice with Bardet-Biedl syndrome type 1. *Invest Ophthalmol Vis Sci* **54:** 6118–6132.

Si-Tayeb K, Noto FK, Sepac A, Sedlic F, Bosnjak ZJ, Lough JW, Duncan SA. 2010. Generation of human induced pluripotent stem cells by simple transient transfection of plasmid DNA encoding reprogramming factors. *BMC Dev Biol* **10:** 81.

Stadtfeld M, Nagaya M, Utikal J, Weir G, Hochedlinger K. 2008. Induced pluripotent stem cells generated without viral integration. *Science* **322:** 945–949.

Sugio A, Yang B, Zhu T, White FF. 2007. Two type III effector genes of *Xanthomonas oryzae* pv. *oryzae* control the induction of the host genes *OsTFIIA*γ*1* and *OsTFX1* during bacterial blight of rice. *Proc Natl Acad Sci* **104:** 10720–10725.

Takahashi K, Yamanaka S. 2006. Induction of pluripotent stem cells from mouse embryonic and adult fibroblast cultures by defined factors. *Cell* **126:** 663–676.

Takahashi K, Tanabe K, Ohnuki M, Narita M, Ichisaka T, Tomoda K, Yamanaka S. 2007. Induction of pluripotent stem cells from adult human fibroblasts by defined factors. *Cell* **131:** 861–872.

Testa F, Maguire AM, Rossi S, Pierce EA, Melillo P, Marshall K, Banfi S, Surace EM, Sun J, Acerra C, et al. 2013. Three-year follow-up after unilateral subretinal delivery of adeno-associated virus in patients with Leber congenital amaurosis type 2. *Ophthalmology* **120:** 1283–1291.

Tucker BA, Scheetz TE, Mullins RF, DeLuca AP, Hoffmann JM, Johnston RM, Jacobson SG, Sheffield VC, Stone EM. 2011. Exome sequencing and analysis of induced pluripotent stem cells identify the cilia-related gene male germ cell-associated kinase (MAK) as a cause of retinitis pigmentosa. *Proc Natl Acad Sci* **108:** E569–E576.

Tucker BA, Anfinson KR, Mullins RF, Stone EM, Young MJ. 2013a. Use of a synthetic xeno-free culture substrate for induced pluripotent stem cell induction and retinal differentiation. *Stem Cells Transl Med* **2:** 16–24.

Tucker BA, Mullins RF, Streb LM, Anfinson K, Eyestone ME, Kaalberg E, Riker MJ, Drack AV, Braun TA, Stone EM. 2013b. Patient-specific iPSC-derived photoreceptor precursor cells as a means to investigate retinitis pigmentosa. *eLife* **2:** e00824.

Wang H, Yang H, Shivalila CS, Dawlaty MM, Cheng AW, Zhang F, Jaenisch R. 2013. One-step generation of mice carrying mutations in multiple genes by CRISPR/Cas-mediated genome engineering. *Cell* **153:** 910–918.

West EL, Pearson RA, Barker SE, Luhmann UFO, Maclaren RE, Barber AC, Duran Y, Smith AJ, Sowden JC, Ali RR. 2010. Long-term survival of photoreceptors transplanted into the adult murine neural retina requires immune modulation. *Stem Cells* **28:** 1997–2007.

Wu Z, Yang H, Colosi P. 2010. Effect of genome size on AAV vector packaging. *Mol Ther* **18:** 80–86.

Wu G, Liu N, Rittelmeyer I, Sharma AD, Sgodda M, Zaehres H, Bleidissel M, Greber B, Gentile L, Han DW, et al. 2011. Generation of healthy mice from gene-corrected disease-specific induced pluripotent stem cells. *PLoS Biol* **9:** e1001099.

Yu J, Vodyanik MA, Smuga-Otto K, Antosiewicz-Bourget J, Frane JL, Tian S, Nie J, Jonsdottir GA, Ruotti V, Stewart R, et al. 2007. Induced pluripotent stem cell lines derived from human somatic cells. *Science* **318:** 1917–1920.

What Is Next for Retinal Gene Therapy?

Luk H. Vandenberghe

Ocular Genomics Institute, Grousbeck Gene Therapy Center, Schepens Eye Research Institute, Massachusetts Eye and Ear Infirmary, Harvard Medical School, Boston, Massachusetts 02114

Correspondence: luk_vandenberghe@meei.harvard.edu

The field of gene therapy for retinal blinding disorders is experiencing incredible momentum, justified by hopeful results in early stage clinical trials for inherited retinal degenerations. The premise of the use of the gene as a drug has come a long way, and may have found its niche in the treatment of retinal disease. Indeed, with only limited treatment options available for retinal indications, gene therapy has been proven feasible, safe, and effective and may lead to durable effects following a single injection. Here, we aim at putting into context the promise and potential, the technical, clinical, and economic boundaries limiting its application and development, and speculate on a future in which gene therapy is an integral component of ophthalmic clinical care.

PROMISE DELIVERED

Three critical components have to be defined and brought together for any therapeutic approach to be successful: target, intervention, and delivery. The target requires the identification of a cell type, tissue, or process relevant to the pathophysiology of the disease. The information on these targets can then be used to devise an intervention through which a disease process can be inhibited, circumvented, or interfered with. The bundling of this intervention with an approach to deliver it to the target within a therapeutic window in a manner that is feasible, safe, and efficient constitutes an attractive treatment paradigm. Over the past two or three decades, efforts of the vision and neuroscience research community have converged with those of the genetics and gene delivery field to lead to the definition of targets, the evaluation of multiple intervention modalities, and the validation of a host of delivery systems.

The first incarnation of this approach was targeting a form of Leber congenital amaurosis (LCA), an early onset form of autosomal recessive retinal degeneration leading to progressive vision loss and nystagmus. *RPE65*, a gene encoding an enzyme pivotal in the recycling of the visual pigment chromophore 11-*cis*-retinal, was identified as one of the genes leading to LCA when mutated on both alleles (Marlhens et al. 1997). The addition of a correct copy of the *RPE65* gene led to the restoration of gene expression in this loss-of-function, single gene disorder (Acland et al. 2001). In parallel, the field of in vivo gene transfer was embarking on evaluating technologies for therapeutic applications, out of which the adeno-associated viral vector (AAV) emerged as a minimally immunogenic vector capable of stably transducing nondividing cells

Cite this article as *Cold Spring Harb Perspect Med* doi: 10.1101/cshperspect.a017442

(Ali et al. 1996). An unconventional surgical route of delivery that layered the gene therapy vector below the retina, adjacent to the therapeutic target cell type, that is, the retinal pigment epithelium (RPE), was proven to be essential for allowing AAV to come to its full potential in terms of gene transfer efficiency, specificity, and safety (Bennett et al. 1994; Ali et al. 1996). Bundled, these pivotal findings led to a demonstration, in a canine model of the disease, that subretinal injection of AAV encoding a promoter driven cDNA of *RPE65* restored objective and behavioral measures of vision (Acland et al. 2001). Validated by three independent groups, clinical trials along this premise yielded promising results with moderate improvements in visual function of patients (Bainbridge et al. 2008; Cideciyan et al. 2008, 2009; Maguire et al. 2008). A successful phase 2 trial (Bennett et al. 2012) justified initiation of a currently active phase 3 study which is aimed at licensure of the first effective gene therapy drug in the United States.

The cumulative research in this area that led to this sequence of events in less than two decades is a model in this era of translational medicine, and has generated an increased interest in gene therapy applications to target ophthalmic disease, particularly for indications in which no treatment options are available or current therapeutic paradigms are inadequate or suboptimal. Moreover, these studies disrupted a prevalent school of thought that experimental treatments such as gene therapy could only be applied in fatal disorders for which no therapies were available.

CARBON COPY?

In 2012, The National Institutes of Health Office of Biotechnological Activities convened several stakeholders in gene therapy. At this meeting, it was suggested that future retinal degeneration therapies could be developed in a streamlined fashion by building on a delivery platform established in the RPE65 studies (O'Reilly et al. 2013). The idea is to use an identical vector type, surgical procedure, and transgene cassette to deliver therapeutic genes for other retinal indications. Indeed, the example that these studies have set, provides a guide for the design and development of gene therapies for other forms of retinal blindness.

The need for streamlining the development of these innovative therapies is high. Treatment options for many retinal blinding disorders are limited to nonexisting yet numerous therapeutic approaches and targets are being pursued preclinically. This requires a multitude of therapies to be developed, for example, there are more than 200 genes causative of inherited retinal disorders when mutated (see https://sph.uth.edu/RetNet/sum-dis.htm#A-genes). Moreover, a variety of different interventions are considered, ranging from gene addition, neuroprotection, and optogenetics. This, added to the targets and intervening modalities in more complex retinal disease, such as age-related macular degeneration (AMD), amounts to a large translational need (Sahel and Roska 2013; Simonato et al. 2013). The time and cost of translating a preclinical proof-of-concept that brings together target, intervention, and delivery is extremely high, and any cost-saving or streamlining of this process would bring transformative therapies to the patient faster.

Since the publication, in 2008, of the results of the early phase studies on the *RPE65* gene therapy trials, extensive efforts have been underway to build on this momentum, and to deliver a second success built on this same mold. In 2014, promising data from a phase 1/2 clinical trial for gene augmentation therapy for choroideremia, an X-linked form of retinal degeneration caused by defects in the REP-1 protein, was presented (MacLaren et al. 2014). These studies used the same vector (AAV2), delivery route (subretinal injection), and promoter (cytomegalovirus [CMV] enhanced chicken β-actin) as two of the RPE65 studies, evidently building on, and adding to, the platform potential of this approach. It is important to highlight also the point of divergence in design of the gene therapy, and its translational path to clinical studies. First, certain design elements of the transgene were added, most notably the woodchuck hepatitis virus posttranscriptional response element (WPRE) known to increase mRNA half-life and thereby lead to enhanced transgene expression. Second, the targeted area for treatment extended, much more than in the RPE65 studies into the macula, the area of the retina where in these patients' most target cells remained viable substrates for gene therapy. In terms of the body of evidence supporting the clinical translation for this second gene target, it appeared less exhaustive animal data was sufficient (Tolmachova et al. 2013). This is an important evolution as animal models of the retinal dystrophies are often lacking, not reflecting human disease, or only demonstrating a slow progressing or mild phenotype within the animal's lifespan (Chang et al. 2002). Also, to take advantage of the clinical validation AAV2 received in the prior studies, improved AAV serotypes that are thought to lead to a more robust expression in photoreceptor cells, next to RPE targets for the gene transfer (Boye et al. 2012; Vandenberghe and Auricchio 2012; Vandenberghe et al. 2011), were not pursued here, possibly limiting the efficacy potential of the study. This highlights an important decision point in the pursuit of developing a novel retinal gene therapy: Does one take advantage of a platform such as AAV2, risking subtherapeutic levels of expression in important target cells, or does one diverge from the validated platform at the risk of complicating the translational path of dealing with more unknowns and higher regulatory hurdles?

A PIPELINE OF PROGRESS

A cadre of clinical studies is currently ongoing, pending, or actively being developed at a preclinical stage (Boye et al. 2013). Many of these studies build on AAV2, but often also chose for a different vector including alternative AAV serotypes or lentiviral systems, either for improved targeting, or to overcome the limited transgene size capacity of AAV. Once results emerge from the clinic, these alternative vector systems may become novel platforms that can be built on. Specifically, trials are ongoing using a lentiviral vector encoding ABCA4 and MYO7A for the treatment of Stargardt disease (Binley et al. 2013) and Usher Type 1B (Zallocchi et al. 2014), respectively. These cDNAs are too large to be packaged in AAV, yet can be accommodated by a lentiviral vector. A concern with this vector system has been the low transduction efficiency for photoreceptor cells, a primary therapeutic target for both these diseases (Auricchio et al. 2001; Bainbridge et al. 2001; Binley et al. 2013). Two clinical studies are underway with a gene therapy approach for durable expression of an antiangiogenic molecule in the treatment of exudative AMD (Maclachlan et al. 2011; Lai et al. 2012). Interestingly, the two trials use similar therapeutic molecules (sFlt1) and AAV2 as a vector, however differ in the surgical delivery of the gene therapy; a group out of Lions Eye Institute in Australia in collaboration with Avalanche Biosciences injects subretinally (Lai et al. 2012), whereas Genzyme/Sanofi is pursuing intravitreal injection (Maclachlan et al. 2011). The outcome of these approaches will inform us on another gene therapy modality: gene transfer for sustained delivery of a secreted therapeutic protein drug. Several gene augmentations approaches are underway clinically: all are AAV2-based, one building on the *RPE65* results but directed at *MERTK* (NCT01482195), a disease-causing gene in retinitis pigmentosa, and another set of studies for Leber hereditary optic neuropathy (LHON) caused by mutations in the mitochondrial gene *ND4* (NCT02161380 and NCT02064569), which is expressed in the retinal ganglion cells that make up the optic nerve. Dozens of other preclinical programs are at various stages of development, for example, AAV5 mediated expression of *GUCY2D* for treatment of another form of LCA, which is soon expected to head to the clinic (Boye et al. 2013).

In short, following a pioneering era of first-in-human, a number of studies are bound to yield results, some building and solidifying the subretinal AAV2 approach, whereas others hopefully will expand the toolset and therapeutic reach for retinal degeneration gene therapies.

IMPROVING ON EFFICACY

In more than a dozen gene therapy clinical trials of several hundreds of subjects, safety endpoints have been met in the absence of significant, drug-related adverse events (Simonato et al. 2013). No phase 3 studies have been completed, and efficacy in a randomized controlled trial has yet to be established for any of the ongoing approaches, although these results are anticipated in the near future for a phase 3 study for one of the RPE65 gene therapies. Reports on efficacy in retinal gene therapy, therefore, have been limited to the phase 1/2 RPE65 and choroideremia (CHM) studies. Data presented there has been promising and demonstrating increased light sensitivity by a variety of measures, and in some subjects improved navigation of a mobility course, indicating not only biological effect of the treatment, but also the potential for clinical benefit. However, based on the remarkable disease rescue observed in dog models following AAV2.RPE65 gene therapy, which appears not as robust as in humans, several hypotheses have been suggested to explain the apparent differences in treatment effect.

Cideciyan and colleagues (2013a) followed treated subjects and compared those to the natural disease progression in dogs and humans as well as the therapeutic effects seen in dogs over time. Using spectral domain optical coherence tomography (SD-OCT) and a novel methodology to model the decay of retinal structure, the investigators concluded that in humans, as opposed to canines, retinal degeneration starts earlier, and the optimal intervention for a gene therapy in this form of LCA is likely before birth (Cideciyan et al. 2013a). Their data suggests treated subjects show stable visual function in the context of ongoing retinal degeneration. To improve both visual function and structural preservation, the investigators propose a combination therapy in which neuroprotective treatment is combined with the gene addition. These results have extensively been argued, over its unorthodox modeling, the limited longitudinal data from patients (as opposed to dogs) following treatment, the small data set with several variables that are unaccounted for in the analysis, and its suggested solution to overcome this concern (Cepko and Vandenberghe 2013; Cideciyan et al. 2013b; Townes-Anderson 2013; Wojno et al. 2013). Moreover, only data from one of the clinical studies was included, making it difficult to assess if the observations can be extended to the other trial designs.

Alternative hypotheses argue that the limitations of the current gene therapy formulations and surgical approaches can be improved on by targeting a larger area of the retina than a subretinal injection can reach, the level of transgene expression is limiting for full treatment effect, or the specificity of expression and stoichiometry of RPE65 in the context of the visual cycle is not in balance, arguing for more specific and regulated expression. These interventions may not have been required in the murine or canine models because of species-specific parameters such as the size of the globe, the procedural difference in terms of surgery, molecular kinetics of vector uptake, transduction, or promoter activity that are possibly distinct in canine versus human retina.

These discussions highlight, in our view, the need to continue to define the therapeutic window for each approach and indication, and to seek to improve the technology and biology of the treatment. Clinical, ethical, and pragmatic boundaries limit us in considering prenatal or neonatal (and before some of these studies, pediatric) gene therapy in ophthalmology, which, at least for now, determines the start of the potential therapeutic window for intervention. The field is in agreement that there is also a clear closing of the window when the therapeutic target cell (often RPE and/or photoreceptors) are atrophied. What is also agreed on, however less defined, is the threshold at which for many of these progressively degenerative diseases, degeneration cannot be stemmed in a cell autonomous fashion. Elucidation and diagnosis of that transition point is essential for identifying the appropriate therapeutic approach for each patient. Technological improvement to gene therapy that can restore gene function in a more physiological manner is likely also to prove important. The prospect of genome editing therapy in this respect is a fascinating one, because this technology may permit the adoption of endogenous regulation of gene expression. Albeit early, and faced with critical hurdles still, the recent advances in this field make this

 Cite this article as *Cold Spring Harb Perspect Med* doi: 10.1101/cshperspect.a017442

approach compelling (Cong et al. 2013; Mali et al. 2013).

While this debate and detailed level of analysis is essential to progress, we cannot lose track of the fact that the noted clinical studies have concluded a biological effect in the absence of harm, with the potential of remarkable, clinically relevant, improvements of visual function. Absent of other treatment options for these patients, this first generation gene therapy is a milestone that can be used as a benchmark for future improvements. It is also important to note that these improvements often can only be validated in cautious, yet pivotal, human clinical studies. The careful translation of this experimental paradigm that has led to the first demonstration of efficacy in the context of safety for in vivo gene therapy is therefore a salute to the need for experimental clinical research to move these important questions forward.

WIDENING THE SPECTRUM

The compelling data from the early clinical trials, and the pipeline of preclinical studies moving to translation, has illustrated, for many, the transformative potential of gene therapy in ophthalmic care. It needs to be noted, however, that the current studies only address very small patient populations, and, at least in the short to mid-term, the prospect of gene therapy alleviating blinding disorders on a wider scale is limited. Several parameters determine this current limitation: (1) LCA, owing to mutations in *RPE65* and *CHM*, only affect few, and many other forms of inherited retinal degeneration will require a different treatment; (2) more common disorders, such as AMD, are currently only in clinical trials in populations at the very late stage of the disease, and even when proven safe and effective in current trials it remains to be seen how these results can be extended to a wider wet AMD population; (3) the therapeutic window for most of the approaches currently in trials is limited to those with remaining target cells and some level of vision; and (4) the prohibitive cost of clinical translation and trial costs for experimental biological therapies.

To broaden the potential of gene therapy for wider patient populations in ophthalmology, progress is made on several fronts. Not unlike the development of this first generation of therapies, the convergence of several fields including genetics, gene delivery, retinal biology, neuroscience, and cell therapy, is leading the charge in this effort. New targets are continuously being identified through gene discovery and studies into the pathophysiology of retinal disease; new disease genes in inherited retinal degenerations are being discovered, as are new targets in AMD and other common-complex retinal disorders. Novel and improved paradigms to intervene are now also more actively considered for vision restoration, in part, because of the traction and excitement spurred by the retinal gene therapy trial success. Specifically, the restoration of vision through gene transfer of an optogenetic switch that is accurately embedded within the neural circuitry of the retina is pursued by several groups and may lead to some level of visual perception in the blind, even in the absence of (endogenous) photoreceptors (Busskamp et al. 2012). Advances in neuroprotection through survival factors, antiapoptotic, or antioxidant agents will be beneficial to other gene therapy strategies, or may be delivered in a sustained fashion via gene transfer (Sahel and Roska 2013). The intersect of gene transfer and genome editing with cell-based transplantation approaches is highly promising to enable visual restoration even when retinal degeneration is extensive, and more traditional approaches of gene therapy are outside of consideration. Finally, progress in the field of gene delivery can further unlock further applications. The limitation on the size of the transgene imposed by the clinically used vector systems currently is not only preventing gene addition in the most common forms of LCA and RP (CEP290 and USH2A, respectively), it also often prevents transgene cassettes to be designed with transcriptional or translational elements (e.g., cell-specific promoters or introns) that would be beneficial, or multiple genes to be transferred in a single vector (e.g., gene replacement combined with a neuroprotective gene). Novel vector technologies like nanoparticle approaches

(Conley and Naash 2010), or methods like genome editing to restore endogenous gene regulation, are expected to have an important impact. To further expand on the paradigm pursued by the pending AMD trials delivering an antiangiogenic protein by gene therapy to achieve long-lived and stable drug delivery to overcome repeat injections in a chronic disease, novel and improved methods to modulate transgene expression will become essential. Somewhat surprisingly, although several methods are available (Zoltick and Wilson 2001), few of them are actively pursued clinically in a gene therapy context, in part due to vector size limitations and the complexity related to translating these systems to human use. Last, efficient and safe targeting from the vitreous would overcome several shortcomings of the subretinal injection route and, certainly, make gene therapy a more routine clinical procedure (Dalkara et al. 2013; Kay et al. 2013).

MEASURING OUTCOME

Shared with other experimental therapeutic strategies in ophthalmology, the ability to measure outcome is pivotal for gene therapy to become a clinical modality in the care of patients. This is primarily of importance to convincingly establish the level of efficacy these therapies bring. Equally important is the quest for early endpoints to assess therapeutic effect to shorten the "bench to bedside and back" life-cycle of the gene therapy development of these cost-heavy trials in often slowly progressing diseases. Because of the advantages that the visual system has in terms of access, diagnosis, and imaging, the measures to establish a biological effect of a treatment are available, and several of those have been used by the different groups pursuing ophthalmic gene therapy clinically. Moving forward, to the extent possible, a standardization of these measures will be beneficial to accurately compare outcomes from different trials and the variables between those. A higher bar to meet is the demonstration of clinical benefit, in part, because of the fact that a sensitive measure of biological effect may not equate to an improvement in quality of life or clinical status. Another aspect, however, is the regulatory definition of clinical benefit in ophthalmology that traditionally has been quite narrow. Because of the onslaught of novel therapeutic approaches for indications for which no treatments options are in current clinical use, disease organizations and clinical researchers continue a dialogue with regulators to establish new endpoint measures for clinical research, and ultimately market approval (Cellular, Tissue and Gene Therapies Advisory Committee 2011, see http://www.fda.gov/downloads/advisor.../ucm259087.pdf). While traditionally, visual acuity, and in limited cases visual field, has been acceptable, the RPE65 phase 3 study currently in progress uses a validated mobility assay as an endpoint (NCT 00999609). Validated surrogate measures such as those obtained via SD-OCT will likely also prove to be extremely valuable (Birch et al. 2013). The availability of a functionally validated biomarker to assess visual function, the stage of a disease process, or the activity of a therapeutic target is generally considered a "Holy Grail" for expediting and quantitation of therapeutic effect in humans. A key requirement for all endpoints, particularly in light of the fact that placebo controlled studies will remain difficult to design in gene therapy, is the availability of natural history studies to outline the disease course by that measure for that particular indication.

ECONOMIC FACTORS

With clinical proof-of-concept established, a delivery platform proposed, and a range of therapeutic targets and intervention of promise in the scientific literature, it may seem surprising and disappointing, particularly to patients and their families, that not more retinal gene therapies reached the clinic. As outlined above, several scientific, biological, and clinical limitations are at cause here. However, economic factors arguably play a primary role. The development of a single gene therapy is a time- and resource-demanding effort. Few centers have all the components under one roof to carry these efforts, and traditionally these have been pursued in academia with, until recently limited, interest from industry. The infrastructure cost to establish a preclinical and particularly a translational gene therapy center is extremely high, and in a declining funding environment, difficult to justify by academic institutions. In the past two years, by the excitement that the first clinical results have generated, fortunately, significant private investment has entered the arena (see http://www.forbes.com/sites/matthewherper/2014/03/26/once-seen-as-too-scary-editing-peoples-genes-with-viruses-makes-a-618-million-comeback/). To sustain this momentum, novel regulatory and economic frameworks are being developed that are tailored to this novel therapeutic domain. One important aspect here is the pricing of a gene therapy drug once on the market, which is expected to determine the incentive for industry to pursue development of these therapies (Brennan and Wilson 2014). Particularly, for gene-specific therapies in rare disorders, these aspects will become vital for continued development as therapies with a larger market are likely more desirable to investors. This is ironic as this field was founded and catapulted to success by demonstrating its potential for very rare disorders. To alleviate this tension, policy and regulatory changes have made orphan drug development more attractive, including extended patent protection, and distinct regulatory paths. The idea to work toward a platform that through clinical experience gains a higher regulatory comfort level is an attractive one, as it is expected to lead to a reduced cost and time of development. To meet this ambition, standardization has to be sought for in vector manufacturing and quality control, clinical trial design, endpoint measures, and clinical follow up. While this is a challenge in an increasingly competitive arena, we argue it is beneficial for both academic and private pursuits in terms of cost-savings and the rate at which therapies can be brought to the patients.

A BRIGHT FUTURE

Gene addition therapy in two forms of inherited retinal degenerations has proven to improve visual function, in some subjects with remarkable success, in the context of a relatively safe procedure and formulation. These results have validated an approach and a technology in a manner that it has the potential to alter the treatment of retinal disorders in the future. Although many aspects in this endeavor remain the subject of research, debate, policy and regulatory adjustments, a light at the end of the tunnel is a driving force for many in the field to pursue, mature, and create novel therapies for vision loss based on this paradigm. The extent to which gene therapy can broaden its impact beyond its current niche applications hinges on scientific and clinical advances, continued funding and investment, and balanced effort between competition and standardization of this promising field.

ACKNOWLEDGMENTS

We thank Livia Carvalho, Heikki Turunen, and Eric Pierce for discussion and manuscript comments. Support for this work was from National Institutes of Health (NIH) Grant DP1-OD008267, Curing Kids Fund, Foundation for Retina Research, Foundation Fighting Blindness, Research to Prevent Blindness, and the Grousbeck Family Foundation. LHV is an inventor on patents related to AAV gene therapy; has served as a consultant and is inventor on technologies licensed to biotechnology and pharmaceutical industry; and is cofounder and consultant to GenSight Biologics.

REFERENCES

Acland GM, Aguirre GD, Ray J, Zhang Q, Aleman TS, Cideciyan AV, Pearce-Kelling SE, Anand V, Zeng Y, Maguire AM, et al. 2001. Gene therapy restores vision in a canine model of childhood blindness. *Nat Genet* **28:** 92–95.

Ali RR, Reichel MB, Thrasher AJ, Levinsky RJ, Kinnon C, Kanuga N, Hunt DM, Bhattacharya SS. 1996. Gene transfer into the mouse retina mediated by an adeno-associated viral vector. *Hum Mol Genet* **5:** 591–594.

Auricchio A, Kobinger G, Anand V, Hildinger M, O'Connor E, Maguire AM, Wilson JM, Bennett J. 2001. Exchange of surface proteins impacts on viral vector cellular specificity and transduction characteristics: The retina as a model. *Hum Mol Genet* **10:** 3075–3081.

Bainbridge JW, Stephens C, Parsley K, Demaison C, Halfyard A, Thrasher AJ, Ali RR. 2001. In vivo gene transfer to the mouse eye using an HIV-based lentiviral vector; efficient long-term transduction of corneal endothelium and retinal pigment epithelium. *Gene Ther* **8:** 1665–1668.

Bainbridge JW, Smith AJ, Barker SS, Robbie S, Henderson R, Balaggan K, Viswanathan A, Holder GE, Stockman A, Tyler N, et al. 2008. Effect of gene therapy on visual function in Leber's congenital amaurosis. *N Engl J Med* **358:** 2231–2239.

Bennett J, Wilson J, Sun D, Forbes B, Maguire A. 1994. Adenovirus vector-mediated in vivo gene transfer into adult murine retina. *Invest Ophthalmol Vis Sci* **35:** 2535–2542.

Bennett J, Ashtari M, Wellman J, Marshall KA, Cyckowski LL, Chung DC, McCague S, Pierce EA, Chen Y, Bennicelli JL, et al. 2012. AAV2 gene therapy readministration in three adults with congenital blindness. *Sci Transl Med* **4:** 120ra115.

Binley K, Widdowson P, Loader J, Kelleher M, Iqball S, Ferrige G, de Belin J, Carlucci M, Angell-Manning D, Hurst F, et al. 2013. Transduction of photoreceptors with equine infectious anemia virus lentiviral vectors: Safety and biodistribution of StarGen for Stargardt disease. *Invest Ophthalmol Vis Sci* **54:** 4061–4071.

Birch DG, Locke KG, Wen Y, Locke KI, Hoffman DR, and Hood DC. 2013. Spectral-domain optical coherence tomography measures of outer segment layer progression in patients with X-linked retinitis pigmentosa. *JAMA ophthalmol* **131:** 1143–1150.

Boye SE, Alexander JJ, Boye SL, Witherspoon CD, Sandefer KJ, Conlon TJ, Erger K, Sun J, Ryals R, Chiodo VA, et al. 2012. The human rhodopsin kinase promoter in an AAV5 vector confers rod- and cone-specific expression in the primate retina. *Hum Gene Ther* **23:** 1101–1115.

Boye SE, Boye SL, Lewin AS, Hauswirth WWA. 2013. A comprehensive review of retinal gene therapy. *Mol Ther* **21:** 509–519.

Brennan TA, Wilson JM. 2014. The special case of gene therapy pricing. *Nat Biotechnol* **32:** 874–876.

Busskamp V, Picaud S, Sahel JA, Roska B. 2012. Optogenetic therapy for retinitis pigmentosa. *Gene Ther* **19:** 169–175.

Cepko CL, Vandenberghe LH. 2013. Retinal gene therapy coming of age. *Hum Gene Ther* **24:** 242–244.

Chang B, Hawes NL, Hurd RE, Davisson MT, Nusinowitz S, Heckenlively JR. 2002. Retinal degeneration mutants in the mouse. *Vision Res* **42:** 517–525.

Cideciyan AV, Aleman TS, Boye SL, Schwartz SB, Kaushal S, Roman AJ, Pang JJ, Sumaroka A, Windsor EA, Wilson JM, et al. 2008. Human gene therapy for RPE65 isomerase deficiency activates the retinoid cycle of vision but with slow rod kinetics. *Proc Natl Acad Sci* **105:** 15112–15117.

Cideciyan AV, Hauswirth WW, Aleman TS, Kaushal S, Schwartz SB, Boye SL, Windsor EA, Conlon TJ, Sumaroka A, Roman AJ, et al. 2009. Vision 1 year after gene therapy for Leber's congenital amaurosis. *N Engl J Med* **361:** 725–727.

Cideciyan AV, Jacobson SG, Beltran WA, Sumaroka A, Swider M, Iwabe S, Roman AJ, Olivares MB, Schwartz SB, Komáromy AM, et al. 2013a. Human retinal gene therapy for Leber congenital amaurosis shows advancing retinal degeneration despite enduring visual improvement. *Proc Natl Acad Sci* **110:** E517–E525.

Cideciyan AV, Jacobson SG, Beltran WA, Hauswirth WW, Aguirre GD. 2013b. Reply to Townes-Anderson. *RPE65* gene therapy does not alter the natural history of retinal degeneration. *Proc Natl Acad Sci* **110:** E1706.

Cong L, Ran FA, Cox D, Lin S, Barretto R, Habib N, Hsu PD, Wu X, Jiang W, Marraffini LA, et al. 2013. Multiplex genome engineering using CRISPR/Cas systems. *Science* **339:** 819–823e.

Conley SM, Naash MI. 2010. Nanoparticles for retinal gene therapy. *Prog Retin Eye Res* **29:** 376–397.

Dalkara D, Byrne LC, Klimczak RR, Visel M, Yin L, Merigan WH, Flannery JG, Schaffer DV. 2013. In vivo-directed evolution of a new adeno-associated virus for therapeutic outer retinal gene delivery from the vitreous. *Sci Transl Med* **5:** 189ra176.

Kay CN, Ryals RC, Aslanidi GV, Min SH, Ruan Q, Sun J, Dyka FM, Kasuga D, Ayala AE, Van Vliet K, et al. 2013. Targeting photoreceptors via intravitreal delivery using novel, capsid-mutated AAV vectors. *PLoS ONE* **8:** e62097.

Lai CM, Estcourt MJ, Himbeck RP, Lee SY, Yew-San Yeo I, Luu C, Loh BK, Lee MW, Barathi A, Villano J, et al. 2012. Preclinical safety evaluation of subretinal AAV2.sFlt-1 in non-human primates. *Gene Ther* **19:** 999–1009.

Maclachlan TK, Lukason M, Collins M, Munger R, Isenberger E, Rogers C, Malatos S, Dufresne E, Morris J, Calcedo R, et al. 2011. Preclinical safety evaluation of AAV2-sFLT01—A gene therapy for age-related macular degeneration. *Mol Ther* **19:** 326–334.

MacLaren RE, Groppe M, Barnard AR, Cottriall CL, Tolmachova T, Seymour L, Clark KR, During MJ, Cremers FP, Black GC, et al. 2014. Retinal gene therapy in patients with choroideremia: Initial findings from a phase 1/2 clinical trial. *Lancet* **383:** 1129–1137.

Maguire AM, Simonelli F, Pierce EA, Pugh EN Jr, Mingozzi F, Bennicelli J, Banfi S, Marshall KA, Testa F, Surace EM, et al. 2008. Safety and efficacy of gene transfer for Leber's congenital amaurosis. *N Engl J Med* **358:** 2240–2248.

Mali P, Yang L, Esvelt KM, Aach J, Guell M, DiCarlo JE, Norville JE, Church GM. 2013. RNA-guided human genome engineering via Cas9. *Science* **339:** 823–826.

Marlhens F, Bareil C, Griffoin JM, Zrenner E, Amalric P, Eliaou C, Liu SY, Harris E, Redmond TM, Arnaud B, et al. 1997. Mutations in *RPE65* cause Leber's congenital amaurosis. *Nat Genet* **17:** 139–141.

O'Reilly M, Kohn DB, Bartlett J, Benson J, Brooks PJ, Byrne BJ, Camozzi C, Cornetta K, Crystal RG, Fong Y, et al. 2013. Gene therapy for rare diseases: Summary of a National Institutes of Health workshop, September 13, 2012. *Hum Gene Ther* **24:** 355–362.

Sahel JA, Roska B. 2013. Gene therapy for blindness. *Annu Rev Neurosci* **36:** 467–488.

Simonato M, Bennett J, Boulis NM, Castro MG, Fink DJ, Goins WF, Gray SJ, Lowenstein PR, Vandenberghe LH, Wilson TJ, et al. 2013. Progress in gene therapy for neurological disorders. *Nat Rev Neurol* **9:** 277–291.

Tolmachova T, Tolmachov OE, Barnard AR, de Silva SR, Lipinski DM, Walker NJ, Maclaren RE, Seabra MC. 2013. Functional expression of Rab escort protein 1 following AAV2-mediated gene delivery in the retina of choroideremia mice and human cells ex vivo. *J Mol Med (Berl)* **91:** 825–837.

Townes-Anderson E. 2013. Increased levels of gene therapy may not be beneficial in retinal disease. *Proc Natl Acad Sci* **110:** E1705.

Vandenberghe LH, Auricchio A. 2012. Novel adeno-associated viral vectors for retinal gene therapy. *Gene Ther* **19:** 162–168.

Vandenberghe LH, Bell P, Maguire AM, Cearley CN, Xiao R, Calcedo R, Wang L, Castle MJ, Maguire AC, Grant R, et al. 2011. Dosage thresholds for AAV2 and AAV8 photoreceptor gene therapy in monkey. *Sci Transl Med* **3:** 88ra54.

Wojno AP, Pierce EA, Bennett J. 2013. Seeing the light. *Sci Transl Med* **5:** 175fs178.

Zallocchi M, Binley K, Lad Y, Ellis S, Widdowson P, Iqball S, Scripps V, Kelleher M, Loader J, Miskin J, et al. 2014. EIAV-based retinal gene therapy in the *shaker1* mouse model for usher syndrome type 1B: Development of UshStat. *PLoS ONE* **9:** e94272.

Zoltick PW, Wilson JM. 2001. Regulated gene expression in gene therapy. *Ann NY Acad Sci* **953:** 53–63.

Index